SUICIDOLOGY

Also Available

Risk Management with Suicidal Patients
*Edited by Bruce Bongar, Alan L. Berman, Ronald W. Maris,
Morton M. Silverman, Eric A. Harris, and Wendy Packman*

Suicidology

A Comprehensive Biopsychosocial Perspective

Ronald W. Maris

Foreword by David A. Jobes

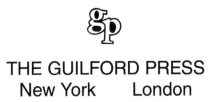

THE GUILFORD PRESS
New York   London

Copyright © 2019 The Guilford Press
A Division of Guilford Publications, Inc.
370 Seventh Avenue, Suite 1200, New York, NY 10001
www.guilford.com

Printed in the United States of America

This book is printed on acid-free paper.

Last digit is print number: 9 8 7 6 5 4 3 2 1

The author has checked with sources believed to be reliable in his efforts to
provide information that is complete and generally in accord with the standards
of practice that are accepted at the time of publication. However, in view of the
possibility of human error or changes in behavioral, mental health, or medical
sciences, neither the author, nor the editor and publisher, nor any other party who
has been involved in the preparation or publication of this work warrants that the
information contained herein is in every respect accurate or complete, and they are
not responsible for any errors or omissions or the results obtained from the use of
such information. Readers are encouraged to confirm the information contained in
this book with other sources.

Library of Congress Cataloging-in-Publication Data
Names: Maris, Ronald W., author.
Title: Suicidology : a comprehensive biopsychosocial perspective / Ronald W.
   Maris ; foreword by David A. Jobes.
Description: First Edition. | New York : The Guilford Press, 2019. | Includes
   bibliographical references and index.
Identifiers: LCCN 2018031472 | ISBN 9781462536986 (hardback)
Subjects: LCSH: Suicide. | Suicide--Prevention. | BISAC: PSYCHOLOGY /
   Suicide. | MEDICAL / Psychiatry / General. | SOCIAL SCIENCE / Social Work.
   | MEDICAL / Nursing / Psychiatric.
Classification: LCC HV6545 .M273 2018 | DDC 362.28—dc23
LC record available at *https://lccn.loc.gov/2018031472*

*To life and the courage to embrace it
in spite of prolonged adversity
and recurring episodic pain,
and to those whose unflinching, compassionate,
overwhelming love provides the will, ability,
and reason to be*

About the Author

Ronald W. Maris, PhD, is Distinguished Professor Emeritus of Psychiatry, Family Medicine, and Sociology at the University of South Carolina (USC). He received his BA, MA, and PhD from the University of Illinois and studied religion and philosophy at Harvard Divinity School. Dr. Maris's eight postdoctoral fellowships included being a National Science Foundation Fellow, National Institute of Mental Health (NIMH) Fellow at Johns Hopkins School of Medicine, World Health Organization Fellow, Yale Foundations Fund Fellow in Psychiatry, Killam Fellow in Psychiatry, Visiting Professor of Psychiatry at the University of Pittsburgh School of Medicine, psychiatric resident at the USC School of Medicine, and intern at the Los Angeles Suicide Prevention Center. He was Assistant Professor of Sociology at Dartmouth College, Assistant Professor of Sociology at Arizona State University, Associate Professor of Psychiatry and Director of the Program in Psychiatry at the Johns Hopkins School of Medicine, Professor and Chairman of Sociology at USC, and Director of the USC Center for the Study of Suicide. For a general overview of his education, training, experience, and certification, see *www.suicideexpert.com*.

Dr. Maris has received suicide research grants from numerous institutions, including the National Institute of General Medical Sciences, NIMH, National Science Foundation, William T. Grant Foundation in New York City, and the USC Provost. His work has been reviewed in *The New York Times, The Wall Street Journal, U.S. News & World Report,* and *The Washington Post,* and he has appeared on *Good Morning America, Court TV,* and *The Dick Cavett Show.* An expert witness in approximately 300 forensic court cases, Dr. Maris has written or edited 23 books, including *Pathways to Suicide: A Survey of Self-Destructive Behaviors; Pillaged: Psychiatric Medications and Suicide Risk; Assessment and Prediction of Suicide;* and *Biology of Suicide;* and has written about 100 articles for such publications as *Oxford Bibliographies, The Lancet, Encyclopedia of Human Biology, American Sociological Review,* and *Journal of Health and Social Behavior.* He has had 10 years of supervised clinical training in psychiatry and suicidology, was certified in forensic suicidology by the American Association of Suicidology, and has Fellow status in the American Academy of Forensic Sciences.

A past president of the American Association of Suicidology, Dr. Maris was editor-in-chief of its journal, *Suicide and Life-Threatening Behavior,* for 16 years. He was voted outstanding teacher and researcher at USC five times; was invited to address the U.S. Congress on veteran suicides; was a consultant to the Columbia University/Food and Drug Administration project to analyze data on the relationship of suicidality and antidepressant treatment in children and adolescents, leading to black-box warnings; was a Deputy Medical Examiner in Baltimore; and has served as consultant and reviewer for grant applications to NIMH, the National Academy of Sciences, and the American Foundation for Suicide Prevention. Dr. Maris helped make the HBO movie *Death by Hanging* and debated Thomas Szasz at Harvard University and Derek Humphry on C-SPAN.

Foreword

I first met Ronald Maris at an American Association of Suicidology (AAS) conference in the mid-1980s. I was a mere graduate student, and Ron was one of the preeminent figures in the field of suicide prevention at the time. With trepidation, I went up to Ron and introduced myself; we shook hands, and he asked me about my research and interest in the field. It was an early star-struck moment that helped fuel my interest in suicidology. Today, as I reflect on the pantheon of suicidologists in the tradition of Edwin Shneidman, Norman Farberow, and Robert Litman, Ron certainly ranks among those who helped create the contemporary field of suicide prevention with his seminal contributions.

The field of suicidology has been graced by many innovative sociologists—Emile Durkheim, David Phillips, Steven Stack, and of course Ron Maris. Ron followed founding editor-in-chief Ed Shneidman as the second editor of the field's first journal, *Suicide and Life-Threatening Behavior,* and he served in that capacity with skill and distinction. While the journal has evolved, the editorial focus, scientific rigor, and overall quality that we see in the journal today were largely the results of Ron's editorial vision and sensibilities. Ron served as president of the AAS, received the AAS Dublin Award in recognition of his many contributions to the field, and has been a leading luminary in suicidology. But the quality that has always impressed me most about Ron is his spectacularly broad, deep expertise, combined with his utter mastery of the field. Ron is as comfortable talking about macro-level sociological forces of suicide as he is musing about the nuances of the biology of suicide. We readers get to be the beneficiaries of this extraordinary scope of knowledge and prowess.

Knowing the extraordinary mind from which it emerges, I would argue that this book is now the most comprehensive, exhaustive, and complete compilation of knowledge about suicide in the history of the field. Although this may sound hyperbolic, a quick look through the table of contents proves the point. This text begins with the field's foundations, and thoughtfully considers theories, scientific data, sociodemographic variables, mental disorders, biology, psychology, religion, history, culture, ethics, clinical care, and special topics. Ron has created *the* authoritative and indispensable scholarly compilation for the field of suicide prevention.

The field of suicide prevention has clearly matured, and it is growing exponentially. There are now several excellent suicide-specific journals; research on suicide is proliferating around the world; major suicide policy initiatives are gaining traction; and grassroots movements of loss survivors and others with lived experience are transforming the field. There are now many books and countless articles pertaining to suicide prevention. Nevertheless, there is no text quite like this one, which covers the field in all its dimensions, nuances, and complexities. I am both touched and honored to be given this opportunity to introduce this worthy addition to our shared cause. I can certainly attest that the next time I teach my "Seminar on Suicide" course, this book will be the text around which I will organize the class, because there is no better collection of suicide prevention knowledge in the literature. Simply stated, *Suicidology: A Comprehensive Biopsychosocial Perspective* is a gift to the field, a tour de force work on suicide prevention, and a fitting capstone contribution by a giant in the field.

DAVID A. JOBES, PhD, ABPP
Professor of Psychology and Director of
the Suicide Prevention Laboratory
The Catholic University of America
Washington, DC

Preface

Suicidology: A Comprehensive Biopsychosocial Perspective is the first interdisciplinary, comprehensive suicide textbook written by a single author. As such, it is unique in presenting a unified general theory and empirical (evidence-based) methodology of self-destruction, suicide, and suicide prevention. Even the best prior suicide textbooks have tended to be edited collections of chapters from specific disciplines, with no overall argument, consistent empirical methodology, or focus. Compared to earlier textbooks, *Suicidology* has several unique features:

1. *An interdisciplinary, international focus.* Most suicide textbooks (and refereed scientific journal articles) are myopic, since they usually focus only on one topic within one academic discipline or field of interest—such as psychiatry (e.g., Simon & Hales, 2012), psychology, counseling, sociology, anthropology, education, public health, medicine, pathology, forensics, criminal justice, biology/neurobiology, pathology, chemistry, religion, or history—and are not especially student-centered. *Suicidology* is intended primarily for interdisciplinary college undergraduates, graduate students, postdoctoral fellows or residents, clinicians, and medical students. Although many of the data presented in this volume come from the United States, we must constantly be aware that suicides in countries like China, India, Syria, Russia, Guyana, South Korea, Egypt, Mozambique, and others (see Chapter 8) often have significant cultural variations that need to be accounted for and explained in any truly general model of suicide.

2. *New chapters and broad scope.* In comparison to my coauthored 2000 text, *Comprehensive Textbook of Suicidology*, this new volume has a greatly expanded coverage. Among the new topics are (a) a more systematic general theory of suicide and self-destructive behaviors (Chapter 28); (b) much greater depth on mental disorder and suicide (viz., the suicidal biogenics of the brain [Chapter 16], major depressive disorder [Chapter 11], bipolar disorder [Chapter 12], schizophrenia and other psychoses [Chapter 13], and personality disorders [Chapter 14]); (c) three chapters covering special topics in the field (suicide in the military [Chapter 20], murder–suicide [Chapter 21], and jail and prison suicides [Chapter 22]); and (d) greatly

expanded discussions of treatment and prevention (Chapters 23–26), covering pharmacotherapy, psychotherapy, and suicide postvention and survivors, as well as a discussion of recent treatment of depression with ketamine (Andrade, 2017; Oaklander, 2017; Nemeroff, 2018). Although I have drawn on the coauthored 2000 text in writing the present book, all of the chapters in this book are new.

3. *Citations of up-to-date research and current scientific literature.* A lot has happened in suicidology since 2000. For example, the *Diagnostic and Statistical Manual of Mental Disorders,* fifth edition (DSM-5), came out in 2013, and the *International Classification of Diseases,* 10th revision (ICD-10), published new code sets in 2015 (ICD-11 is due out in 2019). Furthermore, the U.S. Food and Drug Administration (FDA) and several journal articles reporting clinical trials have issued several new psychiatric drug and suicidality warnings, such as (a) the September 14, 2004, FDA black-box warning on antidepressants and suicidality in pediatric and adolescent samples; (b) the August 31, 2006, FDA suicidality safety review for Ambien, Sonata, and Lunesta; (c) the December 12, 2006, FDA black-box warning for antidepressants and suicidality in adults up to age 24; (d) the January 31, 2008, FDA alert regarding antiepileptics and suicidality; and (e) the adverse effects of Clozaril (Meltzer, 1999). Finally, my assistants and I have scoured the scientific research literature for significant suicide research and clinical trials up to 2018, and I have included that new information here.

4. *Clinically relevant data.* Many suicide texts are exclusively academic and generic. There can be a huge gap between the general principles, data, multivariate statistics, and theories of suicidal behaviors and ideas on the one hand, and the assessment and treatment of particular suicidal individuals on the other. Although I am not primarily a clinician, I have had 10 years of formal psychiatric supervision and training, and was Associate Professor of Psychiatry at the Johns Hopkins School of Medicine, where I directed the MD–PhD Program in Psychiatry. For 16 years I also directed clinical assessment and care at the University of South Carolina Center for the Study of Suicide (with staff members in psychiatry, psychology, nursing, social work, and public health). Over my career I have investigated about 300 forensic suicide cases in great detail, often over several years, and in some of these cases I was involved in the treatment of the persons who eventually committed suicide. Whenever it has been possible and relevant to do so, I have cited and then discussed these specific individual cases in this textbook. Suicides tend to occur one at a time, often in unique circumstances. *Suicidology* includes 53 cases that I have examined carefully, ranging from celebrity cases like Ernest Hemingway, Sylvia Plath, Marilyn Monroe, Philip Seymour Hoffman, Robin Williams, and Kurt Cobain to more ordinary, mundane cases that nevertheless illustrate important aspects of suicide assessment and clinical treatment.

5. *A focus on students.* I often write in the first person and try to engage students or other readers in a participatory or Socratic dialogue. This is similar to what I do in my classes, where I frequently raise questions intended to provoke discussion and further thought, such as these: "Do you or your family/friends have suicidal problems or a positive history for suicide?"; "What are your expectations and concerns

in taking a course like this?"; "Are you currently in psychotherapy and/or taking psychiatric medications, and, if so, can you tolerate this course?"; "Do you know what your local school or university treatment options are?"; and "What is your special interest in the subject of suicide?" I also recommend that class members or readers watch some films and discuss them in class or with others.

Writing this book was a long and arduous task, which I undertook with humility and some trepidation. Although I have an eclectic educational and training background, it is hard for any one person to do justice to all of the specialized areas and detailed aspects of suicide. I welcome your feedback and comments. In particular, instructors using this textbook who are interested in ideas for organizing and deepening their courses and receiving teaching aids can email me at *rwmaris@aol.com*.

Acknowledgments

I am thankful for the supportive criticism and encouragement of the staff at The Guilford Press, especially Jim Nageotte, Seymour Weingarten, Anna Brackett, Marie Sprayberry, Barbara Watkins, and Jane Keislar. I appreciate your believing in me and this project, but still making me "get it right." Thanks, too, to the outside reviewers, endorsers, illustrators, and indexers. As always, I am grateful for the advice and counsel of my four daughters: Elizabeth (an attorney in New York City), Catherine (a dean at Rice University in Houston, Texas), Amanda (a judge in Durham, North Carolina), and Gabriella (a family practice physician in Atlanta, Georgia). Special appreciation and love go to my wife, Beth (a psychiatric social worker), who went through all the good and bad times with me.

Contents

List of Tables, Cases, Figures, and Boxes

Tables

Cases

Figures

Boxes

PART I

FOUNDATIONS

CHAPTER 1

Introduction to Suicidology

Everyone has to die, but no one has to suicide.
—ANONYMOUS

Suicide is not one thing, even though it is one word (Interian et al., 2018). As a scientific discipline, suicidology cuts across many discrete academic departments and specific disciplines. To use a regression model analogy, the total variance in suicide explained by only one academic discipline is minute. We need to go where our subject matter takes us and discard our disciplinary blinders. A way of seeing is always a way of not seeing. The real world of suicide is complex and interdisciplinary and often includes depressive disorders (see Box 1.1). The theoretical approach in the current text is biological, psychological, psychiatric, and sociological. Thus the book's title—*Suicidology: A Comprehensive Biopsychosocial Perspective*.

The Vast Panorama of Self-Destructive Behaviors and Ideas

Suicide can be defined as "intentional self-destruction resulting in your own death by your own action." Sounds pretty straightforward, right? Well, not really. In fact, there is a huge variety of self-destructive behaviors and ideas (Maris, 1991). It follows that assessment, explanation, treatment, and control of suicide are diverse and complex, too. It won't work simply to put antidepressants in the public water supply along with fluoride (however, see Ishii et al., 2015).

It is tempting to conclude that if we could effectively treat the mental disorders involving depression, then we could put a big dent in the annual suicide rate. But there are many people with depressive disorders (about 7% of the U.S. population in 12 months, 17% lifetime; Maris, 2015) and very little suicide (about 1 in 10,000 per year on average). Eighty-five to ninety percent of people with severe depressive disorders never suicide and instead usually die a natural death. The suicide rate in

---

BOX 1.1. Depression and the Black Wolf of Psychiatry

She is always with me, the littermate of depression. She lurks in the shadows by day and her howlings unsettle my sleep at night. Her heaviness sags my back; her wet hot breath blankets the nape of my neck. Her fangs sink deep into my being.

In the best of times, she prances at my side with the pose of a harmless, domesticated pet. But she is always there. And there is no way I can just shake her off, as she might propel crystal pellets of water following a plunge in the black swamp.

I imagine her to be a ponderous, powerful black wolf whose loyalty is inviolate. Oh, how I wish she were a bit less faithful, so I might catch a breath of peace. But this cannot be the lot of a psychiatrist or mental health professional who treats patients with severe and persistent mental illness. The black wolf of psychiatry is suicide.

Source: Stuart Yudofsky, foreword to Simon and Hales (2012, p. xv). Reprinted with permission from *The American Psychiatric Publishing Textbook of Suicide Assessment and Management,* Second Edition. Copyright © 2012 American Psychiatric Association. All Rights Reserved.

---

the United States overall was essentially unchanged (albeit with peaks and troughs over time and with a small but steady increase in the last decade; see Tavernese, 2016) from 1900 to 2017 (see Chapter 25, Table 25.1). Is there a rate below which suicides cannot be reduced? Is the optimum suicide rate really zero, or are we just fooling ourselves?

Figure 1.1 illustrates that the varieties of self-destructive ideas and behaviors exist on a continuum, from totally nonsuicidal thoughts/behaviors to completed suicide. This particular version of the continuum includes 10 types of suicidal ideas and behaviors related to increasing suicidality. As noted just above, only about 1 in 10,000 people in the general population complete suicide each year. When Marsha

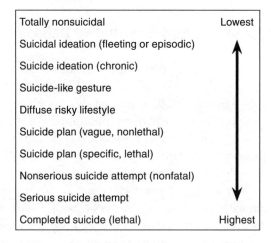

FIGURE 1.1. A continuum of suicidality. *Source:* Maris (1997b).

Linehan asked random samples of shoppers in malls about suicide ideation, maybe 18–24% of the general population had it (Linehan & Laffaw, 1982). Most ideation is fleeting and episodic, and about 80% of the population hardly even thinks about suicide at all.

Columbia University measures suicidality on a 7-point scale (Posner et al., 2007; see Figure 1.2; cf. Interian et al., 2018). One reason for suicidality scales in drug studies of suicide is that drugs result in or cause a miniscule proportion (some say none; Joiner, 2010).

Completed Suicides

The typical suicide completer in most (but not all) of the world is a middle-aged or older white male, who is depressed and abusing alcohol and perhaps pain medications. He is alone (Marchalik & Jurecic, 2018) or socially isolated from his wife and/or family; has few friends (about 50% of my Chicago suicides had no friends); and uses a highly lethal, irreversible method, most often a gunshot to the temple or mouth (see Chapter 9, Figure 9.1; see also Lester, 2012). Over time, he has grown increasingly hopeless and engages in rigid, dichotomous thinking—for instance, "Either I need to be dead, or I will continue to be miserable and have intolerable pain." Often he has some nagging musculoskeletal pain (for which he may be taking narcotics) or physical illnesses, as well as recurring work and interpersonal, marital, and/or sexual problems. About a third of suicides are unemployed when they die (Lee et al., 2018). For some time, he has experienced a series of negative, stressful life events; he may have a first-degree relative who suicided (as the famous novelist Ernest Hemingway's father did; see Case 1.1); and he may come to see suicide as the only real or permanent resolution to his persistent, escalating, intolerable life problems. Almost 90% of typical suicide completers make only one suicide attempt. For example, in my Chicago study, 88% of male suicides age 45 or older made only one fatal suicide attempt (Maris, 1981). In many ways, Hemingway was a typical suicide completer, as detailed in Case 1.1.

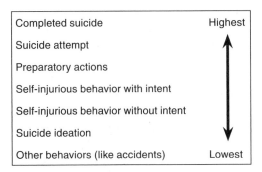

FIGURE 1.2. Columbia classification algorithm for suicide assessment. *Source:* Posner et al. (2007). Reprinted with permission from the *American Journal of Psychiatry.* Copyright © 2007 American Psychiatric Association. All Rights Reserved.

CASE 1.1. Ernest Hemingway

On July 2, 1961, a writer whom many critics call the greatest writer of the century, a man who had a zest for life and adventure as big as his genius, a winner of the Nobel Prize and the Pulitzer Prize, a soldier of fortune with a home in the Sawtooth Mountains, where he hunted in the winter, an apartment in New York, a specially rigged yacht to fish the Gulf Stream, an available apartment at the Ritz in Paris and the Gritti in Venice, a solid marriage, no serious physical ills, good friends everywhere—on that July day, that man, the envy of other men, put a shotgun to his head and killed himself. How did this come to pass? (Hotchner, 1966, p. ix)

Like Sylvia Plath (see Chapter 6, Case 6.1), Ernest Hemingway was a "gifted suicide." His work and sad death are widely known. Hemingway's life exemplifies many of the traits of suicidal careers discussed throughout this book, especially the roles of work problems and alcoholism in self-destruction among males.

Hemingway was born in Oak Park, Illinois, in 1899. His early years do not appear to have been happy, although Hemingway denied this. Hemingway's physician father was a suicide. His mother later sent Hemingway the pistol with which his father shot himself, as a "Christmas present."

"My father died in 1928—shot himself—and left me fifty thousand dollars. . . . When I asked my mother for my inheritance, she said that she had already spent it on me . . . on my travel and education. . . . My mother was a music nut, a frustrated singer, and she gave musicales every week in my fifty-thousand-dollar music room. . . . Several years later, at Christmas time, I received a package from my mother. It contained the revolver with which my father had killed himself. There was a card that said she thought I'd like to have it; I didn't know whether it was an omen or a prophecy." (quoted in Hotchner, 1966, pp. 115–116)

It would not be exaggerating to conclude that Hemingway experienced some relatively early trauma. Although it might be bold to assume that Hemingway's problems with his mother were the cause, it is also well known that he was married four times and had numerous affairs. His relationships with women often seemed to be explosive, compartmentalized, somewhat distant, and not altogether satisfying. However, Hemingway may simply have had great difficulty being close to anyone over long periods of time, regardless of the person's sex.

Hemingway was an active, physical man who loved professional boxing, circuses, bullfighting, horse racing, hunting, and fishing. He once remarked to actress Ava Gardner, "I spend a hell of a lot of time killing animals and fish, so I won't kill myself. When a man is in rebellion against death . . . he gets pleasure out of taking to himself one of the godlike attributes, that of giving it" (quoted in Hotchner, 1966, p. 139).

For an artist, Hemingway had surprisingly little use for the arts. He did not like theatre, opera, or ballet, and rarely attended musical concerts. Of course, those preferences may have been related to his avoidance of people, rather than to an active dislike of some of the things people do. Hemingway went to great pains at times to avoid the public, and one gets the unmistakable impression that most of those who did surround him were unabashed sycophants. As a consequence, he was often alone in the midst of a group of people, and experienced what we have called (perhaps a little too blandly) "negative interaction." Joiner (2005) calls it "thwarted belongingness."

It might be noted that Karl Menninger (1938) has claimed that the ego suffers in direct proportion to the amount of externally directed aggression. If so, Hemingway's paranoia, anxiety, and depression likely were related to his aggressive physical behaviors early in life. For example, he once commented: "In Chicago, where you only used fists, there was this guy who pulled a shiv— . . . a knife and cut me up. We caught him and broke both of his arms at the wrists by twisting them until they snapped" (quoted in Hotchner, 1966, p. 179).

Being a very physical man, Hemingway did not tolerate illness well, although paradoxically his lifestyle seems to have invited poor health and frequent injury. For years Hemingway had problems with his weight, high blood pressure, a high cholesterol level, a chronic bad back, and other physical ailments. Yet he still drank heavily, often did not watch his diet, and continued to be injured, most notably in two small aircraft crashes in Africa in 1953 (see Farah, 2017).

After one particularly bad head injury on his fishing boat in the spring of 1951, Hemingway started talking about being "Black-Ass," or depressed. Like most depressive disorders, Hemingway's recurred periodically throughout his life. They were associated with traits that could possibly be described as mild paranoid schizophrenia (Hotchner, 1966), rigid thinking, and suicidal thoughts. In December 1960, Hemingway had 11 "shock treatments" (as electroconvulsive therapy or ECT was then called) at the Mayo Clinic to help treat his depression and suicidal preoccupation. Subsequently, there were other ECT sessions.

What seemed to bother Hemingway most was his inability to work. A series of statements made to Hotchner indicate the crucial importance of work to Hemingway (compare these to the suicide notes of Harvard physicist Percy Bridgman at Harvard and George Eastman of Eastman Kodak, the latter of whom wrote, "My work is done. Why wait?"):

> "Writing is the only thing that makes me feel that I'm not wasting my time sticking around." (p. 144)
> "When you're the champ, it's better to step down on the best day you've had than to wait until it's starting to leave you and everyone notices it." (p. 262)
> "Hotch, if I cannot exist on my own terms, then existence is impossible. Do you understand? That is how I've lived, and that is how I *must* live . . . because . . . it doesn't matter if I don't write for a day or a year or ten years as long as the knowledge that I *can* write is solid inside me. But a day without that knowledge, or not being sure of it, is eternity." (pp. 297–298)
> "The worst death for anyone is to lose the center of his being, the thing that he really is. Retirement is the filthiest word in the language." (p. 228)

Near the end of his life, Hemingway was increasingly unable to work. His career dipped; at the end, he was developmentally stagnated, frustrated in maintaining achievement in his major life aspiration of writing, hopelessly dissatisfied in other respects, and ill. It seems that his inability to work and his eventual suicide were products of an insidious interactive effect of his early life trauma; basic life values of violence and aggression; unrealistic high aspirations and expectations based on past actual performances; an inability to compromise and be flexible as his life demanded it; his aging and failing physical health; social isolation and negative interaction; recurring depression; hopelessness (Maris, 1981, p. 272); paranoia, delusions, and confused chaotic thought processes; the actual failure of a major novel; and his recent losses and preoccupation with suicide, which he was well equipped to carry out in terms of experience, knowledge, means, and will.

> Basically, Ernest's ability to work had deteriorated to the point where he would spend endless hours with the manuscript of *A Moveable Feast* but was unable to really work on it. Besides his inability to write, Ernest was terribly depressed over the loss of the *finca* . . . His talk about destroying himself had become more frequent. and he would sometimes stand at the gun

rack, holding one of his guns, staring out the window at the distant mountains. (Hotchner, 1966, p. 274)

Finally, in Ketchum, Idaho, in 1961, just after returning from another stay at the Mayo Clinic, Hemingway killed himself with a shotgun in the early morning of July 2. Hotchner remarked that Hemingway had once commented to him that a man can be destroyed, but not defeated.

Sources: Maris (1981, pp. 165–168) and Hotchner (1966).

Not all completed suicides are like Hemingway or have all of the risk factors found in the typical profile I have just described. Although about 78% of all U.S. suicides are male, females account for the remaining 22%, which is not inconsiderable (American Association of Suicidology [AAS], 2015). Most U.S. suicides are committed by whites (90%), but roughly 6% are committed by nonwhites (mainly black males). African American female suicides are extremely rare, accounting for maybe only 1% of all suicides. Although the oldest white males—those age 85 or older—tend to have suicide rates about two to three times as high as those of younger white males, roughly 12% of suicides are committed by adolescents. Suicide rates of the oldest white males have stayed high (or dropped a little from 2006 to 2009), but went back up in 2013 (see Chapter 5, Table 5.1). The absolute highest suicide rates (19.7 per 100,000 in 2013) are among the middle-aged (specifically, those ages 45–54).

The broad category of completed suicides includes probably 15–20 major subtypes (see Table 1.1 and Chapter 2). This is also true of nonfatal attempts, suicide ideations, and indirect self-destructive behaviors. However, the numbers and traits of types of suicide are subjective and arbitrary.

In Table 1.1 several types of suicide are specified (cf. Interian et al., 2018). It needs to be emphasized that these suicide types are somewhat arbitrary. There is no absolute number or correct classification of suicide types. Obviously, there is at least one type of suicide (viz., intentional action by the would-be suicide that results in a person's death). But, depending on your perspective, many different subtypes even of this type could also be posited.

For example, the French sociologist Emile Durkheim (1897/1951; see Chapter 7) thought that suicides were mainly ego-anomic (excessively individuated and/or experiencing normative deregulation). Psychoanalyst Karl Menninger (1938) argued that most completers were depressed, wanting revenge, or guilt-driven. French existentialist Jean Baechler (1979) felt that completed suicides were mainly motivated by escape and/or aggression (with some involving risk taking or sacrificial acts). In earlier work, I (Maris, 1981, 2015) have contended that maybe 75% of all suicides are motivated by the wish for escape, followed by revenge (perhaps 20%; cf. Joiner, 2005, 2010) has claimed that suicide completers have to achieve the ability to suicide (usually over many years and life experiences) and become more fearless of pain and death. He also asserts that they are often experiencing what he calls "thwarted belongingness" and repeated, escalating pain (including "psychache" or emotional pain). Note the disciplinary bias of all of these perspectives on suicide types, which accentuates the need for a more interdisciplinary conceptualization of suicide.

TABLE 1.1. Types of Suicide, from Different Disciplinary Perspectives

Emile Durkheim (1897/1951)—Sociological

    Anomic (sudden normative deregulation)
    Egoistic (excessive individuation)
    Altruistic (insufficient individuation)
    Fatalistic (excessive regulation)

Karl Menninger (1938)—Psychoanalytic

    Revenge (wish-to-kill)
    Depressed (wish-to-die)
    Guilt (wish-to-be-killed)

Jean Baechler (1979)—Existential

    Escape
    Aggressive
    Oblative (sacrificial or transfiguration)
    Ludic (ordeal or game)

Ronald Maris (1981)—Epidemiological

    Escape (perhaps 75%)
    Revenge (roughly 20%)
    Self-sacrificing
    Risk-related

Thomas Joiner (2005), David Klonsky (2015)—Psychological

    Acquired ability to inflict lethal self-injury
    Thwarted belongingness
    Perceived burdensomeness
    Escalating pain

Source: Maris (1997b, pp. 257–259); see also Maris (2017).

One way to delineate major subtypes of completed suicide is to cross-classify sociodemographic traits and motives (Maris et al., 1992). For example, suicides can be subdivided into younger, middle-aged, and older white males; white females (whose rates tend to peak in middle age); black males and females; and Hispanics, Asians, Native Americans, and other racial or ethnic groups. If we assume basic motivations of escape, revenge, altruism, and risk-taking, we could further specify suicidal subtypes. To illustrate, Hemingway can be thought of as an older white male suicide motivated by escape. Often it is useful to distinguish psychiatric patient suicides from suicides in the general population who have never been treated for a mental disorder. Some of the permutation and combination nuances of completed suicide subtypes are considered further in Chapter 3.

Nonfatal Suicide Attempts

It is difficult to accurately measure the incidence or prevalence of nonfatal suicide attempts, since there are no legally mandated registration requirements like the ones for suicidal deaths. One estimate (Drapeau & McIntosh, 2015) found that there were 41,149 completed suicides and 1,028,725 nonfatal attempts in 2013—a ratio of 25:1 (usually the range is between 10:1 and 25:1). Whatever the exact ratio, it is clear that far more people make nonfatal attempts than complete suicide (Maris et al., 2000).

Again to oversimplify, the typical nonfatal suicide attempter in the United States is a younger female with interpersonal problems who overdoses, often four to five times over her life. Females on average make 3–4 suicide attempts for every 1 made by males (Maris et al., 2000; Maris, 2015). Most people (perhaps 85–90%) who make suicide attempts end up dying natural deaths. This lower fatality rate for attempters is a function of both different methods and motives.

There are a relatively small number of people who make nonfatal suicide attempts before completing suicide. In my Chicago survey, 70–75% of all suicide completers made only one attempt—and as noted above, I found that 88% of white males over age 45 made only one fatal suicide attempt (Maris, 1981). Furthermore, 84% of all suicide attempters make only two attempts, and these are mainly younger women (see Chapter 5 and Maris et al., 2000).

Men are much more likely to use firearms and hanging when they attempt suicide, while women are less likely than men to use guns and more likely to take overdoses and poisons. In 2013, the suicide completion rate for white males was 23.4 per 100,000 versus 6.5 for white females, about 3.6 times higher (Drapeau & McIntosh, 2015). Combining those data with the excessive proportion of female suicide attempters versus males (about three to four times higher), we could speculate that if women used more lethal suicide attempt methods, then the male and female suicide rates would be about the same.

Just like suicide completers, nonfatal suicide attempters do not constitute one type, but many. Since fewer suicide attempters by definition do not die, it is tempting to assume that most suicide attempters do not really want to die and choose their attempt methods accordingly. But that is overly simplistic, as the HBO documentary *Cobain: Montage of Heck* (Morgen, 2015), about the frenetic suicidal spiral of Kurt Cobain, illustrates. Among the main motives for nonfatal suicide attempts are these:

- To escape an intolerably painful life situation, even at the risk of death.
- To get even with others, or to punish themselves and/or others.
- To achieve catharsis or tension reduction, or to relieve pressure and demands.
- To "cry for help" (Farberow & Shneidman, 1961) and initiate changes (get treatment, draw attention to themselves and relationships, to transfigure themselves or their life situations, break up an "ice-bound soul," etc.).
- To give in to impulses or take chances; to live on the edge. (However, see Joiner, 2010; also see Gilbert et al., 2011, who found that non-attempters had higher impulsivity scores than did attempters.)

Suicide Ideas and Ideation

Obviously, a lot of people think about suicide, but very few ever even attempt it, let alone complete it. Linehan and Laffaw (1982) speculate that 24% of persons in the U.S. population think about suicide at some time in their lives. In 2013, that would have amounted to 76,800,000 (lifetime) suicide ideators. Combining these data with our earlier U.S. statistics for 2013 (Drapeau & McIntosh, 2015), we get these figures:

- 41,149 completed suicides in the year.
- 1,208,725 suicide attempts (some fatal, most not).
- 76,800,000 lifetime (dividing by 75 mean years, we get 1,024,000 per year) suicide ideators (Mundt et al., 2013, found that patients with suicide ideas and/or prior suicidal behavior were four to nine times more likely to report suicidal behavior prospectively).

As we might expect, there are many different types of suicide ideation. Suicide ideas can be the following:

- Fleeting, episodic, or situational ideas. Beck et al.'s (1979a) Scale for Suicide Ideation includes the timing and strength of the wish to die; scores on this scale range from a low of 0 to a high of 38.
- Chronic and obsessive ideas. For example, the poet Sylvia Plath obsessed about the details of suicide a lot; she thought of a skiing "accident," drowning herself in the ocean, taking an overdose of Seconal, jumping from at least the seventh floor of a building, or gassing herself by placing her head in an unlit oven. (She eventually acted on the last of these ideas; see Case 6.1 in Chapter 6.)
- Ideas including a definite plan (e.g., "I am going to save up my pain medications and then go out in the woods and take them") and a view of suicide as a solution. The philosopher Friedrich Nietzsche said, "The idea of suicide got me through many a difficult night" (quoted in Yalom, 1992).
- Ideas with no plan ("How would you do it?" "I don't know").
- Lethal ideas (involving guns, hanging, jumping from heights, lying on a train track, etc.).
- Nonlethal ideas (a lot of overdosing, cutting oneself, holding one's breath until dead, etc.).
- Ideas involving not only a specific plan, but a schedule for time and circumstances (e.g., "I'll hang myself next weekend, if this pain does not subside").
- Nonspecific and vague plan ("Well, I hadn't really thought about *that*").
- Ideas involving access to lethal means (e.g., actually having a gun and bullets) or not involving such access.
- Ideas involving knowledge about utilizing means (e.g., knowing how to use a gun) or not involving such knowledge.

Many suicide ideas concern problematic interpersonal relationships. For example, de Catanzaro (1992) claims that 64–84% of the variance in suicide ideation is explained by social relations, especially romantic or sexual relations. Suicide ideas also often concern feelings of loneliness and of being a burden to others, which Joiner (2005) calls "perceived burdensomeness."

Having ideas about suicide or death is one of the official psychiatric DSM-5 criteria for diagnosing major depressive disorder. Probably the simplest (and most unreliable) assessment of suicidality is simply to ask patients about their suicide ideation; however, writing "No SI" in a patient's chart is no guarantee that suicide ideas are not present (Silverman & Berman, 2014; Berman, 2018). Patients often are aware that admitting to suicide ideas means running the risks of forced treatment, coercive intervention, and sanctions. There have been cases of military personnel denying their suicide ideas to avoid not being promoted, even though they were actively suicidal (see Chapter 20). In 2015, the copilot of Germanwings Flight 9525, Andreas Lubitz, hid his suicide ideas and plans (for crashing the plane into a mountain) from his superiors in order to be able to carry them out.

Some suicide ideas may be "transformation drives," not actual wishes to die (Hillman, 1977). When Jim Jones and about 914 of his People's Temple followers committed suicide in 1978 in Guyana, South America, Jones had "eschatological" ideas: He thought that the "end of days" was approaching and that the world as we know it was being transformed. He did not think that he and his followers were suiciding, but rather were changing into another type of spiritual life. A similar case was the Heaven's Gate suicide of 39 people on March 26, 1997. The leader of this group, Marshall Applewhite, said that they were undergoing "Chrysalis"—not dying but changing into something else, like a caterpillar becoming a butterfly. Here the idea is not biological cessation as much as it is spiritual transformation. In Theravada Buddhism, the physical body is not considered to be the true self, and through asceticism and yoga it must be renounced to achieve *nirvana*. A similar concept to *nirvana* in classical Hinduism is *moksha*.

Finally, the wish to die is different from the inability to keep living. Linehan (2015) talks about "behavior trumping ideas": A person can wish to keep living but may essentially be unable to because of chronic self-destructive behaviors, which need to be changed.

Indirect Self-Destructive Behaviors

The vast majority of self-destructive behaviors do not result in a discrete suicide attempt or completion. Most self-destructive acts are partial, chronic, and long-term (Menninger, 1938; Farberow, 1980; Maris et al., 2000). Although these actions may contribute to shortening one's life expectancy, as in the case of choreographer and movie director Bob Fosse (Maris, 2015, p. 10), we must remember that completed suicide generally includes a clear intent to die. For example, most cigarette smokers just want to ingest nicotine, not to die, even though they know that their smoking may hasten their death.

As can be seen in Table 1.2, there are many types of behaviors that are not in themselves directly suicidal. They usually do not involve an explicit suicide attempt method, but can be self-destructive over time. Gambling is related to the fact that Las Vegas has the highest suicide rate of any other city in the United States. Gambling is also related to depression, alcohol abuse, and financial problems. Risky sports include race car driving, climbing icy mountains, whitewater rafting, and the like (Klausner, 1968). Many people die under circumstances involving excessive drinking and/or opiate abuse (consider the current epidemic of opioid overdose in the United States). Among celebrities, one thinks of the drug-abuse-related deaths

TABLE 1.2. Indirect Self-Destructive Behaviors

- Pathological gambling
- Risky sports (racing cars, mountain climbing, white water canoeing, etc.)
- Chronic alcohol or substance abuse (especially opiates, cigarettes)
- Dangerous driving (especially while intoxicated)
- Russian roulette
- Unprotected, indiscriminate sexuality
- Obesity or anorexia nervosa
- Self-mutilation, body piercing, excessive tattooing
- Fighting, war

Source: Reprinted from *The Lancet,* Vol. 360, R. W. Maris, "Suicide," pp. 319–326. Copyright © 2002, with permission from Elsevier.

of Philip Seymour Hoffman in 2014, John Belushi in 1982, Elvis Presley in 1977, Janis Joplin in 1970, and many others.

Driving while intoxicated is the number one cause of teenage death, and committing other risky acts under the influence of alcohol or drugs is all too common in this age group. One of my first forensic cases was the intoxication-related death of the son of Dan Chandler and grandson of "Happy" Chandler (a former commissioner of baseball and governor of Kentucky). The grandson had been using cocaine on spring break while watching the movie *Bugsy* about mobster Bugsy Segal, in which Segal plays Russian roulette and survives. He said to his girlfriend, "I can do that," took five of six cartridges out of his .38, spun the cylinder, and promptly shot himself in the head. The family hired me to argue to the medical examiner that there was an 83% chance he would survive, and that the death could be legally ruled an accident. When I brought this up to the medical examiner, he took out a .357 from his desk drawer, put in one bullet, spun the chamber and handed it to me, and said, "Put it to your head and pull the trigger, if you do not think this is suicide."

Indiscriminate sexuality has many self-destructive consequences (Maris, 1972), such as HIV/AIDS and other sexually transmitted diseases—think of former NBA player Magic Johnson. Promiscuity also decreases the chances that a person will have a significant other available when one is needed. For instance, Wilt Chamberlain (also formerly of the NBA) boasted of thousands of lovers, but how can he "be there" for so many partners or they for him?

Most people fail to realize that anorexia nervosa has the highest death rate of any psychiatric disorder. As many as 20% of those with the disorder are dead after about 20 years. One study claimed that persons with anorexia had a death rate 12 times that of those without it. Self-mutilation, excessive tattooing, and body piercing can also be self-destructive. Persons with borderline personality disorder have a penchant for repeated self-cutting. Many felons in jails and prisons are heavily tattooed. There is even a trend toward considering tattoos as fine art: A few persons with exquisite upper-body tattoos have given their consent to be skinned at death and have their skins mounted in frames for posterity (Randall, 2013).

Finally, war and fighting are probably (see Chapter 20) related to increased suicide risk. I have now testified in about a dozen cases of military veteran suicide, most alleged to be related to posttraumatic stress disorder (PTSD). I have addressed the U.S. Congress about this serious problem (Maris, 2008). Finally, do not forget that most suicides are mixed types (Maris et al., 2000).

Definition of Suicide

Now we know that suicide is not just one thing. But how exactly do we define it (Shneidman, 1985)? The word *suicide* in English and French derives from the modern Latin *suicidium* (1651). *Sui* means "of oneself," and *cidium* means "a killing." The idea that an act of suicide is intentional self-murder, and that persons who are suicides kill themselves deliberately, probably first occurred in 1728. The German word for suicide is *selbstmord* ("self-murder" or "self-death"). In Anglo-Latin legal terminology, suicide was called *felo-de-se* (literally "one guilty concerning himself"; Maris, 1993).

According to philosopher David Mayo (1992, 2015), suicide has four basic elements:

1. A death has occurred.
2. The death must be of one's own doing.
3. The ending of life was intentional.
4. The agency of death was active (but occasionally passive).

Let us reflect on each of these four elements.

1. Medically or legally, when a death occurs, the medical examiner or coroner has four choices as to how to certify the manner of death: *natural, accidental, suicidal,* or *homicidal* (these choices are sometimes called the *NASH* classification of death). The manner of death can also be labeled *pending* or *unknown*. The *cause,* or what produced the death, and the *manner* of death are different. Unfortunately, we cannot be certain what criteria medical examiners or coroners may use to determine suicide. For example, do they require a suicide note? The fact remains that to have a bona fide suicide, someone must have died. It is amazing how many scientific articles and books on suicide have been written, but are based on samples without a single actual completed suicide in them (Maris et al., 2000).

If a person dies by someone else's hands, then the death is likely some kind of homicide (or a wrongful death related to medical malpractice). Often contact gunshot wounds (GSWs) indicate suicides, but noncontact GSWs may be homicides or accidents (other things being equal). If a virus, bacteria, or disease kills a person, then the death is natural.

2 and 3. To oversimplify, death can be seen as one of the following:

- Intentional (suicidal).
- Unintentional (accidental).

- Nonintentional (natural).
- Contraintentional (homicidal).

However, since human intention is not pure or constant, determining intentionality can get complicated. People can have both a wish-to-die and a wish-to-live at the same time (i.e., they may be ambivalent). How dominant or pure does the wish-to-die have to be in order for a suicide to occur? Does the suicide wish have to be 100%? Can a suicide wish versus a life wish be 75–25% and the death still be a suicide? Can it even be 51–49%? After all, even most suicide completers have some ambivalence about dying.

4. Suicides are usually active and direct. For example, a person loads a revolver, places it at the temple or puts it in the mouth, and then pulls the trigger. However, some suicides are passive or indirect. Examples might include failing to take life-saving medicine (like insulin) or get life-saving surgery (perhaps for breast or prostate cancer), or failing to move from the path of an oncoming train, bus, or truck. There is also so-called "suicide by cop" when a person provokes a police officer, fully intending for the officer to shoot and kill the provoker.

Edwin Shneidman wrote an entire book just about the definition of suicide (Shneidman, 1985). In that book, he concluded: "Currently in the Western world, suicide is a conscious act of self-induced annihilation, best understood as a multidimensional malaise in a needful individual who defines an issue for which the suicide is perceived as the best solution."

Let's consider some of the ingredients in Shneidman's definition.

1. *"Currently in the Western world":* Although the word *suicide* itself has a timeless essential meaning, suicide has had different connotational nuances in different parts of the world at different times in history. For example, in Chapter 18 I discuss the case of the legendary Greek warrior Ajax, who fell on his sword out of shame during the Trojan War, as depicted on a vase dating back to 540 B.C. By contrast, in the late 20th century in the United States, musician Kurt Cobain's suicide was related to heroin abuse, attention-deficit/hyperactivity disorder (ADHD), and depressive disorder. In ancient India, the concept of *suttee* mandated that a deceased man's widow immolate herself on his funeral pyre. Probably in very ancient civilizations there was not even a word for suicide, given its rarity.

2. *"a conscious act":* Shneidman argues that suicides are a malfunction (catabolic) of our minds, not of our brains. For example, suicidal individuals often have dichotomous, rigid thinking, which leads them to faulty, unnecessary conclusions (such as the need to suicide). When most such persons suicide, they basically know what they are doing and want the outcome.

3. *"a multidimensional malaise":* *Malaise* means an indefinite feeling of debility often preceding the onset of impending illness—a kind of vague funk or *ennui*. Something is perceived as profoundly wrong, but we really cannot understand it. A lot of depressed people suffer from malaise and *ennui*, but are not technically "sick." Since suicide is multifaceted, its etiology is multi-causal and complex. Suicide

is a combined, interactive product of physical, neurobiological, psychological, psychiatric, and social forces, etc.

4. *"a needful individual"*: Notice that each suicide is idiosyncratic or idiographic. No one suicidal individual is exactly like any other. Following Henry Murray (1938), Shneidman claimed that most suicides had unmet (mainly social-psychological) needs or deficits, such as the needs for self-esteem and recognition, security, constancy and predictability, achievement, order, nurturance, and/or control.

5. *"an issue"*: For Shneidman, the dominant suicide issue was repeated, intolerable psychic pain, which he called "psychache (cf. Ducasse et al., 2018)." The most frequently prescribed drug in the United States is a pain medication, hydrocodone. Suicidal pain has both physical and psychic components.

6. *"perceived as the best solution"*: Note that suicidal individuals' perception can be faulty, although not always. Is there an alternative short of suicide that can produce the same result? Most suicides conclude that their pain and suffering are inextricably intertwined with being alive under the best of circumstances (Maris, 1982). Thus, they conclude that the best and perhaps only real solution is to stop living (Shneidman said that *only* is the "four-letter word" in suicidology). All alternative solutions, such as psychiatric medications, psychotherapy, love, money, or religion, are seen as ultimately ineffective. Suicide is viewed as a solution to a problem, but unfortunately the problem may be life itself.

One final caveat: Shneidman's definition of *suicide* really tends to be an explanation, which definitions should not be. We should define something first, then explain it.

Family History and Suicide

Can suicide be genetic, contagious, or modeled after? Is biology destiny? Exactly what do suicides inherit or copy from their families? In this brief final section of this chapter, Figure 1.3 depicts a partial family history of Ernest Hemingway, showing the mental disorders and suicidality of his close relatives. A similar figure for the novelist Virginia Woolf, who also committed suicide, is provided by Jamison (1993). The key in the lower left corner of Figure 1.3 gives the symbols used for suicide and mental disorders. Men are represented by squares and women by circles. In a family tree such as Figure 1.3, usually just first-degree relatives are included (mother, father, siblings, and children). Some aunts, uncles, cousins, nephews, and nieces may also be included if they have clear suicidality or mental disorders.

For example, Hemingway had four suicides in his immediate family (his father, sister, brother, and Ernest himself). Although not depicted in Figure 1.3, Hemingway's granddaughter Margaux Hemingway (a daughter of his son John) suicided at age 41 on July 1, 1996. Several of the Hemingways also had bipolar disorder. Virginia Woolf (who drowned herself) had recurrent depression, bipolar disorder, and cyclothymia in her family tree, but she was the only completed suicide.

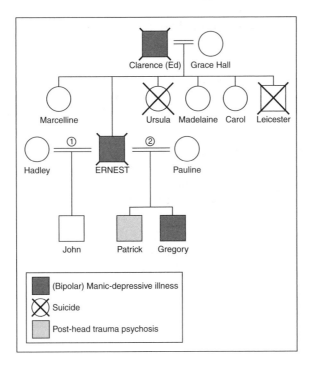

FIGURE 1.3. Partial family history of Ernest Hemingway. *Source:* From *Touched with Fire: Manic–Depressive Illness and the Artistic Temperament* by Kay Redfield Jamison. Copyright © 1993 Kay Redfield Jamison. Reprinted with permission of The Free Press, a division of Simon & Schuster, Inc. All rights reserved.

Here is some additional food for thought:

- Eleven percent of the suicide completers in my Chicago study had suicide in their first-degree families of origin, but none of the natural death controls did (Maris, 1981).
- Family suicide outcomes may be genetic (Roy & Linnoila, 1986: Mann & Currier, 2012) or involve modeling (Phillips et al., 1992).
- Suicides and mood disorders tend to run in families (like Hemingway's).
- An Amish study (Egeland et al., 1987) found that bipolar disorder and suicides were both related to a shared defective narrow portion of chromosome 11.
- From 10 to 18% of alcoholics eventually commit suicide (Roy & Linnoila, 1986; Murphy, 1992).
- Seventy-two percent of suicides in a study in St. Louis (Robins, 1981) were either depressed (47%) or alcoholic (25%). No other single risk factor was present in more than 5% of the St. Louis suicides.
- The fact that a person has a "suicidogenic" family tree does not mean that he or she is doomed to suicide. Eleven percent of family suicides is not even close to 100%.

- Suicides in the Chicago study had a slight tendency to be first-borns (Maris, 1981).
- Early object loss (especially in year 1 to 2 of life) through death or divorce of a parent was more common in the families of suicides than in the families of natural death controls (Maris, 1981, p. 98).
- Suicidal females tended not to be as close to their fathers as nonsuicidal females were (Maris, 1981).
- The problems most prevalent in suicides were exactly those problems present in their families of origin (Maris, 1981).
- First-degree relatives of psychiatric patients have a suicide risk almost eight times higher than the risk in relatives of normal controls (Tsuang, 1983).

I discuss the various questions raised here in later chapters of this book. In Chapter 2, I continue laying the theoretical foundation for suicidology.

CHAPTER 2

The Theoretical Construction of Suicidology

There is nothing more practical than a good theory.
—KURT LEWIN

Suicidology is a specialized academic discipline concerning the scientific study and prevention or control of self-destructive behaviors (Maris, 1993). It is a discipline akin to other academic disciplines, with one important exception: There is no department of suicidology at any extant university or college (although one can get a master's degree in suicidology at Marion College in Wisconsin, and there are some postdoctoral programs). Professionals calling themselves suicidologists can be can be found in a variety of disciplines: psychology, psychiatry, nursing, social work, counseling, sociology, public health, biology, philosophy, religion, and many more.

There are suicidological roots in France through the sociologist Emile Durkheim, in Austria through the psychoanalyst Sigmund Freud, and elsewhere. The modern founder of American suicidology was Edwin Shneidman, a clinical psychologist in Los Angeles. Shneidman coined the word *suicidology* in the late 1960s; started a professional association, the American Association of Suicidology (AAS, *www.suicidology.org*); and founded a scientific suicidological journal, *Suicide and Life-Threatening Behavior*. As the director of a suicide research-funding agency at the National Institute of Mental Health, Shneidman also created a postgraduate suicide training program at the Johns Hopkins University School of Medicine.

The great suicidologists have all had theoretical biases. Durkheim saw suicide as an external and constraining social fact independent of individual psychopathology. Freud and Karl Menninger considered suicide largely a murderous death wish that was turned back on upon oneself ("retroflexed" death, or "murder-in-the-180th-degree"). Edwin Shneidman conceived of suicide as "psychache," or intolerable pain deriving from common frustrated psychological needs (see below and

19

Shneidman, 1987). Psychiatrist John Mann tended to think of suicide as reflecting brain neurotransmitter abnormalities or deficiencies, especially of the serotonergic system in the prefrontal cortex (Maris, 2015; see Chapter 16).

Theory is usually contrasted with practice or empirical foundations (Chapter 3). The suspicion, especially within medicine with its reliance on clinical trials, is that theory is secondary to practice. At worst, theoreticians are seen as web-spinning dilettantes who really lack the practical skills to be able to do much of anything (e.g., prevent a suicide). Practical suicidologists, so the story goes, should pay attention to clinical trial data and neurobiological facts, brain chemistry and function, psychotropic medications (Maris, 2015), and the like.

Yet as Shneidman (1993) argues, theory *is* eminently practical. Theory is both a way of seeing and a way of not seeing. Without theory, one does not even know which facts to pay attention to. Not everything is equally important or attention-worthy. Our theoretical assumptions and biases (usually unstated and often unrecognized) influence what we attend to as well as what we neglect.

Theory can be defined as contemplation; an idea or mental plan for the way to do something; a systematic statement of the principles involved in something; a formulation of apparent relationships or underlying principles of unobserved phenomena that has been verified to some degree; "pure" as opposed to "applied" thought. A *hypothesis,* on the other hand, implies an inadequacy of evidence in support of an explanation, or a need for systematic (usually statistical) tests. Theories often grow out of systems of supported or confirmed hypotheses (see Chapter 28).

More formally, a *theory* can be thought of as set of assumptions, laws, axioms, definitions, concepts, research results, or the like that are deductively related. Table 2.1 presents one ambitious model for constructing systematic suicidological theory. Usually a suicidologist starts out with hypotheses or a causal model of suicide to be tested. The model is normally tested statistically (especially with regression models) in the context of an explicit research or experimental design (see Chapter 3). Sample size and selection, comparison and control groups, false positives (since suicide is rare), power equations, and so on are important considerations in this research process.

If we do our research carefully, we end up with probability estimates that our hypotheses or models are "true"—that is, different from chance associations (note that theories themselves are not true or false). Hypotheses or models that receive this contingent empirical support are often designated as *research results* or *findings.*

However, confirmed or supported hypotheses are only the beginning of formulating a theory, not the stopping point, which many researchers forget. Research results themselves need to be related to each other and to our definitions, postulates, axioms, and concepts, by the use of logic (rules of inference), statistics, or mathematics. Put another way, theory construction transcends model or hypothesis testing.

When research results are inferred deductively from sets of definitions, postulates, axioms, concepts, or laws by using standard rules of inference, they become *theorems* in a systematic theory. One can also proceed backward or inductively (see Table 2.1). Unfortunately for suicidology, very few suicidologists have ever attempted to construct formal theories of suicide (however, see Maris, 1981).

TABLE 2.1. Explanations of Suicidality

Set A	→ Set B	→ Set C (independent variables)	→ Set D (dependent variable = suicidality)
Laws, law-like propositions	Logic	RCTs, experiments, case–control studies	1. Nonsuicidal ideas/ behavior
Axioms, postulates	Mathematics	Research results (risk factors, commonalities, differences)	2. Fleeting suicide ideation
Definitions	Statistics	Empirical generalizations, facts	3. Chronic suicide ideation
Basic concepts	Measurements, scales	Case-control studies, epidemiology	4. Suicide-like gestures 5. Diffuse risk lifestyles 6. Nonlethal, vague plan 7. Specific, lethal plan 8. Nonserious attempts 9. Serious attempts 10. Completed suicides

Note. Set A + Set B + Set C "explains" Set D (here, suicidality). RCTs, randomized clinical trials.
Source: Original table by Maris.

In Table 2.1, what are the Set A propositions? For the most part, Set A propositions concern the assumptions, definitions, and laws or law-like propositions of suicidology's disciplinary or subdisciplinary perspectives. Set A propositions involve overlapping domains thought to be related to suicidal ideas and behaviors. For example, the domains might be biology or neurology, psychiatric disorders, family history and genetics, personality and psychological traits and states, life events, or medical illnesses. Often Set A propositions derive mainly from academic disciplines (psychology, psychiatry, sociology, biology, neurochemistry, neurobiology, economics, public health, etc.).

Disciplinary domain assumptions are of enormous importance in determining how we approach the study of suicide and suicide prevention. While suicidologists give lip service to the multidisciplinary study of suicide, most have very narrow and specialized domain assumptions, usually related to their own professional training and subdisciplinary paradigms.

For example, Shneidman (1993), a clinical psychologist, argued that in essence suicide is primarily a product of what he called "psychache," or repeated, intolerable psychological or mental pain. Shneidman believed (assumed) that suicide springs from an individual's psychic pain, stress, and general agitated *ennui,* which he alternatively called "pain, press, and perturbation," and he showed how the three concepts are interrelated.

Contrast Shneidman's assumptions with those of research neuropsychiatrist John Mann (Mann & Currier, 2012, and see Chapter 12). Unlike Shneidman, Mann tends to see the etiology of suicide in the human brain—most likely in the dysfunctions of the serotonergic system, especially those in the prefrontal cortex. In his lab in Pittsburgh (Mann now works in New York City), Mann and his associates were collecting, freezing, slicing, and examining the brains of suicides and controls in a state-of-the-art biomedical laboratory, while Shneidman was reading Melville's *Moby Dick* and the *Oxford English Dictionary*, wearing ties with whales on them, and interviewing acutely suicidal individuals in Los Angeles.

These two highly divergent, almost diametrically opposed approaches to the study and prevention of suicide grew out of fundamental theoretical differences. To oversimplify, for Shneidman you prevent suicide by getting psychotherapy, and for Mann you prevent suicide with psychiatric treatment, especially psychotropic medications. Theories, explanations, and a general model of suicide are explicated at the end of this chapter.

Key Concepts in Suicidology

Concepts and definitions are the basic building blocks (independent variables) for constructing a theory of suicide (the dependent variable). Although key concepts are presented throughout this text, some are so fundamental that they need to be considered at the beginning. These basic concepts include (1) suicidal careers, (2), lethality, (3) intent and motive, and (4) suicide risk factors.

Suicidal Careers

One central concept in a theory of suicide is the notion of a *suicidal career*, in which suiciding is something worked at, like achievement in a vocation (Joiner, 2005, calls suicide an "acquired capacity;" cf. Klonsky & May, 2015). It is often the result of an extensive accumulation of suicidogenic experiences and conditioning, usually against a backdrop of genetic and constitutional vulnerabilities such as being male and having a positive first-degree family history for suicide and mental disorder (as Ernest Hemingway did; see Chapter 1, Figure 1.3).

Suicides do not usually happen out of the blue, solely as the triggered products of life experiences and often-repeated, intolerable acute stressors. Almost all suicides have relevant biopsychosocial life histories that make them vulnerable to, relatively fearless of, and less protected from suicide. No one suicides in a biographical vacuum. Life histories are always relevant to the final act of suicide. Suicide ability and decisions develop over time and against certain biological, psychological, social, and genetic backdrops. They are never completely explained by acute, situational factors.

The following list (based on Maris, 1993) expands on the basic concept of suicidal careers:

- People are particularly vulnerable to suicide when death, decay, catabolic processes, destruction, and the terror that can accompany them break through their psychic defenses in systematic and patterned ways over a lifetime and dilute the will and ability to continue living (Maris, 1981).
- The concept of suicidal careers implies that it is necessary to conceive of life-threatening behaviors as having relevant life histories. Normally, given

the U.S. death registration and certification system, only a time-of-death profile is constructed, or one based on just a few weeks or months before the death.

- Suicidal deaths are never entirely reactive to present stressors. There is always a relevant set of what we might call "career contingencies," which mediate reaction to stress and help determine which individuals are in so-called "high-risk groups."
- Self-destructive behaviors need to be cast into causal models that span suicidal subjects' lives from birth to death. In addition, adequate samples of cases and controls need to be drawn and analyzed with modern multivariate statistics (such as logistic regression or path analysis).
- It is helpful in the analysis of suicidal careers to specify both direct and indirect causal paths to suicide, and to quantify them both (Maris, 1981).

Other suicidologists have recommended that the core suicide concepts be considered in the context of a person's entire lifespan. For example, Vaillant and Blumenthal (1990) argued that similar suicide risk factors (male sex, depressive disorder, hopelessness, alcoholism, lethal methods, cognitive rigidity, impulsiveness, aging, etc.) appear to operate at various stages of the lifespan of suicides, but that their contributory weights differ (such as beta weights in a regression model or path coefficients in a path model).

Rich et al.(1986) found that under age 30, the primary psychiatric diagnoses of suicides were antisocial personality disorder and substance abuse; from ages 20 to 30, schizophrenia and bipolar disorders predominated; from ages 30 to 50, affective (mood) disorders were central; and over age 50, psychotic affective disorder and organic brain damage were the key diagnoses.

Thomas Joiner (2005, 2010) and his students have introduced the concept of "the acquired ability to inflict lethal self-injury." Joiner (2005; cf. Brown et al, 2018; Klonsky & May, 2015) speaks of the "acquired capacity for suicide" (ACS) indicated by fearlessness about death (FAD) and elevated pain tolerance. Joiner's concept is essentially the same as what I am calling a "suicidal career." Instead of talking about social isolation and negative interaction, Joiner speaks of "thwarted belongingness" and "perceived burdensomeness." David Klonsky (Klonsky & May, 2014, 2015) adds that most so-called "suicide risk factors" are in fact primarily related to suicide ideation, not suicide behaviors. He claims that people tend to move from suicide ideation to suicide attempts and actual suicides if their pain (cf. Bender et al., 2011) and hopelessness persist or escalate and their connectivity fails. When they actually practice self-destruction, they become more expert at it, and thereby increase their capacity to suicide (Anestis et al., 2017).

The life and death of the poet Sylvia Plath constitute one example of a suicidal career. Although Plath gassed herself at age 30, she in fact had a lifelong accumulated experience with suicidogenic forces. Plath suffered from repeated episodes of depressive disorder; had several sessions of electroconvulsive therapy (ECT), which she saw as punishments; and made several suicide attempts, one of which was a very serious attempt with barbiturates. Although she had psychiatric treatment, including antidepressants, it did not relieve her depression or her obsession with suiciding. Finally, at the time of her death, she had a concomitant physical illness (influenza). The concept of a suicidal career emphasizes that multiple biopsychosocial problems such as these interact over a lifetime and synergistically produce the final suicidal outcome. In effect, Plath in the end became capable of suicide at the relatively young age of 30 (she was precocious even in her suicidality!). Plath is discussed in more detail in Chapter 6 (see Case 6.1).

Lethality

Lethality refers to the probability or medical certainty that an action, method, or condition will in fact kill you—that is, lead to a fatal outcome. For example, a high-caliber (.357 magnum or .45 caliber) shot to the brainstem has almost 100% lethality. On the other hand, trying to hold your breath until you die has zero lethality. Giner et al. (2014) talk about violent and serious attempters making more highly lethal attempts.

Although lethality is not restricted to methods of suicide attempts, most measures of suicide lethality refer to this indicator. For example, Card (1974) did an early classic estimate of the most and least lethal suicide methods, listed below in order from most to least lethal:

1. Gunshot
2. Carbon monoxide
3. Hanging
4. Drowning
5. Plastic bag over the head
6. Impact (e.g., blunt force trauma or jumping from heights)
7. Fire (self-immolation)
8. Poison (obviously varies by the type of poison, dose, response, etc.)
9. Drug overdose (often psychiatric or medicine cabinet drugs)
10. Gas
11. Cutting

In a later evaluation of the lethality of suicide methods, the Harvard Injury Control Research Center (2001) found the following fatality percentages by methods:

Rank	Method	% Fatal
1	Firearm	85% (about one-third instantaneously)
2	Hanging/suffocation	69%
3	Fall from height	31%
4	Poison/overdose	2%
5	Cutting	1%

Kar et al. (2014) also have developed a scale for assessing the lethality of suicide attempts.

Aaron T. Beck was one of the first suicidologists to attempt to measure lethality, defined as the medical certainty of death (Weishaar & Beck, 1992). Beck scored lethality as "zero," "low," "medium," or "high." This simple lethality scale is still in use today. However, some suicide scholars believe that we need a lethality scale with 9 or 10 points (not just 4) and better operational definitions and scaling techniques (Smith et al., 1984; Maris et al., 2000).

Others argue that lethality is a function not just of risk factors, but also of protective factors interacting with risk factors. For example, a lethality scale that assesses both risk and protective factors was created years ago by Weisman and Worden (1974). It is aptly designated as the Risk–Rescue Rating Scale. Risk and rescue scores are calculated by assessing the following factors:

Risk factors (A)	Rescue factors (B)
1. Agent or method	1. Location
2. Impaired consciousness	2. Key person
3. Lesions/toxicity	3. Probability of discovery
4. Reversibility	4. Accessibility
5. Treatment required	5. Delay to discovery

Each of the five risk factors is rated from 1 to 3 in severity, and the rescue factors are rated from 3 to 1, according to the strength of the rescue factors. Both totals are then converted to a score of 1 to 5 (e.g., total = 5–6 = 1, 13–15 = 5, etc.). The lethality score itself is then calculated by the formula $A/(A + B) \times 100$. Risk-rescue scores vary from a low of 17 to a high of 83.

A case example will perhaps make the risk–rescue concept clearer. A 36-year-old woman had been drinking heavily and arguing with her husband. She went into her bathroom and ingested from 25 to 90 mg of secobarbital (Seconal) as her husband was leaving for the evening. Upon noting the effects the drug was having on her, she went outside, managed to hail a taxi, and delivered herself to the emergency room. Twenty minutes later, she lapsed into a deep coma; she was sent to intensive care and later transferred to the general hospital for an anticipated stay of more than a week.

Her risk–rescue scoring was as follows: risk score = 5, rescue score = 5, risk-rescue score = 50. Her suicide potential was rated as moderate. Although her behavior was risky, her rescue or protective factors were also high.

Many lethality assessments refer not only to methods of suicide attempt, but rather to other suicide risk factors. Here is a sample of some of the many other lethality assessments (see Chapter 3 for a fuller discussion):

- The American Psychiatric Association has published a *Practice Guideline for the Assessment and Treatment of Patients with Suicidal Behaviors* (Jacobs et al., 2003, 2010).
- The U.S. Department of Veterans Affairs (2012) has created a pocket card template for a Suicide Risk Assessment Guide (see Chapter 20, Box 20.2).
- The AAS has a mnemonic: "IS PATH WARM?" This stands for the following:

ideation, substance abuse, purposelessness, anxiety, trapped feeling, hopelessness, withdrawal, anger, recklessness, and mood changes.

Motive and Intent

Suicide is intentional, not just self-inflicted. In ordinary English, *motive* refers to
one's presumed reason(s) for suiciding (depressive disorder, divorce, hopelessness,
terminal or painful physical illness, shame, guilt, loss, etc.). In suicidology. both
motive (especially) and intent are primary legal concepts (*Black's Law Dictionary*,
2009). In the law, *motive* is the cause or reason that moves the will and induces
action. In other words, motive is that which incites or stimulates a person to do an
act or to produce a result.

Intent is the purpose a person has in using a particular means (e.g., suicide)
to effect a result (e.g., death). Suicidal intent usually indicates that the individual
understood the physical nature and consequences of the self-destructive act. Thus,
for example, very young children may not be able to commit suicide. In the law in
some states, an individual is thought to be able to form suicidal intent, whether or
not he or she is "sane" or "insane." Indeed, most suicide exclusion clauses in life
insurance policies start out: "Whether sane or insane . . ." However, in other states
(such as California, Florida, Kansas, Kentucky, Michigan, Ohio, Oklahoma, Tennessee, and Wisconsin), proof of intent is usually required. The burden of proof is
normally on the plaintiff, since the law assumes that suicide did not occur unless
proven (i.e., more likely not in civil cases). This is a variation on criminal law's
"innocent until proven guilty."

But how does one know an individual's motives or intent, especially after death?
If a suicide attempt is not fatal, there can be direct questioning, or standardized suicide intent scales can be administered. For example, the Beck Suicide Intent Scale
(Beck, 1990) investigates such objective circumstances as isolation, timing, precautions against discovery, acts to get help, final acts, preparations for the attempt,
whether or not a suicide note was left, and communication of intent to others.
In addition, self-reports of purpose, expected fatality, the lethality of the method
used, seriousness of the suicide intent, attitude toward dying, rescue ability, and the
degree of precaution or premeditation are surveyed. Finally, the clinician can measure the attempter's reaction to the attempt, his or her vision of death, the number
of prior attempts (but remember that most older males only make one attempt),
and the involvement of alcohol and other drugs in the attempt.

Some suicidologists (e.g., Jobes et al., 1987) have created retrospective indices
for operationally classifying a death as a suicide when the individual dies from
the attempt. These criteria include not only prior explicit expressions of intent to
kill oneself, such as a suicide note (although up to 85% of suicides leave no note),
but also several indirect indications of suicidal intent. Among these are preparations for death; expressions of farewell, hopelessness, or emotional or physical
pain; efforts to procure or learn about means to die, such as computer searches or
buying the book *Final Exit* (Humphry, 1991/1996); or joining an organization like
the Hemlock Society or its contemporary counterpart, Compassion and Choices.

Preparations can also include precautions to avoid rescue, use of lethal means, and serious mood disorders.

Suicide Risk Factors

A final basic concept related to suicidal outcomes is that of *suicide risk factors,* which are considered throughout this text, particularly in Chapter 3. Their presence increases the probability of a self-destructive outcome, but it can also suggest treatment options. Some of these concepts include depressive and bipolar disorders, alcohol and other substance abuse, hopelessness, access to lethal means, pain, a positive history of self-destructive behaviors, neurobiological dysfunction, social isolation and negative interaction, stress–diathesis, and many others.

Suicide Commonalities and Similarities

Do suicides tend to have some characteristics in common that nonsuicides usually do not have, at least to the same degree? The founding father of American suicidology, Edwin Shneidman, claimed that they do, and that these traits are psychological (Shneidman, 1993). They characterize the suicidal mind, not the brain. Like a suicidological Moses, Shneidman posited 10 common psychological features he claimed are present in human self-destruction. Note that each commonality has two components; they are in effect dichotomies, with 20 total dimensions (e.g., purpose and solution). After listing the commonalities, I comment briefly on each, including their possible implications for suicide intervention or prevention. The commonalities are listed in Table 2.2.

TABLE 2.2. The 10 Commonalities of Suicide

I. The common purpose of suicide is to seek a solution to a life problem.

II. The common goal is cessation of consciousness.

III. The common stimulus is intolerable psychological pain.

IV. The common stressor is frustrated psychological needs.

V. The common emotion is hopelessness–helplessness.

VI. The common cognitive state is ambivalence.

VII. The common perceptual state is constriction.

VIII. The common action is egression.

IX. The common interpersonal act is communication of intent.

X. The common consistency is lifelong coping patterns.

Source: From *Definition of Suicide,* E. Shneidman, 1985. By permission of Regina Ryan Publishing Enterprises, Inc.

I. *The common purpose of suicide is to seek a solution to a life problem* (see Shneidman's definition of suicide in Chapter 1). Most people who commit suicide are in chronically stressful life situations or suicidal careers that seem to demand resolution. Like the chief character in Albert Camus's *The Myth of Sisyphus* (Camus, 1945), suicides experience their lives as painful, intolerable, absurd, meaningless, and perpetual—so much so that suicidal death may seem to be the only way out (Maris, 1982). Of course, one key response to this commonality is that often (not always) there are other solutions short of suicide. As Shneidman once said (personal communication), "Never buy a patient's syllogism," especially not the catabolic conclusion, "Therefore, I must kill myself."

II. *The common goal is cessation of consciousness.* Shneidman claims that suicides want to interrupt their tortured self-consciousness—to stop their mental pain ("psychache") and anguish. Thus it is understandable that analogies to suicide (sleep, anesthesia, psychosis, drug abuse, alcoholic stupor, etc.) all involve alteration or cessation of consciousness. Paradoxically, suicide may be a desperate transformational drive (Hillman, 1977), not necessarily a death wish ("Things have to change, even if I die"). As the lyrics go in the theme song from the classic movie and TV show *M*A*S*H*, "Suicide is painless, it brings on many changes . . ." The challenge to suicide prevention is to facilitate meaningful life change short of death through neurochemistry and psychotherapy.

III. *The common stimulus is intolerable psychological pain.* Shneidman came to see intolerable psychic pain ("*psychache*") as the key commonality is all suicides. He wrote (Shneidman, 1993):

> Nearing the end of my career in suicidology, I think I can now say what has been on my mind in as few as five words: suicide is caused by psychache. . . . Psychache refers to the anguish, soreness, aching psychological pain in the psyche, the mind. It is intrinsically psychological—the pain of excessively felt shame, or guilt, or humiliation, or loneliness, of fear, or anger, or dread of growing old, or of dying or whatever. (p. 51)

One absolutely central question for therapists is to ask their suicidal patients, "Can you tell me where you hurt?" and hope that they know, have insight, and are articulate. Often to prevent suicide, one just has to take the edge off the pain, not eliminate it.

IV. *The common stressor is frustrated psychological needs.* Most suicides have been frustrated in meeting some of their basic psychological needs. These include the 20–30 needs originally listed by Harvard psychologist Henry Murray (1938); examples include achievement, affiliation, autonomy, nurturance, order, play, succorance, and understanding. Or they could just as easily refer to the basic psychological and even physical needs stated by Maslow (1963)—the needs for security, love, self-esteem, shelter, food, sleep, sexual tension reduction, status, and so on. Often meeting psychological needs entails resocialization, ego regression, and even reparenting. Although Shneidman would not admit it, it may also involve "rewiring," or adjusting one's neurochemistry through psychopharmacology (see Mann & Currier, 2012, and the discussion in Chapters 16 and 23).

V. *The common emotion is hopelessness–helplessness.* Suicides are not merely depressed and anxious; as Beck et al. (1985) demonstrated, they tend to have become hopeless that their life quality will *ever* improve sufficiently, and they feel helpless to do anything about it. Therapists need to try to convince their patients, "You can be helped," and "I can and will help you." As psychiatrist Avery Weisman once commented (personal communication), "Suicidal patients need to have at least one significant udder."

VI. *The common cognitive state is ambivalence.* Suicides want to die and to live at the same time. It is common for soon-to-be suicides to make appointments (to play golf or tennis, to take part in a child's or grandchild's birthday or graduation, to take a vacation, to go to a doctor or dentist, etc.) for after their death. Freud claimed that we have both life (*eros*) and death (*thanatos*) wishes (Gay, 1988). All that is required for a suicide is a 51% wish to die. Sometimes therapists justify their interventions on the grounds that they are just responding to their patients' own ambivalence (i.e., reinforcing or supporting the patients' own life wishes).

VII. *The common perceptual state is constriction.* Shneidman used to ask his postdoctoral students at Johns Hopkins School of Medicine, "What is the four-letter word in suicidology?" The answer was *only*—as in "It [attempting suicide] was the only thing I could do." One of the most salient mental traits in depressed, suicidal individuals is the narrowing of their perceived viable alternatives to suicide (i.e., dichotomous thinking; see Weishaar & Beck, 1992). Suicides often think to themselves, "Either I must be miserable, or I must be dead." This perniciously dichotomous logic has led some (e.g., Brandt, 1975) to comment, "Never kill yourself when you are depressed." Cognitive therapy is useful in helping patients to conceive of viable alternatives to suicide.

VIII. *The common action is egression.* Recall some of Ishmael's opening lines in Melville's *Moby Dick* (1851/1981): "Whenever I find myself growing grim about the mouth; whenever it is a damp, drizzly November in my soul; whenever I find myself . . . bringing up the rear of every funeral I meet . . . then, I account it high time to get to sea as soon as I can" (p. 2).

Like Ishmael, suicides flee (fugue, escape) their tormented lives. Most suicides just want their pain to stop, even if they have to die. Many have already tried (repeatedly) alternatives short of suicide (psychiatric medication cocktails, psychotherapies, repeated ECT, alcohol and drug abuse, sexual promiscuity, divorce, religious conversion, overinvestment in work and professional careers, leaving town, taking sick leave, quitting jobs, ending relationships, etc.), but are now faced with the ultimate egression—from life itself. The challenge to suicidologists is to stop or deter the egression, to persuade the would-be suicide that he or she can escape without dying. Sometimes this may mean "Give me the gun [be careful here!] or the pills to hold for you until later on." (Shneidman once said he had a desk drawer full of guns.) Sometimes it means hospitalizations, involuntary commitment, seclusion, restraints—whatever it takes, say some. However, this kind of direct, forceful patriar-chal intervention prompted psychiatrist Thomas Szasz (1985) to say that suicidolo-gists ought to be housed in City Hall, next to the police department.

IX. *The common interpersonal act is communication of intent.* A lot of potential suicides will tell you (or imply) that they are contemplating suicide, if you listen carefully and generally just pay attention, although suicide ideation is not a reli-able indicator of completed suicide. These may not be dramatic cries for help, but rather indirect clues to suicide. Examples might include expressions of hopeless-ness, preparations for death or suicide (getting a gun, taking out life insurance, planning a funeral, writing suicide notes, putting affairs in order), serious/recal-citrant depression, nonfatal suicide attempts, exacerbation of drinking, expres-sions of farewell, inquiries about suicide methods (a person's computer should be checked for searches), isolation, efforts to avoid rescue, and many more. A word of caution: Since completed suicide is relatively rare, most of these clues to suicide will result in false positives (i.e., a suicide is predicted, but there is no suicide). Most clues to suicide are only clear after the suicide, not before.

X. *The common consistency is lifelong coping patterns.* Suicides tend to have what I called above "suicidal careers" and what Joiner (2005) calls "the acquired ability to inflict lethal self-injury." Suicides tend to be chronically self-destructive over long time periods. They have repeatedly exhausted their own adaptive repertoires. Most suicidal crises are only crises because of a long history of partially self-destructive experiences and malfunctioning neurobiology. It follows that suicide intervention cannot be a quick fix of an acute problem in an otherwise healthy, stable individual. Shneidman (1987) said that his 10 commonalities made up a "theoretical cubic model of suicide." In this model, the maximum suicide threat condition occurs when psychache (pain), press (stress), and perturbation (agitation) are all at their maximum levels.

Suicide Differences and Classifications

In spite of the fact that suicides tend to share common traits, clearly not all suicides are alike. For example, while most are middle-aged to older, a considerable number of suicides are younger. Most suicides tend to be males (if white, 72% in the United States), but the number of female suicides is not insignificant (white females make up about 18% of all suicides). A substantial majority (perhaps over 90%) of suicides have a diagnosable mental disorder, according to the American Psychiatric Associa-tion's (2013) *Diagnostic and Statistical Manual of Mental Disorders,* fifth edition (DSM-5), but by no means all do. A little over half of all U.S. suicides use guns (especially men), but others (especially women) tend to employ methods of lesser lethality, like poisons and overdoses. In short, the variability among suicides is great. This complexity, variety, and multidimensionality have some pragmatic consequences for theory construction in suicidology. To be able to understand, assess, or con-trol suicide, we must specify the type of suicide outcome as precisely as possible.

Differentiation and classification of suicide are complex undertakings, which I have gone into great detail about elsewhere (see Maris, 1992b).

A crucial question is this: If suicide is many things, how many? In the extreme, a few clinicians might argue that every individual suicide is unique—that no two suicides are the same. If this were true, then predicting or preventing suicide would be virtually impossible.

Prediction of individual suicides with any accuracy in the short run *is*, in fact, impossible. Logically, if all suicidal careers were unique, then we could only understand what caused *one* suicide and only *after* it happened, which would obviously be too late for treatment or intervention. Fortunately, almost no one believes that all suicides are unique. What is more plausible is that suicides share some traits and states, but not others (see Maris et al., 2000, 51ff.).

If there are too many different types or classes of overlapping suicides (especially given the relative rarity of suicide), then prediction of suicide becomes complex if not impossible (except for group rates over years). For example, in DSM-5 there are 20 types of major mental disorders and about 478 subtypes. Partly because of this, the unreliability and invalidity of psychiatric diagnoses are notorious. Theoretically, we could specify a virtually unlimited number of suicide types or classes, but to do so would be to create differences that really do not make a difference (i.e., specious differences). With this problem in mind, suicidologists usually define three or four basic types of suicide, and perhaps two or three subtypes of each (see Table 2.3 and later in the chapter, Figure 2.1).

Table 2.3 presents a classification of suicidal behaviors that encompasses not only types of completed suicide, but also types of nonfatal suicide attempts, suicide ideation, mixed types of suicidal behaviors, and indirect suicidal behaviors. Most of the subtypes of completed suicides apply *mutatis mutandis* to other forms of self-destructive behaviors and ideas listed in Table 2.3. There are at least as many different types or classes of nonfatal suicide attempters as there are types of completed suicides. One can easily think of suicide attempts that are psychotic versus nonpsychotic, organic versus nonorganic, interpersonal or not, self-harm versus harm to others (such as murder–suicide attempts), altruistic versus narcissistic, risk-taking versus representing a more genuine wish to die, single versus multiple attempts, and so on.

Suicidal ideas or thoughts also need to be differentiated (not from other types, but within the idea types). Most people who think about suicide never make a suicide attempt or complete suicide. Included in this class are individuals who plan and prepare, obsess about suicide, save their pills, consider the circumstances for a suicide attempt (such as painful terminal illness), make living wills, ruminate about suiciding, openly threaten suicide to others, fantasize about suicide, and so on.

Perhaps the largest group of self-destructive behaviors consists of what Farberow (1980) has termed "indirect self-destructive behaviors" (ISDBs). ISDBs include self-mutilation (excessive tattooing and body piercing), deliberate self-harm, parasuicide (such as overdoses where suicide intent is minimal or unknown), participation in risky activities and sports (skydiving, mountain

TABLE 2.3. A Multiaxial Classification of Suicidal Behaviors and Ideation

Suicidal behaviors/ideas	Check (✓)	1. Primary type	2. Certainty	3. Lethality	4. Intent	5. Circumstances	6. Method	7. Sex	8. Age	9. Race	10. Marital status	11. Occupation
I. Completed suicides												
A. Escape, egotic, alone, no hope												
B. Revenge, hate, aggressive												
C. Altruistic, self-sacrificing, transfiguration												
D. Risk-taking, ordeal, game												
E. Mixed												
II. Nonfaral suicide attempts												
A. Escape, catharsis, tension reduction												
B. Interpersonal, manipulation, revenge												
C. Altruistic												
D. Risk-taking												
E. Mixed												
F. Single vs. multiple												
G. Parasuicide												
III. Suicidal ideation												
A. Escape, etc.												
B. Revenge, interpersonal, etc.												
C. Altruistic, etc.												
D. Risk-taking, etc.												
E. Mixed												
IV. Mixed or uncertain mode												
A. Homicide–suicide												
B. Accident–suicide												
C. Natural–suicide												
D. Undetermined, pending												
E. Other mixed												
V. Indirect, self-destructive behavior (not an exclusive category)												
A. Alcoholism												
B. Other drug abuse												
C. Tobacco abuse												
D. Self-mutilation												
E. Anorexia–bulimia												
F. Over, or underweight												
G. Sexual promiscuity												
H. Health management problem, medications												
I. Risky sports												
J. Stress												
K. Accident-proneness												
L. Other (specify)												

Note. Certainty: Rate 0–100%.
Lethality (medical danger to life): Rate zero, low, medium, high (O, L, M, H).
Intent: Rate zero, low, medium, high.
Mitigating circumstances (psychotic, impulsive, intoxicated, confused): Rate zero, low, medium, high.
Method: Firearm (F); poison (solid and liquid) (P); poison (gas) (PG); hanging (H); cutting or piercing (C); jumping (J); drowning (D); crushing (CR); other (O); none (N).
Sex: Male (M) or female (F).
Age: Record actual age at event.
Race: White (W), black (B), Asian (A), other (O).
Marital status: Married (M), single (S), divorced (D), widowed (W), other (O).
Occupation: Manager, executive, administration (M); professional (P); technical worker (T); sales worker (S); clerical worker (C); worker in precision production (mechanical repairer, construction worker) (PP); service worker (SW); operator, laborer (OL); worker in farming, forestry, fishing (F); other (O); none (N).

Source: Maris (1992b, p. 82). Copyright © 1992 The Guilford Press. Reprinted with permission.

climbing, whitewater rafting, race car driving, etc.), pathological gambling, alcoholism and other substance abuse, cigarette smoking, overeating/obesity or anorexia nervosa, overwork or overinvestment in a career, sexual promiscuity or indiscretion, and much more. Completed suicide is the tip of the proverbial self-destructive iceberg. Most self-destructive behaviors never result in an actual suicide attempt or completion.

One final classification category is self-destruction versus all other deaths. Forensically, whether or not a death is a suicide is often determined by a process of elimination. That is, suicide is *not* a natural death, an accident, or a homicide. To make classification difficulties worse, manner of death is often equivocal (the manner of death cannot be determined), pending (the manner of death is not yet known), or overlapping. For example, we may only be able to classify a death as "suicide or accident, undetermined."

Given all the variation in self-destructive behaviors and ideas, the scientific study of suicide (suicidology) would be advanced immensely by the creation of a standardized suicide classification system, similar to DSM-5 or the World Health Organization's (WHO's) *International Classification of Diseases,* 10th revision (ICD-10; WHO, 1992, 2015a). Theoretically, there is no reason why a diagnostic and statistical manual of suicidal behaviors and ideas could not be developed. (O'Carroll et al., 1996, did early work on this topic; cf. Interian et al., 2018.)

In passing, it is important to briefly allude to how suicide is classified in DSM-5 and ICD-10. Since suicide is not a mental disorder per se, there is no DSM-5 code for it. Suicide is an explicit criterion for two mental disorders: major depressive disorder and borderline personality disorder. Suicide risk is also related to a list of other mental disorders. Section III of DSM-5 includes a discussion of "Conditions for Further Study," and a new mental disorder called "suicidal behavior disorder" is proposed there. The criteria for this proposed disorder include a suicide attempt within the past 24 months. One worries that the American Psychiatric Association may end up designating suicide (or attempts) as a new mental disorder, although not all persons committing or attempting suicide are mentally disordered. No doubt the pharmaceutical industry would be pleased if this happens, since it further justifies the use of drugs to treat suicide—and, indeed, to create new drugs (Olfson et al., 2015).

ICD-10 (Cooper, 1994) includes codes for both physical and mental disorders. It and its predecessors have long coded suicidal behaviors. For example, in ICD-10, suicide and intentional self-harm are given codes in the range of X71–X83. Attempted suicide is coded T14.91.

Although Table 2.3 is far from a finished product and has its own obvious shortcomings (such as the lack of parsimony), it is offered as a suicide classification step in the right direction. First, in the far left column, the rater has to decide if a suicidal outcome (just one outcome at a time) is (I) a completion, (II) a nonfatal attempt, (III) ideation, (IV) a mixed or uncertain outcome, or (V) an ISDB. The roman numerals in this column are referred to hereafter as *codes,* and this column as a whole constitutes Axis I of this scheme.

Second, I have assumed (from a prior review of the published scientific literature) that suicidal outcomes are fundamentally either (A) escape, (B) revenge, (C) altruistic, (D) risk-taking, or (E) mixed. If one type is clearly predominant, then it is best not to code the case as mixed. The primary type of suicidal outcome should be checked in column 1.

Third, it is recommend that the rater record the degree of certainty of the type (0–100%) in column 2, the lethality in column 3, the degree of intent to die in column 4, and the presence of mitigating circumstances in column 5. In addition the method, sex, age, race, marital status, and occupational category should be coded for each case (columns 6–11). Code V records all known ISDBs. Code V can be completed for all cases and is not an exclusive code; it also constitutes Axis III of this scheme. However, codes I–IV are mutually exclusive.

In Table 2.3, suicidal outcomes are being coded on three axes: Axis I (outcome and primary type of outcome, recorded in column 1), Axis II (secondary characteristics, recorded in columns 2–11), and Axis III (ISDBs, recorded in code V). For example, the full-length code "IA/75, H, H, M, F, M, 55, W, D, P/A, C, H" would indicate an escape suicide with 75% certainty, high lethality and intent, medium mitigating circumstances, and death by firearm; the individual in this case was a male, age 55, white, divorced, and a professional. The code V subcodes (A C, H) indicate that this man had ISDBs of alcoholism, tobacco use, and health management problems. This classification scheme is incomplete, since it does not rate biological or social types explicitly.

Explanations and Theories

How can the theoretical ingredients described above (definitions, concepts, axioms, postulates, hypotheses, research results, commonalities, differences, facts, randomized clinical trials, experiments, case–control studies, causal models, etc.) all be integrated into a systematic, interactive explanation of suicide?

Explanations or theories are not true or false. Rather, they have *cogency* (or not)—a probability of accounting for outcomes like suicidality. Theory construction in suicidology includes taking hypotheses confirmed statistically by research results (as in what is now called "evidence-based psychiatry") and then converting them into theorems by deducing them logically, mathematically, or statistically from sets of general postulates, axioms, and definitions.

Theory guides us in what to pay attention to. A formal theory of suicide can be thought of as sets (see Table 2.1) of laws or law-like propositions (axioms, assumptions, postulates) and definitions that are related logically or mathematically to hypotheses or models confirmed by empirical research results. To deduce research results from broad-domain axiomatic propositional assumptions is to *explain* them (see Table 2.1).

Hypotheses, as suggested earlier in the chapter, are usually more focused and limited than theories are. A hypothesis, as a statistically testable proposition, implies a statistical test that allows us to accept or reject a null hypothesis under specified conditions and assumptions. One important characteristic of hypotheses is their falsifiability. For example, Durkheim's (1897/1951) hypothesis that suicide rates vary inversely with the degree of social integration (see Chapter 7) was operationalized (as "status integration" by Gibbs & Martin, 1964), tested, and accepted only for occupational statuses.

Causal models tend to predict the relationships of several independent variables (as opposed to hypotheses, which are usually bivariate) to an outcome variable like suicide (Hill, 1965). Causal models are normally operationalized by regression equations (especially logistic regression), but can also include path models, log-linear models, time series models, hazard analysis, and so on.

When hypotheses or causal models receive repeated empirical support in proper research designs in diverse samples and cultures, we tend to regard them as research results (Maris, 1981). Research results are the fundamental empirical regularities of suicidal behaviors and ideas that our theories attempt to explain.

A General Model of Suicide

Alfred North Whitehead said, "Seek simplicity and distrust it." At the risk of oversimplifying or misrepresenting the complexities of suicide, I conclude this chapter with a general model of suicidal behaviors. Not all of the variables discussed above have been included in this model (e.g., preparations for suicide or ISDBs). The model is both an orientation to the study of suicide and a summary, to which I return at the end of this book (see Chapter 28).

Theory should guide research. We should not settle for isolated facts, empirical generalizations, or even confirmed hypotheses. Any bona fide theory of suicide needs to encompass the entire lifespan or suicidal career of a suicide. Suicide requires time and certain experiences. Most suicides represent a gradual nondramatic accumulation of suicide risk factors over many years (about 40 to 60).

Let me clarify some details of the general model of suicidal behaviors in Figure 2.1. In column 1, row 3 (C1, R3), physical and emotional abuse is included and is not limited to one's parents. "Transactional–ecological deficits" (C1, R4) might include cultures, nations, or geographical areas with high suicide rates. "Hopefulness" (C3, R3) would include Linehan's "reasons for living." Finally, in C4, R2, the full phrase for "Low 5-HIAA" (5-HIAA is a serotonin metabolite, 5-hydroxyindoleacetic acid) should read "Low 5-HIAA in the prefrontal cortex and other neurobiological dysfunction."

Some of the salient characteristics of an adequate general model of suicide outlined in Figure 2.1 are now discussed.

- The four rows in the model represent interdisciplinary explanatory domains (viz., psychiatry, biology, psychology, and sociology). These four domains interactively contribute to suicide outcomes. This model of suicide is thus *biopsychosocial*. The ascending or descending lines in the four rows suggest the relative importance of the domains over the lifespan or suicidal career. For example, this model asserts that near the end of the suicidal life cycle, psychiatric and biological forces become more important; personality/psychological forces remains fairly constant; and social factors diminish somewhat in importance. Clearly, there could be more than just these four domains influencing suicide outcomes.

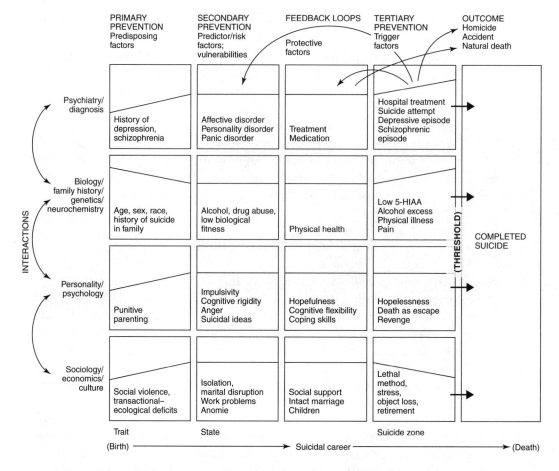

FIGURE 2.1. A general model of suicidal behaviors. Not all interactions are depicted. The figure does not include suicide ideation. *Sources:* Maris et al. (1992, pp. 667–669); Maris et al. (2000, p. 58); Maris (2002, pp. 319–326); Maris (2015, Chapter 8).

- The columns in the model are labeled in at least two ways:
  - First, from left to right, there are (1) predisposing factors (e.g., age, gender, and neurobiology, vs. more acute stressors); (2) predictor, risk, or vulnerability factors; (3) protective factors; (4) trigger, precipitating, or situational factors (note that most suicides are chronically, not acutely or situationally, triggered—healthy people usually absorb or deflect suicide triggers without suiciding); and (5) outcomes (cf. Blumenthal & Kupfer, 1990).
  - Second, columns 1, 2 and 4 remind us that suicide prevention varies over the life cycle. Gerald Caplan (1964; see also Maris et al., 2000) defined three types of prevention: *primary prevention* (which reduces incidence—i.e., it keeps suicide from ever developing), *secondary prevention* (which reduces prevalence or total cases), and *tertiary prevention* (which detects and limits damages of late-occurring disease processes—here, suicidality).

- Note that column 4 in the model can be thought of as a "suicide zone." Predisposing and suicide risk factors over time can interact, compound, and potentiate each other (e.g., in so-called "kindled depression"), leading either to suicide or (most likely) to "feedback loops" resulting in various treatments, interventions, or recurring episodes of suicidal disorders. Litman (1992) created the concept of the suicide zone with its heightened suicide risk, but he also suggested that for perhaps every 100 people who enter the suicide zone, only 1 or 2 ever commit suicide.

- There is also a "threshold" between heightened suicide risk (column 4) and completed suicide (column 5), or feedback loops (this is a dynamic model) into treatment and/or recurring suicidal disorder). Jerome Motto (1992) argues that everyone has a personal threshold of pain tolerance beyond which suicide is likely, even necessary. Shneidman (1993) and Joiner (2005) add the concepts of "psychache" and repeated painful life experiences, leading to the "acquired ability" to breach the suicide threshold.

- The vast majority of individuals in the suicide zone never commit suicide; rather, they enter feedback loops into psychotherapeutic and/or pharmacological treatment (and/or into further suicide episodes and experiences). One big challenge in suicidology is to identify those individuals and the unique suicide risk factors that might encourage them to cross the suicide threshold. Most suicidal individuals eventually die natural deaths.

- The particular suicide risk and protective factors listed in the various cells of Figure 2.1 are defined and discussed in the chapters that follow. Do not forget that there are many different types of suicide careers, each with its own dynamics, salient features, and idiosyncrasies. Suicidal careers are not linear, simple, or consistent. Most such careers have many starts, stops, reversals, feedback loops, and restarts. Suicidal people can get better and even opt out of suicidal careers altogether (even if they fit the model at one time).

Having laid the theoretical foundation of definitions, key concepts, and models that explain suicide and suicidality in Part I (Chapters 1 and 2), in Part II (Chapters 3 and 4) I turn now to a consideration of data, research, and assessment. In these chapters, I operationalize the definitions, types of information, research methods, and empirical evidence (evidence-based suicidology) that are used to determine some of the key variables in explanations of suicide and suicidality.

PART II

DATA, RESEARCH, ASSESSMENT

CHAPTER 3

Grounding Suicidology in Empirical Evidence

Give me a man's actual findings, so long as he has taken some
pains about his methods of reaching them, and I care not what
obviously silly theory he may have incorporated them into.
—GEORGE CASPAR HOMANS

In Chapters 1 and 2, I have defined *suicide* and *suicidality,* and have also reviewed some of the commonalities and differences of suicides. In this chapter and Chapter 4, let us consider how to use data to build a theory of suicide, incorporating previously stated variables and definitions (cf. Nock, 2018). This chapter gives an overview of some of the basic descriptive statistics for suicide in the United States and the world; many more statistics will be coming later.

An important question is this: How do we measure suicide risk factors and other key independent variables in building our theory of suicide? For example, how do we reliably and validly measure depression, hopelessness, alcoholism, psychic pain, suicidality, and so on? Some measurements are fairly obvious and straightforward (like those of age, sex, race, marital status, or occupation), but others are not (like those of depression and hopelessness). Another way of putting it is that variables like depression, hopelessness, suicide risk, personality, and so forth often require the use of scales, inventories, and clinical checklists or standardized criteria, such as the Beck Depression Inventory–II (BDI-II), the Hamilton Rating Scale for Depression (HAM-D), DSM-5, ICD-10, the Minnesota Multiphasic Personality Inventory–2 (MMPI-2), Linehan et al.'s Reasons for Living Inventory, Beck et al.'s Scale for Suicide Ideation, and many others. Measurement issues and the use of scales are illustrated with two cases: that of Van Watson (Case 3.1) and that of Antwan Sedgwick, the subject of the HBO documentary film *Death by Hanging* (Zabihyan, 1998). (Readers may wish to view an introduction to the film at *www. suicideexpert.com/videos,* or purchase the film at Amazon.com, and discuss it.)

Emile Durkheim was fond of saying, "These being the facts, what is their explanation?" In 2015, I was called by the mass media about the Germanwings murder–suicide plane crash in the French Alps, committed by co-pilot Andreas Lubitz. Reporters asked me to give them an explanation of why it happened. The problem was that I had almost no facts upon which to base my opinion. The word *empirical* means being guided by data and practical experience, and not just hunches, speculations, and ungrounded generic theories. We need to strive to have evidence-based psychiatry and suicidology, such as the use of psychotropic drugs based on randomized clinical trials (RCTs; Maris, 2015: Mann & Currier, 2012).

To be concerned about facts and systematic observations implies quantification, paying attention to numbers, data, counting, sampling, measurement, statistical analysis, appropriate methods, and research design (Nock, 2018). Typical empirical propositions in suicidology often take the following forms:

"In this large simple random sample of completed suicides, 72% were male, and the mean age was 47 years."
"The mean BDI-II score was 21, and the mean HAM-D score was 24."
"The 5-hydroxyindoleacetic acid (5-HIAA) level in the cerebrospinal fluid (CSF) was 92.5 nm/liter."
"Age, sex, race, history of major depressive episode, prior suicide attempt, and alcohol or other substance abuse explained 65% of the variance (R^2) in suicide outcome."

Any bona fide science attempts to be objective, universal, impartial, and culture-free (or culture-specific), and to have valid, reliable, sensitive, and specific propositions based in careful measurement and analysis.

What Are the Major Data Sources in Suicidology?

Where do our empirical building blocks come from (Mann & Rudd, 2018)? Suicide is rare (1 in 10,000 per year on average in the United States, as noted in Chapter 1), and those who suicide cannot respond to our questioning—they are dead. These two conditions complicate the study of suicide. For example, most studies of suicide have to be in large cities or counties in order to get enough random data to sample. Always ask: Does the sample represent the population being studied? Who or what is being left out? Also, if you wait until a suicide has already occurred, then obviously you cannot interview the person who suicided. Other informants may give biased or even false information about the person after the death.

Among the major data sources for the study of suicide are these (see Anestis et al., 2017, on what they call "Big Data," and see *www.gartner.com/it-glossary/big-data*):

1. Surveys, case–control studies, and epidemiological studies.
2. Vital statistics, death certificates and records, and coroner/medical examiner records, including toxicology reports.
3. RCTs or experiments, especially psychopharmacological studies.

4. Treatment records, hospital charts, and clinical interviews.
5. Psychological autopsies.
6. So-called "soft" data (diaries, notes, letters, poems, history, art, computer searches, phone records, etc.).

Surveys

Once funded, surveys start with getting a list of names and addresses of all suicides from a county, state, or national vital statistics office. Early in my career, for example, I studied 2,153 completed suicides and controls in Cook County (Chicago), Illinois, which represented a systematic simple random sample of 5 years of Chicago suicides (Maris, 1969, 1981). Survey design must always include appropriate controls, and for those I used natural deaths and nonfatal suicide attempts. Most suicides in Chicago were older white males, and when I knocked on their doors, the respondents were typically their spouses—mainly older white females. For each suicide, I tried to get two to three (multiple) informants who likely had differing perspectives on the suicide. Surveys of suicide are necessarily retrospective (after the fact). Longitudinal studies (like those done by Beck) are better, but it takes many years to gather the data. I used a standardized, precoded interview schedule. The interview data were entered into a computer file and then analyzed by comparing suicide cases and controls through various means: percentages, rates, tests of statistical significance, odds ratios and relative risks, regression and analysis of variance, and a procedure called *multivariate nominal scale analysis* (Maris, 1981). I then wrote two books on the Chicago data (1969, 1981).

Vital Statistics

Everyone reading this will eventually have a death certificate filled out on him or her. What will be the most important single item on your death certificate (the date, cause of death, manner of death, whether you are still married or not, etc.)? Figure 3.1 depicts a standard U.S. death certificate. It contains basic incident data (when the death occurred, where, the informant, body disposition, etc.). It also includes a lot of sociodemographic information (age, sex, race, marital status, usual occupation, education); questions about the cause of death (primary, secondary, and tertiary causes) and manner of death (natural, accidental, suicidal, homicidal—the so-called NASH classification, mentioned in Chapter 1); data on certification and pronouncement of death (time); registration and/or census data (such as whether or not the decedent was Hispanic); injury data; a question related to being female (i.e., pregnancy status); and a question about tobacco use.

The empirical investigation of suicide based upon death records has a rich history, dating back at least to Durkheim (1897/1951), Henry and Short (1954), Gibbs and Martin (1964), myself (Maris, 1969, 1981), Phillips (1974), Stack (1982), and Pescosolido and Georgianna (1989), among others later on. Using death records is not without controversy, however. For example, how accurate are vital statistics? We often do not know what criteria coroners and medical examiners use to certify a suicide. If a suicide note is required, then suicides could be undercounted by 75–85%

LOCAL FILE NO.   STATE FILE NO.

NAME OF DECEDENT — For use by physician od institution

To Be Completed/Verified By: FUNERAL DIRECTOR

1. DECEDENTS LEGAL NAME (Include AKA's if any) (First, Middle, Last) | 2. SEX | 3. SOCIAL SECURITY NUMBER

4a. AGE-Last Birthday (Years) | 4b. UNDER 1 YEAR — Months / Days | 4C. UNDER 1 DAY — Hours / Minutes | 5. DATE OF BIRTH (Mo/Day/Yr) | 6. BIRTHPLACE (City and State of Foreign Country)

7a. RESIDENCE STATE | 7b. COUNTY | 7c. CITY OR TOWN

7d. STREET AND NUMBER | 7e. APT. NO. | 7f. ZIP CODE | 7g. INSIDE CITY LIMITS? ☐ Yes ☐ No

8. EVER IN US ARMED FORCES? ☐ Yes ☐ No | 9. MARITAL STATUS AT TIME OF DEATH ☐ Married ☐ Married, but separated ☐ Widowed ☐ Divorced ☐ Never Married ☐ Unknown | 10. SURVIVNG SPOUSE'S NAME (If wife, give name prior to first marriage)

11. FATHER'S NAME (First, Middle, Last) | 12. MOTHER'S NAME PRIOR TO FIRST MARRIAGE (First, Middle, Last)

13a. INFORMANTS NAME | 13b. RELATIONSHIP TO DECEDENT | 13c. MAILING ADDRESS (Street and Number, City, State, Zip Code)

14. PLACE OF DEATH (Check only one: see instructions)

IF DEATH OCCURRED IN A HOSPITAL ☐ Inpatient ☐ Emergency Room Outpatient ☐ Dead on Arrival | IF DEATH OCCURRED SOMEWHERE OTHER THAN A HOSPITAL ☐ Hospice facility ☐ Nursing home/Long term care facility ☐ Decedent's home ☐ Other (Specify):

15. FACULTY NAME (If not institution, give street & number) | 16. CITY OR TOWN, STATE, AND ZIP CODE | 17. COUNTY OF DEATH

18. METHOD OF DISPOSITION: ☐ Burial ☐ Cremation ☐ Donation ☐ Entombment ☐ Removal from State ☐ Other (Specify): | 19. PLACE OF DISPOSITION (Name of cemetery, crematory, other place)

20. LOCATION-CITY, TOWN, AND STATE | 21. NAME AND COMPLETE ADDRESS OF FUNERAL FACILITY

22. SIGNATURE OF FUNERAL SERVICE LICENSEE OR OTHER AGENT | 23. LICENSE NUMBER (Of Licensee)

ITEMS 24-28 MUST BE COMPLETED BY PERSON WHO PRONOUNCES OR CERTIFIES DEATH | 24. DATE PRONOUNCED DEAD (Mo/Day/Yr) | 25. TIME PRONOUNCED DEAD

26. SIGNATURE OF PERSON PRONOUNCING DEATH (Only When applicable) | 27. LICENSE NUMBER | 28. DATE SIGNED (Mo/Day/Yr)

29. ACTUAL OR PRESUMED DATE OF DEATH (Mo/Day/Yr) (Spell Month) | 30. ACTUAL OR PRESUMED TIME OF DEATH | 31. WAS MEDICAL EXAMINER OR CORONER CONTACTED? ☐ Yes ☐ No

To Be Completed By: MEDICAL CERTIFIER

CAUSE OF DEATH (See instructions and examples) | Approximate interval: Onset to death

32. PART I. Enter the chain of events–diseases, injuries, or complications–that directly caused the death. DO NOT enter terminal events such as cardiac arrest, respiratory arrest, or ventricular fibrillation without showing the etiology DO NOT ABBREVIATE. Enter only one cause on a line. Add additional lines if necessary.

IMMEDIATE CAUSE (Final disease or condition resulting in death) → a _____
Due to (or as a consequence of):

Sequentially list conditions, if any, leading to the cause listed on line a. Enter the UNDERLYING CAUSE (disease or injury that initiated the events resulting in death) LAST
b _____
Due to (or as a consequence of):
c _____
Due to (or as a consequence of):
d _____

PART II. Enter other significant conditions contributing to death but not resulting in the underlying cause given in PART I | 33. WAS AN AUTOPSY PERFOMED? ☐ Yes ☐ No
34. WERE AUTOPSY FINDINGS AVAILABLE TO COMPLETE THE CAUSE OF DEATH? ☐ Yes ☐ No

35. DID TOBACCO USE CONTRIBUTE TO DEATH? ☐ Yes ☐ Probably ☐ No ☐ Unknown | 36. IF FEMALE. ☐ Not pregnant within past year ☐ Pregnant at time of death ☐ Not pregnant, but pregnant within 42 days of death ☐ Not pregnant, but pregnant 43 days to 1 year before death ☐ Unknown if pregnant within the past year | 37. MANNER OF DEATH ☐ Natural ☐ Homicide ☐ Accident ☐ Pending investigation ☐ Suicide ☐ Could not be determined

38. DATE OF INJURY (Mo/Day/Yr) (Spell Month) | 39. TIME OF INJURY | 40. PLACE OF INJURY (e.g. Decedent's home; construction site; restaurant; wooded area) | 41. INJURY AT WORK? ☐ Yes ☐ No

42. LOCATION OF INJURY: State | City or Town. | Street & Number. | Apartment No.: | Zip Code

43. DESCRIBE HOW INJURY OCCURRED. | 44. IF TRANSPORATION INJURY, SPECIFY ☐ Driver/Operator ☐ Passenger ☐ Pedestrian ☐ Other (Specify)

45. CERTIFIER (Check only one)
☐ Certifying physician-To the best of my knowledge, death occurred due to the cause(s) and manner stated.
☐ Pronouncing & Certifying physician-To the best of my knowledge, death occurred at the time, date, and place, and due to the cause(s) and manner stated.
☐ Medical Examiner/Coroner-On the basis of examination, and/or investigation, in my opinion, death occurred at the time, date, and place, and due to the cause(s) and manner stated.

Signature of certifier. _____

46. NAME, ADDRESS, AND ZIP CODE OF PERSON COMPLETING CAUSE OF DEATH (Item 32)

47. TITLE OF CERTIFIER | 48. LICENSE NUMBER | 49. DATE CERTIFIED (Mo/Day/Yr) | 50. FOR REGISTRAR ONLY–DATE FILED (Mo/Day/Yr)

To Be Completed By: FUNERAL DIRECTOR

51. DECEDENT'S EDUCATION-Check the box that best describes the highest degree or level of school completed at the time of death.
☐ 8th grade or less
☐ 9th - 12th grade; no diploma
☐ High school graduate or GED completed
☐ Some college credit, but no degree
☐ Associate degree (e.g., AA, AS)
☐ Bachelor's degree (e.g., BA, AB, BS)
☐ Master's degree (e.g., MA, MS, MEng, MEd, MSW, MBA)
☐ Doctorate (e.g., PhD, EdD) or Professional degree (e.g., MD, DDS, DVM, LLB, JD)

52. DECEDENT OF HISPANIC ORIGIN? Check the box that best describes whether the decedent is Spanish/Hispanic/Latino. Check the "No" box if decedent is not Spanish/Hispanic/Latino.
☐ No, not Spanish/Hispanic/Latino
☐ Yes, Mexican, Mexican American, Chicano
☐ Yes, Puerto Rican
☐ Yes, Cuban
☐ Yes, other Spanish/Hispanic/Latino (Specify) _____

53. DECEDENT'S RACE (Check one or more races to indicate what the decedent considered himself or herself to be)
☐ White
☐ Black or African American
☐ American Indian or Alaska Native (Name of the enrolled or principal tribe) _____
☐ Asian Indian
☐ Chinese
☐ Filipino
☐ Japanese
☐ Korean
☐ Vietnamese
☐ Other Asian (Specify) _____
☐ Native Hawaiian
☐ Guamanian or Chamorro
☐ Samoan
☐ Other Pacific Islander (Specify) _____
☐ Other (Specify) _____

54. DECEDENT'S USUAL OCCUPATION (Indicate type of work done during most of working life DO NOT USE RETIRED).

55. KIND OF BUSINESS/INDUSTRY

FIGURE 3.1. U.S. standard certificate of death.

(since suicides leave a suicide note only about 15–25% of the time). Douglas (1967) argued that there are as many official statistics as there are officials (i.e., death records are not very accurate).

Another issue is the measurement of the socioeconomic status of suicides. Suicides tend to be stigmatized deaths, so one question that arises is whether or not the families of upper-status decedents can avoid having the deaths certified as suicides, resulting in an undercount of suicides in such decedents. We shall see later that suicide rates tend to be higher at lower socioeconomic levels, but is the upper-status undercount phenomenon real?

Another issue is the kind of data that we can get from death records. One of the most outspoken critics of using death records to study suicide has been Jack Douglas (1967). He insisted that we need what he called "situated subjective meanings of suicide," and that these can only be obtained by interviewing serious suicide attempters who survive, not by acquiring retrospective data on decedents. Furthermore, many of the data from death certificates are dull and bland, and perhaps not very clinically relevant.

Clinical Trials and Experiments

In an experiment or clinical trial, the researcher directly manipulates one or more independent variables and then measures the effects on a dependent variable, such as suicidality or depression score outcomes (but usually not completed suicide, since the number of cases would need to be gigantic to detect suicides). There are not many suicide experiments, for obvious reasons (however, see Shneidman, 1967). For example, it is unethical to randomly deny possibly life-saving treatment to members of the placebo group. I sometimes fantasize that my tombstone will read "Ronald William Maris, placebo group member." People who have made a suicide attempt or are significantly depressed often cannot even be included in a clinical trial. Thus clinical trials are testing the wrong people (Maris, 2015).

Consider the experimental design illustrated in Figure 3.2. Many conditions are not specified in this figure, to keep it simple. Sixty subjects each are randomly

Study Groups	Baseline		Treatment					Follow-Up	
Experimental Group ($n = 60$, fluoxetine)									
Control Group #1 ($n = 60$, placebo)									
Control Group #2 ($n = 60$, imipramine)									
	1	2	3	4	5	6	7	8	9–12
				Weeks					

FIGURE 3.2. Clinical trial design for fluoxetine, imipramine, and placebo. *Source:* Adapted from Maris et al. (2000, p. 73). Copyright © The Guilford Press. Adapted with permission.

assigned to experimental or control groups. Most trials are *double-blind,* meaning that neither the subject nor the experimenter knows who is getting which treatment. All 180 subjects undergo a *washout* period to clear their systems of other drugs. A preexperiment baseline set of measurements is taken. Starting with week 3, the experimental group gets 20 mg of fluoxetine (Prozac) per day, control group 1 gets an inert placebo, and control group 2 gets 150 mg of imipramine (Tofranil) for a total of 6 weeks.

At the end of the 6-week experimental period (the end of week 8), posttreatment measures (e.g., the HAM-D, the Covi Anxiety Scale, adverse effects, biological markers, electrocardiograms [EKGs]) are taken. The three groups are then tested statistically for significant differences. After a follow-up period of 4 weeks after the end of treatment, the same measures are taken and the same tests are conducted at the end of week 12.

Treatment Records

Much of the information about suicide completers and attempters is, in effect, obtained from so-called "convenience samples" of the patients of psychiatrists, psychologists, social workers, counselors, nurses, and medical records. Clearly such data tend to be biased and not very scientific, since the data were normally gathered for treatment, not research, purposes. Treatment records are thus normally obtained on small, biased samples of single individuals or small groups of patients or forensic cases. It is like the old mantra, "I know a man or woman who [is suicidal]." How does one know that specific patients are representative of anything in particular or what their ad hoc data may indicate? Remember, too, that patient data are usually about living people who may not be very suicidal at all. Suicide completers, by definition, are dead. For example, although I have now investigated about 300 forensic suicide cases, I am certain that what I have learned from them is hardly representative of suicides in general. The focus of these documents and data is on treatment (often alleged bad treatment or malpractice) or litigation (especially seeking compensation), not research.

Hospital records for suicidal patients include some of the following types of data:

- Admission and discharge summaries (the later are especially informative).
- Social histories, often taken by social workers.
- Progress notes (sometimes verbatim) made by the patient's treatment team.
- Mental status examinations or psychiatric evaluations.
- Medication and pharmacy records.
- Vital sign charts.
- Psychological testing records.

Discharge summaries are particularly helpful for understanding individual suicidal patients. Discharge data include (1) admissions and discharge dates; (2) discharge DSM diagnostic codes and mental status; (3) the chief complaint, or reason for admission; (4) course of stay in hospital, procedures, and treatment; (5) history of present mental disorder and prior hospitalizations; and (6) the treatment plan, discharge medications, and follow-up appointment or referrals.

Although I routinely do my own psychological autopsies (see the "Forms" section of my personal website, *www.suicideexpert.com/forms*), many of the data needed for a psychological autopsy can be gleaned from a good social history taken by a social worker or other health care professional. Among other data, these histories often include a family tree highlighting psychiatric disorders, copies of prior psychiatric treatment records, and much more. A social history of a patient can provide valuable data on a suicidal career. Progress notes provide logged and dated verbatim quotes by both the patient and the staff about suicide ideation and plans, crucial events, mental status, and so on

A mental status exam by a psychiatrist is similar to a physical exam by an internist and needs to be done each time the patient is seen. Some of the items evaluated include motor activity, hygiene, eye contact, mood, perception, orientation (date, day, year, season, person, place), memory, calculations, reading and writing capacity, attention, visual–spatial ability, abstraction, and insight. A lot of physicians use something called the Mini-Mental State Exam (Folstein et al., 1975; see Maris et al., 2000; see also the Montreal Cognitive Assessment in Nasreddine et al., 2005). In response to a series of questions, the patient can score a maximum of 30 points. A score below 20 may indicate cognitive impairment.

Since a lot of psychiatrists (see Maris, 2015) consider psychiatric treatment to be virtually synonymous with giving psychotropic medication (psychiatrists seldom do psychotherapy any more), the patient's medication records, prescriptions ("scripts"), and doctors' orders become crucial data. These records include information about which drugs were prescribed, when, how much, discontinuations, changes in scripts (increases or decreases in dosage), multiple scripts at the same time, and so on.

Some of the medication- and suicide-related questions might include these:

- Do the medications match the diagnosis (such as a mood stabilizer for bipolar disorder)?
- Was the dosage appropriate? (Doctors often "start low and go slow," but in doing so they can undermedicate patients—e.g., give an inadequate dose of an antidepressant.)
- Were any of the psychotropic medications potentially suicidogenic (such as antidepressants in young patients, or drugs based on gamma-aminobutyric acid [GABA] like Neurontin or Valium)?
- Were adverse effects, especially serious ones, monitored closely? (Was the patient reminded to come back to the emergency room, if having adverse effects? Were contact numbers and addresses given?)
- How soon was drug treatment started or discontinued?
- Was the patient on an inappropriate drug cocktail (including interaction effects)?
- Was the dosage mindlessly increased, when it perhaps ought to have been discontinued or changed?

Psychiatric nurses keep detailed dated charts of patients' vital signs, such as these:

- Sleep charts.
- Weight gain or loss.
- Eating records.
- Libido fluctuations.
- Urine voiding or bowel movements.
- Pulse, respiration, and temperature.
- Personal grooming and hygiene.
- Activity notes (such as exercise, physical therapy).

As far as suicide risk goes, clinicians pay special attention to patients' vital signs that might represent changes in what are called *vegetative symptoms* (such as sleep, libido, and diurnal rhythms). Vegetative symptom changes (e.g., in response to antidepressant treatment) often occur before mood symptoms improve, thereby energizing patients and giving them a window of opportunity to act out persistent suicide ideation or previous suicide plans. In my Chicago research (Maris, 1981), I also found that terminal insomnia (such as awakening in the last third of the sleep cycle and being unable to fall back to sleep) was a unique risk factor for suicide. Subsequent research has replicated this finding (Petersen, 2016b).

There is usually a psychologist on a patient's treatment team (especially if the patient is getting psychotherapy), who may administer a variety of psychological tests to aid in DSM diagnosis or assess the patient's personality. The MMPI-2 has historically been the most widely used psychological test (although imagine giving a depressed patient over 500 questions to answer!). However, no psychological test profile consistently discriminates suicidal from nonsuicidal patients (Eyman & Eyman, 1992).

Psychological tests (and there are many more than those listed below) that might be in a patient's file include the following:

- The MMPI-2.
- The HAM-D or BDI-II.
- The Rorschach (an inkblot projective test, not used much today).
- The Thematic Apperception Test (TAT).
- The Millon Clinical Multiaxial Inventory–IV (MCMI-IV).
- The California Personality Inventory (CPI).
- The Structured Clinical Interview for DSM-5 (SCID-5).
- The Schedule for Affective Disorders and Schizophrenia (SADS).
- The Diagnostic Interview Schedule (DIS).
- The Suicide Probability Scale (SPS; Cull & Gill, 1982).

Psychological Autopsies

When I am retained to take a legal case involving suicide issues, I almost always insist on doing a psychological autopsy (again, see *www.suicideexpert.com/forms*)—although given my theoretical perspective, it is more of a biopsychosocial autopsy. A *psychological autopsy* can be defined as a procedure for reconstructing an individual's psychological life after the fact of death, particularly the person's lifestyle, thoughts, feelings, and behaviors manifested during the weeks just preceding the death, in order to better understand the psychological circumstances contributing to the death (Clark & Horton-Deutsch, 1992). One major reason I insist on psychological autopsy data is that the standard data from treatment records described above simply do not give sufficient information about suicide and suicide risk factors. Official suicide data (e.g., the information from death certificates) have a gap or lacuna in them that needs to be filled by doing a psychological autopsy (Maris, 2015; Snider et al., 2006; Silverman & Berman, 2014). Note that psychological autopsies may have different formats for clinical, research, or legal purposes. There is no one standard psychological autopsy (however, see *www.suicidology.org* for a psychological autopsy certificate training program).

My own psychological autopsy takes about 2 hours to administer. I prefer to do the psychological autopsy myself, interviewing multiple informants face to face or on the phone. Among the types of data that can be collected are these:

- Biodemographic overview.
- Suicide event/incident description.
- Social and family history.
- Medications involved.
- Medical examiner/coroner reports (including toxicology, autopsy, and other lab reports).
- Drug mechanisms of possible suicide etiology.
- Changes after ingesting psychotropic drugs.
- Police incident reports.
- My personal list of 15 suicide risk factors, presented later in this chapter and discussed in Chapter 4 (or other risk factor lists, like that of Jacobs et al., 2003, 2010).
- Suicide risk scales (such as a suicide risk score of 1–10 based on the old Los Angeles Suicide Prevention Center [LASPC] scale).
- DSM criteria for major depressive disorder.
- Suicide protective factors.
- Personal documents.
- School records.
- Work/military records.
- List of possible witnesses.
- Private investigator reports (if any; insurance companies often do these).
- Pictures of the deceased and family members (to put faces to the file).
- Other information volunteered by family members or other clients.

"Soft" Data

So-called "soft" data can consist of diaries, suicide (and other) notes, letters, CDs or DVDs, pictures, wills, desk calendars, poems written, books read recently, tattoos, internet searches, phone and text records, and history and art (see Chapter 18). My very first forensic case involved a man accused of embezzling. He was found dead, but his manner of death was listed as equivocal by the coroner. On his forearm was the tattoo "Death Before Dishonor." The jury concluded that his manner of death was suicide. Although often confusing and unclear, this kind of data can prove very helpful, even if not decisive.

Survivors or investigators should always search the decedent's personal computer for documents and online searches. The police usually also do this; they also collect pill bottles, and the like. For example, I had a case of a Harvard student who did multiple computer searches for how to use dry ice and a Hefty bag to asphyxiate himself. In another case, the decedent's cell phone had videos of him practicing a Russian roulette suicide attempt. In a third case, a young honors student's journal writing showed him to be obviously psychotic. About 5% of individuals with schizophrenia eventually kill themselves, so this was helpful information.

On the other hand, soft data can be ambiguous and inconclusive. There is almost never a desk calendar that reads, "Kill myself next Tuesday at 4 P.M." In fact, known suicides often have plans on their calendars for *after* they intend to suicide. Suicides tend to be ambivalent about dying and often plan to die and live at the same time. It is not uncommon for someone to plan to commit suicide on Tuesday, but also write that he or she is going to, say. a daughter's college graduation the following Saturday.

You might think that suicide notes are "windows to the soul" (Shneidman's phrase) of the would-be suicide, but they often are not. Believe it or not, some suicides may not even be aware that they are suicidal. I imagine people needing to remind celebrities such as John Belushi or Kurt Cobain, "You know, if you keep living like that, you will be lucky to make it until age 40," and this being something that the soon-to-be-dead individuals never really thought or cared much about. Also remember that up to 85% of suicides do not even write suicide notes (although they may leave other clues).

Soft data may also include the bedside books being read by decedents. Although Derek Humphry's (1991/1996) *Final Exit* (a *New York Times* best-seller on how to kill yourself) will probably not be among them, often there are books with depressing, violent, or disturbing themes. For instance, was a young female who died reading Sylvia Plath's poems, her novel *The Bell Jar,* or other depressing literature? This is soft information that probably would not be admissible in court, but every bit of evidence helps (especially when taken altogether).

Suicide Rates in the United States

Major data components in the empirical foundation of suicidal behaviors are suicide rates. A *suicide rate* is a measure of suicide in relation to the population in general during some specified time period. One common computing formula for suicide rates is this:

$$\text{Suicides/population} \times 100{,}000 = \text{Suicide rate}$$

We use suicide rates in part because frequencies can be misleading. For example, black males have higher suicide rates than white females, even though white female suicides are more frequent. Rates standardize for population size. Some of the fundamental empirical regularities for U.S. suicide rates in 2013 are depicted in Table 3.1 (cf. Tavernese, 2016).

In 2013 (see *www.suicidology.org/resources/facts-statistics* or *https://afsp.org/about-suicide/suicide-statistics* for more recent data), there were 41,149 U.S. suicides, or a rate of 13 per 100,000; this indicates that completed suicide is a very rare event. For every 10,000 people, there was about 1 suicide per year. In the United States, 90% of all suicides were committed by whites (70% by white males). The relative risk for suicide of males versus females was 3.5. Nonwhite females made up only 2.6% of all U.S. suicides. Suicides constituted 1.6% of all annual deaths. Suicide was the 10th leading cause of death (but the 2nd for 15- to 24-year-olds, after accidents).

The ratio of elderly suicides (those age 65+ years) to young suicides (those ages 15–24 years) was 1.5. Although the old made up 14.1% of the U.S. population, they made up 17.5% of the suicides. The middle-aged (those ages 45–54 years) had the highest suicide rates, 19.7 per 100,000. Between 2003 and 2013 (and beyond), middle-aged suicide rates increased from 15.9 to 19.7. I have more to say in Chapter 5 about why this change occurred. Still, generally speaking, the older people get, the higher the suicide rate becomes (certainly for males).

Firearms were the leading suicide method (51.5% overall in 2015; 51.8% for males, 38.3% for females in 2013 [see Table 9.2 in Chapter 9; data by gender are not shown in Table 3.1]). Women tended to use less lethal methods than men did. For men, the three leading suicide attempt methods were firearms, hanging, and carbon monoxide poisoning, in that order. For women, the firearm and overdose suicide methods were the first and second methods, with hanging third.

From 2003 to 2013 there was a slight increase in the U.S. suicide rate (10.8 to 13.0; Tavernese, 2016), but if we step back and take in the bigger picture over a longer time, we see that U.S. suicide rates on average have hovered around 12 per 100,000 for the last 100 years (see Figure 25.1 and Table 25.1 in Chapter 25). One wonders whether about 12 per 100,000 is the lowest possible (not the best, but the most likely) suicide rate, instead of 0, as many suicide preventers claim (e.g., as the American Foundation for Suicide Prevention [*www.afsp.org*] seems to suggest). Finally, note that there are about 25 nonfatal suicide attempts each year for every 1 completed suicide. This results in roughly 1 million new suicide survivors each year.

It can also be concluded from Table 3.1 that 90% of all suicides in the United States in 2013 were committed by whites. Black suicides constituted only 2,353 of the 41,149 total U.S. suicides that year, or about 18% (mostly by black males; 1,891 of 2,353, or 80%). Compared to U.S. whites, blacks have low suicide rates. For example, white males have a suicide rate of 23.4, but black males only have a rate of 9.7. White females have a suicide rate of 6.5, versus 2.0 for black females. One exception to low black suicide rates occurs in black males ages 20–35 in urban areas (Gibbs, 1997). Black males have relatively high suicide rates from about ages 25 to 34, as do Native American males in that same age group (see Chapter 8 for other ethnic and racial group suicide rates).

TABLE 3.1. U.S. Official Final Data on Suicide, 2013

	Number	Per Day	Rate	% of Deaths	Group (Number of Suicides)	Rate
Nation	41,149	112.7	13.0	1.6	White male (28,943)	23.4
Males	32,055	87.8	20.6	2.5	White female (8,211)	6.5
Females	9,094	24.9	5.7	0.7	Nonwhite male (3,112)	9.7
Whites	37,154	101.8	14.9	1.7	Nonwhite female (883)	2.6
Nonwhites	3,995	10.9	6.0	1.1	Black male (1,891)	9.0
Blacks	2,353	6.4	5.4	0.8	Black female (462)	2.0
Elderly (65+ yrs.)	7,215	19.8	16.1	0.4	Hispanic (2,865)	5.3
Young (15–24 yrs.)	4,878	13.4	11.1	17.1	Native Americans (521)	11.7
Middle-Aged (45–64 yrs.)	15,756	43.2	19.0	3.1	Asian/Pacific Islanders (1,121)	6.0

Fatal Outcomes (Suicides): a minimal rate increase was seen from 2012 to 2013, continuing the recent rate increases after long-term trends of decline.

- Average of 1 person every 12.8 minutes killed themselves
- Average of 1 old person every 1 hour and 13 minutes killed themselves
- Average of 1 young person every 1 hour and 48 minutes killed themselves. (If the 395 suicides below age 15 are included, 1 young person every 1 hour and 40 minutes)
- 10th-ranking cause of death in U.S.—2nd for **young** →
- 3.5 male deaths by suicide for each female death by suicide
- Suicide ranks 10th as a cause of death; Homicide ranks 16th

Nonfatal Outcomes (Attempts) (figures are estimates):

- 1,028,725 annual attempts in U.S. (using 25:1 ration); 2013 SAMHSA study: 1.3 million adults (18 and up)
- Translates of one attempt every 31 seconds (based on 1,028,725 attempts) [1.3 million = 1 every 24 seconds]
- 25 attempts for every death by suicide for nation (one estimate); 100–200:1 for young; 4:1 for elderly
- 3 female attempts for each male attempt

Leading Causes of Death 15–24 yrs		
Cause	Number	Rate
All Causes	28,486	64.8
1-Accidents	11,619	26.4
2-Suicide	4,878	11.1
3-Homicide	4,329	9.8
10–14 yrs	386	1.9
15–19 yrs	1,748	8.3
20–24 yrs	3,130	13.7

Exposure to Suicide ("know someone who died by suicide") and Suicide Loss Survivors (those bereaved of suicide):†

* Recent (Cerel, 2015) research-based estimate suggests that for each death by suicide → 115 people are *exposed* (4.7 million annually), and among those, 25 experience a major life disruption (*loss survivors*)

- If each suicide has devastating effects and intimately affects 25 other people, there are over **1 million loss survivors a year**
- Based on the 825,832 suicides from 1989 through 2013, therefore, the number of survivors of suicide loss in the U.S. is 20.65 million (1 of every 15 Americans in 2013); number grew by 1,028,725 in 2013
- If there is a suicide every 12.8 minutes, then there are 25 new loss survivors every 12.8 minutes as well.

Suicide Methods	Number	Rate	Percent of Total		Number	Rate	Percent of Total
Firearm suicides (1st)	21,175	6.7	51.5%	All but firearms	19,974	6.3	48.5%
Suffocation/hanging (2nd)	10,062	3.2	24.5%	Poisoning (3rd)	6,637	2.1	16.1%
Cut/pierce	783	0.2	1.9%	Drowning	397	0.1	1.0%

U.S.A. Suicide Rates 2003–2013
(Rates per 100,000 population)

Group/Age	2003	2004	2005	2006	2007	2008	2009	2010	2011	2012	2013
5–14	0.6	0.7	0.7	0.5	0.5	0.6	0.7	0.7	0.7	0.8	1.0
15–24	9.7	10.3	10.0	9.9	9.7	10.0	10.1	10.5	11.0	11.1	11.1
25–34	12.7	12.7	12.4	12.3	13.0	12.9	12.8	14.0	14.6	14.7	14.8
35–44	14.9	15.0	14.9	15.1	15.6	15.9	16.1	16.0	16.2	16.7	16.2
45–54	15.9	16.6	16.5	17.2	17.7	18.7	19.3	19.6	19.8	20.0	19.7
55–64	13.8	13.8	13.9	14.5	15.5	16.3	16.7	17.5	17.1	18.0	18.1
65–74	12.7	12.3	12.6	12.6	12.6	13.9	14.0	13.7	14.1	14.0	15.0
75–84	16.4	16.3	16.9	15.9	16.3	16.0	15.7	15.7	16.5	16.8	17.1
85+	16.9	16.4	16.9	15.9	15.6	15.6	15.6	17.6	16.9	17.8	18.6
65+	14.6	14.3	14.7	14.2	14.3	14.8	14.8	14.9	15.3	15.4	16.1
Total	10.8	11.0	11.0	11.1	11.5	11.8	12.0	12.4	12.7	12.9	13.0
Men	17.6	17.7	17.7	17.8	18.3	19.0	19.2	20.0	20.2	20.6	20.6
Women	4.3	4.6	4.5	4.6	4.8	4.9	5.0	5.2	5.4	5.5	5.7
White	12.1	12.3	12.3	12.4	12.9	13.3	13.5	14.1	14.5	14.8	14.9
Non-white	5.5	5.8	5.5	5.5	5.6	5.7	5.8	5.8	5.8	6.1	6.0
Black	5.1	5.2	5.1	4.9	4.9	5.2	5.1	5.1	5.3	5.5	5.4
45–64	15.0	15.4	15.3	16.0	16.7	17.5	18.0	18.6	18.6	19.1	19.0

15 Leading Causes of Death in the U.S.A., 2013
(total of 2,596,993 deaths; 821.5 rate)

Rank and Cause of Death	Rate	Deaths
1 Diseases of the heart (heart disease)	193.3	611,105
2 Malignant neoplasms (cancer)	185.0	584,881
3 Chronic lower respiratory diseases	47.2	149,205
4 Accidents (unintentional injury)	41.3	130,557
5 Cerebrovascular diseases (stroke)	40.8	128,978
6 Alzheimer's disease	26.8	84,767
7 Diabetes mellitus (diabetes)	23.9	75,578
8 Influenza & pneumonia	18.0	56,979
9 Nephritis, nephrosis (kidney disease)	14.9	47,112
10 Suicide [Intentional Self-Harm]	13.0	41,149
11 Septicemia	12.1	28,156
12 Chronic liver disease and cirrhosis	11.5	36,427
13 Essential hypertension and renal disease	9.7	30,770
14 Parkinson's disease	8.0	25,196
15 Pneumonitis due to solids and liquids	5.9	18,579
-All other causes (Residual)	170.0	537,554
16 Homicide	5.1	16,121

- Old made up 14.1 % of 2013 population but 17.5% of the suicides • Young were 13.9% of 2013 population and 11.9% of the suicides • Middle Aged were 26.3% of the 2012 population but were 38.3% of the suicides • 1,169,291* Years of Potential Life Lost Before Age 75 (37,728 of 41,149 suicides below age 75)

*alternate YPLL figure: 1,166,172 using individual years in calculations rather than 10-year age groups as above.

Many figures appearing here are derived or calculated from data in the following *official data sources:* downloaded 6 July 2015 from CDC's website: *http://www.cdc.gov/nchs/data/nvsr/nvsr64/nvsr64_02.pdf* and the multiple cause data file at *http://www.cdc.gov/nchs/data_access/Vitalstatsonline.htm.* Some figures derived or calculated from data at the CDC's WISQARS Fatal Injuries Report site: *http://www.cdc.gov/injury/wisgars/fatal_injury_reports. html*, downloaded 22 Jan 2015.

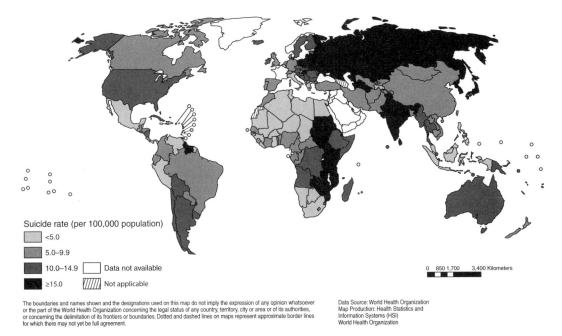

FIGURE 3.3. World age-standardized suicide rates (per 100,000 population), both sexes, 2012. *Source:* World Health Organization (2012b). In public domain.

World Suicide Rates

To prevent basing a theory of suicide on only data from the United States (which has only about 5–6% of the world's suicides), Figure 3.3 presents an overview of the World Health Organization's (WHO's) worldwide data (2012b) on suicide rates. The WHO warns readers that international suicide rates are not strictly comparable, given the vagaries of reporting and coding differences—so *caveat emptor.*

If world suicide rates are grouped as "high" (≥ 15 per 100,000), "moderate" (11–12) and "low" (≤ 4), then suicide rates in the United States are moderate. In Figure 3.3, the countries of the former Soviet Union, India, South Central Africa, and Guyana have among the highest suicide rates.

The WHO itself ranks countries with the highest (≥15 per 100,000) suicide rates. Some of the *highest*-ranked countries include the following (roughly in this order): Greenland, Lithuania, South Korea, Guyana (where the Jonestown suicides occurred), Kazakhstan, Slovenia, Japan, Hungary, Ukraine, Poland, Finland, and

SAMHSA 2013 study (2014): Substance Abuse and Mental Health Services Administration [SAMHSA], Center for Behavioral Health Statistics and Quality. (2014, September 4). *The NSDUH Report: Substance Use and Mental Health Estimates from the 2013 National Survey on Drug Use and Health: Overview of Findings.* Rockville, MD: SAMHSA. *http://store.samhsa.gov/shin/content//NSDUH14-0904/NSDUH14-0904.pdf*

Cerel, J. (2015, April 18). *We are all connected in suicidology: The continuum of "survivorship."* Plenary presentation at the 48th annual conference of the American Association of Suicidology, Atlanta GA. [data from Cerel, Brown, Maple, Bush, van de Venne, Moore, & Flaherty, in progress]

†Cerel, J., McIntosh, J. L., Neimeyer, R. A., Maple, M., & Marshall, D. (2014). The continuum of "survivorship": Definitional issues in the aftermath of suicide. *Suicide and Life-Threatening Behavior, 44*(6), 591–600.

Suicide rate = (number of suicides by group/population of group) × 100,000   Suicide Data Page: 2013
Prepared for AAS by Christopher W. Drapeau, M.A., & John L. McIntosh, Ph.D.   7 January 2015 • Revised 22 January 2015 & 24 April 2015
Source: Drapeau and McIntosh (2015), for the American Association of Suicidology (AAS).

Austria (which is interesting, since Austria is mainly Catholic, and most Catholic countries have low suicide rates).

Countries with *moderate* (10–14.9 per 100,000) suicide rates include the United States, Cuba, Germany, Sweden, Norway, the United Kingdom, and Canada. The countries with the *lowest* (≤5) worldwide suicide rates include Mexico, the Philippines, the Bahamas, Pakistan, Egypt, and Syria (many of these are Catholic or Muslim countries). See Chapter 8 and Wasserman and Wasserman (2009) for much more detailed data on international variations in suicide rates.

Measurement Scales

This section begins the transition to measurement of data, which continues in Chapter 4. For example, a DSM diagnosis of (say) major depressive disorder is often not enough for determining severity or suicidality. One problem is that psychiatric diagnosis is notoriously unreliable and varies among different psychiatrists. Another problem is that psychiatric diagnosis is hard to quantify. For example, do clinicians just count DSM criteria? Even with a consensus diagnosis, the question might remain, "Well, how depressed is the patient?"

A *scale* is a continuum resulting from objective, standardized procedures combining one or more measurements, in order to form a single score that is assigned to each individual. For example, many psychiatric drug manufacturers use a score of less than 7 on the HAM-D to indicate remission of depressive symptoms (due to their drug, it is implied).

There are a great many scales for a large variety of variables and purposes. Since measuring depressive disorder is critical for the study of suicide, I focus here on just two depression scales: (1) the HAM-D (Hamilton, 1960) and (2) the BDI-II (Beck et al., 1996). One has to be careful here, since there are numerous versions and revisions of each scale and other entirely different scales (for example, see Gananca et al., 2017).

On the 17-item HAM-D scale (there are different versions), scores vary from a low of 0 to a high of 50. Severity of depression is measured as follows:

> 25+ = severe depression
> 18–24 = moderate depression
> 7–17 = mild depression
> > 7 = not depressed, resolved, in remission

The BDI-II (I used the original BDI in my Chicago suicide surveys; Maris, 1981) has 21 items and scores ranging from 0 to 63, with the following severity ranges:

> 29+ = severe depression
> 20–28 = moderate depression
> 14–19 = mild depression
> 0–13 = no depression

Beck also created a scale for measuring hopelessness (Beck et al., 1974a; see Maris et al., 2000). Having separate scales for depression and hopelessness, as well as suicide intent, allows us to determine how these three factors are related to each other; hopelessness may be predictive of suicide ideas or intent, but not of suicide attempts (Qiu et al., 2017). Table 11.4 in Chapter 11 presents Beck and colleagues' correlation matrix of depression, hopelessness, and suicide intent. In Table 11.4, we see the following:

- Hopelessness has a higher correlation with suicide intent (+.68) than depression does (+.57).
- Hopelessness has a higher negative correlation (–.74) with wish-to-live than does depression (–.57).
- The relationship between depression and suicide intent is due in part to hopelessness.
- Thus hopelessness is more "predictive" of suicide intent than depression is.

We see now how scales can be very useful in data analysis and theory construction, more so than mere psychiatric diagnoses.

A Case Example Utilizing Scales

In Case 3.1, I utilized several scales related to suicidality to help me resolve a manner-of-death controversy (name, place, and other details have been changed to protect the family). Van Watson was a 45-year-old white male from a major city, who was found dead in his garage from carbon monoxide poisoning. The issue in the legal case was whether his death was a suicide or an accident.

CASE 3.1. Van Watson

Van Watson was a 45-year-old white male from a major city who died of carbon monoxide poisoning in his garage at home. He had been washing and waxing his wife's car. Watson was a heavy drinker, and his business as a certified public accountant (CPA) was near bankruptcy. His death was initially listed as an accident by the local medical examiner. But Watson's insurance companies were suspicious and refused to pay out some of his recent life insurance policies, claiming that his death was a suicide. Both sides retained lawyers and experts. At issue was Watson's manner of death. Eventually the wife and the insurance companies settled the case without going to trial.

It had been a hot summer morning when Watson washed the car in the driveway. After finishing washing the car, he pulled it into the garage and shut the door, presumably to wax it out of the sun. He left the motor running and the car radio on, but had a fan going in the garage. When Watson was found by his brother-in-law later that morning, he was sitting in a canvas lawn chair next to the car. There were water buckets, wax, and rags near his feet. His body had turned a bright reddish-orange. One hypothesis was that he had gotten faint or dizzy after washing the car outside and sat down for a minute, intending to shut off the car motor after closing the garage door. Instead, he lost consciousness and never recovered. Of course, a more cynical hypothesis is that he was deeply in debt and just staged his own death to look like an accident.

Other relevant facts were that Watson had no suicides in his family and had made no prior suicide attempts. He had been married once and had two sons, the older of whom had a history of depression and suicide ideation. After his death, Watson's estate totaled $7–10 million. He had been having an extramarital affair just before his death; his girlfriend had called him at home, and his wife answered and found out about the affair. She responded by going to the beach and leaving Watson at home alone. Watson was a very successful CPA (one of his clients was a National Football League team). He was in good physical health and condition, and weighed about 215–220 pounds. He had never seen a mental health counselor in his life. The week Watson died, nothing much unusual had happened, other than his girlfriend's calling his home and his burning his leg on his car exhaust pipe.

Source: Adapted from Maris et al. (2000). Copyright © The Guilford Press. Adapted with permission.

The death was investigated, since Watson's insurance company denied payment of his life insurance proceeds. A "suicide clause" is found in most life insurance policies: If a person takes out a life insurance policy and then suicides within 2 years (usually) of its issuance, the insurance company does not have to pay the face value of the policy, just the premiums paid. Watson took his policies out within 2 years of dying. Was his death a suicide?

The investigation used several measurements to help form and support an opinion as to whether Watson's death was an accident or a suicide. A lot was at stake, since the wife had to declare bankruptcy and her sons were forced to drop out of college. She was allowed to keep the family home. Since Watson was dead, the data came from third parties, and this introduced unknown possible bias into the data; for example, would the family members tell the truth, since they desperately needed the insurance money? The scales that were used included the following (see also Rothberg & Geer-Williams, 1992; note that some of these scales and some of the ones in the next list are now outdated, given the age of the case):

- My own 15 suicide risk factors (see below and Chapter 4); Watson had 7 of these 15, or 47%.
- Cull and Gill's (1982) SPS (scores of 15 and 11 by two raters indicated "mild" or even "low" suicide risk).
- The original BDI. Watson had scores of 2, 4, and 6 by three raters, and the mean BDI score for known suicides on the original BDI is 21.
- The Tuckman and Youngman (1968) suicide rate scale. Watson had 7 high-risk items, but also 7 low-risk items.
- The Motto Clinical Instrument to Estimate Suicide Risk (see Motto, 1992). Watson's score of 408–435 put him in the sixth decile, or at "moderate" suicide risk.
- The Los Angeles Suicide Prevention Center Scale (Beck et al., 1974b). Watson scored 7.4 out of a high of 10.

The following were considered but not used:

- Weisman and Worden's (1974) Risk–Rescue Scale.
- The MMPI-2 (see Maris et al., 1992, for a discussion).
- Lettieri et al.'s (1974) Suicide Death Prediction Scales (for young and old females and young and old males).

Based on all these measurements and clinical interviews, with the surviving family members and business partners using my psychological autopsy, I concluded that Watson's death was "equivocal"; that is, there was insufficient empirical evidence to clearly support either a suicidal or an accidental manner of death.

Note that a medical examiner is not required to certify a death in a Procrustean (i.e., forced) manner as either natural, accidental, suicidal, or homicidal. For example, the examiner in Watson's case could have certified Watson's manner of death as "unknown" or "pending." After reading my expert report, hearing other testimony, and reviewing documents (such as the toxicology report), the medical examiner persisted in ruling Watson's death as "suicidal." There was no empirical basis for me to disagree. The insurance company nevertheless settled with the wife and sons (all three of whom had large life insurance policies on Watson).

The Case in the HBO Movie *Death by Hanging*

By way of transition to Chapter 4 and its consideration of suicide risk factors, readers are invited to view the HBO movie I have mentioned at the start of this chapter, *Death by Hanging* (Zabihyan, 1998; see also *www.suicideexpert.com/videos*). The movie is about 1 hour and 40 minutes long.

In July 1996, I was asked by BBC/HBO producer Kimi Zabihyan to come to Hampton, Virginia for a week to investigate the hanging death (on October 3, 1995) of a 20-year-old black male, Antwan Sedgwick, and to be in the HBO movie she was filming. The information that follows was presented in the HBO movie (no confidential information is cited).

The police said that Sedgwick hanged himself by his belt from a set of monkey bars in a park near the Hampton Coliseum downtown, but the family believed that the police killed Sedgwick and then suspended his body from the bars. It was clear from the beginning that this was an explosive, divisive case. It also seemed likely that the producer hoped the investigation would support her belief that the Hampton police possibly murdered Sedgwick and then staged his death to look like a suicide. This was a high-profile case in which Jesse Jackson and the FBI got involved.

The Sedgwick death occurred in the early morning (4:10 A.M.) of the day O. J. Simpson was acquitted. A local clergyman, the Reverend Harris, said that the mood at the time of the black community and Antwan Sedgwick was jubilant, not depressed. Antwan's father, Clarence, reported that recently Antwan had confronted two white police patrol officers parked in the neighborhood, and that one of the officers had threatened Antwan.

No one witnessed Antwan's death or even saw him in the hours just before he died (only about 1–2% of suicides are witnessed). Even though the death site was very public, few people were up and about at 4:10 A.M. The family said that Antwan had been upbeat recently and not depressed; however, he had had a recent argument with a pregnant girlfriend and was found with cocaine in his body at the time of death.

The presence of cocaine suggests that Antwan's death could have been an auto-erotic asphyxiation, in which an individual partly strangles himself while masturbating and then accidentally dies. Was he murdered, perhaps in a drug deal gone bad? The crime scene did not show any signs of a struggle or any defensive wounds (e.g., from trying to fend off an attacker or attackers. He was found hanging with his pants down around his ankles, with some urine and feces underneath him (the body often purges itself when someone is hanged), and with a trickle of blood from his nose (did he snort the coke?).

Antwan seemed attractive, bright, sociable, and athletic. He was regarded as a leader among his friends, and he was trying to get his general equivalency diploma (GED). The FBI investigated the Sedgwick case, and concluded on August 2, 2000 that there was insufficient evidence to support the family's claims of murder. There was never a trial. Let us examine some of the issues raised in the Antwan Sedgwick case.

Suicide Risk Factors

Chapter 4 makes it clear that some states and/or traits occur statistically more commonly in suicides than in nonsuicides. Generally, the more risk factors one has, the higher one's suicide risk. My own list of suicide risk factors (Maris, 1981) numbers 15. Since no psychological autopsy was done, information about several of these important risk factors was lacking.

Maris suicide risk factors	Present in Sedgwick?
Mental disorders, especially mood disorders	+ (depressed over girlfriend)
Alcohol or other substance abuse	+ (cocaine)
Ideas of suicide or death	? (don't know)
Prior self-destructive acts or attempts	0 (or don't know)
Social isolation or negative interaction	?
Love, romantic, or family problems	+ (pregnant girlfriend)
Work problems or unemployment	+ (school dropout)
Hopelessness and cognitive rigidity	?
Being an older white male	0
Use of a lethal method to attempt suicide	+ (hanging)
Aggression, anger, irritability, impulsivity	?
Stress, negative life events	+ (an argument with cops)
Physical illness and chronic pain	0
Family history of suicide or mental disorder	?
Repetition of the factors above—suicidal career	+ (about 20 years)

Thus Sedgwick had at least 7 of 15 risk factors, or 46%—about a 5 on a 10-point suicide risk scale. Should all of the question marks become positives, then Sedgwick would have 11 of 15 suicide risk factors—a 7 on a 10-point scale (73%). If "low" = 0–3 risk factors, "moderate" = 4–7, and "high" = 8–10, then Sedgwick had a moderate suicide risk. Hendin (1969) pointed out that although the suicide rate among blacks is low in general, it tends to be equal to or higher than that of white males in the 20- to 35-year age group. We need to be careful here, however, because just counting suicide risk factors does not determine suicidality.

Physical Evidence

Often physical evidence from the police and/or medical examiner carries the day. Was a wound a contact wound (which is typical for suicides, but there was no gun here)? Did the deceased have alcohol in his blood (about a third of suicides are intoxicated at death) and at what level? Were there other drugs detected (such as Sedgwick's cocaine)? Was there a suicide note left? Did the scene indicate a struggle?

Contrary to the logo on the T-shirts the Sedgwick family had made up, "Black Men Don't Hang Themselves," young black males do commit suicide. Hanging is the second most common suicide method for men, second only to firearms.

Homicide was a possible manner of death for Sedgwick and is very common among black males. A black American male has a 5% chance of dying of homicide up to age 45. Antwan was physically fit. Where were the signs of a struggle? Could he have been killed in a drug incident gone bad? If so, he likely would have been shot or stabbed, not hanged.

Often the physical evidence by itself does not tell us the manner of death. Normally a psychological autopsy also needs to be done with the survivors. Even though the Hampton police investigation could have been better, I doubt that that a better physical investigation would have told us whether Sedgwick's death was a homicide or a suicide.

Blame and Responsibility

Any time a young person dies unnaturally, there is a tendency to blame someone. However, in Antwan Sedgwick's case, there may not have been any evil, racist perpetrator. Sometimes bad things just happen. Since members of minority groups tend not to control their own lives as much as those in majority groups do, it is often assumed that they do not control their deaths either. If this case concerned a middle-aged white professional, we might be more likely to think that he hanged himself. It is tempting to conclude, "Someone must have done this to Antwan," considering all of the prior discrimination and violence that he and other African Americans have been subjected to.

There was a certain amount of hysteria surrounding the Sedgwick case. No doubt something awful happened to Antwan and the Sedgwick family. The surviving family members still have to cope with their profound grief. However, the undeniable fact that the family was and still is hurting does not make Antwan's death a homicide.

Antwan had been arrested before for car theft, had fathered a child out of wedlock, and had had an argument with his pregnant girlfriend about the child shortly before he died. He had cocaine in his body at the time of death; he was unemployed; he had dropped out of high school; he had had some conflict with his parents; at least some witnesses said that he had been depressed recently; and there may have been other suicidogenic factors that we just do not know about. All of this could have gotten to Antwan on Tuesday, October 3, 1995. Suicides tend to occur early in the week. He could have decided to escape from all of his problems.

One could argue that HBO should not, in effect, have tried this case in the mass media. It certainly polarized the Hampton community. The best alternative would have been a trial. Sometimes the best situation in equivocal cases is to ask 12 jurors to hear the evidence and then vote on a verdict. But trials cost money. Was Sedgwick's death was a homicide or a suicide? What other evidence would have made a difference?

Experts need to make every effort to remain scientific and objective. The film producer was disappointed that the investigation found the manner of Sedgwick's death to be equivocal. However, the real issue is what really happened with a focus on facts and reasonable probabilities. Let the attorneys take sides. That being said, the grief of the Sedgwick family was palpable. In Chapter 4, I continue to examine measurement issues and operational definitions of suicide risk factors.

CHAPTER 4

Measurement
Risk Factors and Risk Assessment

The objective and measurable observations that would accurately
determine the risk of suicide in one person may have very different
significance for another, or no relevance at all for a third.
—JEROME A. MOTTO

It is important to strive for empirical or evidence-based suicide risk factors. Looking at risk factor or suicide assessment documents, one can sometimes feel disoriented and "lost at sea." For example, the American Psychiatric Association's *Practice Guideline for the Assessment and Treatment of Patients with Suicidal Behaviors* (Jacobs et al., 2003, 2010) lists over 60 suicide risk factors, and they all seem equally important. Does everything cause or contribute to suicide? Are not some factors more suicidogenic than others? Which factors are weighted most heavily in which regression models?

When I derived my own 15 suicide risk factors in Chicago, they were evidence-based. That is, they only included factors that were statistically significant for completed suicides in research comparing them to natural death and nonfatal suicide attempt control groups (Maris, 1981). Furthermore, the rank ordering of these risk factors was roughly based on their prevalence and statistical differentiation among completed suicides. For example, mental (especially mood) disorders were ranked first, alcohol and other substance abuse was ranked second, and so on. Robins (1981) did much the same thing in St. Louis. He reported that 47% of all suicides there had a depressive or other mood disorder, and 25% had an alcohol or other substance abuse problem. No other suicide risk factor was present in more than 5% of all his suicides.

This chapter discusses (1) suicide risk factors and (2) individual suicide risk assessment. Suicide risk factors are often generic and concern groups over long time frames (e.g., 5 or 10 years), whereas suicide assessment is usually specific and focused on individuals (*idiographic*) in shorter time frames. Of course, these two measurements overlap (like circles in Venn diagrams).

61

For example, with risk factors, one might conclude after examining empirical evidence in groups of individuals and controls that over 95% of all suicides have some diagnosable mental disorder at the time of their death (Joiner, 2005). With a suicidal individual, the empirical and clinical assessment might focus on how likely and under what circumstances the person might engage in self-harm next weekend, if he or she is not hospitalized this Friday, started on a trial of psychotropic medication(s), or given ECT.

Empiricism needs to be counterbalanced with clinical judgment. All of the empirical and statistical evidence might suggest a conclusion of (say) low suicide risk, but the clinician's gut might indicate that, in spite of the numbers, the patient actually has a high suicide risk and something needs to be done (besides just counting things). While empiricism tends to be dry, impersonal, and mechanical, individual suicide assessment in large part rests on the therapeutic relationship with the patient. Does the clinician convey to the patient that he or she is competent and actually cares whether the patient lives or dies, or does the clinician display what Rudd (2012) and Maltsberger (1992) call "countertransference hatred"?

People usually die by suicide one at a time. While it is important to have good science about generic suicide risk factors, in the end the question is always this: Can the clinician help this one human being she or he is sitting with at the moment? Everything else is irrelevant, if it does not inform the exigencies of a particular individual standing (trembling) at the suicide threshold.

Let us return to some of the implications of Jerome Motto's statement, used as the epigraph for this chapter (see Motto, 1992). While it may be true that no three suicides are exactly alike, they do share some commonalities (see Shneidman, 1993; see also Chapter 2 and Table 2.2 of this book). Motto's approach runs the risk of engendering predictive futility and nihilism. Suicide cannot be predicted, so why bother? In fact, Motto says that we should eliminate the word *prediction* from our suicidology vocabulary. Trying to create predictive precision is like trying to clear a path through a swamp, he says. We just cannot do it. Instead, we should estimate or "assess" suicide risk (Pokorny, 1992).

Motto claims that we can only (even with the best science and data) predict group suicide risk over fairly long time frames (like 5–10+ years), not individual risk in short time frames (like next Saturday). For Motto, the key issue in suicide assessment (see also Shneidman, 1993; Joiner, 2005; Klonsky, 2015; Ducasse et al., 2018) is tolerance of psychic pain, or what Shneidman calls "psychache" (see Chapter 2, Figure 2.1, column 4). Motto claims that all of us have a pain tolerance threshold beyond which suicide is more probable, and sometimes *perhaps* even necessary. When clinicians assess a suicidal individual, they should always ask, in effect: "Tell me, where do you hurt?" Is it not interesting that hydrocodone is the number one prescribed drug in the United States (Maris, 2015; see also Chapter 15, Table 15.1)?

Motto reminds us that statistical significance is not the same as clinical significance. Put differently, empirical risk assessment via scales is not the same as clinical judgment. Motto also cautions us to pay attention to timing issues. Suicide risk varies over time. Exactly when is someone suicidal? Is the risk acute or chronic, and under what circumstances? Can protective factors compensate for suicide risk factors? For example, can a person have a host of painful suicide risk factors and still not be able or likely to suicide? Why, for example, do black women have higher rates of depressive disorder than white women do, but lower suicide rates (Walker et al., 2018)?

Sensitivity, Specificity, and Predictive Value

Pokorny (1983, 1992) has argued that since suicide is very rare (1 in 10,000 in the general population each year), we tend to get what are known as *false positives* when we try to predict it. That is, we predict a suicide, but get a nonsuicide. In his research, Pokorny got on average about 30% false positives. If we predicted "no suicide" every time, we would almost always get it right and look like mavens.

Epidemiological predictions can be either true or false, positive or negative (Rothman et al., 2012). For example, a *false negative* would be a prediction of no suicide when the outcome is in fact a suicide. Two related statistical concepts are *sensitivity* and *specificity*. *Sensitivity* means roughly correctly identifying true positives. It is calculated with the following formula:

$$TP/(TP + FN) \times 100$$

Specificity means roughly correctly identifying true negatives. Its formula is this:

$$TN/(FP + TN) \times 100$$

Most suicide assessment scales have low sensitivity.

Pokorny (1992) claims that the biggest problem in suicide prediction is false positives. Imagine the treatment implications of predicting that 30% of inpatients at a psychiatric hospital were suicidal. The institution could hardly afford to put 30 of (say) 100 patients on 24/7 close suicide watch. This is not to say that false negatives are not a problem too. Failure to detect a suicide leads to many a medical malpractice lawsuit. Nevertheless, Pokorny singles out false positives as the biggest predictive problem. The ultimate issue here is predictability. For example, using the 15 suicide risk factors described below and briefly discussed in Chapter 3, how many times would we correctly predict suicide? *Predictive value* is calculated as follows:

$$TP/(TP + FP) \times 100$$

Pokorny says that even when our predictive scales are both highly sensitive and specific, we only predict suicide right about 1% of the time. Put differently, we have a 99% error rate. This is hardly impressive. In an actual predictive study (Pokorny, 1992, p. 121) with lower sensitivity and specificity scores, the suicide predictive value was only 2.8%. This means that there was a 97–98% error rate.

Pokorny (1992, p. 127) concludes: "We do not possess any item of information or any combination of items that would permit us to identify to a useful degree the particular persons who will commit suicide." Those of us who work in suicide prevention certainly have our work cut out for us!

Causation versus Association

It gets worse. Not only is suicide rare, and not only does prediction tend to result in false positives, but also statistical association is not the same as causation (Maris, 2015). For example, the wind velocity in Chicago could be associated with the birth rate in New Delhi, but no one in his or her right mind would think the relationship was causal.

When the U.S. Food and Drug Administration's (FDA's) pharmacological advisory committees reviewed the statistical data for nine antidepressants and their association with suicidality, it was clear that for patients up to age 24, taking any of the nine antidepressants on average doubled the patients' suicidality risk (Maris, 2015). After getting a strong majority committee vote, the FDA decided to require a black-box warning (the strongest available) on the product description that taking any of these antidepressants increased suicidality risk for individuals up to age 24. Interestingly, one committee member abstained from voting, saying that statistical association is not the same as causation.

So what is a *cause*? *Cause* refers to an antecedent condition's producing an effect (*Black's Law Dictionary*, 2009), like one billiard ball's striking another. A patient takes a pill (or has another antecedent condition) and then commits suicide shortly thereafter; *post hoc ergo propter hoc* ("after this, therefore because of this"). Note that causes are usually substantial and proximate, although they can be indirect.

In the law, causation is often measured by the nine criteria created by a British statistician, Sir Austin Bradford Hill (1897–1991). These criteria (Hill, 1965), adapted for suicidality and with the relationship between suicidality in youth and antidepressant medications as an example, are as follows:

1. Strength of association (suicidality is roughly twice as likely in younger patients taking antidepressants as in control groups).
2. Consistency (which concerns how common the result is; suicidality is twice as common in young people taking antidepressants).
3. Specificity of association (psychiatric medications are not specifically related to suicidality, since suicide often has other, more relevant risk factors).
4. Temporality (the cause must come before the effect).
5. Dose–response effect (usually the larger the dose, the larger the response).
6. Biological plausibility (it is plausible that antidepressants elevate suicide risk, since they affect serotonin levels in the prefrontal cortex, which in turn affect aggression).
7. Coherence with other knowledge (many clinical trials show increased suicidality in youth after ingestion of antidepressants, but some do not).
8. Experiments (there are very few, if any, confirming or disconfirming suicide experiments, since we cannot ethically withhold treatment from the control groups or test seriously depressed or suicidal patients).
9. Analogy (animal experiments [e.g., cats on high doses of Prozac] show increases in aggression and violence after ingestion of antidepressants).

One wonders how clear and definitive even Hill's criteria are. For example, he did not say whether all or just some (and if just some, which ones) of the criteria are required to establish a causal relationship. Can causality only be suggested? Hill implied that the greater the number of criteria met, the more likely it is that the relationship is causal. Are some criteria more important than others? How are his criteria operationally defined; that is, how are they measured?

In court, it is often argued that an antecedent factor (such as a suicide risk factor) may make a "substantial proximate contribution" to a suicide outcome, without clearly being a cause. The law does not require that a risk factor be the one and only cause of a suicide outcome. As we have seen, suicide has many interacting antecedent causes. A risk factor may be a "necessary" condition (without which suicide would not occur), but may not be a "sufficient" condition (the one and only required condition). The concept or definition of cause can vary from state to state.

Suicide Risk Factors

Given all of the measurement problems described to this point, I proceed to a consideration of suicide risk factors with some caution (Feigelman et al., 2018). *Risk factors* are states, traits, or conditions that are significantly more common among eventual known suicides than they are in nonsuicidal populations, or in suicide completers versus nonfatal suicide attempters or suicide ideators.

Suicide risk factors may be utilized, in part, to try to whittle down the number of people at risk for suicide to a more manageable or preventable size. For example, to be able to go from 1 in 10,000 (in the general population) to 10 or 15 in 100 (among those hospitalized for major depressive disorder who eventually suicide) is a big improvement. It gives us some indication of which persons to pay closer attention to; it also makes us more able to do so, since there are fewer of them.

An important question here is this: What do risk factors tell us about the probability of a suicide outcome and in what time frame? For example, Ernest Hemingway (see Chapter 1, Case 1.1) had all 15 of the suicide risk factors described below, and did in fact kill himself at just over age 60. Unfortunately (for prediction), most people with suicide risk factors die natural deaths; for example, even 85–90% of depressed patients die natural deaths, and the risk is never more than about 1% a year. Suicide risk factors are not very reliable or valid in indicating a suicide outcome (see Ribeiro et al., 2016).

So-called "high-suicide-risk" groups are *really not at very high risk* for suicide at all. Furthermore, one protective factor or one individual's coping strength can nullify several suicide risk factors. What is needed is some way to assess risk and protective factors interactively and arrive at a unique, ad hoc suicide risk score for a particular individual in particular circumstances.

How many suicide risk factors are there? Whose scale of risk factors should be used for measurements, and what specific risk factors should be included? Below, 15 empirically derived suicide risk factors are examined. The American Psychiatric Association (Jacobs et al., 2003, 2010) lists over 60 risk factors, many of which are not on my own list (such as the patient's strengths, specific plans and preparations, history of sexual abuse, etc.). Yet another list of suicide risk factors (Feinstein & Plutchik, 1990) lists 62 risk factors, including impulsivity, suspiciousness, rebellious-ness, strong sex drive, cynicism, and low cholesterol. Which list are you going to believe, and what risk factors are you going to include? There is recent evidence that samples for risk factors tend to focus on white young adults and to underreport racial, ethnic, veteran, and lesbian/gay/bisexual/transgender (LGBT) status (Cha et al., 2018).

We should always strive for parsimony, but not to foolish extremes; in other words, we should adopt the motto (after Whitehead), "Seek simplicity and distrust it." Many of the American Psychiatric Association's and of Feinstein and Plutchik's risk factors are, in effect, specifying and unpacking subcategories of my own 15 risk factors, like those for mental disorders (Maris et al., 2000). Thus these three suicide risk factor lists (and there are many more than three, of course) are actually not all that different. Let us now look at each of my 15 risk factors in some detail. Note that many of these risk factors are elaborated in entire chapters that follow later.

Table 4.1 specifies these 15 common single risk factors for suicide. Of course, this dodges the problem of interaction among multiple risk factors. For one exam-ple of how to calculate interactive suicide risk factors, see Maris (1981, p. 324), in which one model of risk factors resulted in 62% (R^2) of the variance explained in suicide outcome.

Mental Disorders

Almost all individuals who commit suicide have a "diagnosable" mental disor-der (see Chapters 10–14). Joiner (2005) says that 95% do, but most suicides never

---

TABLE 4.1. Common Single Risk Factors for Suicide

1. Mental disorders (especially mood disorders).
2. Alcohol and other substance abuse (especially cocaine and opiate abuse).
3. Suicide ideation, talk, and preparations.
4. Prior suicide attempts (but the typical suicide completer tends to make only one attempt).
5. Use of lethal methods to attempt suicide (such as a firearm to the head).
6. Social isolation and negative interaction, (being profoundly alone), recent interpersonal loss.
7. Hopelessness and cognitive rigidity.
8. Being an older white male (middle-aged to elderly).
9. Family history of suicide or mental disorder.
10. Work, occupation, and unemployment.
11. Marriage/children, sexuality, and family pathology.
12. Stress and diathesis.
13. Aggression, neurobiological dysfunction, anger, impulsivity.
14. Physical illness/chronic pain (including psychache) and its treatment.
15. Suicidal career (acquired ability to inflict lethal self-injury).

Sources: Adapted from Maris (1992b). Copyright © The Guilford Press. Adapted with permission.

get diagnosed or treated. When Tanney (2000) broke down the mental disorders reported among suicides in one set of studies, he found that 61% of the suicides had affective (mood) disorders, 41% substance use disorders, 42% personality disorders (mostly borderline and antisocial), 10% anxiety disorders (Rothschild, 2017), and 6% one of the schizophrenias or other psychotic disorders.

Among the mood disorders, both major depressive disorder and bipolar disorders are prominent in suicides. Tanney (2000) said that major depressive disorder was cited in nine studies and bipolar disorders in two. But Baldessarini et al. (2012) claim that bipolar disorders are slightly more common in suicides than unipolar depressive disorders. My own research using the original BDI found that several specific depressive items occurred more often in completed suicides (cf. Green et al., 2015): sleep disturbance, hopelessness, wanting to die, and feelings of dissatisfaction (Maris, 1981).

One has to be careful when speaking about mental disorder as a suicide risk factor. Clearly, not all suicides are "crazy," acting under an irresistible psychiatric impulse; nor are all suicides irrational. Suicide itself is not a mental disorder as defined by DSM. Suicide is an explicit diagnostic criterion only for major depressive disorder and borderline personality disorder.

I have long argued (Maris, 1982; see also Chapter 19) that suicide can be and often is "rational." Suicide can make sense in that it solves a problem, even though it is an extreme solution and normally not the preferred or best one. Suicides are not necessarily confused, severely depressed, or psychotic at the time they commit suicide.

Alcoholism and Other Substance Abuse

In most studies (Robins, 1981), alcohol abuse is the second most important single suicide risk factor (see Chapter 15; Maris, 2015; Bagge & Borges, 2017). Note that ethanol itself is a depressing substance. Roy and Linnoila (1986) found that on average, 18% of all those with alcoholism eventually die by suicide; Murphy (1992) says that the lifetime alcoholic suicide risk is more like 10%. Some (Ballenger et al., 1979) argue that alcohol is self-medicating, since in the short run it transiently raises brain serotonin. However, in the long run alcohol lowers brain serotonin and increases depression risk.

Alcoholic suicides are mainly men (88%), have a mean age of 47 years, and have had alcoholism for about 25 years before they suicide (Maris, 1981). Karl Menninger (1938) viewed alcoholism itself as a slow substitute for suicide (he called it "partial" suicide). Alcohol increases suicide risk through disinhibition, agitation, impulsivity, irritability, violence/aggression, disruption of social and economic support and interpersonal relationships, and hopelessness (Mack & Lightdale, 2006).

Other substances abused by suicides include opiates, barbiturates, stimulants, cocaine, Adderall and other ADHD medications, hallucinogens, and household chemicals and pesticides (Maris, 2015). These nonalcoholic substances can be a special problem for younger female suicides, who often overdose on them. For example, Marzuk et al. (1992) found that about 29% of New York City suicides ages 21–30 tested positive for cocaine.

Suicide Ideation, Talk, and Preparation

In clinics, hospitals, jail, and prisons, often the only risk factor for suicide considered is the person's response to the question of whether he or she is currently thinking about suiciding. One major problem with this approach is that completed suicides are often more likely to deny suicide ideation than they are to admit it (Silverman & Berman, 2014; Berman, 2018). Thus responses about suicide ideation are not very predictive of suicide.

A lot of people think about suicide at some time in their lives—Nock (2009, 2014) estimates that 12-14% do so, and Linehan and Laffaw (1982) say 20% or more—but very few ever actually commit suicide. From 12 to 20% of the population have suicide ideation, but only 1 in 10,000 a year actually suicide. Clearly, merely asking about suicide ideation is not enough. Clinicians should also inquire about specific plans, access to lethal means (Lester, 2012), and other preparations to attempt suicide. Remember that the Columbia suicidality scale (Figure 1.2) also measures preparatory actions to suicide.

Even if people are insightful, honest, and forthcoming about their suicide ideas, the relationship among suicide ideas, suicide attempts, and suicide completions is complex and not well understood. Klonsky and May (2014) claim that we do not know how to differentiate suicide ideators or nonfatal attempters from suicide completers well (see also Caine & Mann, 2017). Many of the risk factors for suicide ideation are not clearly related to either suicide attempts or completions. Klonsky and May recommend the work of Joiner (2005) and O'Connor (2011) as to which additional risk factors may suggest who actually suicides. Millner et al. (2017) argue that the pathway from a suicide idea to a completion is also complex. For example, they point out that while the median onset for a suicide idea before an actual attempt is 1–5 years, 86.5% of proximal planning steps take place within 1 week of attempting, and 66% within 12 hours.

One might think that suicide ideas expressed in suicide notes would tell us why someone suicides. But most notes are discovered too late to help save the persons who actually wrote them. Furthermore, only about 10–25% of all suicides write suicide notes. Paradoxically, some people who kill themselves may have no explicit ideas about doing it. For example, did the comedian John Belushi think much about suicide when he overdosed? (His death may have been accidental.)

Prior Suicide Attempts

Most studies show that nonfatal suicide attempts have a strong positive correlation with completed suicide (Maris et al., 1992; Isometsa & Lönnqvist, 1998). Among completers, about 70% make only one suicide attempt, 13.8% make two attempts, 4.8% make three, 3.9% make four, and 3.3% make 5 or more attempts before completing suicide (Maris et al., 2000). Very few completers make more than five nonfatal attempts before they suicide, and almost all of these attempts are by younger women. Probably, if women used more lethal attempt methods (as men do), then on average they too would likely make fewer attempts than they actually do. One very important fact, which I have mentioned in Chapter 1 and come back to later, is that of white male suicides over age 45, 88% make only one fatal suicide attempt (at least in my Chicago survey; Maris, 1981).

From 10 to 20% of nonfatal suicide attempters eventually go on to complete suicide at some time during their lives, but this also means that 80–90% do not ever commit suicide (Maris et al., 2000). Nonfatal suicide attempts outnumber completed suicides by about 10:1 to 25:1. Many first-time suicide attempters get treatment that they would not ordinarily get, if they had not attempted suicide. Thus low-lethality suicide attempts can be reinforcing or even a protective factor against completed suicide.

Joiner (2005) has argued that suicide attempters are in effect "practicing" for completed suicide—that is, gaining experience that allows them to be *able* to suicide later on. He said that suicides need certain kinds of experiences repeated over time to "achieve" suicide. Suiciding is not easy to do. As he puts it, one has to acquire the ability to inflict lethal self-injury. It is somewhat problematic for Joiner's theory that his own father only made one fatal suicide attempt, as do the vast majority of other prototypical white male suicides. But people can get the experience they need to commit suicide other than by making multiple suicide attempts.

Use of Lethal Methods to Attempt Suicide

Obviously, if people use a method that is likely to kill them, then they are at a greater risk to suicide (Giner et al., 2014). It follows that a clinician should always ask a would-be suicide about the planned method and try to limit access to lethal means (Lester, 2012).

Most suicides in the United States use firearms to suicide; which is fairly unique among countries. In 2013, 51.5% of all completed suicides used firearms. The second most common method was hanging (24.5%, which is also highly lethal). Poisoning, especially with carbon monoxide from cars, was the third most preferred suicide attempt method (16.1%) (Drapeau & McIntosh, 2015; see Chapter 3, Table 3.1).

In the United States, the use of lethal methods differs by gender. For example, note that the rank order of suicide attempt methods for men in Table 4.2 is as follows: (1) firearms, (2) hanging, and (3) poisons, but for women the order is (1) firearms, (2) poisons, and (3) hanging. In other earlier findings (e.g., McIntosh, 2002) and some recent data, women's use of firearms and poisons to attempt suicide were virtually tied (about 33% each). Given their preference for firearm methods, it is

TABLE 4.2. Suicide Attempt Methods by Gender

	Men	Women
Firearms	56.4%	31.2%
Hanging	25.2%	23.5%
Poisoning	11.2%	36.2%

Source: Centers for Disease Control and Prevention (2018). Data in public domain.

no surprise that male suicide rates typically exceed those of females by a factor of three or four.

Recently, there has been new interest in attempts at restricting lethal means (Lester, 2012). Some simple changes can reduce suicide rates dramatically (if individuals do not just switch to other methods). Among the method changes that have been proposed (or, in some cases, already implemented) are these:

- Gun control (but this is complicated by Second Amendment rights in the U.S. Constitution).
- Square vehicle exhaust pipes that hoses will not fit over.
- Jump restraints on bridges (like fences or barriers).
- Various methods of pill control (reducing prescription size, wrapping pills individually, monitoring large prescriptions, using harder-to-open bottle tops and safety seals on bottles—see the recent Tylenol bottling and packaging changes).
- Control of pesticides (which are often used in rural China and India by young females in suicide attempts).
- Detoxifying home gas (as was done in the United Kingdom some time ago).
- Not building structures over two to five stories high (40% of suicides in New York City are jumpers).
- Not allowing ropes, belts, drawstrings or shoestrings, and phone or computer cords in jails, prisons, or hospitals.

Social Isolation and Negative Interaction

Social isolation and negative interaction are suicidogenic (see Chapter 7). Sadly for suicide prevention, one of the most influential suicide management textbooks (Simon & Hales, 2012) does not have a single chapter among its 34 on the social relations of suicides. Isolation raises irritability and aggression, at the same time that it reduces targets of aggression to the suicidal person alone.

Joiner (2005) speaks of "thwarted belongingness" and "perceived burdensomeness." In my Chicago study (Maris, 1981), almost 50% of completed suicides had no close friends (cf., Feigelman et al., 2018). Among other things, friends can encourage would-be suicides to focus attention outside themselves, which can distract them from their suicidal agenda.

What is there about social isolation that increases suicide risk? For one, fewer people will notice a suicide attempt or preparations for it, which increases its lethality. When Sylvia Plath (see Case 6.1 in Chapter 6) made a serious suicide attempt with an overdose of barbiturates, she went down in her basement and hid behind a woodpile. She almost died when those searching for her could not quickly find her.

Many suicides feel that no one cares whether they live or die. Part of the genius of the U.K. group known as the Samaritans, founded by Chad Varah, is the concept of "befriending." The Samaritans' emphasis is not on professional competence, but rather on just "being there." Suicidal individuals often need a relationship like that of a nurturing, nursing mother, with her noncontingent support and love. My colleagues and I sometimes talk about the importance in suicide prevention of having at least one "significant udder." Corny, but apt.

When a person is alone, by definition, she or he has no counterbalancing perspective or sounding board for decision making. The person may decide to suicide, and there is no one there to say: "You know, you don't have to do *that!* Let's consider some alternatives that might have the same result."

With negative interaction, a person is not alone, but the significant udder, in effect, has poisoned milk. Joiner (2005) speaks of an incident in which internet viewers of a person who was threatening to overdose actually encouraged him to go ahead and suicide. One also thinks of punitive parenting, prolonged physical and sexual abuse, having alcoholic parents, and a multiproblem family of origin as suicidogenic. In all these cases, social interaction is not absent, but is negative and destructive.

Hopelessness and Cognitive Rigidity

As discussed in Chapter 11 (see especially Table 11.4), hopelessness correlates more highly with suicide intent than depression does (however, see Qiu et al., 2017). Beck et al. (1974a) constructed a Hopelessness Scale consisting of 20 true–false questions. Ten years later (Beck et al., 1985), they followed up one of their studies of 165 patients hospitalized with suicide ideation. Of those who had suicided over those 10 years, 91% had Hopelessness Scale scores greater than 9.

Hopelessness often involves seeing no alternatives to suicide: It is a kind of rigid thinking or "tunnel vision" (with the cynical belief that any light at the end of the tunnel is probably on a freight train). Hopeless individuals not only perceive life as painful and intolerable, but also believe that it is never going to improve; for them, the only (that word again) escape from their pain is to stop living by suiciding.

Being an Older White Male

One striking trait of suicide completers in most of the world is that roughly 70% of them are older males. In 2013 in the United States, the elderly made up 14.1% of the population, but 17.5% of suicides (Drapeau & McIntosh, 2015; see Chapter 3, Table 3.1).

Some (e.g., de Catanzaro, 1992) have suggested that maleness itself is related to premature death in general and to suicide in particular. Except for diseases related to female physiology and reproduction (like breast and ovarian cancers), men tend to have higher death rates than do females, even *in utero*. The deaths are not just from suicide, but also, for example, from heart disease and lung cancer. We know that it is not just maleness, chromosomes, or biology that causes elevated male suicide rates, since (for example) African American male suicide rates level off in middle age (but may rise later in life), much as suicide rates of white females do.

Many suicidologists do not realize that the celebrated rise (up to 300%) in adolescent suicide rates in the United States in the late 1960s and early 1970s was almost exclusively among young males (Maris, 1985). More recent data (2013; again, see Table 3.1) reveal that the white male suicide rate is higher for those ages 45–54 or older.

Only about 22% of all U.S. suicides are committed by white females, and very few black females suicide. In fact, African American women are almost immune to suicide. In most places in the world (except in China, India and a few other countries), male suicide rates exceed those of females by a ratio of 3:1 to 5:1.

Family History of Suicide or Mental Disorder

Suicides and mood disorders tend to run in families, as I have noted in Chapter 1 with regard to the family histories of Ernest Hemingway and Virginia Woolf (see Jamison, 1993). Eleven percent of the Chicago suicides I studied had a first-degree relative who suicided, but none of the natural death controls did (Maris, 1981).

Family history and suicide may be related through either biology and genetics (Roy et al., 1991) or modeling of prior family suicides (Phillips et al., 1992). This is especially true for adolescents. For example, adolescent suicide rates rose 6.9% in the 7–10 days after adolescent suicide stories were on New York City's three major television networks (CBS, NBC, and ABC). But adult suicides only went up 0.5% under the same circumstances. Suicide by contagion is much more likely if the person is younger.

There can also be sociobiological family factors. For example, having young dependent children to care for may discourage suicide, but being beyond the reproductive years can encourage older suicides. As biological fitness wanes, people are less likely to have more children, and they do not need to support adult children as much. Some may then think, in effect, "Why hang around?"

Work, Occupation, and Unemployment

In general, work and productive life activities tend to protect against suicide, and not working or not having meaningful hobbies aggravates the suicide rate. Remember that suicide rates are high in the elderly, who are often no longer working. As noted in Case 1.1, Ernest Hemingway said, "Retirement is the filthiest word in the language" (quoted in Hotchner, 1966, p. 228). Harvard Nobel laureate physicist Percy Bridgman committed suicide as soon as he finished work on his collected papers (he had metastatic cancer), and Eastman Kodak founder George Eastman (who suffered from a painful spinal condition) left this simple suicide note: "My work is done. Why wait?"

Although many occupations do not contribute much to the suicide rate, some do (Maris et al., 2000; Maris, 2010). Occupational groups for which high suicide rates are typical include dentists, physicians, physical or manual laborers, artists (notably poets), and military veterans (see Maris, 2008). Groups with low suicide rates include the clergy, pilots, elementary school teachers, and clerical workers. One problem with occupations and suicide rates is that high and low rates can be found within each of the U.S. Census occupational categories. For example, among physicians, psychiatrists have high suicide rates, but pediatricians and surgeons have low suicide rates. Interestingly, *The New York Times* reported (Sanger-Katz, 2016) that surgeons were mainly Republicans and psychiatrists were mainly Democrats.

Business cycles and stock market variations are also correlated with the suicide rate (Henry & Short, 1954). Durkheim (1897/1951) claimed that suicide rates are highest when social norms are suddenly disrupted (such as during stock market collapses). He called this socioeconomic condition *anomie* (literally, "without norms"). Note that about 33% of suicides are unemployed at the time they suicide, compared to just 6% (in 2015) of the general population.

Marriage/Children, Sexuality, and Family Pathology

Marriage and having a family are usually associated with lower suicide rates (see Chapter 6, Figure 6.1). Suicide rates are almost always highest among the divorced and widowed, especially for men. Even though widowhood and divorce are highly suicidogenic for men, being widowed is actually slightly protective for suicide in white women. Women have always been force-fed the idea that marriage and childbearing are good for them. But are they really?

Freud viewed sexual energy as a large portion of life energy. Being young and fit includes having reproductive possibilities, and being able to use sexuality to cope, such as orgasmic pleasure to counter pain, reduces tension, and distract oneself. Therefore, we would expect suicidal people on average to have more sexual dysfunctions. Some sexual diversities, particularly those that have historically been regarded by mainstream culture as deviant, may also be associated with higher suicidality. For example, homosexual males have a suicide rate about twice that of heterosexual males (see Chapter 6).

Family pathology among eventual (later) suicides can include early object loss; early maternal separation; physical, sexual, and emotional abuse; incest; young adult sexual promiscuity; and even frequent family residential moves (which are especially likely in the military). Sexual abuse as a child is related to abnormal hypothalamic–pituitary–adrenocortical (HPA) function later in adulthood (Mann & Currier, 2012).

Stress and Diathesis

In the present context, *diathesis* refers to biological givens, early life experiences, or behavioral traits (like impulsivity) that contribute to a predisposition to suicide, in combination with normally chronic (sometimes acute) stressful life circumstances (Mann & Currier, 2012). An overly simplistic example might be provided by a cognitively rigid, aging male going through a second divorce. To be sure, there are many other interacting suicide risk factors.

Stress, on the other hand, includes both excessive negative (and even positive) life events that tend to strain our adaptability, and that can thus change our neurobiology or ability to cope. Most suicides experience multiple stressors over very long time periods. Repeated stress has psychological, developmental, neurobiological, and social consequences.

Is suicide "triggered"? In the general model of suicide presented in Chapter 2 (see especially Figure 2.1, column 4), I suggest some possible "triggers" of suicide (see also Maltsberger et al., 2003). However, my theory of suicide is that usually most suicides are the result of complex, prolonged stress coupled with diathesis. The vast majority of individuals do not respond to even extreme stress or negative life events by suiciding, especially if the stressors are acute and time-limited. Those individuals who do make a suicidal response to stress have chronic vulnerabilities, including diathetic behavioral traits, life experiences, and repeated psychic pain.

Suicides are not triggered in the sense that the immediate precursors of suicide are very different from the individual's long-term stressors. For the most part, the same factors seem to be operating in the weeks just before a suicide as were there all along, although they may summate qualitatively, and intensify near the end. As Motto (1992) suggests, there is a gradual, lifelong repetition and accumulation of stressors that breaches an adaptive threshold in some vulnerable individuals. Friends and relatives of the suicide often do not notice anything special going on just before the suicide, and may express surprise that the suicide occurred when it did (or even that it occurred at all).

Aggression, Neurobiological Dysfunction, Anger, and Impulsivity

Never forget that suicide is a violent act that requires some minimal aggressive energy (Giner et al., 2014). Hopelessness and depressive disorder by themselves are usually insufficient to cause a suicide. In fact, aggression may be more basic in suicide than depression is, since aggression occurs in all species (animal and human) at all ages, but depression does not. The aggressive catalyst in suicide can include anger, irritability, frustration, hatred (murderous rage), dissatisfaction, desperation, and anxiety.

Animals tend to behave aggressively under specific conditions, including (1) predation for food or sex, (2) between-male rivalries, (3) fear, (4) irritability, (5) territoriality, (6) maternal protection of the young, and (7) instrumentality (i.e., committing an act to obtain another end, like escape from perceived threats or danger).

Suicide is just one of several aggressive malfunctions of the brain (especially of the serotonergic and, to a lesser degree, dopaminergic systems). Others include sleep difficulties, impulsivity, disinhibition, headaches, mood volatility (labile mood), poor peer relationships, and glucocorticosteroid abnormalities (our adrenal glands sit on top of the kidneys and produce dopamine, norepinephrine, and epinephrine hormones, which protect us against stress; see Brown et al., 1992, on the functioning of the HPA axis). Those who have committed violent suicides tend to have lower levels of CSF serotonin (and its metabolites) in the prefrontal cortex of the brain (see Chapter 16 and Maris, 2015).

Do not forget that Freud and Menninger saw suicides as displaced or disguised murders. For example, Menninger (1938) called suicide "murder in the 180th degree." Hate or the wish-to-kill is usually stronger in younger suicides and often involves interpersonal dynamics (e.g., see Sylvia Plath's [1966] poem "Daddy"). In older suicides, anger is frequently directed more at the terms of life and a deteriorating human condition (Maris, 1982)—a kind of protest of pain, decay, decline, atrophy, and failure, rather than a grievance with other people.

The frustration–aggression hypothesis (Henry & Short, 1954; Dollard et al., 1939) generally assumes that the more frustration, the more aggression. There are also, of course, murder–suicides (see Chapter 21 and Joiner, 2014). The perpetrators of these are typically men killing women and then themselves. Some murder-suicides can result from unexpended aggressive energy—such as hopelessness and a diffuse concept of self, requiring the murder of others in order to kill oneself (see my discussion of Jim Jones and Jonestown in Chapter 17)—or from guilt.

Physical Illness/Chronic Pain and Its Treatment

In and of itself, physical illness is not highly associated with suicide; there are a lot of sick, older people who never suicide. For example, in my Chicago study, the natural death controls had far more physical illness than the suicides did; they were about 20 years older on average, too (Maris, 1981). Most physically ill individuals do not suicide because of that fact alone. It takes other suicide risk factors interacting with aging and physical illness to increase suicide rates.

On the other hand, since suicides tend to be older, there is a positive association of some physical illnesses with suicide (O'Neill et al., 2018). Some of the physical illnesses found to be more common in suicides than in controls (this is not a complete listing) include epilepsy (Maris, 1986), malignant neoplasms or cancers (Quan et al., 2002), chronic pulmonary disease, AIDS, gastrointestinal disorders, and musculoskeletal disorders (Goldblatt, 2000; Berman & Pompili, 2011). Among the musculoskeletal disorders are arthritis, spinal stenosis, hip and knee deterioration, and the chronic pain often associated with these.

Many of my forensic suicide cases are related to the drug treatment of chronic pain, such as the use of opiates and gabapentin. Neurontin is a GABA agonist, which many think decreases brain serotonin and epinephrine (which are monoamines). Any drug that reduces monoamines tends to increase both depressive disorder and suicide risk. The same is true for benzodiazepine tranquilizers, which are also GABA-based.

Suicidal Career

Most people bear up surprisingly well under acute insults to their adaptive repertoire. Bad things happen routinely, and most of us cope and eventually move on with our lives, albeit with some scars and compromise. Those who do not cope well, are not resilient, and eventually commit suicide tend to have lifelong patterns of stress–diathesis traits and states that help make them more vulnerable to suicide. As noted in Chapter 2, Joiner (2005) calls such a lifelong pattern "the acquired ability to inflict lethal self-injury." I call it a "suicidal career" (Maris, 1981).

In the very young, there is almost no suicide. But suicide rates increase dramatically with age, almost in a straight line over the lifespan, for white males. In 2013, the age group with the highest average suicide rate consisted of 45- to 54-year-olds, at 19.7 per 100,000 (Drapeau & McIntosh, 2015; see Table 3.1). The mean age of suicides in my Chicago sample was 51 years (Maris, 1981). The suicide rate stays high or even climbs after midlife among white males.

What does this tell us? In general, the longer the suicidal career, the greater the suicide risk (other things being equal). Most suicidal careers are long (about 50–70 years), although at times episodically intense. Shorter, less intense suicidal careers tend to have a lower probability of ending in suicide. Often we need to try to weight various risk factors in suicidal careers. One or two risk factors may be salient and determinative, overpowering the other risk and protective factors, such as a late life, recurring depressive episodes, or chronic alcoholism with accompanying abandonment by sources of social support. Once again, risk factors cannot just be counted to determine suicide risk. Usually suicide risk factors are multiple and interactive, waxing and waning over long time frames or careers.

Risk Factors Applied to a Suicide Case

CASE 4.1. Silvia Suarez

Silvia Suarez was a 30-year-old unmarried female of mixed Hispanic–Asian ethnicity. She committed suicide in April 2006 in her apartment in a major southwestern U.S. city by cutting herself multiple times on the throat, arms, and thighs with a straight-edged razor. In May 2004, she had been diagnosed with an anxiety disorder (panic disorder) and given the antidepressant paroxetine (Paxil; 20 mg every morning). The police found two empty Paxil prescription bottles (each for 30 pills and dated March 15 and April 10, 2006) in her apartment. She had collected her own blood in bowls and placed them on the kitchen counter.

Silvia had graduated from college and received a BA in 1999. Her job at the time of her suicide was as a mental health technician at a local university hospital. In the summers, she worked at Yellowstone Park in a program for autistic women. Silvia was athletic; she played soccer, rode her trail bike, hiked, and went fishing with her dad. She was outgoing and had a good sense of humor. At age 30, however, she had never had a serious romantic relationship. There was some question among her survivors that she might be a lesbian, although she had never discussed the matter with them. Just before her death, she had moved into her own apartment.

Silvia had never had a diagnosis of depression or schizophrenia, and had never reported any suicide ideation or nonfatal attempts. She drank alcohol about three times a week, but did not smoke. Other than for her anxiety disorder, Silvia seldom went to doctors. One of her doctors reported that she was "grossly overdue for health care maintenance."

There seemed to be an acute mental health issue about 3 days before Silvia died. She called her sister early Monday morning and sounded confused and paranoid. She asked her sister if the family was keeping secrets from her, and said that she felt that something bad was about to happen. She also reported that she was having problems about missing work and pestering one of her coworkers. In her phone calls to this coworker, Silvia's conversation was described as "weird"; she was talking at length about life energy and religion. Her coworker reported Suarez to an administrator on the Wednesday morning of the suicide. By late Thursday, the family became very concerned about Silvia, went to her apartment, and found her lying dead on the floor, exsanguinated.

Source: Maris. The case is based on data presented publicly in court, but all identifying information has been fictionalized to protect the individual and family.

Silvia Suarez clearly had only 3 of the 15 risk factors just discussed: #1, a mental disorder (an anxiety disorder); #12, stress and diathesis; and #13, aggression and irritability, possibly aggravated by serotonin flux from her antidepressant treatment. It is possible that she also had #6, social isolation (but she had strong family support), and #10, work problems. Thus, altogether, she had 3–5 suicide risk factors and would have scored 2–3 on a 10-point suicide risk scale.

Generally, 1–3 risk factors indicate low suicide risk, 4–6 factors indicate moderate risk, and 7–10 suggest high suicide risk (other things being equal). Based on this simple risk factor analysis alone, Silvia's suicide would not have been predicted, but she did in fact suicide. She was a false negative, to use Pokorny's terminology.

Two other suicide risk factors in the case of Silvia Suarez included (1) a possible misdiagnosed and untreated schizophrenic disorder, and (2) an adverse reaction to her antidepressant medication, Paxil (especially if she overdosed on it). If she had schizophrenia, then she should have received an antipsychotic and perhaps should even have been hospitalized. Schizophrenic suicides tend to use bizarre methods to attempt suicide, and Silvia's collecting her own blood in bowls was undoubtedly bizarre. If she were having an adverse antidepressant effect, then her prescriber should have probably stopped the Paxil or switched her to another antidepressant and monitored her closely. In any event, we see with this case how hard it is to use suicide risk factors reliably and validly to correctly assess an individual suicide outcome—a topic to which I now turn.

Suicide Risk Assessment of Individuals

Individual suicide risk assessment is a major topic that cannot be adequately considered in a few pages. For example, the Simon and Hales (2012) textbook devotes five entire chapters to suicide assessment. The focus here is on how a clinician assesses a suicidal individual in a clinical interview. Remember the quotation from Motto at the start of this chapter. Suicide risk factors for different, unique individuals may themselves need to be considered *ad hominem*; assessment does not mean going mechanically through a checklist of generic risk factors.

Sometimes an individual needs to be admitted (even involuntarily) as an inpatient to a psychiatric hospital, given a thorough in-house assessment, watched 24/7 for several days, and *perhaps* started on a cocktail of powerful psychiatric medications and a series of cognitive therapy treatments. Clinicians cannot do therapy with a cadaver. How do they know which individuals to put into this treatment group? This is not a trivial question, since such treatment can be coercive and is frequently resisted.

As discussed earlier, most suicide risk assessment results in false positives. That is, it tends to identify patients as suicidal who are not in fact seriously at risk for suicide (especially in the short run). On the other hand, there are patients like Silvia Suarez, who are false negatives: They may be assessed as not acutely suicidal when they actually are. Accurate individual suicide assessment is difficult, but it is crucial to do such an assessment as well as possible.

One of the best clinical interview protocols for suicidal patients is that of Rudd (2012; see also Simon, 2012). Rudd gives a detailed list of assessment procedures to follow. Among the aspects of assessment that Rudd emphasizes as critically important are the following:

1. Establishing a therapeutic relationship or alliance with the patient (see Maltsberger & Stoklosa, 2012), and having a treatment "captain" who is in charge of the treatment team.
2. Not being afraid to foster short-term dependency (Shneidman).
3. Being sensitive to and avoiding what has been called "countertransference hatred" by Maltsberger (1992; Maltsberger & Buie, 1989; see below).
4. Conducting a thorough examination of the patient's suicide ideation, including rating it on a severity scale, such as from 1 (low) to 10 (high).
5. Going over the patient's specific suicide plans: What method would be used; does the patient have the means to suicide by that method; in what circumstances would the patient actually do it; and so on?
6. Taking a thorough psychiatric history and recording all past suicide attempts.
7. Examining the patient's psychiatric medications carefully. Are they appropriate for the diagnosis? Could they interact or have serious adverse effects?
8. Reviewing a standard list of suicide risk factors like that of the American Psychiatric Association (Jacobs et al., 2003, 2010) or my own (Maris, 2015), giving special attention to hopelessness and impulsivity.
9. Listing the counterbalancing suicide protective factors and determining how they interact with the suicide risk factors.
10. Doing a careful mental status exam and a thorough psychiatric examination repeatedly. Maltsberger and Stoklosa (2012, p. 309) provide a list of specific mental status items to monitor.
11. Combining the suicide assessment with a good, thorough physical examination by an internist or family practitioner (including possibly lab tests, x-rays, and perhaps some imaging or scans), and getting a medical history. One needs to rule out conditions like thyroid malfunction, tumors, drug and/or alcohol abuse, and other diseases (AIDS, other sexually transmitted diseases, hepatitis, etc.) that can cause psychiatric symptoms.

Let me now elaborate on some of Rudd's points.

• Transference and countertransference issues are important. Is the clinician able to establish a therapeutic relationship with the patient? If not, what is the clinician going to do about it? Does the patient need a physician or psychotherapist with particular characteristics (male or female, young or old, straight or LGBT, etc.)? If there is a treatment team, who is the "go-to" person on the team?
• Can the clinician tolerate patients who are at their worst, allow them to regress (if need be) or to make excessive demands, and permit them to be dependent on the clinician for a while?

- Maltsberger and Buie (1980) speak of "countertransference hatred" (therapists' expressing malice to their patients, ending sessions early, being late for appointments, taking phone calls during sessions, canceling appointments, etc.). Again, awareness and avoidance of this are essential.

- Suicide ideation should not be assessed via "yes–no" questions. Ask instead: "How would you rate your suicide ideation on a scale of 0 ('I have no intent at all') to 10 ('I will act on my thoughts as soon as possible')?"

- What are the patient's plans and other preparations for suicide attempts? Has the patient taken out life insurance, made funeral plans, and/or bought a gun and practiced shooting it? Has he or she written suicide notes, done computer searches? Under what circumstances would the patient attempt suicide?

- How many times has the patient attempted suicide in the past? What triggered those past suicide attempts, if anything? What exactly did he or she do then, and when (how often)? How did people react to those suicide attempts?

- Pay special attention to the patient's medications (Maris, 2015). Do the medications fit the diagnosis? How many psychiatric medications has the patient taken, and what were they? Did the patient ever experience adverse medication effects? Is the patient taking medications for chronic pain? If so, what are they? Does the patient take prescribed psychiatric or pain medications irregularly?

- Does the patient live alone? How many close friends does he or she have? Do you have contact information for these friends? Are any friends themselves suicidal? Does the patient have children or pets? If children, how many, and what is the patient's relationship with them? Is the patient actively religious? Does the patient have a decent job and enough money? How satisfied is the patient with his or her life, say, on a scale of 1–10? How is the patient's sex life? Is the patient currently in treatment?

- Rate the mental status of the individual. In addition, rate hopelessness, anguish, rage, aloneness, anxiety, self-hate, dissociations, feeling entrapped, anhedonia, suicide ideation preoccupation, and impulses to self-harm. If the patient admits to self-harm impulses, ask, "How would you do it—cutting, drugs, guns, what?"

The next chapter is the first of five chapters in Part III on sociodemographic issues. It starts by looking more closely at specific suicide risk factors. Among the most important of these by far are aging and what I call the "suicidal career"; therefore, I begin by discussing these factors in Chapter 5.

PART III

SOCIODEMOGRAPHIC ISSUES

CHAPTER 5

Age, Lifespan, and Suicidal Careers

What does a man care about? Staying healthy, working good.
Eating and drinking with his friends. Enjoying himself in bed.
I haven't any of them.

—ERNEST HEMINGWAY

Clearly, aging has an important relationship with suicide (see Table 5.1). Young children are virtually immune to suicide, in part because they lack a mature concept of death. As people age, the suicide rate goes up as well, especially for males. Obviously, suicide meanings and dynamics change with age. The very notion of a suicidal career suggests that over time, with certain kinds of life experiences, suicidality varies.

Suicide risk factors vary with age. Wanting to die when you are 5 is very different from when you are 85. Depressive disorders, alcohol abuse, use of lethal methods like guns, living alone, loss of social support, hopelessness, work and money problems, irritability, and physical illness all tend to increase as we age. If the suicidal career theory is right, then eventual suicides need time and certain kinds of life experiences in order to acquire or achieve the ability to inflict lethal self-injury.

In the contemporary United States, on average, males live to be about 75 years old and females to about 80, other things being equal. Traditionally, suicidologists have examined the suicidality of the following age groups:

- *Children,* roughly from birth to puberty. Very few children under ages 5–9 suicide. In fact, most U.S. vital statistics for suicide start at age 5.
- *Adolescents,* beginning with puberty to young adulthood. Early adolescents are roughly ages 12–17; later adolescents are ages 18–22.
- *Middle-aged,* ages 35–55.
- *Elderly,* traditionally over age 65, but people are living longer. Ages 65–74 are now often called the *young-old,* ages 75–84 the *old-old,* and ages 85+ the *oldest-old.*

All these age categories are capricious and arbitrary. We could just use census-like age categories, such as those in Table 5.1 (5–14, 15–24, 25–34, 35–44, 45–54, etc.). Especially early in life and as we age, there are different developmental tasks and expectations (e.g., see the works of Jean Piaget, 1929; Erik Erikson, 1963; and Sigmund Freud, 1917/1957), which are probably related to suicide risk factors. If people become developmentally stagnated as they age chronologically—for example, if they fail to make the transition from adolescence to young adulthood or from middle-aged to elderly—their risk of suicide may go up.

If we do not intentionally interfere with the life cycle (say, by suicide or homicide), have a fatal accident, or early illness, then our lives end naturally with catabolic diseases (mainly cancers, stroke, and heart diseases) or injuries. We do not have to do anything, and eventually our lives stop in about 27,000 days (75 years × 365 days) after birth. It doesn't seem like a very long time, does it?

It stands to reason that if life is painful, stressful, or otherwise problematic (especially repeatedly and over long time periods), then a person might choose to hasten his or her death in order to avoid a prolonged, painful existence with no real hope of improvement. But if there is some kind of life after biological death (such as the continued existence of a soul, or an afterlife in heaven or hell), then suicide may not resolve the person's problems. For example, if suicide offends God, then the suicide may be punished longer than the human life cycle—indeed, for eternity, in a place like Dante's Inferno or a Hieronymus Bosch painting.

Some Fundamental Questions about Age and Suicide

Readers should think about answers to the following age-related questions.

* How young can a person be and still commit suicide?
* If a person is old and sick, should or could he or she hasten death? What is your own opinion about physician-assisted suicide? See the HBO movie *You Don't Know Jack* (Levinson, 2010), with Al Pacino playing Jack Kevorkian.
* Why do older white males have the highest suicide rates generally?
* What about the *Sleeping Beauty* phenomenon of dying young and leaving an attractive corpse? Does such a romantic view of suicide distort or cover up the ugliness of suicide?
* Near the end of life, how could suicide resolve life problems? As noted in Chapter 1, the philosopher Friedrich Nietzsche once said, "The thought of suicide has got me through many a dark night."
* Why is the suicide rate actually relatively low (about 1 in 10,000 per year in the United States), especially among the young? Do we "have it backward" trying to understand suicide rates as too high?

Generalizations on Age, Race, and Suicide

The most recent available age data for suicide (at the time I wrote this writing) are those for 2013 (generated in 2015, see *suicidology.org*). Take a look at Table 5.1

TABLE 5.1. U.S. Suicide Rates by Age, Sex, and Race

Group/ age	2003	2004	2005	2006	2007	2008	2009	2010	2011	2012	2013	Group/ age
						U.S. suicide rates, 2003–2013 (Rates per 100,000 population)						
5–14	0.6	0.7	0.7	0.5	0.5	0.6	0.7	0.7	0.7	0.8	1.0	5–14
15–24	9.7	10.3	10.0	9.9	9.7	10.0	10.1	10.5	11.0	11.1	11.1	15–24
25–34	12.7	12.7	12.4	12.3	13.0	12.9	12.8	14.0	14.6	14.7	14.8	25–34
35–44	14.9	15.0	14.9	15.1	15.6	15.9	16.1	16.0	16.2	16.7	16.2	35–44
45–54	15.9	16.6	16.5	17.2	17.7	18.7	19.3	19.6	19.8	20.0	19.7	45–54
55–64	13.8	13.8	13.9	14.5	15.5	16.3	16.7	17.5	17.1	18.0	18.1	55–64
65–74	12.7	12.3	12.6	12.6	12.6	13.9	14.0	13.7	14.1	14.0	15.0	65–74
75–84	16.4	16.3	16.9	15.9	16.3	16.0	15.7	15.7	16.5	16.8	17.1	75–84
85+	16.9	16.4	16.9	15.9	15.6	15.6	15.6	17.6	16.9	17.8	18.6	85+
65+	14.6	14.3	14.7	14.2	14.3	14.8	14.8	14.9	15.3	15.4	16.1	65+
Total	10.8	11.0	11.0	11.1	11.5	11.8	12.0	12.4	12.7	12.9	13.0	Total
Men	17.6	17.7	17.7	17.8	18.3	19.0	19.2	20.0	20.2	20.6	20.6	Men
Women	4.3	4.6	4.5	4.6	4.8	4.9	5.0	5.2	5.4	5.5	5.7	Women
White	12.1	12.3	12.3	12.4	12.9	13.3	13.5	14.1	14.5	14.8	14.9	White
Nonwhite	5.5	5.8	5.5	5.5	5.6	5.7	5.8	5.8	5.8	6.1	6.0	Nonwhite
Black	5.1	5.2	5.1	4.9	4.9	5.2	5.1	5.1	5.3	5.5	5.4	Black

Source: Drapeau and McIntosh (2015), for the American Association of Suicidology (AAS).

(which is actually an enlargement of a section of Table 3.1 in Chapter 3) and at Figures 5.1 and 5.2, and note the following generalizations about age and suicide.

- Consider Table 5.1 and Figure 5.2 (as well as Table 25.1 in Chapter 25). Over the years 1900–2013, the suicide rate has remained fairly constant—with some peaks (the suicide rates went up steadily in the last 10 years) and troughs—at about 11 to 13.2 per 100,000. This raises an interesting question: What is the optimum suicide rate, 0 or 11–13.2 per 100,000? Is the suicide rate (like the death rate) about as low as we can expect it to go? The only places with a suicide rate of 0 are fictional Utopias, like the World State in Aldous Huxley's (1932) *Brave New World* (cf. Marchalik & Jurecic, 2018).

- Compare the data in Table 5.1 from 2003 to 2013. Observe:

  o There were no very statistically significant increases in the suicide rates of those ages 15–24 and 25–34, although both rates have gone up a little in recent years. When the FDA black-box warnings for the use of antidepressants with young adults were issued in 2004 and 2006, the suicide rates for those age groups stayed about the same or even went down somewhat. Some had worried that not giving young people antidepressants might increase their suicide rate.

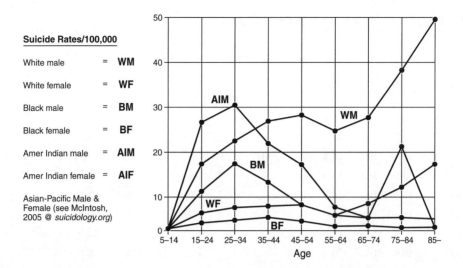

FIGURE 5.1. U.S. suicide rates by age, sex, and race. Not all results are graphed here, in order to avoid clutter and make the graph readable. (For all the data, like Asian-Pacific Americans, see McIntosh, 2005.) *Source:* McIntosh (2002), for the American Association of Suicidology (AAS).

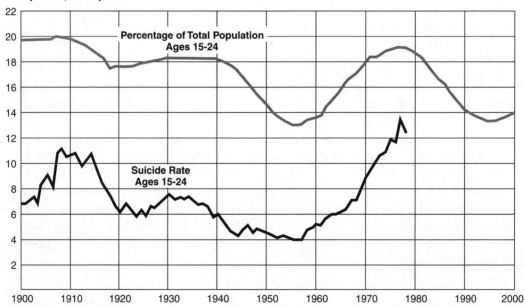

FIGURE 5.2. Percentage of the total population and suicide rate for 15- to 24-year-olds. *Source:* Figure 16-9: U.S. Suicide Rates, Total Population and Males 15–24, from *Suicide in America; New and Expanded Edition* by Herbert Hendin. Copyright © 1995, 1989 by Herbert Hendin, M.D. Used by permission of W. W. Norton & Company, Inc.

○ From 2003 to 2013 there were increases in the suicide rate of the middle-aged (45-54). Since 2006, the highest suicide rates have been among the middle-aged, although those over 85 years have very high suicide rates, too.

○ The suicide rates of the elderly (65+) were essentially unchanged from 2003 to 2013 (up slightly in the last few years).

• Figure 5.1 shows that only the suicide rates of white males go up in virtually a straight line as they age. Their age curve is slightly bimodal, with another peak in middle age.

• In data not presented here, from 1950 to 1996 there was a striking increase in the suicide rates of 15- to 24-year-olds, from about 4 to 12 per 100,000. The peak year was in 1977. The increase over that time period was 317% and led to Congressional hearings on the problem of adolescent suicide. I found the increase to be 237% from 1960 to 1977 (Maris, 1985). Almost all of that teen suicide increase was among males (however, lately there has been a significant rate increase among young girls; Plemmons et al., 2018). Even with the dramatic increase in adolescent suicide rates, they never went above the mean not controlling for age (i.e., 12 per 100,000).

• The highest U.S. suicide rates have been and still are for those over age 45. The population over age 65 makes up 14.1% of the U.S. population, but 17.5% of the suicides (2013).

• Female suicide rates tend to peak at around ages 45–54 (see Figure 5.1), then decline slightly with advancing age. Why is that: Menopause? Children leaving home?

• Very few people commit suicide under age 14 (however, see Tishler, 1980). Usually their suicide rate is less than 1.0. In my Chicago study (Maris, 1981), suicides under age 21 made up just 2% of all Chicago suicides. Why is suicide virtually nonexistent in the very young?

• The median (average) age (not the rate) for suicide was about age 51 in Chicago (Maris, 1981).

• The ratio of male to female suicide rates is about 3:1 to 4:1, except for those over age 65, where it is 5:1 or 6:1 (especially for African Americans).

• African American suicide rates for males tend to peak early (ages 25–34) and then decline until about age 65, after which they go back up again (Figure 5.1). Why do black male suicide rates resemble the female age patterns (until after age 65), unlike those of white males?

• White suicide rates, regardless of gender, exceed those of blacks by a ratio of about 2:1.

• African American female suicide rates are very low throughout the life cycle. What could the almost nonexistent suicide rates of black females teach us about how to prevent suicide (Nisbet, 1996; Walker et al., 2018)?

• Easterlin (1987) claimed that the spike in the adolescent suicide rate mentioned above was a function of the birth cohort size. Figure 5.2 shows that the birth cohort size for 15- to 24-year-olds from 1900 to 1980 mirrored the suicide rate for that age group. The theory is that the greater the cohort's competition for scarce opportunities (work, sex, marriage, education, etc.), the higher the adolescent suicide rate.

• Native American male youth/young adults have elevated suicide rates, particularly from ages 25 to 34 (see Figure 5.1). Factors for this ethnic group include unemployment, poverty, alcohol and other substance abuse, family stress and disruption, poor health, and stagnant development opportunities. Not all tribes/nations share in the elevated suicide rates. All of the original alarm about Native American suicide focused on data from just one tribe in one area (a Shoshone reservation). Other groups, like the Navajo Nation, universally condemn suicide. Apaches, on the other hand, tend to be very aggressive and use lethal methods to attempt suicide. Still other tribes, like the Dakota and Cheyenne, display a pattern of deliberate headlong rush into death, which they sometimes refer to as "Crazy-Dog-Wishing-to-Die" (similar to "suicide by cop"). In short, not all Native American suicides are alike.

• Yale psychologist Daniel Levinson has argued (see Levinson et al., 1978, for men, and Levinson with Levinson, 1996, for women; also Sher, 2015, and Able & Ramsey, 2017) that suicide rates tend to increase at points marking age group transitions (childhood to adolescence, adolescence to young adulthood, young adulthood to middle age, and middle age to elderly status), especially if there has been developmental stagnation at earlier life stages as one ages (abortive transitions).

• So-called "cluster suicides" (at least two to three suicides close in time and place) tend to occur largely among teenagers. Suicide contagion affects about 6–7 % of adolescents, but only about 3% of adults (Phillips, 1974).

• Although young and old suicides share some traits (such as depression, hopelessness, using a gun to attempt, isolation, escape motives), they differ on others: Younger suicides are more likely to be females; to have more revenge motives; to exhibit more substance abuse; to have made more nonfatal, multiple suicide attempts; and to have more divorce in their families (see Table 5.2, below).

• There is greater use of firearms as a suicide attempt method as one ages especially among males.

• Divorced people tend to have higher suicide rates as they age (see Chapter 6).

• According to my own work (Maris, 1981) and Joiner's (2005), it takes time (certain kinds of aging) to become suicidal. It's an "acquired ability." My notion of a "suicidal career" refers to the fact that the ability to commit or achieve suicide requires development over many years.

• Societies age, too. For example, modern humans have existed for about 200,000 years, but one of the earliest graphic representations of suicide (that of the legendary Greek warrior Ajax; see Chapter 18) is dated as late as 540 B.C.

- Shiang et al. (1997) have studied Asian American versus European American suicides in San Francisco. They found a higher female-to-male suicide ratio (similar to the ratio in China) among Asian Americans (1:2) than among European Americans (1:3). They also found a much higher Asian American suicide rate among very elderly females, and a much greater use of hanging in attempts. European Americans were more likely to use firearms and overdoses to attempt suicide. Chinese hangings often had revenge motives, since the dead, when hanged, are thought to return to haunt the living.

- In addition, Shiang et al. (1997) found that alcohol and drugs had much less prominence in Asian American suicides than in European American suicides (8% vs. 31%). Asian American suicides also had better mental health and higher average socioeconomic status than the European American suicides did. A major factor in Chinese American suicides in particular was the perceived failure of the younger family members to care for or support their aged suiciding parents.

Children and Adolescents

A Google search of the usual databases for articles and book chapters on *child suicide* yields disappointing results. Ash (2012) and Price (2010) are the most notable exceptions. There is little scientific information on child suicide, and one reason is that child suicide is rare (but see Tishler, 1980). For example, in 2005, out of a total U.S. population of 295 million, there were only 272 suicides for 5- to 14-year-olds. Take a look at Figure 5.1 and Table 5.1, which show that the suicide rate of 5- to 14-year-olds is virtually 0 (that is, less than 1 in 100,000 per year).

Although suicide is rare in children, some youngsters do commit suicide (Pfeffer, 1986). Below age 5, children probably lack the ability to conceive of death as final biological cessation. Thus most of them cannot form the intent to suicide. However, the extremely low suicide rate of children deserves some thought. It is inappropriate to say that there are not very many of them and just move on. Child suicide (like that of African American women) might suggest some answers to adult suicide prevention.

For example, most young children lack access to and knowledge of lethal means to suicide. If 50–60% of suicides use guns, then the very young are likely to have a lower suicide rate due to lack of access to lethal means. Interestingly, Shaffer (1974) found that more child suicides than nonsuicidal children tended to have IQs over 130. A lower prevalence of depressive disorder, substance abuse, and greater familial support also likely protect young children from suicide.

As older suicides are, child suicides are more likely to be male—Ash (2012) says five times more likely. Perhaps young boys are more also likely to be impulsive and aggressive than young girls are, but we have to be careful here. In Asian countries like China, suicide rates are comparable among boys and girls, with the suicide rates of girls even exceeding those of boys in some countries.

Although suicide is rare in children, partial self-destruction is not. Blumenthal and Kupfer(1990) reported that in 1 year 12,000 children were admitted to U.S.

emergency rooms for suicidal behaviors, but that only 1% of those were classified as "suicidal." Therefore, childhood self-destruction and suicide may be undercounted.

As in adults, depressive disorder is a major risk factor for child and adolescent suicides (Pfeffer, 1989). Although diagnosing personality disorders in very young children is discouraged, male children who are suicidal tend to be antisocial, such as having conduct disorder; female suicidal children have symptoms similar to adult borderline personality disorder (Ash, 2012).

Finally, suicidal children tend to have multiproblem families of origin (Ash, 2012; Maris, 1981). These problems include parental alcoholism, affective (mood) and anxiety disorders, child physical and sexual abuse, higher rates of divorce, domestic discord, financial problems, and chaotic and unpredictable family events. The challenge is how to convey a sense of hope and possibility to helpless and often isolated suicidal children. Also, although suicide rates may be low among children, this provides little comfort to families that have lost a child to suicide.

Although child suicide is rare, adolescent suicide rates rise dramatically by ages 15–24 in the United States (see Figure 5.1; cf. Annor et al., 2018). The highest suicide rates in the 15–24 age group are those for (1) Native American males, (2) white males, (3) black males, (4) white females, and (5) black females, in that order. In 2013, there were 4,878 adolescent suicides out of 41,149 total suicides, or 12% of the total.

The suicide rate of 11.1 per 100,000 (2013) among 15- to 24-year-olds was a little below the national average of 13 per 100,000 (see King, 1997). Remember that even when the adolescent suicide rate tripled from 1950 to 1977, it never rose above 12. For the years 2003 to 2013, adolescent suicide rates hovered between 9.7 and 11.1 per 100,000 (Table 5.1), going up slightly over that time.

Although suicide is the 10th leading cause of death overall (about 1.6% of all deaths each year), for 15- to 24-year-olds suicide is the 2nd leading cause of death, just after accidents (mainly in cars) and just ahead of homicides. We must keep in mind, however, that young people seldom die of heart disease, cancers, or other illnesses. That is, it is not so much that their suicide rate is high, as it is that the alternative causes of death have not had time to "kick in" yet.

When adolescent suicide was at its zenith and the public uproar it caused was at a maximum, I wrote an article called "The Adolescent Suicide Problem" (Maris, 1985; cf. Berman et al., 2006). In that article, I took my 5-year simple random sample of all Chicago suicides and subdivided the groups at either end of the age spectrum into "younger" (age 21 or under) and "older" (age 65 or older). Those data are presented in Table 5.2.

Younger and older suicides in Chicago shared several traits: Mean scores on the original BDI for both groups were in the lower 20s; both groups had high Beck Hopelessness Scale scores (85%); both tended to use a firearm to attempt suicide (61%, if older); about two-thirds of both groups had no close friends or only one; and 82–90% saw death as a way to escape their life problems.

On the other hand, younger suicides were different from older suicides in these respects: Younger suicides were more likely to be women (frequency is different from rates); 70% of older suicides made one suicide attempt, and 70% of younger suicides made multiple attempts; and death was twice as likely to be seen as revenge (50% vs. 25%) in younger suicides (perhaps suggesting a greater role for

TABLE 5.2. Younger and Older Suicides Compared (Chicago Sample)

A. Younger and older suicides: SIMILAR traits

	Younger	Older
Depression	$\overline{X} = 24$	$\overline{X} = 21$
Hopelessness	85%	85%
Most common method	Gun	Gun (61%)
0–1 close friends	66%	67%
Death seen as escape	90%	82%

B. Younger and older suicides: DIFFERENT traits

	Younger	Older
Percent female	87%	45%
Death seen as revenge	50%	25%
Working full time	7%	23%
Suicide in family	38%	11%
3–5 drinks, when drinking	36%	19%
Parents divorced	45%	13%
Achieve most important goal	0%	61%
Dissatisfaction	73%	42%
Irritability	75%	61%
Low self-esteem	75%	53%
Only one suicide attempt	29%	68%

Source: Maris, Ronald W. with Bernard Lazerwitz. *Pathways to Suicide: A Survey of Self-Destructive Behaviors.* Copyright © 1981 The Johns Hopkins University Press. Reprinted with permission of Johns Hopkins University Press.

interpersonal dynamics). About 40% of younger suicides had had another suicide in their family, but only 11% of older suicides did; younger suicides tended to drink (and abuse nonalcoholic substances) to excess about twice as much as older suicides did (36% vs. 19%). Younger suicides were more dissatisfied, were more irritable, and had lower self-esteem than older suicides, and there was about three times more parental divorce (45% vs. 13%) in the families of younger suicides. Finally, younger suicides were less likely to be working or to have achieved their life goals, since they were younger.

Before we can hope to understand adolescent suicide, however, we have to understand adolescence itself as a developmental life stage. We tend to forget that in preindustrial societies, adolescence was not recognized as a life stage. Children went directly into adulthood after puberty. Marriage tended to be early, and children worked mainly on farms.

Only recently have childhood and adolescence emerged as full-blown life stages characterized primarily by dormancy, latency, and prolonged preparation for adulthood. Adolescence is marked by marginality, confusion, and ambiguity. The greatest problem many adolescents have today is their own sense of uselessness until they become adult professionals or find other meaningful employment (Maris, 1985).

Adolescents are expected to delay sexual gratification (or at least marriage) and meaningful employment (working at McDonald's or being a law clerk runner does not count). Unemployment and other forms of economic disenfranchisement are particularly acute among teenagers (notably American blacks). Children are expected to stay in school much longer than at the turn of the 20th century. This is probably good for their development, although attending college means that they often go into deep debt. It also leads to profound isolation of the young from larger society (Coleman, 1962). Both physical and sexual abuse of pubescent children who stay around home longer than before can also contribute to suicidality.

Substance abuse is a special problem in teen suicides (see the recent epidemic of opiate overdose deaths; Sarasohn, 2017). One could argue that adolescents' being shut out from meaningful participation in society for long periods of dormancy contributes to the problem of alcohol and other substance abuse. Little wonder, then, that adolescents in contemporary society tend to have a special set of social problems, including teen suicide. Of course, adolescent suicide is not just the result of socioeconomic conditions (Berman et al., 2006; Maris et al., 2000).

Harold: A Fictional Case of an Adolescent Male Suicide

Harold and Maude (Ashby & Higgins, 1971) is a classic dark comedy film starring Bud Cort as 16-year-old Harold and Ruth Gordon as soon-to-be-80-year-old Maude. They meet at a funeral in which neither of them knows the deceased. Major themes of the film include learning how to live and the contrast between two very different types of mothering: one by Harold's cold, narcissistic, domineering biological mother, and the other by his surrogate mother, altruistic, free-thinking Maude. Harold and Maude are idiosyncratic examples of an adolescent male and an elderly female suicide. (I discuss Maude's suicide later in this chapter.)

Harold is depressed and isolated. He has little will to live (the movie starts with his faking hanging himself), much anhedonia (his inability to take pleasure is clear), and an apparent obsession with dying (e.g., he goes to funerals of people he does not know). When his mother gives him a Jaguar sports car, he converts it into a hearse. His father is dead; he has no siblings; and he is very quiet and introverted. He makes multiple feigned suicide attempts that are good examples of what Menninger (1938) called "murder in the 180th degree"; that is, they are thinly disguised efforts to hurt his mother and get her attention.

Indeed, Harold's cold, controlling mother hardly notices him. In the opening scene of the film, his mother walks into her parlor to make a hairstyling appointment, sees Harold hanging, goes ahead and makes her phone call, and then comments to Harold on the way out, "Harold, dinner at 8 P.M., and try to be a little more lively."

Harold's mother seems incapable of love. She is the epitome of narcissism. A swimming pool scene is reminiscent of the Greek god Narcissus seeing his reflection in a pool of water and falling in love with himself. As her affected French suggests, the mother is superficial, selfish, and materialistic. Her main values are money, social status, and self-aggrandizement, with underlying low self-esteem. Such parents can be murderous of their children.

Harold's first simulated suicide attempt occurs when he is in a prep school chemistry lab explosion. His mother is told that he is dead, but in fact he is upstairs in the hallway at home witnessing his mother fainting at being told. This is the first time he has ever gotten any reaction out of his mother. After this incident, he begins a series of fake suicide attempts in front of his mother.

The film suggests that adolescent male suicide is in part a product of pathological mothering, and that Maude, as a more appropriate surrogate mother, might be able to save Harold. While worth considering, this hypothesis is overly simplistic, since it fails to account for other suicide risk factors (biology, psychiatric disorder, social isolation, etc.) that have less to do with family or socialization.

Middle-Aged Suicides

Until recently, suicidologists have argued that the older people get, the higher their suicide risk or rate becomes (this is the basis for what Joiner [2005] calls "acquired risk" and I (1981, 2015) call a "suicidal career"). While this is still generally true (especially for white males), since 2006 the highest absolute suicide rates have been found in 45- to 54-year-olds (e.g., 17.2 in 2006 and 19.7 in 2013; Kuehn, 2014). The mean (average) suicide rate has been for those in their 40s since about the 1980s. One has to wonder why suicide rates are peaking earlier than before. One possibility is that the increase could be, in part, a cohort effect. Thus far, this chapter has examined suicide in children, adolescents, and the elderly (and I discuss the elderly further below), but not so much middle-aged suicide.

Midlife is normally a time when power peaks. By age 40, most of us are what we are ever going to be. Erikson (1963) claimed that stagnation versus generativity is the main development task of midlife. Yale psychologist Levinson (Levinson et al., 1978; Levinson with Levinson, 1996) argued that between ages 40 and 55 we need to appraise the past and rid ourselves of prior illusions. Often in middle age there are major changes in life structure (such as divorce, job plateauing or loss, children leaving home, diminished energy, and incipient or actual illness). In midlife, many people turn more inward and are less concerned with the mastery of the external environment.

Four polarities may be involved with midlife individuation: (1) young–old, (2) destructive–creative, (3) masculine–feminine, and (4) attached–separated (Levinson et al., 1978). For example, many midlife males need to become more appropriately old, creative, feminine, and separated. Midlife is a time when men and women need to modify their dreams and realize that occupational success does not necessarily entail happiness. For example, when I retired as editor of the *Suicide and Life-Threatening Behavior* journal, I was given a baseball cap by Mort Silverman with this inscription: "Never confuse having a career with having a life."

More than routine developmental problems occur in middle-aged suicides. Suicide can be thought of as the ultimate in developmental stagnation. There may be no perceived life good enough to allow continued living. Some middle-aged people cannot survive their midlife crises and make a transition to old age. For example, they cannot survive a divorce, can no longer take pleasure in their life work, and/ or cannot give up the tyranny of youthful illusions—especially if they have chronic physical illnesses, recurring depressive episodes, alcohol or other substance abuse problems (including abuse of prescription opiates), and minimal economic, emotional, and spiritual resources.

For men, midlife may mean living without alcohol, advancement at work, and sexual acting out. Some midlifers kill themselves in part because they do not believe it is possible to change their young adult lifestyles. If you will, their "middle-lescence" does them in, as it did Hemingway (see also Styron, 1990).

Robins (1981) claimed that the distinctive traits of midlife male suicides (vs. midlife nonsuicides) include the following: (1) loss of spouse, usually through divorce; (2) years of heavy drinking (most alcoholic suicides are males); (3) high depression risk; (4) personal experiences with other suicides, perhaps in their own families; (5) and facing debilitating old age without psychological compromises or diversions. Occupational loss is another male midlife suicide risk factor (e.g., stagnated job mobility, job loss, or downward job mobility). Sometimes middle-aged suicide note writers display less affect than younger note writers and are less likely to give a reason for their suicides. This can reflect a kind of Darwinian inability to go on with life in general, rather than a failure to overcome any specific life obstacle.

Midlife suicide treatment often involves ameliorating biological imbalances or dysfunctions. Many midlife suicides have undiagnosed, untreated, or undertreated mood disorders (Østergaard, 2018). Clinicians may need to consider aggressive medications (including MAOIs) in sufficient doses. Alcohol abuse is often a complicating biological condition in midlife suicide. ECT is another valuable tool for those at risk for midlife suicide. I once met a Harvard chemistry professor at a professional meeting who swore that ECT saved his life.

Creativity in the face of chronic suicide risk factors involves building a life more appropriate to being middle-aged. A lot of middle-aged people suicide because they cannot compromise. In midlife males may need to become more appropriately old and feminine, more psychologically flexible and less cognitively rigid; they may need to become able to let their big dreams go in favor of more modest aspirations. Resignation, humor, and reorganization can be important midlife therapy objectives. In midlife one is usually no longer in a pattern of ascendancy, even if one was at younger ages. A central question may be this: "Is there a good enough future for me, or am I just in a pattern of stagnation or entropy until natural death?"

Isolation can be a special problem in midlife; this is what Joiner calls "thwarted belongingness" and "perceived burdensomeness," and what I call "social isolation and negative interaction." In my Chicago survey (Maris, 1981), 50% of older suicides had no close friends at all (cf. Marver et al., 2017). In midlife, men may discover that their work disappoints them and cannot save them. Like the hamster on its exercise wheel in John Updike's novels, midlife men may be working as hard as they can just to stay even.

Men may find out too late that their spouses or partners, children, and grandchildren are better sources of peace and immortality than more money, jobs, sexual relationships, or material acquisitions. It is nice to have fine cars, a beach or lakefront house, or a mountain cabin, or to take trips to exotic places—but "everywhere you go, there you are."

Elderly Suicides

Earlier in this chapter, I have separated the elderly into three groups: the young-old (ages 65–74), the old-old (ages 75–84), and the oldest-old (ages 85+). In 2013, as one progressed through these elder age groups, the suicide rate went straight up from 15 to 17.1 to 18.6 per 100,000 (see Table 5.1). The suicide rate of the oldest-old (18.6) is second only to the rate for those ages 45–54 (19.7). Elder suicide is somewhat like increased natural death rates as people age (Yin, 2006). In both cases the life cycle runs its course, but with suicide, elders probably "nudge it" a little to avoid pain and the effort that aging requires just to keep going each day. Note, too, that the proportion of elders in the total society is increasing. From 1995 to 2050, the proportions of those ages 75–84 and those ages 85 years and older will grow dramatically. Thus we should also expect suicide to grow in those age groups. Table 5.1 shows that there was a slight drop in the suicide rate for those ages 65–74 from 2006 to 2009, but that from 2010 to 2013 the rate for this age group went up a little.

Conwell and Heisel (2012) claim that older adults have the highest suicide rates of any age group. One important question, of course, is why. Go back to Chapter 4 and look at Table 4.1, which lists the 15 common single risk factors for suicide. You will see that parts or all of 10 of the 15 suicide risk factors are more prevalent in the aged:

- Mood disorders. Conwell and Heisel (2012) point out that depression is often undiagnosed and untreated or undertreated in elders, but that three-fourths of elders see their family doctors within 30 days of suiciding; thus there are opportunities to treat them. In one study (Benson et al., 2018), 78% of suicides were men, but only 35% of the men got antidepressant treatment, compared with 54% of the women. In another study (Szanto et al., 2018) of patients over age 50 with major depression, the cluster with personality pathology had the highest suicide risk.
- Alcohol abuse (Maris, 2015; Murphy, 1992).
- Use of lethal methods. Conwell and Heisel (2012) say that most elders use guns, and that aging, being alone, and having a gun are a lethal combination.
- Isolation and being alone through loss of friends and family, especially of a spouse.
- Hopelessness and cognitive rigidity. Clark (Roger Clark, personal communication, 1993) notes the relative inability of the aged to compromise and the resultant character fault.
- Being an older white male.
- Work problems. Conwell and Heisel (2012) point out particular difficulties in coping with retirement. Remember the suicide notes of George Eastman and Percy Bridgman, mentioned earlier (see Chapter 4).
- Heightened irritability and anger, often at the human condition itself (Maris, 1982).
- Physical illness, pain, and the use of opiates to try to manage pain.
- Suicidal careers. The longer a person lives, the more likely he or she is to acquire the ability to inflict lethal self-injury.

The aged are likely to have experienced significant multiple losses, such as widowhood and retirement, as well as the loss of memory, physical health, financial resources, and mental health. It has been estimated that about one-third of all patients with Alzheimer's disease have major depressive disorder. One might suspect that for aged persons who live in a geriarchy (like China, or Asia in general), the suicidal effects of aging might be mitigated. On the other hand, South Korea has one of the highest suicide rates in the world (see Chapter 3, Figure 3.3).

Go back to the general model of suicide in Chapter 2 (Figure 2.1), if you will. Look at the suicide risk factors in column 2 and the trigger factors for suicide in column 4, just before the suicide threshold. In this model for suicide, many suicide risk factors are more likely as we age:

- Hospitalization (Desjardins, 2016; Lee et al., 2018).
- Having a depressive episode.
- Alcohol excesses (Bagge & Borges, 2017).
- Physical illness and pain.
- Feelings of hopelessness and helplessness (dependency but fewer resources).
- Seeing death as escape from life problems.
- Probability of utilizing lethal methods to attempt.
- Multiple object losses.
- Retirement.

There was one particularly poignant case of mine, an aging white male I'll call John. John was a 67-year-old retired railroad worker in the southeastern United States (Maris et al., 2000). At the time he suicided, he was divorced and alcoholic. He initially shot himself in the face with a shotgun, but did not die and "just" lost his lower jaw. After surviving this serious suicide attempt, John was placed in a psychiatric hospital. He had managed to save a lot of money and had written a power-of-attorney agreement that if he was declared incompetent or died, the money would all go to his ex-wife. When his face shot did not kill him, and he was committed to the psychiatric hospital, the agreement went into effect. The ex-wife then refused to give John any money back. Because of his facial prosthesis, he continually drooled on himself. The *coup de grace* for John was magnetic resonance imaging (MRI) showing him to have brain tumors that required brain surgery.

John's last psychiatric inpatient progress notes read as follows:

4/18/89   10 P.M.   Put on close observation for suicide.

4/19/89   1:30 A.M.   "Let me die soon."

5/16/89   9:30 P.M.   "My wife don't want me home. I've got no place to go. I'm at the end of the road. I have played a lot of checkers in my life. This is my last move."

5/18/89   8:10 A.M.   I entered the room. Client found hanging by cotton belt from a ceiling sprinkler pipe.

Maude: A Fictional Case of an Elderly Female Suicide

Finally, let's consider the character of Maude from the film *Harold and Maude* (Ashby & Higgins, 1971). Maude in many ways is the opposite of Harold's mother. She is a fierce individual (like the daisies in a field she points out to Harold that just *look* the same), asocial (she steals cars from priests), altruistic, and giving. She is free-thinking and not bound by law, custom, or propriety (e.g., she often spends her day letting animals out of their cages at pet shops); she is not repressed sexually (she does nude modeling at the age of almost 80). In fact, there is a bedroom scene that may test your stomach. (Harold's psychiatrist says, "I know people sometimes wish to sleep with their mother, but with their grandmother?!") Harold's first smile in the entire movie is when he is with Maude, using her olfactory machine. She lives in an abandoned railroad car.

Maude is a former Austrian Jew, living alone in the United States. Although most elder suicides are males and use a gun to suicide, Maude, like most female suicides, overdoses near the end of the movie. Being fiercely independent, she tells Harold that after age 80 she may not be competent and autonomous enough to decide about her own suicide, and so she is suiciding while she is still clear-headed and in charge of her own life. Do others have the moral and legal right to force us to keep living? On the surface, Maude seems to be in good health and fine spirits. She seems to be in good shape both physically and intellectually (she has a very quick, optimistic mind) and to lack many of the traditional suicide risk factors.

However, later in the movie, we notice that Maude has tattoos on her forearm, which indicate that she was in a Nazi concentration camp during World War II. Although the details are not clear, it is implied that she lost her entire family in the camp. One has to wonder what scars remained from that horrific trauma as a young woman. She also tells Harold that she does not miss the kings and queens in Vienna, but she does miss the pomp and circumstance. This suggests that she is somewhat romantic and idealistic. Furthermore, as part of her radical social protests, she puts herself above the law. In fact, she is a car thief and pet business saboteur—basically a self-absorbed narcissist, and in this respect rather like Harold's mother. In short, Maude is not entirely healthy and problem-free, even though she is funny and cute.

The movie hints that while Harold's suicide would be inappropriate, Maude's suicide might be either appropriate and reasonable or irrational. What do you think? Her overdose certainly crushes Harold. It seems selfish of her to do that to him. How could she know he would survive? Basically, Maude decides all on her own that it is a good time to die. Do our lives belong just to us?

In Chapter 6, I consider the role of sex, gender, and marital status as risk factors in suicide. One striking fact is that about 78% of all U.S. suicides are by males, and 70% by white males).

CHAPTER 6

Sex, Gender, and Marital Status
A Phallocentric Focus

> Men, eternally awestruck by women's ability to create life,
> consoled themselves by creating death.
> —FRANK PITTMAN

It is clear from the data presented so far that sex and gender make a huge difference in suicide outcome. U.S. male suicide rates exceed those of females at all ages (see Chapter 5, Figure 5.1). Black females in the United States have extremely low suicide rates, even though they have high rates of other suicide risk factors (e.g., depressive disorder, as do white females; Walker et al., 2018). Table 5.1 has shown that from 2003 to 2013, male-to-female suicide ratios in the United States ranged from 3.6:1 to 4.09:1. Moreover, the male excess suicide rate is observed virtually worldwide. For example, in Lithuania the ratio is 5.9:1, and in Greece it is 6:1. Only in some Asian and some Muslim countries does the male-to-female suicide ratio go lower. For example, in South Korea, it is 1.8:1; in India, it is 1.7:1; in Bahrain (which is 80% Muslim), it is 1.1:1; and in China, there is actually an excess female suicide rate ratio (0.92:1). Among 15- to 24-year-olds who suicided in 1990 in the United States, the male-to-female sex ratio was 5.3:1. This chapter asks why male suicide rates on average are usually about four times higher than those of females; it also poses other questions about the roles of sex, gender, and marital status in suicide.

Sex and gender are different concepts. *Sex* refers to biological differences, such as those in the genitalia and reproductive organs, average birth weight, hormones, chromosomes, neurochemical processing, and brain anatomy. Of the 46 human chromosomes, the 23rd pair are the sex chromosomes; 99% of all humans are clearly XX (female) or XY (male), with a few chromosomal aberrations like XYY, XXY, XXX, XO, and YO. Chromosomal sex is set at conception, but development is initially the same for embryos of both sexes until initially some with female characteristics (genitalia) differentiate into males. Thus, in a sense, we all start out as female or neuter. Puberty is marked in large part by first ejaculation in boys and

98

first menstruation in girls; it also includes striking biological changes related to sex drive, sexual capabilities, and aggression.

Gender, on the other hand, refers more to male and female socialization, sexual stereotypes, cultural expectations, and sex roles (Maris et al., 2000; Able & Ramsey, 2017). For example, in a Human Area Relations File (at Yale University) study of 185 societies, 94% of these societies considered hunting predominantly a male activity, and 92% saw cooking as a female activity. More pertinent to suicide, boys are often socialized to be more aggressive, impulsive, and risk-taking, and to become more familiar with and to own guns or other weapons.

Other considerations include issues of *gender identity*—that is, whether one identifies as male, female, or other. When biological sex and gender identity do not match, a person may identify as transsexual or transgender (American Psychological Association, 2015). Another issue is *sexual orientation,* which is one's sexual and romantic attraction to male or female partners or to both, such as being lesbian, gay, bisexual, or transsexual (LGBT). Some of these gender issues (which are partly related to biology and partly to socialization) are more highly related to suicide outcomes than others are.

One of the more important gender differences related to suicide outcome is that men and women tend to use different methods to attempt suicide. These varying attempt methods differ dramatically in lethality (the medical probability that, if a method is used, the result will be fatal). Men on average use more lethal methods (especially firearms in the U.S.). This is noteworthy because although the suicide rates of males are about four times higher than those of females, females make about three to four times more suicide attempts than males do. Thus, if lethality of attempt were constant, male and female suicide rates would be about the same.

As shown in Table 6.1, males and females both prefer the use of firearms to attempt suicide; it's the number one method (51.5% in 2013 overall; see Chapter 3, Table 3.1). However, firearms were used in 2006 by about 51.8% of men, but only 38.3% of women (Table 6.1). Although the data are not presented in Table 6.1 (see Chapter 9, Figure 9.1), men are more likely than women to shoot themselves in the head. Most data show that drug and medication overdoses are the second method of choice for women, but hanging is second for men. In one year (McIntosh, 2002), for women, firearms and overdoses were virtually tied (33% each) as the method of choice. Note that overdoses tend to have lower lethality, take longer to kill, and allow more chances for life-saving intervention. Hanging, on the other hand, is very lethal; death usually takes only 4–5 minutes, through anoxia of the brain and cardiac arrest.

Carbon monoxide poisoning is the third and fourth preferred method for men and women, respectively (depending on the year sampled). Normally, carbon monoxide poisoning is the third-ranked method for men, and in recent years hanging has ranked third for women. Jumping from a high place is the fifth preferred method for both men and women. Why do men and women use the suicide attempt methods they do? A more complete answer to this question will have to wait for Chapter 9 (on suicide methods). But on average, men tend to be more aggressive and violent (Giner et al., 2014), and (as noted above) are more likely to own guns or other weapons and be familiar with their use, than women are. Most women also tend to have greater ambivalence about dying and self-mutilation than men do.

TABLE 6.1. Suicide Methods by Gender: Percentages and Ranks

Method	1990		1996		2006	
	Male	Female	Male	Female	Male	Female
Firearms	64.0 (1)	39.8 (1)	63.5 (1)	38.5 (1)	51.8 (1)	38.3 (1)
Drugs/meds.	5.2 (4)	25.0 (2)	5.5 (4)	24.0 (2)	6.9 (3)	22.0 (2)
Hanging	13.5 (2)	9.4 (4)	16.6 (2)	16.0 (3)	23.1 (2)	15.6 (3)
Carbon monoxide	9.6 (3)	12.6 (3)	6.0 (3)	6.7 (4)	5.6 (4)	6.4 (4)
Jumping	1.8 (5)	3.0 (5)	1.7 (5)	3.2 (5)	5.2 (5)	5.7 (5)
Cutting/piercing	1.3 (6)	1.4 (8)	1.4 (6)	1.3 (7)		
Drowning	1.1 (7)	2.8 (6)	0.9 (7)	2.0 (6)		
Poisons	0.6 (8)	1.0 (9)	0.5 (8)	0.7 (9)		
Other	3.4	5.0	2.2	8.2	7.4	12.0
Totals	100	100	100	100	100	100

Note. Ranks are given in parentheses. Wound sites: Temple (62%), mouth (7%), frontal/forehead (7%), chest (16%), abdomen (2%). Place of suicide attempt: House (78.9%), public area (16.9%), business (1.9%), hotel (1.9%). See more recent methods and gender data throughout the book.
Sources: Maris et al. (2000), Callanan and Davis (2011).

Sexuality and Suicide

At first blush, sexuality and suicide seem like strange bedfellows. What do libido, passion, and Eros have to do with depression, anhedonia, and Thanatos? Sigmund Freud thought that sexual energy (Eros and libido) was in fact life energy. Think about it. When you are seriously ill, you are often asexual—so much so that the return of sexual interest and drive is often a sign that health is improving and normal life is returning. Biologically, being young and fit includes reproductive possibilities and sexual defenses, such as using sex to cope, to achieve orgasmic pleasure and tension reduction, and to increase social involvement with sexual overtones. de Catanzaro (1986) argues that when men (especially) age, become less biologically and sexually fit, and have fewer offspring to support (cf. Joiner, 2005), then they become more vulnerable to suicide. That is, biologically, they have less reason to stay around and keep living.

We would expect that depressed, suicidal people would tend to have various sexual dysfunctions. These might include a loss of interest in sexuality (especially for women); loss of social boundaries and normal sexual proprieties; a view of sex as a quasi-religious form of salvation (a form of apotheosis, consisting of seeing your lover as godlike; remember also that the Muslim afterlife is very sexual for *jihadists*); or even the loss of the ability to have sex. Remember, too, that sexual activity is like a drug; it needs to be repeated to be effective (i.e., there is a dose–response factor).

Promiscuous sexuality attempts, in effect, to deny the finitude, atrophy, and decay essential to being human (Becker, 1973). That is, as an ephemeral and temporary pleasure, sexual activity in part attempts to deny death, pain, the powerlessness, and lack of control that we have over our finite human condition. Note as well that sex and suicide are both preemptory drives, "primitive forces that are difficult to deny" (Weisman, 1967), often acted upon impulsively and passionately with intent to decrease tension.

Low-lethality suicide attempts and sexual acting out are only partially self-destructive (Maris, 1972). For some people, they may even make life possible and sustainable. Repetitive suicide attempts may represent a kind of "vocation," a way of staying alive through partial self-destruction and psychic surgery. (See Case 6.1, describing the poet Sylvia Plath and her sadomasochistic relationships with men.)

Much sexual activity is aggressive. For some men, sex indicates power over women, and as such is not all that much about sex itself—so much so that if a woman agrees to have sex, the man may lose interest. (The current #MeToo movement is a large-scale societal response to such men.) I comment here on aggression and sexuality, because aggression is clearly related to suicide outcomes. Murder–suicide (Joiner, 2014) most often involves males killing women, either spouses or lovers (see Chapter 21 for a fuller discussion).

In the film *Whose Life Is It Anyway?* (Badham & Clark, 1981), Richard Dreyfuss plays a man who cannot have sexual intercourse at all, due to spinal injuries sustained in a car accident. Since his quadriplegia makes him in effect sexless, he also becomes more suicidal and wants to die. Yet throughout the movie he obsesses about sex, in feeble attempts to maintain some semblance of normality and be able to keep living. He even fantasizes about his attorney's having proxy sex for him with his female physician. I discuss this film at greater length in connection with the ethics of assisted suicide in Chapter 19.

Data on Gender and Suicide

As emphasized throughout this book, my theory of suicide rests on empirical building blocks (evidence-based suicidology). Some recent data on suicide and gender (see especially Gold, 2012) include the following:

- Nearly 80% of all completed suicides are committed by males (78% in the United States in 2013). Yet women have higher rates of depression and suicide attempts. Major depressive disorder has about a prevalence of 6–11% in women (still, they have a lower suicide rate), but only 2.6–5.5% in men. Women tend to make three to four times more suicide attempts than men do, but male suicide rates exceed those of females by four times. This leads to what has been called the "gender paradox in suicide" (Canetto & Sakinofsky, 1998). Given all their suicide risk factors, it is paradoxical that women (this is especially true for black women in the U.S.) have much lower suicide rates than men do.

- After mood disorders, alcohol or other substance abuse is a very important suicide risk factor. But, once again, these data are heavily weighted toward men. About 88% of alcoholic suicides are older males, mainly white males. When alcohol was controlled in Russia during Gorbachev's *perestroika,* the national suicide rate went down (Pridemore & Spivak, 2003).

• Males use more lethal methods than women do to attempt suicide. One estimate of gun ownership is that 16–19% of the U.S. population own guns, but that 26–30% of gun ownership is by males versus only 7–8% by females (Gold, 2006, 2012).

• The best biological marker for suicide is low brain serotonin (5-HT) and its metabolite, 5-HIAA, especially in the prefrontal cortex (Maris, 2015). In John Mann's laboratory in Pittsburgh, when suicidal and nonsuicidal brains were compared, most of the brain samples with these markers came from men (Mann & Currier, 2012).

• All these data raise the interesting question of what keeps women alive. Do females have counterbalancing suicide protective factors? The short answer is yes. For one thing, suicidal women are more likely than men to see physicians and get treated (Benson et al., 2018). For another, suicide has more interpersonal connotations and implications for women than it does for men. Women also tend to show more adaptive and flexible (are less rigid) coping than men do (Kaplan & Klein, 1989; Gold, 2012). For a lot of male suicides, the first time we learn anything about their problems and the ways they coped (or did not cope) with them is when they are found dead.

• A suicide risk factor more prevalent in women is sexual abuse. About 20–25% of women report lifetime sexual abuse, but only 5–10% of men do (Gold, 2006, 2012). Sexual abuse has all kinds of suicidogenic properties, including changes in the brain (Mann & Currier, 2012). Yet, in spite of this, women have lower suicide rates than men do.

• As we will see shortly, marriage, children, and family tend to protect women from suicide, in spite of postpartum and other depressions (Gold, 2012). What is not widely known is that marriage protects men from suicide, far more than it does women. As noted above, murder–suicide mainly involves men killing their female lovers or spouses. Filicide–suicide (in which a mother kills first her children, then herself) is the second most common type of murder–suicide (Gold, 2012).

• Women who are suicidal are much more likely to have borderline personality disorder, while suicidal males tend to have antisocial personality disorder. This is worth mentioning, since most of those diagnosed with borderline personalities make low-lethality cutting and self-mutilation suicide attempts, whereas males with antisocial personalities are much more violent, aggressive, and lethal in their suicide attempts, often with firearms. (See the final section of this chapter, and Chapter 14, for further discussion.)

• Physician-assisted suicides tend to involve male physicians killing females. For example, the first 8 of Jack Kevorkian's assisted suicides, and 12 of his first 15, were *females* (Maris et al., 2000, p. 468). After Oregon's Death with Dignity Act was passed in 1997, men and women were about equally likely to request lethal overdoses—but one wonders what this means, since men on average have suicide rates four times higher than women do (mostly with firearms, not drugs).

- Race and gender suicide rate ratios (United States, 2013, not controlled for age) are as follows:

    - White males vs. black males = 2.6:1
    - White males vs. white females = 3.6:1
    - White males vs. black females = 11.7:1
    - White females vs. black females = 3.3:1
    - White females vs. black males = 0.7:1
    - Black males vs. black females = 4.5:1

- Sher (2015) found that the male gender role, unwillingness to get help, and higher testosterone levels were related to increased suicide risk in men.

Most explanations of suicidal behavior are based on data from white males, not on data from females and especially not from black females. I refer to this male preponderance as a "phallocentric bias," which is a barrier to adequately understanding female suicides. What we know about gender and suicide is based almost entirely on white male data (see Chapter 5, Figure 5.1). The phallocentric bias penetrates even the descriptions of suicidal behavior. For example, men "succeed" at or "complete" suicide, but women "fail" at or "attempt" suicide. The next section takes a closer look at this phallocentric perspective (Canetto, 2008). It is almost as if women are seen as lacking what it takes to be suicidal (see Durkheim, 1897/1951, on female suicides).

A Phallocentric Perspective on Suicide

Our current understanding of what causes suicide depicts it as essentially a male phenomenon. Most of the data for examining suicide come from countries in which men have higher suicide rates than women do. Many of these data come from English-speaking industrialized countries like the United States, Great Britain, Canada, Australia, or New Zealand. Patriarchal countries like Russia also have high suicide rates, with male suicide rates that exceed those of females by 6:1 to 7:1 (Lee et al., 2015). In Russia, male suicide rates are in the 70s per 100,000, versus about 21.1 per 100,000 in the United States (in 2014). High male rates are also found in Austria.

The entire explanatory gestalt for suicide tends to be masculine or phallocentric. High suicide rates are seen to result from essentially male traits, such as untreated and undiagnosed depressive disorders, alcohol abuse, ownership and use of guns, work problems, social isolation, stress from work, a tendency toward aggression (based in part in testosterone levels), chronic physical illnesses that include musculoskeletal pain, and the like. Obviously, a lot of these risk factors are simply not relevant (or at least less relevant) to female suicides.

Durkheim thought that women were incapable of deliberate suicide (cf. Canetto, 2008). The phallocentric perspective distorts our understanding of female suicides. Female suicides may be misclassified as nonsuicides due to this phallocentric and cultural bias. Female suicides also may be hidden, and their true rates underestimated, since they are just assumed not to happen that often.

A Gynocentric Perspective on Suicide

Female suicide needs to be seen in its own right, not as a pale reflection of a male disorder or disease. Obviously, the science of female suicidology should not just be based on male suicides and what we know about them. It is possible that the low rates of female suicide and the presumed male dominance of suicide are not even real (Canetto & Sakinofsky, 1998), although that position seems extreme and unlikely.

Suicidology needs to look at countries in which female suicide rates exceed those of males and try to figure out why. In China, for example, female suicide rates exceed those of males (0.92:1), as noted earlier. Female suicide in China is often a cultural strategy for influencing others when women are otherwise power-less. Indeed, female suicide is often expected (i.e., it is not just a matter of personal intent) under certain circumstances. For example, when women are child-less or fail to give birth to a son, they may be seen as a failure and even expected to suicide. For women in China, then, suicide is often a social or cultural act; it is not so much about private individual psychopathology or neurobiological dysfunction. In rural China in particular, suicide is a lot like homicide; that is, women are culturally driven to take suicidal action under some conditions (see Chapter 8, Box 8.1).

Remember, too, the classical form of Indian female suicide called *sati* or *suttee* (see Chapter 18, Figure 18.4). When a married woman's husband died, often she was expected to be burned on his funeral pyre along with his other possessions, or to drown herself in the Ganges River. Her own intent was irrelevant. There was little debate about what she might have felt about being burned alive or drowning herself. Even in more recent years in India, when a family lacks the required dowry for a daughter to get married, the daughter is often found burned to death (Hitch-cock, 2001).

Another example of a gynocentric perspective on female suicide is the work of Kaplan and Klein (1989). They argue that female suicides in the United States are more about interpersonal relationships than male suicides are. Women are thought to be more likely than men to try to preserve relationships, especially with their own children. Kaplan and Klein maintain that women tend to have lower suicide rates than males do, since it is harder for women to abandon those who need them, no matter how much they may be suffering personally—even though female depression rates are about twice those of males. Employment tends to protect women from suicide more than it does men, and being married protects men from suicide more than it does women (see Figure 6.1, below). Social involvement is much more of a protective factor for women (especially black women) than it is for men (Nisbet, 1996; Walker et al., 2018).

Typically, black females in the United States have very low suicide rates. This is both paradoxical and enigmatic (Burnett-Zeigler, 2018). Black females have a multitude of suicide risk factors, such as social, economic, and psychological stress, frustration, and adversity. Black females tend to be poor and socially mar-ginalized, often raise large families by themselves, and have relatively high rates of depression. White female depression rates exceed those of white males by a factor of about two, but black female depression rates exceed those of black males by a factor of about four. Yet black females have low suicide rates. Why is this?

One obvious answer is that they have counterbalancing suicide protective factors. As a consequence of residing in larger households, they have an increase in supportive family ties. For example, I (Maris, 1969) found that in Chicago, a higher population per household was related to a lower suicide rate. Areas with high suicide rates had on average 2.5 people per household, but there were on average 3.7 people per household in areas with low suicide rates (these differences were statistically significant).

Black females attempt suicide at about the same rate as white females do, but they are more protected from completing suicide. Furthermore, black females have other suicide protective factors, such as religious involvement and values that consider suicide as sinful or otherwise inappropriate. George Murphy claims (personal communication) that the adversity of black females tends to *temper* and protect them from suicide (much as iron is tempered by fire). Note, too, that in a single-parent household, suicide by a black mother means potentially much greater damage to her dependent children.

The Paradox of the Self-Destructive Female

When I was a postdoctoral fellow in psychiatry at Johns Hopkins, I noticed that a lot of the female suicide attempters that I was treating in the emergency room were obviously also sexually deviant or diverse. These women seemed fairly healthy and were, aside from their suicide attempts, doing fairly well. For example, a woman I'll call Pat was a PhD student who lived in downtown Baltimore with three other female college students and a retired male engineer in a luxury hotel penthouse. In exchange for occasional sex and companionship with the four women, this man paid their room and board, took care of their university tuition, and gave them credit cards and expense money.

Another example of seemingly healthy women using sex in exchange for money (call girls) was provided by the "Mayflower Madam," Sydney Biddle Barrows, at Brown University (see Barrows with Novak, 1986), who had organized a group of attractive, bright female students to be in her call girl organization. After all, when a woman is bright but poor, somehow she has to pay the high (then $40,000) annual tuition at Brown. Follow-up studies of these women did not find them to be unsuccessful, unhappy, or dead by suicide.

I interviewed and gave a research questionnaire to 48 consecutive female Johns Hopkins Hospital emergency room admissions for suicide attempts, and then compared their data with data on female suicide completers in Baltimore in the same year. Without going into detail (Maris, 1972), the results are presented in Table 6.2. There was a cluster of interrelated variables that were positively associated with female suicide attempts, but negatively correlated with completed suicide.

TABLE 6.2. Characteristics of Female Suicide Attempters, Baltimore, Maryland, 1969–1970

	1	2	3	4	5	6	7	8	9	10
1. Multiproblem family	1.000	.465	.307	.523	.439	.440	.203	.420	.233	−.550
2. Isolation–rejection		1.000	.371	.331	.413	.346	.222	.430	.308	−.318
3. Narcissism			1.000	.376	.465	.244	.291	.360	−.068	−.387
4. Depression				1.000	.533	.459	.075	.357	.101	−.832
5. Sex deviance					1.000	.439	.068	.445	.280	−.574
6. Marital problems						1.000	.388	.442	.193	−.416
7. Drug abuse							1.000	.315	.237	−.202
8. Stigma								1.000	.455	−.378
9. Suicide attempts									1.000	−.130
10. Suicide completions										1.000

Note. An *r* of ±.235 is statistically significant at the .05 level.
Source: Maris (1971).

Could sexual deviance, drug abuse, and nonfatal suicide attempts in women be operating to enhance, preserve, and maintain life, rather than to end it? If so, then the behavior of the women described above and in Table 6.2 was "paradoxical," since one would expect that such sexual deviance would cause them serious harm and increase their suicide risk. Partial self-destruction toward the end of making their lives possible (given what they had to work with) might prove fatal, but was intended by these women to be problem-solving. They were simply using their best interactive assets to achieve aims that most of us share. The coming together of male and female genitalia (the exchange is more than just that) can be seen as an economic exchange. Were these apparently self-destructive females often just exchanging the best, most rare, and valued interactive assets that they had available?

There can be social as well as individual benefits of sexual deviance. Such deviance can serve to define normative boundaries (Erikson, 1969). Homans (1974) argues that deviant institutions that persist over time (such as prostitution) ultimately have payoffs for both individuals and the larger society. This is not to argue that sexual deviance is the preferred coping mechanism for women. It certainly has costs and associated risks. But it is at least paradoxical. One can be partially self-destructive in order to cope or improve one's life, rather than to end it.

The Case of Sylvia Plath

A female suicide (gynocentric) worth looking at is that of poet Sylvia Plath, who died from a gas overdose in her London flat at the age of 30 on February 11, 1963. Like Ernest Hemingway, Plath had a long history of depressive disorder. Both were given ECT, and both were angry and aggressive. Unlike Hemingway, Plath was young, had multiple interpersonal problems, and did not have a lot of Hemingway's suicide risk factors.

CASE 6.1. Sylvia Plath

Sylvia Plath was a bright poet who suicided at age 30 after a tortured young adulthood. We know a great deal about Plath from her poetry, especially the poems in *Ariel* (Plath, 1966); her semiautobiographical novel, *The Bell Jar* (Plath, 1963/2005); Rosenstein's (1973) doctoral dissertation, a critical biography; the initial chapter in Alvarez's (1971) *The Savage God*; and her friend and biographer, Lois Ames (see Ames's biographical note at the end of *The Bell Jar).*

Plath was raised in Winthrop and Wellesley, Massachusetts, the daughter of a Boston University biology professor (Otto Plath, a Harvard PhD) who studied bees, and a mother (Aurelia Schober) who taught shorthand and typing. Plath was an excellent student, graduating *summa cum laude* from Smith College in 1955. After her junior year at Smith, Plath received a guest editorship award from *Mademoiselle* magazine. This experience seemed to trigger an acute depressive illness with serious suicidal episodes, and resulted in psychiatric hospitalization and ECT. Later in London, Plath was treated with antidepressants, probably tricyclics.

In 1956 Plath received a Fulbright fellowship to Cambridge University, where she met and married poet Ted Hughes. In 1957 Plath and Hughes moved to the United States, and Plath accepted an instructorship in English at Smith College. In 1958 they moved to Beacon Hill in Boston, where they both wrote. In 1959 they returned to England, where Plath met Al Alvarez, poetry editor for *The Observer,* and had an affair with him (which he describes in his book *The Savage God).*

A daughter, Frieda, was born in April 1960, and a son, Nicholas, in January 1962. Nicholas himself committed suicide by hanging in 2009. About the time her son was born, Plath published *The Bell Jar* in England, under the pseudonym Victoria Lucas. Plath suffered repeated depressive episodes, and she and her husband separated in the summer of 1962 when Hughes left her for another woman. The children remained with Plath.

After a bitterly cold winter in London and a frenzy of writing disturbing poems, including some of her *Ariel* poems, Sylvia Plath suicided by gassing herself in her kitchen. Home gas was later detoxified in Great Britain, and the national suicide rate went down and stayed down. Plath had been depressed (Hughes later said she had an adverse reaction to her antidepressants), lonely, burdened by the care of two small children, and periodically ill with the flu.

In an attempt to understand Plath better, let us back up a little. Plath had a love–hate relationship with her father, Otto. When Plath was 8 years old, Otto died of a long and difficult diabetic illness, which had required that his leg be amputated. It seems that she never fully worked through her feelings about her father and did not mourn his death until she was an adult (see Plath, 1963/2005, pp. 135–137). Some of her ambivalence was captured in her poem "Daddy" ("Daddy, I have had to kill you./You died before I had time . . ."; Plath, 1966, p. 49). This suggests what Litman (1989) might have called "ego splitting," in which a hated external object is internalized, and then the death wish for the external object is turned back on the ego.

Plath also had very negative feelings for her mother, Aurelia (who was Otto's second wife), verging on hatred (see Plath, 1963/2005). Biographer Rosenstein comments (1973, p. 48), characterizing Esther Greenwood in *The Bell Jar* as a proxy for Plath herself: "Does she like anything? Not men, not children, few if any women."

What Rosenstein fails to notice with sufficient clarity and compassion was Plath's ultimate contempt for herself. Plath's early experiences, like Esther's (Plath, 1963/2005), led to a basic feeling of subjective inadequacy. All of her later achievements, straight-A grades, prizes, fellowships, publications, and awards could not substitute for her felt loss of early love and noncontingent approval. Mother love is freely given or withheld, without regard to merit. You do not earn it. It is either there or not. Nothing can substitute for early noncontingent acceptance.

This inability to accept herself and others led inexorably to social isolation. Esther becomes (and Plath became) intensely, painfully, critical of herself and others, compulsive, perfectionistic, and rigid. She lacks animal vitality (including sexuality). Often Esther cannot do anything, is unable to make up her mind, and becomes virtually paralyzed (Plath, 1963/2005). In one of the more poignant metaphors of *The Bell Jar,* Esther pictures herself sitting in the crotch of a ripe fig tree starving, but unable to pick which fig to eat. The figs are symbolic of life opportunities forgone.

Men are not tolerable once Esther gets to know them. The ultimate isolation and logical conclusion of her rigidity is the closed world of the "bell jar." Esther shuts herself off from people, new experiences, reality (as opposed to fantasy), and finally from life itself. The symbolism of the bell jar is closure of a life never fully lived because of depressive psychosis. A very similar metaphor is provided by the fetus in the jar of formaldehyde Esther sees in the gross anatomy laboratory of Buddy Willard, her premedical student boyfriend.

Plath's early familial conflict and rigidity as an adolescent led to further negative interactions and sexual problems as a young adult. Rosenstein (1973, p. 49) notes that Plath's sexual repression was closely intertwined with her general difficulty with human relationships (a lot of sexual relationships are not really about sex at all): "That sexuality contaminates is merely an extension of Esther's (Plath's) notion of human relatedness. It's not just kisses that stick, it's people." In the novel, as Plath did in life, Esther enters into a series of doomed, often sadomasochistic sexual relationships with men. Her college sweetheart, Buddy Willard, is safe. He is a relatively unaggressive, well-mannered, Yale premedical student who never seems to have much in common with Esther's dark, artistic side.

Later in the novel, Esther decides to be "relieved" of her virginity and chooses a summer school Harvard math professor (Plath, 1963/2005). When the encounter goes awry, Esther blames the seduced Harvard professor and demands that he pay the emergency room bill for treatment of her hemorrhaging. Sex and children seem to be viewed as "experiences" (remember Joiner's [2005, 2010] theory of the "acquired ability" to suicide) that might make her a better writer, than as gratifying in and of themselves.

Even Esther's initially positive therapeutic relationship with her female psychiatrist, Dr. Nolan, becomes ambivalent when Dr. Nolan gives her unexpected ECT. At least, however, this second course of ECT goes better than Esther's first, ordered by a male psychiatrist named Dr. Gordon. Plath herself felt betrayed when she was given unanticipated ECT. She likened it to the electrocution of the Rosenberg spies.

Plath's real-life sexual involvement with Alvarez turned out poorly, too. After Plath's death, Alvarez confessed that he let Plath down, knowing that she was suicidal (he later made a suicide attempt himself while on sabbatical at Princeton):

> She must have thought I was stupid and insensitive. Which I was. But to have been otherwise would have meant accepting responsibilities I didn't want and couldn't, in my own depression, have coped with. When I left about eight o'clock to go to my dinner-party, I knew I had let her down in some final and unforgivable way. And I knew she knew. I never again saw her alive. (Alvarez, 1971, p. 48)

It would be a disservice to Alvarez and to Plath's complex suicidal career to suggest that Alvarez was responsible for Plath's suicide. However, once again Plath had become involved with someone who seemed to contribute to her undoing rather than to her growth and well-being.

Plath's parental conflicts, rigidity, lack of positive social interactions, and isolation (of which sexual problems were just one facet) made her life become unacceptable—not just unsatisfying, but intolerable. The depression that had hounded her all her life turned into hopelessness. In *The Bell Jar* (1963/2005, p. 130), Esther describes herself as "incurable" in the days leading up to her suicide attempt, and expresses doubts even near the novel's end: "How did I know that someday . . . the bell jar, with its stifling distortions, wouldn't descend again?" (p. 197).

As described by Alvarez (1971) and Ames (see the biographical note in Plath, 1966/2005), the final suicide attempt with toxic oven gas had a kind of quiet desperation about it. It was cold; there were two young children to care for; Plath had been physically ill; she had recently separated from Hughes; she was very lonely; and Alvarez had been unable to help her.

Yet all of Plath's attempts were ambivalent. Plath wanted to die and live at the same time. Plath left a note for her *au pair* girl to call Plath's doctor, and even gave her the phone number. When the babysitter could not get into the flat (which had been the flat of the poet William Butler Yeats earlier), and no neighbors could be roused (the gas had knocked out Plath's neighbor, too), the *au pair* left for a few hours before trying to get in again. By then Plath was already dead.

Source: Adapted from Maris, Ronald W. with Bernard Lazerwitz. *Pathways to Suicide: A Survey of Self-Destructive Behaviors.* © 1981 The Johns Hopkins University Press. Adapted with permission of Johns Hopkins University Press.

Compare Case 6.1 with the more phallocentric suicide of Hemingway (Chapter 1, Case 1.1). Are the same risk factors present? Could Plath's suicide be explained just on the basis of what we know about Hemingway? For example, Plath did not abuse alcohol; she did not shoot herself; she made many nonfatal suicide attempts; she did not have a long suicidal career (Hemingway lived about twice as long as Plath did); her work (although morbid) was going fairly well; and (as just noted) she had a lot of interpersonal problems. Hemingway seemed more angry at life and the human condition, and not so much at other people.

Family, Marital Status, and Suicide

Families can cause or contribute to suicides. We have already seen in Chapter 1 (Figure 1.3) how suicides tended to be overrepresented in Ernest Hemingway's family. (See other genealogies of artists' family suicides in Jamison's 1993 book, *Touched with Fire.*) This suggests that genetic predispositions contribute to mood disorders, (although the concordance is never 100%), as well as modeling and contagion from family suicides. Suicide can be in a family's problem-solving repertoire.

Families of suicides tend to be overrepresented with traits like marital dysfunction, child abuse, marital separation, divorce and broken homes, rigid and controlling parents, frequent moving of residence, unemployed parents, financial difficulties, substance abuse, and psychiatric disorder (Maris, 1997a; Maris et al., 2000; Bongar et al., 2000).

On the other hand, in general marriage and family protect against suicide. This is especially true for men, but not so much for women. Take a look at Figure 6.1. Marital and family status and suicide look mainly like this:

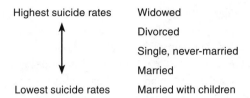

Widowhood and divorce are particularly suicidogenic for men. Marriage does not protect women as much against suicide. It is more complicated to unravel why marriage and family tend to be protective against suicide. Obviously, married people with children are less socially isolated; if they do become suicidal, it is more likely that someone will notice and get them treatment. Also, in a sense, not having children is a little like suicide, since you fail to propagate your genes. Having family members gives people another reason to be other than just themselves, as well as the attendant socialization, nurturing, and economic responsibilities. However, it is also true that pathological marriage and family relationships can be suicidogenic, not protective.

Suicide and the LGBT Population

Now that we have examined suicide and heterosexuality in heterosexuals of both genders in some detail, what about lesbians, gays, bisexuals, and transsexuals (the

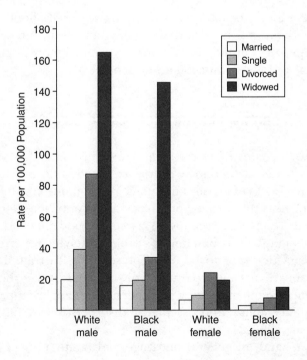

FIGURE 6.1. U.S. suicide rates by marital status, race, and sex, 1996. *Source:* Maris et al. (2000, p. 223). Copyright © The Guilford Press. Reprinted with permission.

LGBT population)? Do members of this diverse population have elevated suicide rates, and if so, how much and why (Maris et al., 2000; Cha et al., 2018)?

The answer is complicated and concerns much more than sexual orientation and gender identity. Considering all of the studies, on average, gay men probably have a suicide rate about twice that of heterosexual males (Maris et al., 2000). Gay males (this is less true of lesbians) can have tumultuous interpersonal lives, hundreds of lifetime sexual partners, and the threat of getting AIDS. LGBT individuals also have to live in a homophobic, hostile larger society, filled with condemning far-right religious conservatives and lots of stigma. This stress is compounded if their families of origin are also rejecting and critical.

Many LGBT individuals thus suffer from loneliness, anxiety, increased depression, lowered self-esteem, and increased alcohol and other substance abuse, as well as (and probably as consequences of) familial and social rejection. All of these traits tend to raise suicide risk. Even though there is now better, more effective, and less expensive treatment for AIDS, some studies have found that a diagnosis of HIV (with its prospect of premature death) raised the suicide risk to about 36 times that of white heterosexual males without an HIV diagnosis.

Empirical research on LGBT suicide risk has come to diverse conclusions. An early study by Saghir and Robins (1971) found that 23% of homosexual males had made at least one suicide attempt, versus 5% of heterosexual males (a relative risk of about 4:1). When Hendin (1982) studied male suicidal students at Columbia University, he found that about 20% of them were homosexual (vs. about 1–3% of the general population). A study of gay street youth (Yates et al., 1988) claimed that 53% had attempted suicide.

One study of LGBT youth by Gibson (1989), funded by the U.S. government, claimed that suicide was the leading cause of death among gay males, lesbians, bisexuals, and the "transgendered" (note that this last category included both transsexuals and transvestites). However, Gibson was soundly criticized for his poor research methods.

More recent research on the LGBT population and suicide has found that gay men have a suicide risk two to five times higher than that of heterosexual males (Simon & Hales, 2006), or simply that there is an unspecified elevated suicide risk in homosexual men (Simon & Hales, 2012). Some recent research (Cramer et al., 2014) claims that much of the increased LGBT suicide risk is due to Joiner's (2005) traits of thwarted belongingness and perceived burdensomeness.

Two HBO comedy specials by two lesbians (Wanda Sykes and Rosie O'Donnell) made some important points. Sykes said that being homosexual is like being black (which she is); it is not a matter of choice. O'Donnell said to a white heterosexual male heckler in her audience, "I won't hold it against you; you were born that way."

Maleness, Aggression, and Violence

The prototypical sexual act is a somewhat aggressive penetration of a female by a male, and aggression is related to suicide (Maris et al., 2000). All suicidal acts involve some minimal aggressive action. Aggression is more basic to suicide than depression is, and it is mainly a male trait. Like sex, suicide requires energy, needs an aggressive catalyst, and is usually initiated and engaged in by a male. When young males are at their prime ages for sexual activity (say, ages 15–24), their leading causes of death are all violent and aggressive: accidents, suicide, and homicide. Also, early life adversity is related to adult antisocial behavior and increased impulsivity, especially in males. In particular, there are brain changes with child sexual abuse: Early sexual abuse is associated with abnormal HPA axis function in adulthood (Mann & Currier, 2012).

There are some important gender-related hormonal and neurobiological differences. Women have lower testosterone levels that males do; testosterone is associated with aggression; and aggression is associated with increased suicide risk. As noted earlier, male suicides tend to have lower levels of prefrontal cortex 5-HT and its metabolite 5-HIAA, especially if the suicidal act was violent (Mann & Currier, 2012). Suicide is in part an aggressive malfunction of the 5-HT system.

When there are murder–suicides, they almost always involve males murdering females, also as noted earlier. In fact, when females are violated sexually (raped), they may kill themselves, but not the violent perpetrators. See the ancient historical examples of Lucretia and Dido in Chapter 18.

Taking a view based on quantitative evolutionary biology, de Catanzaro (1986, 1992) notes that women's suicide rates peak at about the time they go into menopause (ages 45–54). His current work at McMaster University concerns the reproductive impact of estrogens. For the most part (unless they take extreme medical measures), menopausal women are not biologically able to reproduce; nor do they especially need to nurture their current offspring. Thus menopausal women are relatively unfit reproductively and have less reason to continue living—and, other things being equal, more reason to suicide. Men stay sexually and reproductively fit until late in the life cycle, but their suicide rate goes up for every 5–10 years that they become less reproductively fit. So, as men age, they (too) have more reason to suicide.

Autoerotic Asphyxia

Autoerotic asphyxia is a usually private male masturbatory behavior involving bondage. Normally an adolescent or young adult male (cross-dressed as a females about 20% of the time, but usually just nude) attaches a rope or ligature around his neck (and sometimes around his genitals) to restrict blood flow, heighten sensation, and induce altered consciousness while masturbating. Suicide (intent is questionable, so the correct manner of death may be accident) can result if the combination of blood flow loss and ejaculatory distraction causes rapid unconsciousness and anoxic brain damage (which can happen in just a few minutes; Maris et al., 2000).

You will remember that I considered autoerotic asphyxia as one possibility in the case of Antwan Sedgwick (see Chapter 3). I had a verified case of autoerotic asphyxia in which the perpetrator had a fail-safe device requiring him to kick a 2 × 4 release board mechanism, but he missed and ended up videotaping his own self-induced death. A famous case of autoerotic asphyxia involved David Carradine, an actor famous for the *Kung Fu* TV series and two of the *Kill Bill* movies. On June 5,

2005, at age 72, Carradine was found nude and dead with a nylon rope around his neck and genitals in a Bangkok hotel.

Erotic asphyxia does not have to be self-administered. One partner often partially strangles the other during sex to intensify the recipient's orgasmic experience. There was a well-known mystery movie titled *Rising Sun* (Kaufman, 1993) about this topic, starring Wesley Snipes and Sean Connery.

Bob Fosse: *All That Jazz*

All That Jazz was a 1979 film directed by Bob Fosse (who also produced the stage musical *Chicago*). It was semiautobiographical (like Sylvia Plath's novel *The Bell Jar*). For example, like the film's protagonist, Joe Gideon, Fosse abused drugs, was a workaholic, and died at the relatively young age of 60 of a heart attack. The themes of the film are living on the edge, narcissistic pursuit of one's life work, sexual promiscuity, substance abuse (especially stimulants, including speed and cigarettes), risk taking, and premature death by self-induced heart disease (in Fosse's case, a kind of slow suicide). What can we learn about suicidogenic forces in self-absorbed, aggressive, sexually promiscuous males like the film's Joe Gideon?

In the film, Roy Scheider (of *Jaws* fame) played Joe Gideon; Jessica Lange played Angelique, an angel of death. Since Fosse sexualized everything, both life and death were sexualized. Sandahl Bergman portrayed the lead dancer, and John Lithgow played a competing musical director. The film opens with dancers on a stage auditioning for a Joe Gideon musical, but most of them get rejected. One spurned dancer says, "Fuck him!", and another answers, "I did, and he still won't pick me." Even in the sensate world, many attempt but few succeed. It is as if after a long torturous internal debate, you decide to sell your body for sex, but then nobody will make you an offer.

Gideon is a perfectionist. His comments are always qualified, he is never satisfied, and nothing (work, women) is ever good enough. Gideon is uncompromising in his efforts to "get it right." In the end this dissatisfaction, striving, and stress cause his heart to explode. One of the themes is promiscuity versus commitment. Does faithfulness to one woman equal finitude and death? Gideon cannot even remember the names (a kind of sexual universalism) of his lovers and invites some of them over to his apartment at the same time by mistake. The idea is that sexual exuberance is deadly, empty, fleeting narcissistic gratification, and that one cannot be saved by sexual activity. When people like Gideon get sick and are dying, there is no one who cares enough to hold their hand.

In the movie Gideon has his nonfatal heart attack while everyone is sitting around a table rehearsing the script; the sound shuts off, and just the picture remains. This reminds us that the death of self is different from the death of others. He is feeling unique pain and illness, and everyone else (unaware) is laughing and uninvolved from him. Narcissists die and suffer alone. Joe Gideon is in interpersonal bankruptcy. Like Hemingway, he is alone in the midst of a crowd.

For Gideon it is always work before play, narcissism before altruism, self before family. Gideon often forgets to even pick up his own daughter for weekend custody.

Angelique, the angel of death, asks Gideon, "Work?" To which he replies, "All there is."

In the film, Gideon is clearly getting sick and in fact is slowly dying, but he ignores his health. He keeps chain-smoking and abuses Dexedrine. He gets extra second and third chances, but ignores them. How many chances do we get to do the right thing, to be forgiven? How many times can we remarry and start over? In spite of multiple warnings about the unhealthiness of his morbid lifestyle, he is rigid and compromising. Ben Vereen, as the character O'Connor Flood, says, "The only reality [boundary] for this cat is death."

Other Gender-Related Self-Destructive Behaviors

There are other gender-related self-destructive behaviors that I only have space to allude to briefly here. For example, personality disorders (Black & Andreasen, 2014) tend to be very different for suicidal women and men (see Chapter 14). Many suicidal females suffer from borderline personality disorder and frequently cut themselves. In fact, major depression and borderline personality disorder are the only two psychiatric disorders that have suicidal behaviors or thoughts as one explicit criterion.

Borderline personality disorder is characterized by a pervasive pattern of mood instability, unstable and intense interpersonal relationships, impulsivity, inappropriate intense anger, lack of control of anger, recurrent suicidal threats and gestures, self-mutilating (often cutting) behavior, marked and persistent identity disturbance, chronic feelings of emptiness, and frantic efforts to avoid real or imagined abandonment (Black & Andreasen, 2014; Maris et al., 2000).

Many (especially younger) suicidal males, on the other hand, tend to have antisocial personality disorder, characterized by unlawful behavior, irritation/aggression (often leading to fights), impulsivity, disregard for safety of self and others, lack of remorse or empathy, and irresponsibility (especially at work). Note that many of the traits for both borderline and antisocial personalities are suicidogenic. I should also at least mention self-mutilation other than that associated with borderline personality, particularly in male jail and prison populations (Maris et al., 2000; Favazza, 1996).

In Chapter 8, I have much more to say about gender and suicide variations in other countries. First, however, Chapter 7 turns from sexual relations to social relations in general. The sociology of suicide is often neglected, given the psychiatric and psychological focus of most suicidologists.

Social Relations, Work, and the Economy

Social versus Individual Facts

> The private experiences usually thought to be the proximate causes
> of suicide have only the influences borrowed from the victim's
> moral disposition . . . his sadness comes to him from without.
>
> —EMILE DURKHEIM

Most theories of suicide focus on *idiographic* states, or traits of specific suicidal individuals. For example, how serious is a person's depressive disorder? Is it being effectively medicated? Has the person formed a specific lethal plan to attempt suicide, and under what circumstances would he or she do it? Does the person own a gun? Does he or she abuse alcohol, live alone, have meaningful satisfying daily routines?

But how can we understand and control the suicide rates of *collectivities,* not of individuals (cf. Mayhew, 1983)? As we shall see shortly, suicide rates are external to and constraining of suicidal individuals. Durkheim (1897/1951) argued that suicide rates are what he called "social facts." That is, they are qualitatively different from individual suicides. Social facts like suicide rates require *nomothetic* propositions—ones involving abstract, general, universal laws, such as "The suicide rate varies inversely with the degree of social integration" (Durkheim, 1897/1951). The high male suicide rate in Russia, or the high female suicide rate in China, requires a different level of explanation than do the individual facts of a particular suicide.

This chapter considers broad social, economic, and occupational factors in suicide (cf. Feigelman et al., 2018). For example, how do social isolation, lack of social support, negative interaction, stress, and what Joiner (2005) calls "thwarted belongingness" and "perceived burdensomeness" affect suicide outcomes? Under what broad social conditions are suicide rates higher? For example:

- Durkheim explained social disintegration, anomie, and egoistic individuation versus altruistic and fatalistic social forces in suicide.
- Gibbs discussed an operational measurement of social integration, which he called "status integration."

- Henry and Short talked about the interaction of external and internal restraint in economic business cycles and frustration–aggression theory.
- Douglas emphasized the situated social meanings of highly suicidal groups (e.g., serious suicide attempters).
- Phillips discussed suicide contagion and suggestibility, including the 12% suicide rate rise in the United States 7 to 10 days after the suicide of Marilyn Monroe.
- I considered ecology and suicide variation in census tracts in Chicago.
- Stack outlined sociological work on suicide, especially the effect of celebrity suicides on others.

Overview of Social Relations and Suicide

On the surface, suicide seems like one of the most private and asocial of all human acts. Horton (2006) claimed that "although suicide seems like a personal and individual act, it is also paradoxically a public event, a tear in the social fabric" (cf. Stack, 1982). Most suicides occur in private, not in public places (e.g., 78.9% occur at home; see note to Table 6.1 in Chapter 6). Other people are seldom present at the time of a suicide. Maybe just 1–2% of suicides are witnessed by others. There is further social isolation, since suicides are rare (about 1 in 10,000 in the general population per year in the United States, as noted throughout this book) and stigmatized. People usually do not talk about suicides in their families, and they tend not to know much about other suicides. Thus most of us do not have firsthand experience with suicide or even death very often. When was the last time you saw a dead body?

The privacy and isolation of suicide does not mean that it is asocial. Indeed, a major theory of suicide is that it results in part from perceived burdensomeness, thwarted, or failed social relations (see Joiner, 2005). Social relations can basically be either (1) absent (almost 50% of my Chicago suicides had no close friends when they died; Maris, 1981; however, see Marver et al., 2017: friendship quality not quantity predicted suicide attempts at a 1-year follow-up; for each point of friendship impairment, the risk of suicide increased by a factor of 1.8) or (2) negative (present but negative, like Harold's interactions with his narcissistic mother in the movie *Harold and Maude,* as described in Chapter 5).

As I have said earlier, in order to live (or certainly to live well), each of us needs at least one significant other or "significant udder"—one crucial, sustaining relationship, which could be with God or with another person. Friends and family give us a reason (and a resource) to be (see the dedication to this book). Imagine not having a mother or father, brothers or sisters, grandparents, a spouse or partner, best friends, or a church/temple/mosque community. Social interaction also distracts us from ourselves and our own problems. Social interaction gives us meaningful responsibilities—for example, when we take care of our aging grandparents or parents, raise our children, help friends through crises, and so on.

Sometimes social relations can be present but negative and suicidogenic. For example, young people may copy the self-destructive lifestyles of friends (e.g., suicide pacts). Parents can be destructive and narcissistic; including verbal, sexual or physical abuse. Alcoholism, mood disorders, and violence tend to run in families. See the description of Hemingway's suicidogenic family in Chapter 1 (Figure 1.3 and Case 1.1).

Sexual activities, considered in Chapter, 6 are social relations in a special sense. Obviously if people were totally asocial, then human beings would not be propagated and would disappear. Maybe this is one reason why sexual activities are normally so pleasurable (in part to guarantee the propagation of the human species). Clearly, sex and procreation require some minimal social activities, at least for a short time. From these brief comments, it should be apparent that social relations are important factors in suicidality.

History of the Sociology of Suicide

The following is an overview of the history of the sociology of suicide (see Maris et al., 2000, for more detailed coverage; Maris, 2017). As stated at the start of the chapter, the French social philosopher Emile Durkheim argued that suicide rates are social facts, and as such are external to and constraining of suicidal individuals. The social aspect is qualitatively different from an individual suicide. The whole (the suicide rate) is not just the sum of its parts (of individual suicides), any more than a Rolex watch is just its unassembled individual parts lying on a watchmaker's workbench. Broad social facts determine the suicide rate; among these are *anomie,* or literally existence without norms (e.g., the sudden disruptions of economic constraints in the United States in 1929 and 2008). Another is *egoism,* meaning excessive individuation, whereby certain individuals are not well protected by normal social constraints (examples include conditions of high divorce rates, homelessness, or social isolation). High suicide rates are the joint interactive products of minimal social regulation and maximal individuation. According to Durkheim, most suicides are "ego-anomic" (see Figure 7.1).

To Durkheim's theory of external restraint, Henry (a psychiatrist) and Short (a sociologist) in 1954 added the concept of *internal restraint* (similar to the Freudian concept of a punitive superego or guilt); they also extended the theory to include homicide rates. Their frustration–aggression hypothesis (based on Dollard et al.'s [1939] work at Yale) contended that suicide is the result of summated frustration and stress directed toward the self. Directed toward others, this frustration and stress become homicide or assault. At issue is what conditions determine the target for aggression. Business cycles can generate both frustration and failed external restraint. Suicide rates are highest when there is strong internal restraint and weak external restraint. Homicide (or assault) rates are highest when there is weak internal restraint (such as in sociopathy) and strong external restraint (see Figure 7.2).

Sociologists Gibbs and Martin (1964) argued that Durkheim's concept of social integration was not operationally defined, and thus that his theory was untestable. Gibbs went to great lengths to measure what he called "status integration"–for example, the proportion of individuals occupying a status set, such as a certain combination of age, sex, race, and occupation. The status integration theory of suicide maintains that less frequently occupied status sets (e.g., young widowed males)

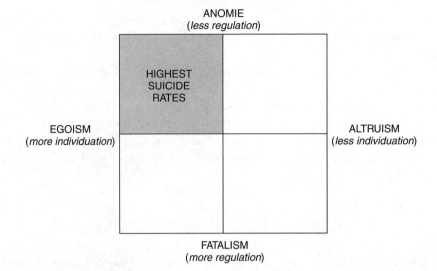

FIGURE 7.1. Durkheim's typology of suicide. *Source:* Original graphic by Maris.

imply more unstable and disrupted social relations, more role conflict, and more incompatible statuses, and (thus) should have higher suicide rates.

For example, Gibbs (1994) presented some data on marital status integration, including the following statistics in which marital status is cross-tabulated with age, sex, race, occupation, religious affiliation, and parental status (Maris et al., 2000, p. 246):

Single   = .92 (proportion occupying the marital status set)
Married   = .06
Widowed = .01
Divorced = .015

	Strong Internal Restraint	Weak Internal Restraint
Weak External Restraint	Suicide—Self-Aggression	Unpredictable
Strong External Restraint	Anxiety or Conflict	Homicide—Other-Aggression

FIGURE 7.2. Henry and Short's aggressive responses to frustration. *Source:* Adapted from *Suicide and Homicide* by A. F. Henry & J. Short. Copyright © 1954 by The Free Press. Copyright renewed © 1982 by Mary H. Bloch & James F. Short. Adapted with permission of The Free Press, a division of Simon & Schuster, Inc. All rights reserved.

Although one would need to look at all of the data and all the measures of status integration, these data fit with the status integration theory of suicide for the most part. The data would predict higher suicide rates for the widowed and divorced compared to the married (which is true). The only anomaly here is for single persons.

Douglas (1967) was a Princeton sociologist (specifically, an ethnomethodologist) who argued that the study of suicide could not be founded in official or vital statistics data, since (for one thing) suicide rates are unreliable and invalid. For example, some officials require that a suicide note be found in order to certify a death as a suicide, which occurs in only 10–25% of all suicides. Unlike the NASH classification (natural, accidental, suicidal, homicidal) on death certificates, suicide does not have one clear, consistent meaning, but rather many "situated subjective meanings" that we could discover by intensively studying living serious suicide attempters. Douglas contended that it is not possible to predict individual suicides by using abstract concepts like anomie or egoism. See Box 7.1 for more on Douglas's critique of Durkheim. Suicidology needs intensive observation of living individuals who have actually engaged in self-destructive behaviors, not retrospective death records of decedents assumed to be suicides.

I (Maris, 1969, 1981, 2015; Maris et al., 2000) have argued that suicides are not so much acute or triggered by current stressors, as they are reflections of what I call "suicidal careers." Suicide is like an achievement in a vocation and usually takes many years to develop; as I see it, this is one reason why suicide rates tend to be highest late in the life cycle. Suicides need to be studied interdisciplinarily.

BOX 7.1. Excerpts from Douglas's Critique of Durkheim

- What Durkheim is doing is assuming his socialistic theory of suicide is correct and then explaining away any data that is contrary to it.

- Official statistics cannot be expected to have any significant value in constructing or testing sociolog[ical] theories of suicide.

- There are as many official statistics as there are officials.

- The more socially integrated an individual is, the more he and his significant others will try to avoid having his death categorized or classified as a suicide, assuming that suicide is judged negatively.

- The more integrated the deceased individual is . . . the more officials responsible for deciding what the cause of death is will be favorably influenced . . . by the preferences of the deceased and his significant others.

- The most important error involved in the use of official statistics . . . is the assumption that "suicidal actions" have a necessary and sufficient universal meaning throughout the Western world.

- A basic reorientation of sociological work on suicide in the direction of intensive observation (ethnomethodology), description, and analysis of individual cases of suicide seems to be necessary.

Suicidology is not organized like academic departments in universities. We need at least a biopsychosocial model of suicide to even hope to understand or control it. Suicidology also needs sophisticated measurements, data gathering with controls, and regression analyses across academic disciplines, so that under controlled conditions we can try to specify the amount of variance explained by combinations of antecedent variables in particular subsets of suicides. See also the ecological analysis of suicide rates in community areas in my Chicago study (Maris et al., 2000, p. 249). Actual suicides, survivors, and controls need to be given psychological autopsies (e.g., see my autopsy form at *www.suicideexpert.com/forms*). Durkheim focused too exclusively on social factors in suicide.

Phillips (1974; Phillips & Carstensen, 1986), a Princeton sociologist, criticized Durkheim further for claiming that suicide was not contagious or copied. For instance, in a series of carefully done demographic studies, Phillips showed that 7–10 days after the suicide of actress Marilyn Monroe, the U.S. suicide rate went up by 12%. He discovered that in general, suicides were more contagious in the young (6–7%) than in older adults (3%), and that suicide rates rose after most celebrity suicides. The more a suicide was covered on the front pages of a major newspaper such as *The New York Times* or *Los Angeles Times* the more the suicide rate increased, in a kind of dose–response phenomenon (see Table 7.2, below). Phillips (1974) went on to discuss what he called the "Werther effect," after Goethe's fictional character in *The Sorrows of Young Werther* (1774). Werther shot himself over unrequited love, and many copycat suicides resulted. Another interesting finding came from Phillips's (1970) doctoral dissertation on what he called the "death-dip": He showed that people routinely postponed even their own natural deaths until after important social events like their birthdays or the Apollo moon shot. Over his career, Phillips has looked empirically at a wide range of possible contagions (murder–suicides followed by airplane crashes by pilots, heavyweight boxing fights and murders, suicide rates after soap opera suicides, etc.). Some of these suggested relationships strain credulity (Maris et al., 2000, p. 248).

Sociologist Steven Stack, who coauthored an interesting empirical book titled *Suicide Movies* (Stack & Bowman, 2011), studied the strange correlation between car radio stations tuned to country music (when left for car repair) and the suicide rates of the owners, and did several studies on contagion and suicide. Wasserman (1989), studying the economy and suicide, determined which occupations had the highest suicide rates (such as sheep herders, dentists, hairdressers, female physicians, and laborers) and which had the lowest suicide rates (such as airline pilots, clergy, naval officers, building contractors). Pescosolido (1994), a sociologist at Yale, argued that the study of suicide needs to be couched in what she called a "network theory." She maintained that disintegrating network ties deny individuals both integrative and regulative protection from suicide. She claimed that moderate levels of social integration and regulation are optimal in protecting individuals from suicide.

There must be at least 20 other sociologists worldwide currently doing important recent work on suicide. I can only mention a few of them here (my thanks to Steven Stack for helping me create a list of some of them). In an *American Sociological Review* article, Abrutyn and Mueller (2014) wrote that although Durkheim claimed strong social relationships protect individuals from suicide, they can also increase suicide vulnerability when there is exposure to suicidality. For example, suicide attempts of role models can trigger suicide ideation and some suicide attempts (especially in girls; see Plemmons et al., 2018, and the popular 2018 Netflix series *13 Reasons Why*). Milner et al. (2013) wrote an article on long-term unemployment and how it can increase suicide rates.

Jie Zhang has been doing important work for many years on the social psychology of suicide. He has published over 100 articles, many in leading psychiatric journals (e.g., Zhang et al., 2004). Thomas Niederkrotenthaler, an MD/PhD in Vienna, Austria, is doing major work on the media, contagion, and suicide (Niederkrotenthaler, 2015). He is also affiliated with the International Association for Suicide Prevention (IASP). Jonathan Scourfield (of Cardiff University in Wales) and his colleagues do qualitative work on gender and suicide. See their interesting book, *Understanding Suicide: A Sociological Autopsy* (Fincham et al., 2011).

Social Isolation and Thwarted Belongingness

What is suicidogenic about being alone? Could not isolation be peaceful and calming? Think of religious ascetics, meditation, and yoga. In Buddhism, *nirvana* involves dissociating from your physical body as the "not-self." *Samsara* in classical Hinduism entails changing your physical embodiment, transmigration of souls, and reincarnation. The Christian heaven is a spiritual population of souls, not a physical afterlife for most. Could not your private home or residence be your oasis or castle in a troubled world?

On the other hand, social isolation could:

• Deny people needed social support and intervention. Consider a newborn infant, nursing and totally dependent on the mother, who loses his or her mother. One significant other in this case is crucially different from none (Asch, 1955). Suicide rates of the married are almost always lower than those of the single, widowed, or divorced. Who is going to make sure that a person takes psychiatric medications or keeps doctors' appointments? Who is going to call 911 or drive the person to the emergency room for treatment after a suicide attempt?

• Reduce targets for aggression. Suicide is often the leading cause of death in jails and prisons (see Chapter 22). They tend to house young, aggressive males, with a history of substance abuse and violent offenses. Whom are they going to aggress against in solitary confinement? Self-mutilation short of suicide is a related problem (Favazza, 1996) in incarcerated populations.

• Lead to greater impulsivity and fewer constraints against poor judgment. In large families or among people with many friends, there are more people around to say, "You're going to do *what!?*" Checks and balances are important, especially when people are depressed, confused, psychotic, and/or desperate. If a person cuts his or her wrists in a large African American family, chances are good that someone will drive the family member to the emergency room for stitches. If the person is an isolated older white male, good luck to him!

* Enhance depression. When people are repeatedly alone, they tend to be more depressed. Depression increases the probability of suicide. Joiner (2005) has claimed that thwarted belongingness increases the desire for death.

* Increase the chances that you will die by yourself (alone). When you die, the world does not die. People can love you, celebrate your life, and mourn your passing, but they cannot die for you. Among the many horrible things about the atomic bombs dropped on Hiroshima and Nagasaki in World War II was the fear that all people (even survivors) and nature itself had been poisoned by radiation and were doomed (Lifton, 1983). Dying by suicide or even naturally is an isolating event.

There is a lot of research on the relationship of social isolation to self-destruction. For example, having just one supportive significant other can be enough for a person to persist in what he or she knows is sound judgment (e.g., not making a suicide attempt). Asch (1955) showed two cards to groups of 10 people: card A with a short line, and card B with both a short and a longer line. They were then asked: "Which line on card B is the same length as the line on card A?" The answer was obvious. But if all 9 of the other subjects in each group (the 10th subject was designated as the experimental subject) said that the longer line on card B was the correct one, then the experimental subject agreed with them on the wrong answer. If only 1 of the 9 said it was the short line, then the subject tended to persist in saying that the two short lines matched. Having only a single supportive other made the difference.

Sainsbury (1955), working in London, said that there was a higher suicide rate if people lived alone, lived in just one room, lived in a hotel room, or were divorced. In Chicago, I found much the same thing (Maris, 1969). The higher the population per household in 76 community areas, the lower the suicide rate (the correlation was –.72 and was statistically significant). One has to be careful here and not commit what is called the "ecological fallacy." That is, analysis of data about groups living in a community area or census tract cannot be used to draw reliable conclusions about individual suicides in that same area. But these data at least suggest that social isolation raises rates of self-destruction and suicide.

One of my graduate students (Nisbet, 1996; cf. Walker et al., 2018) tried to determine why African American females had such low suicide rates in spite of having high rates of depression, lots of poverty, more absent fathers in raising their children, and other adversities. What Nisbet found was that larger average family or household size, and more kinship relationships, were related to lower suicide ideation among these women.

When I did my 1981 survey of suicide in Chicago, I asked informants (mostly wives of deceased husbands who had either suicided or died naturally) about the decedents' close friends. Even though the natural death control groups were on average 20 years older than the suicides, the natural death controls had about twice as many close friends as the suicides did. I also asked whether the decedents had three or more close friends at the time of death. The answers were as follows; those dying natural deaths (29% yes), nonfatal suicide attempters (35% yes), and suicide completers (11% yes). Finally, I asked if the decedents had no close friends at all; 49% of the suicides had no close friends, versus 33% of the older subjects dying natural deaths (the quality, not just the quantity, of a relationship was also important, cf. Stanley et al., 2008).

One important caveat about social involvement and suicide: If a group's norms favor of suicide, then social involvement *increases* suicide potential. Examples of pro-suicide groups include Jim Jones's Guyana religious cult, *kamikaze* pilots in World War II, *jihadists,* and the Heaven's Gate cult (see Chapter 17).

Joiner (2005) speaks of "thwarted belongingness" in much the same sense I speak of social isolation. He asks if connectivity can make suicide impossible. Unfortunately, the answer may be no: In a case where I provided postventive care (see Chapter 26), a distraught husband and father hanged himself from a rafter in his garage, and his wife and two young children saw his body when they came home from school and pushed the garage door opener. Horrible as it is, sometimes suicidal pain and depression trump connectivity.

Joiner (2005) also mentions a case in San Francisco described by Jerome Motto. The young man left a note in his apartment saying, "I'm going to walk to the [Golden Gate] bridge. If one person smiles at me on the way, I will not jump." No one did, and the man jumped. Joiner also says that depressed people tend to lack eye contact, which is a manifestation of not belonging. In addition, suicidal poets (versus nonsuicidal poets) use the "we" pronoun less in their poems.

As we've seen, single people have higher suicide rates than married people (Joiner, 2005, p. 124). Also, pregnant women have lower suicide rates than women who are not pregnant. (Of course, the suicide of a pregnant woman is usually in effect filicide–suicide, which is the second leading type of murder–suicide.) In addition, immigrants (especially first-generation immigrants) typically have higher suicide rates than those who stayed in their mother countries (Joiner, 2005, p. 127).

By contrast, most national tragedies tend to unite and connect people, and during these tragedies the suicide rate tends to go down. For example, when President John F. Kennedy was assassinated on November 22, 1963, there were no suicides in the United States from the 22nd to the 30th. On September 11, 2001, national suicide prevention crisis hotline calls dropped from an average of 600 a day to just 300 a day (Joiner, 2005, p. 128).

Communities also have lower suicide rates when their sports teams are winning and are ranked higher nationally (Joiner, 2005, pp. 129–130). In general, the higher-ranked a college team is, the lower the suicide rate is in its fan base. Moreover, if Monday is the day of the week with the highest suicide rate (which I found in Chicago), then Joiner (2005, p. 135) suspects that this might be in part because feelings of being burdensome and not belonging may intensify as the work week starts.

In general, Joiner concludes than the more isolation, the greater the desire for death. Yet one needs to remember that thwarted belongingness, perceived burdensomeness, and the acquired ability to inflict lethal self-injury are all by themselves fairly anemic concepts. It is when they result in extreme pain and the desire or need for relief from it in vulnerable individuals that they gather the power to increase suicide risk dramatically.

Stress, Negative Interaction, and Perceived Burdensomeness

If isolation and thwarted belongingness are one side of the social relations coin in suicidology, then the other side is stressful, negative interpersonal relations. In the first case, social relations are absent; in the second case, social relations are present but negative, stressful, and suicidogenic. Stress or negative life events are abundant adverse social events, relationships, or ties that paradoxically push or drive the individual toward self-destruction and suicide.

In Chapter 4, I have spoken of stress and diathesis as constituting a suicide risk factor. The word *diathesis* comes from the Greek for "disposition" and designates a constitutional predisposition to a particular abnormal state or diseased condition. This predisposition consists of factors along the lines of temperament, rather than personality (Leamon & Bostwick, 2012); these factors include genetic or biological givens, early life experiences, or behavioral traits (like impulsivity) that predispose one to suicide under conditions of stress (Yufit & Bongar, 1992). Felner et al. (1992) say that diathesis indicates genes or environmentally acquired trait-like individual-level vulnerabilities (cf., Mann & Currier, 2012). For example, as noted in earlier chapters, early life stress or abuse can lead to an abnormal HPA axis in adulthood (Mann & Currier, 2012).

Stress, on the other hand, means more state-like negative interactions, events, and relationships. Stress can occur throughout the life cycle (see the general model of suicidal behaviors, Chapter 2, Figure 2.1). Thus there can be early, midlife, and late-life stress (including suicide-triggering stress in vulnerable individuals). Diathesis and stress interact to increase suicide risk.

In my Chicago suicide surveys (Maris, 1969, 1981), I defined "negative interaction" as interpersonal relationships that were painful, unpleasant, rejecting, or isolating. Negative interaction included early life separation from or rejection by parents, not feeling close to one's mother or father, having siblings with major problems, having marital and sexual (including abuse) problems as an adult, experiencing job and work troubles, getting arrested, and conceiving of your own death as getting even with someone. All of these variables and others were operationalized and converted into a negative interaction scale.

Overall, in Chicago (Maris, 1981), nonfatal suicide attempters and completers had higher negative interaction scores that the natural death controls did (34.6 for attempters, 20.5 for completers, and 18.5 for those dying natural deaths). The attempters probably had higher scores, since they were drawn from psychiatric patient groups and the completers and natural death controls were not.

One has to be careful here. Stress is more than just negative interaction. Having excessive *positive* social interactions, commitments, and responsibilities can also cause stress. For example, in the Holmes and Rahe (1967) Social Readjustment Rating Scale, a test of stress (see Table 7.1), some of the stressful life events (like getting married, achieving a marital reconciliation, or having an outstanding personal achievement) are positive, not negative. Many artistic or musical performers are hospitalized while on tour. Too much of a good thing can be bad for us, too.

House (1986) defines *stress* as what occurs when an individual confronts a situation in which his or her usual modes of behavior or coping are insufficient and the consequences of not adapting are serious. Stress and related problems (like depression and hopelessness) tend to compound until the only perceived resolution may be to escape from life itself through suicide.

The Holmes and Rahe (pronounced "Ray") test in Table 7.1 measures the adjustment time needed for 43 life events. In setting up this scale, Holmes and Rahe asked subjects, "If getting (say) married takes you 50 days to adjust, how many days would these other 42 events take you to adjust?" These average adjustment days are listed after each of the life events in Table 7.1 (50 for marriage and so on). Then, armed with average life change event values, other subjects were asked to circle all the life events they experienced in the last calendar year before taking the stress test. The circled scores were added up to give a summary stress number. Readers may wish to pause and actually take the test themselves. The summary score should be between 0 and 300+. Holmes and Rahe defined a minor life crisis as any summated score of 150 total life change units, and a major life crisis as 300+ points.

Holmes and Rahe went on to argue that the greater the summated score of life change units, the more vulnerable a person would be to having an illness or injury in the same prior 12 months as the stress. Stress is almost always significantly associated with recent illnesses and injuries.

To extend this argument to suicide (which Holmes and Rahe did not), the greater the summated stress score, the greater the vulnerability to suicide attempts or completions. The higher the stress test score, the more likely suicidality is when combined with diathetic factors. Note that most individuals do not respond to stress or negative life events by suiciding. Those who do tend to have diathetic vulnerabilities and are repeatedly stressed. Motto (1992) claims that everyone has a pain threshold (lower for vulnerable individuals) beyond which stress becomes intolerable.

In a study by Dean et al. (1996), negative life events were significantly positively associated with depression ($r = .48$), hopelessness (.25), and suicide ideation (.30). Scores on Linehan et al.'s (1983) Reasons for Living Inventory were significantly negatively correlated with suicide ideation (–.64).

"Perceived burdensomeness" is a special kind of negative interaction. For example, among the Yuit of St. Lawrence Island (Leighton & Hughes, 1955), a nomadic hunting and gathering society, family members who could no longer hunt or travel (often elderly, infirm males) could become a burden to the well-being or even survival of their families. If such an infirmed family member asked his relatives three times to kill him (a kind of altruistic suicide), then the family was morally obligated to honor his wish by shooting him (usually a man's wife did this) or hanging him (the entire family usually did this). The man would turn his parka inside out first (Maris, 1981).

In speaking of perceived burdensomeness, both Joiner (2005) and I (Maris et al., 1992) cite the work of quantitative evolutionary biologist Denys de Catanzaro (1992). de Catanzaro (1992, p. 609) has argued for what he calls the "Ψ [psi] coefficient," which indicates an individual's residual capacity to promote inclusive fitness or representation of his or her genes in subsequent generations. A negative Ψ value means that the individual's continued existence is a detriment to his or

TABLE 7.1. Holmes and Rahe Stress Test (Social Readjustment Rating Scale)

Rank	Life event	Mean value of life change units
1	Death of a spouse	100
2	Divorce	73
3	Marital separation	65
4	Jail term	63
5	Death of a close family member	63
6	Personal injury or illness	53
7	Marriage	50
8	Fired at work	47
9	Marital reconciliation	45
10	Retirement	45
11	Change in health of family member	44
12	Pregnancy	39
13	Sex difficulties	39
14	Gain of new family member	39
15	Business readjustment	39
16	Change in financial state	38
17	Death of close friend	37
18	Change to different line of work	36
19	Change in number of arguments with spouse	35
20	Mortgage over $100,000	31
21	Foreclosure on mortgage or loan	30
22	Change in responsibilities at work	29
23	Son or daughter leaving home	29
24	Trouble with in-laws	29
25	Outstanding personal achievement	28
26	Wife begin or stop work	26
27	Begin or end school	26
28	Change in living conditions	25
29	Revision of personal habits	24
30	Trouble with boss	23
31	Change in work hours or conditions	20
32	Change in residence	20
33	Change in schools	20
34	Change in recreation	19
35	Change in church activities	19
36	Change in social activities	18
37	Mortgage or loan less than $100,000	17
38	Change in sleeping habits	16
39	Change in number of family get-togethers	15
40	Change in eating habits	15
41	Vacation	13
42	Christmas	12
43	Minor violations of the law	11

Note. To get your own stress score, just circle all the numbers that apply to you in the last year and add them up. If you are not married, you may need to consider dating relationships. And you may want to adjust the $100,000 value in items 20 and 37 upward, since mortgages for that amount are fairly common nowadays.

Source: Holmes and Rahe (1967, p. 216). Reprinted with permission.

her inclusive fitness. Thus the lower the Ψ score, the more likely suicide or self-destruction becomes.

Joiner (2005) found that the suicide notes of those who actually died had more themes of perceived burdensomeness in them than the notes of attempters who didn't die had, and that perceived burdensomeness predicted the use of a more lethal method to attempt. Rightly or wrongly, suicides tend to see themselves in very negative terms. Suicidal children often see themselves as expendable.

de Catanzaro (1992), in fact, has claimed that some suicides could produce an adaptive advantage for their significant others. Think about typical older suicides. They are less likely to have new or young children to nurture or support. Their existing children (each of whom has 50% of each parent's genes) are themselves less in need of support and nurturance from their aging parents. With advanced aging and increasing infirmity, the parents can become a hardship for the surviving kin to care for. In effect, aged parents can be a burden for their children. Biologically speaking, the parents' genes might be better off if the parents died. This sounds harsh and cold, but it follows from de Catanzaro's thesis.

Joiner (2005) concluded that most suicides are mistaken when they view themselves as burdens. Joiner's father was a suicide, as was my own father—who abandoned me, my sister, and my mother (his wife), went off to Alaska, and drank himself to death at age 43. However, one way of viewing my father's death is similar to de Catanzaro's views: When my uncle got my dad's death certificate, my mom was able to receive Social Security benefits, and we got our first television set. I did not think of my dad as a burden, but the Social Security monies were indeed a newfound benefit; if he had not killed himself, we would never have gotten them (or at least not that soon).

Contagion, Imitation, Suicide Clusters, and Suicide Pacts

The vast majority of all suicides are committed by only one person, usually in the privacy of the home. The event is asocial, in the sense that no one else is there is most cases. However, there can be exceptions: witnessed suicides, perhaps 1–2% of all suicides (McDowell et al., 1994); suicide pacts, probably fewer than 1% of suicides; cluster suicides, usually in young people; copycat or imitation suicides, like those following Marilyn Monroe's suicide (cf. Summers, 1985); and even some mass suicides like Jonestown, which involved as many as 914 suicides (Chapter 17 considers mass suicides). These rare cases of multiple suicide victims raise questions about their social relations. How did one suicidal individual persuade, coerce, or otherwise influence others to suicide as well?

Suicide Contagion and Imitation

Copying another's suicide seems odd, even preposterous. Why throw away a perfectly good life, just because someone else did or is about to do? Common sense tells us that people who copy other suicides are peculiar in some way, vulnerable, or "prepped" to imitate other suicides.

Copying a suicide in part is determined by cultural surroundings and expectations. When I lived in Vienna, Austria, themes of death and suicide seemed to be everywhere. For example, when I went to the Opera, the characters frequently killed themselves. On the Ringstrasse, there was a petting museum with dead baby animals, of all things. At the zoo, the attendants clubbed live rabbits and tossed them to vultures as the paying customers and their kids watched. It may be a lot easier to consider suicide when cultural surroundings such as these seem to suggest a "death culture"—and indeed, even though Austria is mainly Roman Catholic (a religion in which suicide was formerly prohibited and is still strongly discouraged), it has a high suicide rate. On the other hand, the Tiv of Nigeria have almost no suicides to copy, and their suicide rate is very low.

Contemporary sociology (see the work of Niederkrotenthaler in Vienna, 2015; Mueller and Abrutyn in Memphis, 2015; and Stack in Detroit, 1987) seems almost obsessed with suicide contagion, imitation, modeling, suggestibility, and so on. This was not always true. Durkheim had little use for contagion. He wrote:

> Contagion [or] imitation never seems to propagate [suicide] so as to effect the social suicide rate. . . . It is inadmissible that a social fact is merely a generalized individual fact. . . . Most untenable of all is that this generalization is due to some blind contagion. . . . Imitation is not an original factor in suicide. (1897/1951, p. 140)

Some roots of the concept of contagion can be traced to public health, epidemiology, and epidemics. *Epidemiology* is the study of the distribution and determinants of a diseases and injuries (here, suicides) in human populations (Mausner & Bahm, 1985; Rothman et al., 2012). An epidemic is an occurrence in a community or region of a group of illnesses of similar nature (here, suicides), clearly in excess of normal expectancy.

Contagion also reminds us of the research on stimulus and response, such as the classical conditioning of Pavlov's dogs, or B. F. Skinner's instrumental or operant conditioning of pigeons in a Skinner box. From this and similar research, we can specify some of the factors in the variation of modeling a stimulus suicide event:

• The more similar the copying individual is to the stimulus suicide, the more likely copying is. For example, Table 7.2 shows that in the month (especially the 7–10 days) after the suicide of Marilyn Monroe on August 6, 1962, the U.S. suicide rate rose 12% over the control years at the same time. We would expect that the rise in copied suicides would be highest in age 30-something white females (who were more like Monroe).

• Table 7.2 also shows that there is a dose–response relationship: The greater the exposure to the stimulus suicide story, the greater the probability of copying. The more days Monroe's suicide story ran on the front page of *The New York Times,* for instance, the greater the copycat response. Note that in the cases of possible suicides who may copy, publicity and First Amendment rights of free speech can conflict with suicide prevention considerations.

• The more the stimulus suicide is glorified, romanticized, praised, or otherwise depicted favorably, the more likely the copying is. After World War II, for example, defeated Japanese officers were expected to suicide in response to the shame of defeat in battle, and often did so *en masse*. It was considered heroic and dignified and culturally appropriate for the officers to apologize through suicide to the enlisted men for failing them and the Empire.

• Young people and teenagers are more likely to imitate or copy a stimulus suicide. Most studies show about a 6–7% rise in teen suicides after a teen suicide stimulus. Only about 2–3% percent of adults copy other suicides. Hallinan (2014) reports that about 5% of teen suicides are the result of contagion.

As discussed earlier, by far the most seminal work on suicide and contagion has been done by Phillips (1974; see Maris et al., 2000). Table 7.2 (from Phillips, 1974, p. 344) demonstrates that, contrary to Durkheim, U.S. suicides rose (by a total of 1,298.5) in the month after front-page coverage in *The New York Times,* especially for the stories of actress Marilyn Monroe and of Stephen Ward, a prominent figure in the 1963 Profumo scandal in Great Britain. Phillips found the suggestibility effect to be significant but small (about 2.5%). Wasserman (1984) only found a contagion effect among celebrity suicides. Stack (1987) also found that the suicide imitation effect held only for entertainers and celebrities, not for artists, villains, or the economic elite.

Finally, Gould and Shaffer (1986) found a statistically significant increase in teen suicide attempts and completions 2 weeks after the broadcast in the greater New York area of four television movies from October 1984 to February 1985. This was ironic, since the movies were intended to be suicide prevention movies.

Suicide Clusters

Suicide clusters can be defined as three or more linked suicide events in a series, in a common space (like a school or community), and usually in a limited, contiguous time frame (7–10 days, 2 weeks, a month or two, etc.). Maybe 5% of all adolescent suicides occur in clusters (Velting & Gould, 1997). Joiner (2005) has argued that cluster suicides share "assortatively related" suicide risk factors. In other words, the relatedness among the people in the cluster is not random, but is based on shared interests or problems like substance abuse.

One example of a cluster suicide occurred on May 4, 1990, in Sheridan, Arkansas (Maris et al., 2000, p. 253ff). Thomas Smith, age 17, stood up in his American history class, told a girl in his class that he loved her, then pulled a .22 pistol from his pocket and shot himself in the forehead. He died 4 hours later. That evening, between 10 and 11 P.M., a friend of Smith's at Sheridan High School, Thomas Chidester, 19, shot himself in the head with a .45 and died immediately. The next day, Jerry McCool, a classmate of Smith and Chidester, shot himself at home with a .22. Earlier (March 28, 1990), Ronald Wilkinson had shot himself. So, in Sheridan, there were four related suicidal deaths in 2 months—three of them in just 2 days.

TABLE 7.2. Rise in the Number of U.S. Suicides after Suicide Stories Were Publicized on the Front Page of *The New York Times*, 1948–1967

Name of publicized suicide	Date of suicide story	Observed no. of suicides in mo. after suicide story	Expected no. of suicides in mo. after suicide story	Rise in no. of U.S. suicides after suicide story
Lockridge (author)	Mar. 8, 1948	1,510	1,521.5	–11.5
Landis (film star)	July 6, 1948	1,482	1,457.5	24.5
Brooks (financier)	Aug. 28, 1948	1,250	1,350	–100.0
Holt (betrayed husband)	Mar. 10, 1949	1,583	1,521.5	61.5
Forrestal (ex-secretary of defense)	May 22, 1949	1,549	1,493.5	55.5
Baker (professor)	Apr. 26, 1950	1,600	1,493.5	106.5
Lang (police witness)	Apr. 20, 1951	1,423	1,519.5	–96.5
Soule (professor)	Aug. 4, 1951	1,321	1,342	–21.0
Adamic (writer)	Sept. 5, 1951	1,276	1,258.5	17.5
Stengel (N.J. police chief)	Oct. 7, 1951	1,407	1,296.5	110.5
Feller (U.N. official)	Nov. 15, 1951	1,207	1,229	–22.0
LaFollette (senator)	Feb. 25, 1953	1,435	1,412	23.0
Armstrong (inventor of FM radio)	Feb. 2, 1954	1,240	1,227	13.0
Hunt (senator)	June 20, 1954	1,458	1,368.5	89.5
Vargas (Brazilian president)	Aug. 25, 1954	1,357	1,321.5	35.5
Norman (Canadian ambassador)	Apr. 5, 1957	1,511	1,649.5	–138.5
Young (financier)	Jan. 26, 1958	1,361	1,352	9.0
Schupler (N.Y.C. councilman)	May 3, 1958	1,672	1,587	85.0
Quiggle (admiral)	July 25, 1958	1,519	1,451	8.0
Zwillman (underworld leader)	Feb. 27, 1959	1,707	1,609	98.0
Bang-Jensen (U.N. diplomat)	Nov. 27, 1959	1,477	1,423	54.0
Smith (police chief)	Mar. 20, 1960	1,669	1,609	60.0
Gedik (Turkish minister)	May 31, 1960	1,568	1,628.5	–60.5
Monroe (film star)	Aug. 6, 1962	1,838	1,640.5	197.5
Ward (implicated in Profumo affair)	Aug. 4, 1963	1,801	1,640.5	160.5
Heyde & Tillman (Nazi officials)	Feb. 14, 1964	1,647	1,584.5	62.5
Lord (N.J. party chief)	June 17, 1965	1,801	1,743	58.0
Burros (KKK leader)	Nov. 1, 1965	1,710	1,652	58.0
Mott (American in Russian jail)	Jan. 22, 1966	1,757	1,717	40.0
Pike (son of Bishop Pike)	Feb. 5, 1966	1,620	1,567.5	52.5
Kravchenko (Russian defector)	Feb. 26, 1966	1,921	1,853	68.0
LoJui-Ching (Chinese army leader)	Jan. 21, 1967	1,821	1,717	104.0
Amer (Egyptian field marshal)	Sept. 16, 1967	1,770	1,733.5	36.5
Total				1,298.5

Source: David P. Phillips, "The Influence of Suggestion on Suicide: Substantive and Theoretical Implications of the Werther Effect," *American Sociological Review*, Vol. 39, No. 3 (Jun., 1974), Table 1, pp. 344. Reprinted with permission.

In March 1987, there was a much-publicized suicide cluster incident of four teenagers (two boys and two girls) in Bergenfield, New Jersey. They all poisoned themselves in a garage with carbon monoxide. All four had signed a suicide note on a paper bag, saying that they wanted a common wake and burial. One of the four, Thomas Rizzo, had witnessed the death of James Majors, who died in September 1986 after falling or jumping off Englewood Cliffs. Majors had been dating Lisa Burress, one of the four cluster suicides.

Joiner (2005) has mentioned some other cluster suicides. For example, in London in a psychiatric hospital (Haw, 1994), there were 14 suicides in just 12 months. There was also a website that promoted suicide and spawned about 24 suicides. Joiner also wonders whether Nirvana musician Kurt Cobain's suicide was copied. Jobes et al. (1996) says no, as would Gould and Shaffer (1986). More recently, there was concern that the suicide of comedian Robin Williams in August 2014 would be copied.

Suicide Pacts

A *suicide pact* often involves older spouses or partners who voluntarily agree to die together, rather than having one partner (usually the female, in a heterosexual couple) continue to live after the other partner suicides. In these suicide pacts, the wishes of the male partner seem to prevail, even if the female is young and healthy.

One such suicide pact was that of Arthur Koestler (author of *Darkness at Noon*; Koestler, 1940) and his (third) wife, Cynthia Jeffries, in March 1983. Koestler was vice-president of the Voluntary Euthanasia Society in London. (See Chapter 21, Case 21.6; see also Mazower, 2000, who notes the curious possible relationship of Koestler's hypersexuality and suicide.) After Koestler contracted Parkinson's disease and leukemia, he and his wife overdosed on barbiturates. He was 78 and ill, but she was only 55 and healthy.

A variation of the suicide pact theme occurs in the classical Hindu ritual of *sati* or *suttee,* in which a deceased husband's wife is expected to be burned alive on his funeral pyre after he dies (Maris et al., 2000; see Chapter 18, Figure 18.4). This is a death or suicide pact between husband and wife, as well as a cultural obligation or expectation of the wife to commit suicide.

Another interesting suicide pact involved the parents of Derek Humphry's second wife, Anne Wickett. Humphry wrote the best-seller *Final Exit* (Humphry, 1991/1996) and founded the Hemlock Society, first in Great Britain and then later in the United States. Wickett's parents were the first two members of the Hemlock Society. In her book *Double Exit,* Wickett (1989) describes the suicide pact of her father (age 92) and mother (age 78), both of whom suffered from serious illnesses with poor prognoses. Wickett herself later suicided alone, wandering off in the woods of Eugene, Oregon on her horse. Humphry was soundly criticized for abandoning her when she got breast cancer. He had helped his first wife die by suicide (as described in *Jean's Way;* Humphry, 2003) after she got breast cancer.

Suicide pacts are fairly common in traditional Japan. A Yukio Mishima (1960/2012) short story, "Patriotism," involves a young couple having passionate sex (again, note the strange sex-and-suicide connection), and then the man stabbing his partner and committing *seppuku*. Mishima in fact later had himself beheaded in a pact with one of his officers after his private army took over a Japanese military base. Mishima chided the soldiers at the base for not being proper Samurais. However, suicide pacts are rare in the United States (Fishbain et al., 1984). In Dade County, Florida, for instance, there were only 20 suicide pacts out of 5,895 suicides over 25 years.

Work, Occupation, Socioeconomic Status, Mobility, and Unemployment

In earlier chapters I have discussed the importance of work, especially for men like Ernest Hemingway, Percy Bridgman, and George Eastman (see the 10th suicide risk factor in Chapter 4, Table 4.1; see also Maris, 1981). We all need some meaningful activity most days to impart structure and purpose to our lives. One of the first questions people ask at social events is "What do you do?" Most people do not have endowments and need to work to pay the bills.

Work is about more than money. Not being able to get a job or the right job, being demoted, losing a job, or even retiring can create major stress and challenges to one's self-image. This is not to claim that all work or too much work is good, suicidologically speaking. Remember the case of Bob Fosse, considered in Chapter 6. Indeed, some jobs (like dentistry) can increase suicide risk for up to six times the norm for all workers. Take a look at the article "Suicide within the Dental Profession" (Maris, 2010). Even though work discourages suicide, some work nevertheless is associated with a higher suicide risk (Lee et al., 2018).

Occupation and Suicide

Can some jobs or professions increase your suicide risk? Yes, but remember that Chapter 2's theory of suicide is multifactorial. One suicide risk factor seldom accounts for much variance in suicide outcome. For example, even the vast majority (85–90%) of hospitalized depressed patients die natural deaths. When jobs are associated with elevated suicide risk, the risk is normally small and due to other variables connected with the job (access to guns or opiates, alcohol abuse, divorce, etc.), and not the job itself.

Nonetheless, the popular media and the internet never seem to tire of talking about jobs with the highest suicide rates. For example, Pamela Kulbarsh (2014) asks, "Who is likely to take their own life?" Her rank-ordered answers are (1) physicians, (2) dentists, (3) finance workers, (4) lawyers, and (5) police officers. For women, being a police officer is the third riskiest occupation for suicide. Being a female physician is also near the top, and for black men, being a police officer is the riskiest occupation for suicide (2.55).

The *New Health Guide* (July 14, 2015) has ranked professions by suicide risk as follows:

Profession	More likely to suicide than average
1. Physicians	1.87
2. Dentists	1.67
3. Veterinarians	1.54
4. Finance workers	1.51
5. Heavy-construction workers	1.46
6. Lawyers	1.33
7. Farm managers	1.32
8. Pharmacists	1.29

In regard to farm managers, you may want to take a look at a movie I helped make on suicides in this group ("Green Blood, Red Tears," 1995). Excerpts from this film can be found on a page of my website (*www.suicideexpert.com/videos*).

Yet another source on suicide and occupations is a paper by Hope Tiesman and colleagues (2015) on workplace suicides. Tiesman et al. found that the three occupations with the highest suicide rates were (1) police officers (5.3 per million suicide risk); (2) those working in farming, fishing, and forestry (5.1); and (3) installation and repair technicians (e.g., auto mechanics; 3.3). A more detailed list of suicide rate risk for occupations can be found in Roberts et al. (2013).

Stack's (2000) occupational relative suicide risk data are presented in Table 7.3. Stack has told me (personal communication, 2015) that more recent data (after 1990) are not readily available for the U.S., but that there are more recent Danish and U.K. data. Stack's occupations with the highest relative suicide risk are as follows:

1. Dentists (4.45)
2. Artists (2.12)
3. Carpenters (2.00)
4. Doctors (1.94), especially female physicians.

His occupations with the lowest risk are these:

1. Elementary school teachers (–0.44)
2. Postal workers (–0.38)
3. Clerks (–0.25)
4. Executives and managers (–0.03)
5. Nurses (–0.01)

An article for *Newsweek* (Peterson, 1997) examined the suicide of John Curtis, Jr., the chief executive officer (CEO) for Luby's Cafeterias. He stabbed himself to death just before a board meeting in which he had to announce a profit margin decline and lay off 1% of Luby's workforce nationwide. At the time, I commented that with CEOs, no one is "guarding the guardians." If a CEO gets depressed and anxious, who is going to tell him or her to get treatment?

**TABLE 7.3. Relative Risk Ratios of Suicide
for Selected Occupations, Relative to the Working-Age
Population in 21 States: United States, 1990**

Occupation	Relative risk ratio
Managerial/professional	
Executives/managers	−0.03
Doctors	1.94*
Dentists	4.45*
Lawyers	1.44
Professors	1.13
Accountants	1.17
Engineers	1.21
Mathematicians and scientists	1.85*
Artists	2.12*
Nurses	−0.01
Social workers	1.41
Elementary school teachers	−0.44*
Clerical	
Bookkeepers	−0.28
Clerks	−0.25*
Postal workers	−0.38*
Service	
Police	−0.07
Private security	1.14
Cooks	−0.16
Bartenders	1.25
Agricultural and extractive	
Farmers	0.08
Farm workers	1.13
Miners	1.33*
Skilled manual	
Machinists	1.63*
Auto mechanics	1.41*
Electricians	1.32*
Plumbers	1.63*
Carpenters	2.00*
Semi-/unskilled manual	
Welders	1.46*
Laborers	1.31*
Truck drivers (heavy equipment)	1.09

Note. More recent occupational suicide risk data are not available in the United States.

*$p < .05$.

Source: Stack (2000). Copyright © 2000 The Guilford Press.
Reprinted with permission.

Socioeconomic Status and Suicide

What if we look not at jobs and suicide, but at socioeconomic status (SES) and suicide (Maris et al., 2000, pp. 194–197; Maris, 1981, pp. 136–169)? Durkheim argued that suicide rates should be highest at upper levels of SES, since persons at these levels have fewer social constraints, less social integration, and more anomie and egoism. But Durkheim was wrong (Stack, 2000, p. 194). Most data show that as one goes up the SES ladder, suicide rates tend to fall; that is, SES and suicide rates overall have an inverse or negative relationship.

When I examined occupational SES in my Chicago survey (Maris, 1981), it was clear that suicide rates in lower-SES occupations were higher than those in the middle- and upper-SES occupations. For example, the average rate for lower-SES laborers was 50.6 per 100,000, for middle-level service workers was 46.4, and for clerical workers was 13.0. The rate for professional and technical workers was 14.8 per 100,000.

Stack (2000) reported that the suicide rate for laborers was 94.4 per 100,000, eight times the national average. The reasons for this inverse relationship are unclear. Stack opines that it might be due to higher divorce rates in lower-SES groups. It could also be a product of poverty and increased alcohol abuse.

Social Mobility

What if the more pertinent issue in regard to suicide is not SES per se, but rather movement or mobility among SES levels (Maris, 1969)? Mobility can be intergenerational (e.g., father to son), intragenerational (e.g., son's or daughter's first to last SES), or geographic (such as changing jobs or regions).

Earlier research (Porterfield & Gibbs, 1960; see Maris et al., 2000, pp. 210–213) found that suicides had twice the downward intragenerational mobility of nonsuicidal controls. Breed (1963) said that 53% of suicides were downwardly mobile. Shepherd and Barraclough (1980) claimed that suicides had more unemployment, more job changes, and more work absences that non-suicides did.

When I studied SES changes in Chicago (Maris, 1981), I did not find much, if any, downward intergenerational mobility for suicides themselves. As for intragenerational mobility, I discovered three patterns (looking at first job, last job minus 5 years, and last job): (1) no changes (for 33% of suicides); (2) downward mobility, then up (18%); and (3) upward mobility, then plateauing (12%). Suicides were more likely than nonsuicides to have no SES change.

The Chicago suicides tended to have erratic work histories, more unemployment, and more SES stagnation than the nonsuicides. However, overall, work mobility did not seem to contribute much to suicide outcome. The SES data were thus inconclusive as to their influence on suicide.

Unemployment

If work protects against suicide, then not working ought to aggravate the suicide rate (see Lee et al., 2018). Unemployment not only erodes personal income; it also

reduces self-esteem, increases anxiety and poor mental health, increases hopelessness, adds to marital strain, and increases alcohol abuse—not just for unemployed
individuals, but also for their families and communities, if there is a high rate of
general unemployment.

Research in New Orleans (Breed, 1963) found that about one-third (33%) of
suicides were unemployed at the time of death, versus just 5% of nonsuicidal controls. Platt (1984) said that the suicide rate for the unemployed in the United Kingdom was 78.4 per 100,000, compared to 14.1 for the general population. In Austria,
Schony and Grausgruber (1987) claimed that the suicide rate for the unemployed
were 98.3 per 100,000, versus 25 in the general population. Cullen and Hodgetts
(2001) said that 50% of suicides had job problems, compared to 18% of nonsuicides.

One impressive study (Nordt et al., 2015) discovered that nearly 31,250 suicides
each year in 63 WHO countries resulted from or were associated with people's
being unemployed. The rise in the suicide rate lagged 6 months behind the rise in
unemployment. The same study also showed that after financial austerity measures
were implemented in Greece in 2012, the country had the highest months of suicide
in 30 years.

The next chapter, Chapter 8, is a reminder that the United States is not the center of the suicidological universe. To hope to understand suicide, we must not just
focus on the suicide of older white males in the West. Suicide and self-destruction
vary by race, gender, culture, and ethnicity.

CHAPTER 8

International Variation, Ethnicity, and Race in Suicide

One has to be constantly on guard against suicidological ethnocentrism. The United States only has 5–6% of the world's suicides, but China and India together have 68%. The world is only 32% Christian and 28% white. There are about 800,000 suicides worldwide each year, but only 41,149 of them occurred in the United States in a recent year (2013).
    —RONALD W. MARIS, summarizing World Health Organization (WHO) and other data

One glance at the WHO world map in Chapter 3 (Figure 3.3) should assure us that any science of suicidal behaviors based solely on U.S. suicides is seriously deficient. The WHO (2012b, 2015c) estimates that there are about 800,000 suicides worldwide each year. This means that the roughly 44,193 annual (2015) suicides in the U.S. make up only about 6% of the world's suicides. In Table 8.1, the suicide rates for 38 of 170 countries are ranked and listed for both males and females. The epigraph to this chapter argues that international variation in suicide rates is an important component of an empirically grounded suicidology.

Suicide varies by race, ethnicity, culture, and religion (among other factors). In this chapter, the focus is on international variation, ethnicity, and race in suicide rates; Chapter 17 examines culture and religion. However, this division is arbitrary. Some overlap with culture and religion in the current chapter is unavoidable—for example, in discussing suicides in Muslim or Roman Catholic countries.

One of the goals of this chapter is to avoid suicidological ethnocentrism and myopia. Although suicides share some traits and states worldwide, there is also considerable international variation. For example, in Russia and the United States the focus is on older white males, who have the highest suicide rates; but in China and India the focus shifts to younger females, who have the highest rates there. Most likely one explanation of suicide does not fit all. Given the space limitations, some countries are not discussed in this chapter and are not included in Table 8.1. To find more information on international suicide variation, take a look at Wasserman

TABLE 8.1. Suicide Rates for 40 Selected World Countries

Rank	Country	Both sexes	Male rank	Males	Female rank	Females
1	**Guyana**[a]	44.2	1	70.8	1	22.1
2	**South Korea**	28.9	5	41.7	5	18.0
3	**Sri Lanka**	28.8	3	46.4	7	12.8
4	**Lithuania**	28.2	2	51.0	29	8.4
5	**Suriname**	27.8	4	44.5	11	11.9
6	**Mozambique**	27.4	8	34.2	2	21.1
7	**Tanzania**	24.9	13	31.6	4	18.3
7	**Nepal**	24.9	17	30.1	3	20.0
9	**Kazakhstan**	23.9	6	40.6	21	9.3
11	India	21.1	22	25.8	6	16.4
14	Russia	19.3	7	35.1	46	6.2
16	Hungary	19.1	12	32.4	34	7.4
17	Japan	18.5	20	26.9	17	10.1
21	Sudan	17.2	33	23.0	12	11.5
24	Poland	16.6	15	30.5	98	3.8
27	Kenya	16.2	26	24.4	29	8.4
33	Finland	14.8	34	22.2	32	7.5
50	United States	12.1	46	19.4	61	5.2
54	Austria	11.5	53	18.2	54	5.4
56	Cuba	11.4	50	18.5	78	4.5
58	Sweden	11.1	63	16.2	48	6.1
63	Australia	10.6	65	16.1	61	5.2
70	Canada	9.8	70	14.9	73	4.8
77	Germany	9.2	72	14.5	89	4.1
81	Norway	9.1	84	13.0	61	5.2
94	China	7.8	128	7.1	24	8.7
105	United Kingdom	6.2	101	9.8	119	2.6
110	Israel	5.9	101	9.8	127	2.1
128	Italy	4.7	121	7.6	137	1.9
137	Mexico	4.2	128	7.1	141	1.7
144	United Arab Emirates	3.2	155	3.9	141	1.7
150	Philippines	2.9	146	4.8	154	1.2
153	Haiti	2.8	159	3.3	123	2.4
158	Bahamas	2.3	154	3.6	151	1.3
162	Libya	1.8	163	2.2	148	1.4
163	Egypt	1.7	160	2.4	154	1.2
163	Iraq	1.7	166	1.2	132	2.1
166	Jamaica	1.2	165	1.8	164	0.7
170	Syria	0.4	170	0.7	170	0.2
170	Saudi Arabia	0.4	171	0.6	170	0.2

Note. Rates are per 100,000 population. Countries ranked in the top 10 are given in boldface. A total of 172 countries were ranked.

[a]Other sources list Greenland as number 1 (83.0 for both sexes, 116.9 for males, 45.0 for females).

Source: World Health Organization (WHO) (2015c). Data in public domain.

and Wasserman's (2009) encyclopedic suicidology textbook, which examines suicide in a great many other countries.

Some of the countries with high, moderate, and low suicide rates, in descending order, are as follows:

High suicide rates (18+ per 100,000)	Greenland, Guyana, South Korea, Sri Lanka, Lithuania, Mozambique, Tanzania, Kazakhstan, India, Russia, Hungary, Japan
Moderate suicide rates (7.8–13 per 100,000)	United States, Austria, Cuba, Sweden, Australia, Canada, Germany, China
Low suicide rates (<4.3 per 100,000)	Mexico, United Arab Emirates, Philippines, Haiti, Bahamas, Libya, Egypt, Iraq, Jamaica, Syria, Saudi Arabia

A huge word of caution is in order in considering international variation in suicide, however. Durkheim (1897/1951) said, "These being the facts, what is their explanation?" It is not scientifically sound to go around trying to explain "facts" that may not even be true and that are certainly not clear. For example, why was Greenland's suicide rate ranked first in 2009, but not even listed in the WHO (2012b) data? Probably there were no reliable data for Greenland in 2009, but they were reported anyway.

Can we even believe the high suicide rates in east and south central Africa—South Sudan, Mozambique, Kenya, Tanzania, Zambia? I asked David Lester, past president of the International Association for Suicide Prevention (IASP), that question. His reply was this: "I doubt that those nations report mortality statistics. They are typically estimated. I mean, really, Sudan knows its suicide rate?" I posed the same question to sociologist Steven Stack. His answer was this: "I believe that many of the approximately 180 nations with 'data' are actually estimated based on neighboring countries, GNP, etc. Hard data points are not available for most of these nations."

Having stated this important *caveat emptor,* I now speculate on some of the data. For example, consider Greenland. It has only 50,000 people (be careful of small numbers, from which unsound conclusions are often drawn), is one of the least populated countries in the world, and relies heavily on coastal fishing and hunting industries. Before 1930 Greenland had virtually no suicides, but presumably by 1986 it had a suicide rate of 83 per 100,000. Most Greenland suicides are committed by teenagers and young adults, not by the typical older adults. Some speculate that weather-related disruption of diurnal rhythms in the winter cause lower brain serotonin, sleeplessness, and depression, but most of Greenland's suicides occur in the summer months. It is hard to know exactly what is happening in Greenland, if anything noteworthy.

Suriname and Guyana, both among the top five countries in suicide rates in Table 8.1, are physically contiguous coastal countries in northeastern South America. Guyana is infamous for the 900+ mass suicides in Jonestown. A lot of suicide in Suriname and Guyana involves the hardships of life in poor rural areas and the use of farm pesticides to attempt suicide (Graafsma et al., 2006). There is also con-siderable alcohol abuse. In a recent year, there were only 10 psychiatrists in all of Guyana.

Sri Lanka, also among the top five countries listed in Table 8.1, is an island country off the coast of India. It too has high rates of poverty, debt burdens, jobless-ness, and alcoholism rates.

In the remainder of this chapter, I investigate several groupings of countries that have more reliable and valid suicide data, like South Korea, Russia, Lithuania, India, one Muslim country, and one Catholic country, as well as a few African coun-tries with questionable data, to try to determine why their suicide rates are high or low.

Concepts of Ethnicity, Race, and Culture

Ethnicity refers to any group that can be set off by national origin or religion. Eth-nicity usually connotes national origin and language variations. In any given coun-try, there can be many different ethnic groups.

Even though I do not say much about race per se and focus instead on ethnicity and culture, it's helpful to offer a definition of *race* at this point. According to the American Sociological Association (n.d.), " 'Race' refers to physical differences that groups and cultures consider socially significant, while 'ethnicity' refers to shared culture, such as language, ancestry, practices, and beliefs." Templeton (2013) states: "Biologically, there are no objective criteria for choosing one adaptive trait over another to define race. . . . Humans have much genetic diversity, but the vast major-ity of this diversity reflects individual uniqueness and not race." Of course, there could be hundreds of races worldwide, depending on which traits one chooses to specify. Anthropologist Marvin Harris (1971; Harris & Johnson, 2006) has argued that it is impossible to set a limit on the number of races that could be identified.

Culture (see Chapter 17) is an acquired way of life of a particular group of people (Harris, 1971, p. 136; Harris & Johnson, 2006). Language is an especially important component of culture. Tylor's (1871) classical definition of culture is this: "a complex whole that includes knowledge, belief, art, morals, law, custom, and any other capabilities and habits acquired by humans as members of society." Finally, a *minority* is any group of people who, because of their physical or cultural character-istics, are singled out for differential and unequal treatment by the majority group in a culture, and who are thus objects of collective discrimination (such as racism). A minority group may actually be a numerical majority (e.g., blacks in South Africa, females in the United States).

Several times I have traveled (sometimes as a WHO Fellow) and lived in coun-tries with high suicide rates for months, in an effort to immerse myself in their cul-tures and daily routines—a kind of suicidological osmosis, if you will. For example, I lived in Vienna, Austria; West Berlin, Germany (in the 1970s, before the Berlin Wall came down); Calgary, Alberta, Canada; and Helsinki, Finland.

Some of these countries tend to have a somber death ambience, if not a sui-cide culture. Among other things, I was struck by the stuffed dead baby animal museum (not really a "petting" museum, but you could touch the animals) on the Ringstrasse in Vienna (mentioned in Chapter 7) and being chastised by the natives to stay off the grass in Peter-Jordan-Strasse Park. In the winter, Helsinki was a land of almost perpetual darkness, Finlandia Vodka, and the manufacture of icebreaker ships. West Berlin had an excessive number of aged widows and widowers. About 80% of the buildings were still scarred with shrapnel from World War II, and the city shared the same somber death culture that I experienced in Austria. Calgary was a boom-and-bust oil city with many suicidogenic anomic factors and a macho, cowboy, gun-oriented mentality.

Russia, Lithuania, and Kazakhstan

Russia

In Table 8.1, Russia's suicide rate is ranked 14th highest in the world overall (see also Chapter 3, Figure 3.3). The Russian male suicide rate exceeds the female rate by 6:1, compared to roughly 4:1 in the United States. There is a Russian male suicide rate excess over U.S. males at all ages. Russian male suicide rates for men in their 50s are almost five times higher than for U.S. men in their 50s.

Most Russian scholars (e.g., Pridemore & Spivak, 2003; Wasserman & Varnik, 2001; Nemtsov, 2003) have argued that alcohol consumption plays a major role in Russian suicides. Notice in Figure 8.1 that a striking change occurred in Russian suicide rates circa 1985. Mikhail Gorbachev, the Soviet Union's final leader, initiated an antialcohol campaign in May–June 1985 as part of *perestroika*. Alcohol prices were increased, and production was cut. The results were less alcohol consumption and a 40% drop in suicide rates in Russia in a year or two (see Figure 8.1).

However, the *perestroika* campaign proved very unpopular (like Prohibition in the United States) and was defunct by October 1988. By the mid-1990s, Russian suicide rates had returned to their 1985 levels or higher (a kind of "challenge–dechallenge–rechallenge" research design). Nemtsov (2003) found that Russian suicides with positive blood alcohol levels at autopsy were highly correlated ($r = .98$) with changes in Russian alcohol consumption as a whole. The number of suicides among sober people did not change much during *perestroika*.

The Russian experience with alcohol seems to parallel the American temperance movement and the ratification in 1919 of the 18th Amendment to the U.S. Constitution (Maris, 1988, p. 326), which restricted the sale of alcohol. (The 18th Amendment was repealed by the 21st Amendment in 1933.) But I have not tried to determine whether Prohibition affected the U.S. suicide rate (and if so, how much).

There have also been large-scale economic, political, and other social changes in Russia that have probably played a part in the hard rebound of the Russian suicide rates in the late 1980s and early 1990s—for example, higher unemployment rates, conversion to capitalism, the fragmentation of central control, and the resulting rise of anomie (Pridemore & Spivak, 2003, p. 144). According to Karl Marx, life was supposed to improve during Communism; thus rising suicide rates could be seen as a failure of Communism. Apparently the Russian government realized this, and from 1974 to 1986 there were no suicide data available in the U.S.S.R.

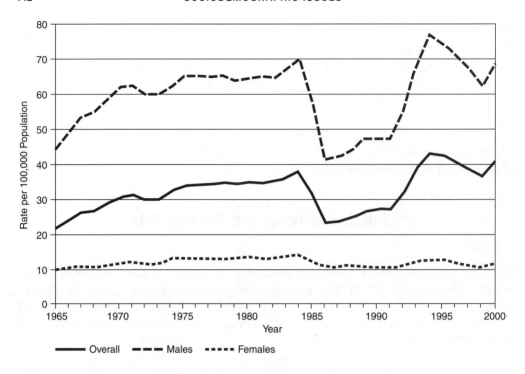

FIGURE 8.1. Suicide rates in Russia, 1965–1999. *Source:* "Patterns of Suicide Mortality in Russia" by W. A. Pridemore and A. L. Spivak, *Suicide and Life-Threatening Behavior,* 33(2), 132–150. Copyright © 2003 by the American Association of Suicidology. Reproduced with permission of John Wiley & Sons, Inc.

Lithuania

Lithuania is on the Baltic Sea, nestled among Latvia, Poland, and Belarus. In 2003 it had a population of about 3.5 million. From 1924 to 1939, in an independent Lithuania, the suicide rate was modest—about 8.1 per 100,000. However, in 1940 Lithuania was occupied by Soviet forces and became part of the Soviet Union (Gailiene, 2004). The next year, Lithuania was occupied by Nazi Germany, and the Nazis remained until early 1945, when the Soviets retook the country. From 1940 to 1953, 33% of the Lithuanian population either was killed by the Soviets (or in other conflicts), was deported to Siberia, or emigrated to other countries. During the Soviet occupation from 1940 to 1984, Lithuania's suicide rates rose 4.5 times, from about 8 to 36 per 100,000.

There was a respite in the increased suicide rates from about 1986 to 1990, with the advent of *perestroika* and its antialcohol campaign. But by 1991 the Lithuanian suicide rate began to rise again, and in 2015 it had the fourth highest suicide rate of any country in the world (Table 8.1). The Lithuanian increase in suicide rates was correlated with the collapse of the Soviet Union and Lithuania's regaining political independence. The pre-Soviet-occupation low suicide rates did not return.

The Lithuanian suicide rate increase was especially marked among rural males, who tended to hang themselves. The most likely general explanations for the high

Lithuanian suicide rates are the long-lasting effects of the Nazi and Soviet occupations (anomie, social and economic disruption, hopelessness, etc.), binge drinking, and an indifferent attitude toward suicide prevention.

Kazakhstan

Kazakhstan is a geographically large country in central Asia. Independent since 1991, it, like Lithuania, had been part of the Soviet Union. Table 8.1 lists its suicide rate as the 9th highest in the world. Suicide by teenagers and young people is a big issue in the country. Kazakhstan has the highest number of recorded suicides among girls ages 15–19, and for boys it is the second highest after Russia. A UNICEF report in 2009 stated that between 1999 and 2009 the number of suicides among young people in the country increased by 23%.

Hungary, Austria, and Germany

For many years, the countries of the old Hapsburg Empire (dissolved in 1918) or contiguous to it had the highest suicide rates in the world (Maris et al., 2000). The capital of that empire was Vienna, Austria. One reason I sought fellowships to go to Vienna and West Berlin was to study their high suicide rates. From 1960 to 2006, Hungary had the world's highest suicide rates. Budapest was the most studied site, although Moksony (1997) also studied 600 Hungarian villages. In 1993, Austria was 10th, Germany 17th, and Poland 20th in the world suicide rankings.

Then something remarkable happened: In 2015 (see Table 8.1), Hungary dropped to 16th (still high but much lower), Austria to 54th, and Germany to 77th in the world suicide rankings. Only Hungary at 16th and Poland at 24th stayed relatively high. And even in Hungary, the suicide rate dropped 46% from 1983 until 2006. The obvious questions are these: Why did these declines occur, and could we use this information to help prevent suicide in other countries?

The best recent study I could find on Hungary's suicide decline was that of Rihmer et al. (2013). Rihmer and colleagues found that employment, low alcohol and tobacco consumption, and treatment of depressive disorder, especially with modern antidepressants (Maris, 2015), were all significantly negatively correlated with the Hungarian suicide rate. That is, the more unemployment, alcohol/tobacco consumption, and lack of treatment of depression, the higher the Hungarian suicide rate. When Moksony (1997) studied Hungarian suicides in the late 1990s, he found that socioeconomic backwardness and a "subculture of suicide" were associated with their high suicide rates.

Austria is somewhat of a suicidological anomaly. It is mainly a Catholic country, and Catholic countries tend to have low suicide rates because of the religion's former proscription (and continuing disapproval) of suicide. However, Austria has a much more aged population than, say, Mexico does. While in Vienna for a year, I studied with Professor Erwin Ringel (see his *Das Leben Wegwerfen?*, Ringel, 1978). Ringel argued that Vienna had a "presuicidal syndrome" that increased its population's suicidal vulnerability and included constriction of thought, aggression turned

inward, and suicidal fantasies that are evident in their operas and the local literature. Farberow (1975) compared Viennese suicides to those in Los Angeles; he
found that Viennese suicides were more likely to use domestic gas to attempt suicide (38%), and that far fewer of the Los Angeles suicides left notes (18%, vs. 46% in
Vienna). In post-World War II Austria, many suicides were older widows who were
alone and socially alienated.

After World War II, Germany also had an aged population, especially elderly
widows. The German character was suicidogenic as well. Some of these suicidogenic traits included inflexibility, rigidity, preoccupation with death, high alcohol
consumption, and depressive tendencies. When Kushner (1989) studied German
immigrants, he found that they had a propensity to high suicide rates. For example,
he found that in New York City, 43% of all suicides were committed by German
nationals. Schmidtke et al. (2004) have continued the research on German suicides
in particular and European suicides in general.

Scandinavia: Norway, Sweden, Denmark, and Finland

Scandinavia has exhibited the same declines in suicide rates that Hungary and Austria have. Whereas Finland, Sweden, and Norway were ranked 7th, 18th, and 21st in
world suicide rates in 1993, by 2015 these rates had declined to 33rd, 58th, and 81st,
respectively. In Hendin's (1964) classic book *Suicide and Scandinavia,* he observed
that Norwegians had lower suicide rates than other Scandinavian countries. That
difference continues today. Hendin attributed the lower Norwegian suicide rate to
a more open expression of anger and less internalization; to Norwegians' not being
as competitive as other Scandinavians, with success and achievement not being
that important; and to alcohol consumption's being regarded more negatively in
Norway. Also, he claimed that Norwegian females were more involved with their
children and less involved with their husbands.

Hendin saw Swedes, on the other hand, as preoccupied with success and
performance. Failure to reach overly ambitious goals led to more depression,
and work was inordinately important. There was early separation from mothers.
Females were often angry over male infidelity and abandonment. Maternal control
of females went well into adulthood, and there was a cultural preoccupation with
death (as evidenced in the films of Ingmar Bergman, such as *The Virgin Spring* and
The Seventh Seal). Danes disciplined their children through guilt, in Hendin's view,
and children were markedly dependent on their parents. There was a high level of
depressive disorder; suicide was not taboo, and there was a fantasy of reunion with
loved ones after death (cf. Østergaard, 2018).

Much of the classical work on Finnish suicides has been done by Ächte and
Lönnqvist (see their work in Farberow, 1975, and elsewhere). According to them,
Finns tend to be industrious and introverted, are often sulky, have drinking habits
associated with violence (especially of vodka), are prone to depressive disorder,
have a masculine ideal of supermen who do not reveal their feelings, have high rates
of violence in general, and experience unfavorable climatic conditions affecting

depression and diurnal rhythms. One might wonder why the Finnish suicide rate has dropped so dramatically, since obviously the weather in Finland did not change much from 1993 to 2015. But perhaps the treatment of depression with antidepressant medications has increased.

Finally, one has to be careful in attributing suicide rates to national character. For one thing, suicides may or may not share in their nation's character. For another, Hendin and Ächte were both psychiatrists and tended to neglect nonpsychiatric variables.

Africa: Mozambique, Tanzania, and Sudan/South Sudan

For many years, the WHO did not list African suicide rates. Presumably there were no data, or at least no reliable data. For example, in 1987 and in 1993 (Maris et al., 2000), no African countries were ranked for suicide rates. Yet in 2012–2015, Mozambique, Tanzania, Sudan, and Kenya all had relatively high suicide rates (see Table 8.1). African suicide is poorly documented and poorly understood (however, see Bohannan, 1960). As noted earlier, often the WHO has only estimates of suicide rates, not hard data and not explanations of the varying rates.

Mozambique

Keeping in mind these caveats about the unreliability of African suicide data, I nevertheless discuss these data for a few African nations, such as Mozambique. In 2011 there were 2,667 suicides in Mozambique, for a suicide rate of 18 per 100,000 and a world suicide rank of 19th. It was ranked 6th in 2015 (see Table 8.1). Yet suicides made up only 0.9% of all deaths in Mozambique (vs. 1.6 % in the United States). By far the leading cause of death was HIV/AIDS, and HIV disease itself is correlated with a higher suicide rate. Most of the east central African countries with high suicide rates have been plagued by civil war, ethnic conflicts, famine, drought, and deadly AIDS epidemics. Note that Hungary, Austria, Germany, and Poland also had high suicide rates in the years after war had ravaged their countries. Mozambique ranks lowest in Africa in per capita gross national product, high in inequality, and low in life expectancy—all suicidogenic factors. The official language is Portuguese, and most of the 24 million people are Bantu.

Tanzania

In 2001 there were 3,420 suicides in Tanzania, and 70% of these were committed by men. Its suicide rate was ranked 7th in the world by the WHO in 2015, as shown in Table 8.1. Most of the recent increase involves youth ages 15–25. Tanzania also has high rates of HIV/AIDS, which (as just noted) increase the suicide rate. In Tanzania there is widespread ignorance of clinical depression, and one typically does not go to doctors or psychiatrists when depressed.

Sudan and South Sudan

Sudan has been racked by civil war since 1955. More than 2.5 million people have been killed, and many more have become refugees. South Sudan became independent of Sudan on July 9, 2011. Due to the constant civil war, weapons are readily available to use for suicide. Suicide is high (the second leading cause of death) in Sudanese young people 15–29 years old. Many young people in east central Africa can easily become hopeless for their future and just opt out of life itself. The most common suicide methods are firearms, hanging, and pesticide ingestion. Sudan has also had many droughts and floods. The Sudan suicide rate ranked 21st in the world in 2015.

In South Sudan, suicide is a criminal offense and thus is likely to be under-reported. South Sudan has about 8–10 million people, of which about 2,000 committed suicide in 2012, roughly twice as many men as women (Koang, 2014). About three-fourths of suicides were in poor or lower-middle income groups. Slavery and the slave trade also have a long history in Sudan.

Asia: Japan, China, India, and South Korea

Asia encompasses many diverse countries, such as China (Fang et al., 2015), Japan, South Korea, Singapore (Loh et al., 2012), Vietnam, Taiwan, the Philippines, Sri Lanka, Burma, Mongolia, Laos, Malaysia, and India, as well as Near Eastern countries like Pakistan, Iraq, and Iran. Given this diversity, Asian suicides are not uniform.

Of the suicide rates for 71 WHO countries in 1987 (Maris et al., 2000), only Japan's was ranked near the top (at 12th); Singapore's was 29th, South Korea's 31st, and Hong Kong's 32nd. In 2015, South Korea had moved way up in the world suicide rankings to 2nd, India to 11th, and Japan to 17th; China was ranked 94th (see Table 8.1).

An important qualification is that some Asian suicide rates do not show as much of a male excess (if any) as those in the West. As we have seen in Chapter 6, the Chinese male-to-female suicide ratio is actually 0.92:1 (i.e., women have higher suicide rates than men). In 2015 (see Table 8.1), the Chinese male suicide rate ranked 128th worldwide, but the Chinese female rate ranked 24th. In general, the male-to-female ratios of suicides are generally lower in Asian societies than in the West: Hong Kong, 1.1:1; Singapore, 1.3:1; Japan, 1.8:1; Taiwan, 1.5:1; India, 1.4:1; the Philippines, 1.5:1; and South Korea, 2.2:1. It is believed that Confucian values (especially in China), which are considered to be the cultural foundation of many Asian societies, may partially explain the suicide risk for young Asian women (however, see Lam, 2014).

Japan

Asian suicides in general, and Japanese suicides in particular, tend to have more of what Durkheim called "altruistic" characteristics. That is, they tend to result from "insufficient individuation," moral obligations, duty, or self-sacrifice, such as in the Japanese cultural traditions of *hara-kiri* or the *kamikaze* pilots of World War II. My uncle was a B-29 pilot in World War II and took pictures of Japanese officers committing *hara-kiri* in front of their enlisted men for the shame of losing the war.

In other cases, suicides tend to be what Durkheim called "anomic." Japanese suicides are often the result of intense competition, high expectations, rigid and unrealistic conceptualizations, rapid social change, or sudden deregulation. In Japan suicide is permissible or even appropriate in some circumstances, as just noted (*hara-kiri*).

I add a few words here about the exhibitionistic, ritual suicide of Yukio Mishima (for a detailed case presentation, see Maris et al., 2000). Mishima was a famous Japanese novelist and playwright who expected to win the Nobel Prize in Literature in 1967 or 1968 (it was in fact won by fellow countryman Yasunari Kawabata in 1968). As a child, Mishima was raised primarily by his grandmother, who dressed and treated him as a girl. He was physically frail and led a protected life, mainly indoors. As an adult, Mishima was homosexual and a fierce bodybuilder, a champion of Samurai warriors, and a devotee of Emperor worship. He became a celebrated movie actor, made millions of dollars, and even created his own private army. Mishima believed that one should die in the prime of life (his own death occurred when he was 45). On November 11, 1970, Mishima and a few members of his private army captured a Japanese general and forced him to assemble his troops; then Mishima dropped leaflets and lectured the troops on Samurai values, urging them to overthrow the government. Finally, he committed *hara-kiri* in front of the troops before having himself beheaded with a sword by one of his own lieutenants.

China

In 2010, China and India, with their massive populations, had averages of approximately 300,000 and 187,000 suicides, respectively per year. China's rate was 7.8 per 100,000; India had a rate of 21.1 per 100,000. Their combined total of suicides, 487,000 in 2010, represented about 60% of the world's suicides (J. Zhang, personal communication, July 31, 2015). We should also remember that the majority of Asia's (and the world's) population is Buddhist, Hindu, or Muslim, not Christian.

I have noted above that in Asian countries, there is often greater parity of male and female suicide rates than is found in the West. In an influential *Lancet* article, Phillips et al. (2002) claimed that female Chinese suicide rates were 25% higher than those of males. Table 8.1 indicates that in 2015 they were actually 80% higher, although the overall rate has dropped. Much of the female–male differential is explained by very high rural Chinese female suicide rates at young ages (see Box 8.1). Chinese suicide rates among young rural women were 66% higher than among young rural men (Phillips et al., 2002). In fact, Phillips et al. argued that 56% of all female suicides in the world are from China.

Of course, the big question is this: Why the high rate in this particular group? Unfortunately, we lack good Chinese individual suicide data. Phillips et al. contend

BOX 8.1. Suicide and Chinese Rural Young Women

Suicide rates in China are now relatively low, but they used to be among the highest in the world. A study published in 2002 reported suicide as the fifth leading cause of death, with a mean annual rate of 23 per 100,000, for a total of 287,000 suicide deaths per year (3.6% of all deaths) in China. By 2012, however, China ranked 94th in suicides out of 170 countries. Why were they so high, and why did they fall?

The demographic pattern of suicide in China was different from that reported in Western countries. China had rural rates two- to threefold greater than the urban rates, and female rates higher than the male rates. In the West, rates in urban and rural areas are roughly equivalent, and rates of suicide in men are two- to fourfold higher than the rates in women. The age pattern of Chinese suicide was generally a bimodal one with peaks in young adulthood and among the elderly. Among young adults 15–34 years of age, suicide was the leading cause of death, accounting for 19% of all deaths in this age group. With a large population base in rural areas of China, rural young female suicides made a substantial contribution to the then-high rate of suicide and the total number of suicides in China. Reduction of the Chinese rural young female suicide was the key to lowering the overall rates of suicide in China.

One unique aspect of Chinese rural young female suicide lay in the effects of traditional marriage and love relations. Among Chinese rural young women, being married was not necessarily a protective factor, as it is found to be in the West. Dating or being in love created suicidal risk for Chinese rural young women. A wife traditionally lived with the husband's family, where the wife's mother-in-law ruled the home. The majority of familial conflicts took place between the wife and her husband or in-laws. In traditional Chinese culture, when problems arose in the family and marital arena, women were usually the first to be blamed and held responsible. Therefore, Chinese rural young women, with a low social and familial status, were more likely to feel suppressed and helpless in this patriarchal society and to go to extremes to escape.

The so-called "strain theory" of suicide accounts for the high risk of suicide by Chinese rural young women, and explains why Chinese rural young women were so likely to commit suicide. The strain theory of suicide postulates that strain, resulting from conflicting and competing pressures in an individual's life, usually precedes suicidal behavior. The assumption of the theory is that strain, in the form of psychological suffering due to conflicting pressures of which a victim may or may not be consciously aware, is so unbearable that the victim finds a solution to release or stop it. Different from simple pressure or stress, which is a single-variable phenomenon, a strain consists of at least two pressures or variables.

The theory describes four types of strain derived from specific sources, each of which consists of at least two conflicting social facts:

1. *Conflicting values.* When two conflicting social values or beliefs are competing in an individual's daily life, the person experiences value strain.
2. *Reality versus aspiration.* If there is a discrepancy between an individual's aspiration and the reality the person has to live with, the person experiences aspiration strain.
3. *Relative deprivation.* In the situation where an extremely poor individual realizes that other people of the same or similar background are leading a much better life, the person experiences deprivation strain.
4. *Deficient coping.* Facing a life crisis, some individuals are not able to cope with it, and thus they experience coping strain.

(continued)

BOX 8.1. *(continued)*

The married rural young women in China may have experienced value strain in daily life. On one hand, they were confined by traditional Confucian ideology, in which women are treated as being of less value; on the other hand, they were being told by the Communist government that women and men are equal. Those women who internalized both sets of values may have experienced an unbearable strain, a psychological frustration. If they gave up either the Communist egalitarian gender value or the Confucian traditional sexism, this value strain would disappear. An unmarried rural woman may have experienced less frustration, due to less traditional pressure from the marital relationship.

By 2012, however, the suicide rate in China had dropped to 8 per 100,000 from 23 per 100,000 in the 1990s. Although rural young female suicides made a substantial contribution to the high rates of suicide in China more than 20 years ago, greatly reduced suicide rates in this female population have contributed to the overall decrease of suicide rates in China. These young women are dealing with less psychological strain as they move into cities, have increased individual freedom, and are liberated from the traditional rural family.

Source: Jie Zhang (personal communication, July 31, 2015).

that rural females who suicide have low social status and limited opportunity to improve their life situations. Zhang et al. (2004; see also Box 8.1) remind us that traditional Confucian values degrade the status of women.

There are no strong religious or legal prohibitions against suicide in China, particularly for low-status women. Two major Eastern religions (Hinduism and Buddhism) value asceticism and extinction of the physical body (as reflected in the concepts of *moksha* and *nirvana,* respectively). As in Japan, suicide is often acceptable in conditions of shame or defeat; it can even be self-actualizing, since in the East the true self is not found in one's physical body.

It seems that mental disorder diagnoses do not play as prominent a role in Chinese suicide attempts as in the West; severe acute stress seems to be more of a suicidogenic factor. Only 38% of Chinese suicide attempters had a diagnosable mental disorder (Phillips et al., 2002), versus up to 90% of U.S. suicide attempters.

In a study by Pearson et al. (2002) of 147 women under age 35 in rural China who made a suicide attempt, the most common precipitants were unhappy marriage (65%) and financial problems (43%; cf. Box 8.1). Often these suicide attempts were impulsive: About half of Pearson's attempters said they had thought about harming themselves for less than 1 day before acting.

In rural China, the vast majority of female suicides have ready access to potent, toxic pesticides (such as dichlorvos and parathion) in their homes. Pesticides tend to be used for suicide, instead of hanging. I would imagine that such suicide methods are slow and painful (self-punishing?). Finally, there is a scarcity of well-trained medical personnel available in rural China to treat self-poisonings. In a patriarchal society that in the past has practiced female infanticide and aborted female fetuses, one wonders how enthusiastically medical personnel might work to save female suicide attempters.

India

India is similar to China in many respects. They both have very large, highly dense populations (Maris, 1988), with relatively low female status, a higher female-to-male suicide ratio than the West, rural suicides involving the use of pesticides, and self-abnegating religious traditions (Hindu or Buddhist). However, India's suicide rate is higher than China's: 21.1 versus 7.8 per 100,000 in 2015 (see Table 8.1).

Sridhar (2001) points out that suicide rates are much higher in southern India, especially in Puducherry, than in other parts of India. In an article *in The Lancet*, Aaron et al. (2004) provide shocking data on young rural female suicides in southern India. For young women ages 10–19 years, suicide accounted for 50–75% of all deaths. The average suicide rate for young women was 148 per 100,000, 2.6 times higher than that of young men.

As in China, the purported causes of young female suicides include family conflicts, domestic violence (including murder), academic failure, unfilled romantic ideals (including dowry suicides), mental illness, the low status and devaluation of women, and the easy availability of farm pesticides (Aaron et al., 2004).

A few aspects of female suicides in India deserve closer attention. Widows practiced *sati* or *suttee* until it was outlawed in 1829 by the British. In this custom, as noted in earlier chapters and described in Chapter 18, a widow climbed onto her deceased husband's funeral pyre before it was lit (or even lit it herself), and was burned herself along with him (Tousignant et al., 1998). One justification for this practice was that her husband was the wife's main reason for living, and his death rendered her future life meaningless. There were also other suicide methods, like drowning in the Ganges River.

A similar low regard for women can be seen in the customs of so-called "dowry death," including dowry suicide. If a young woman and her family lack the financial resources to allow her to get married, the problem may be solved by her suicide. Bride burning, another form of dowry death, is murder by the husband or his family when the wife's family refuses to pay additional dowry. The Indian parliament estimates that of the 11,259 dowry deaths from 1988 to 1990, 4,038 or 35% were suicides. Probably many *satis* and dowry deaths were in fact murders (Tousignant et al., 1998).

South Korea[1]

In South Korea, suicide was the 4th leading cause of death in 2014, compared to the 10th or 11th cause of death in the United States. The total number of deaths from suicides was 13,836, comprising about 5.2% of total deaths. The suicide rate of South Korea tripled from 9.1 per 100,000 in 1985 to 27.3 in 2014. South Korea has undergone incredible economic development and industrialization since the 1960s, and its economy now stands as the 11th largest in the world. In addition, since the 1980s South Korea has democratized, after more than two decades of oppressive

---

[1] The South Korean suicide data have been contributed by Eui-Hang Shin (personal communication, November 12, 2015), unless otherwise noted.

authoritarian rule. What are the factors that account for the unprecedented rise in the suicide rate, in spite of South Korea's impressive record of economic development and political transformation? The observed trend in the suicide rate may be a classic example of Emile Durkheim's modernization thesis. Durkheim asserted that the suicide rate of a society is influenced by the extent to which individuals are integrated into their society and regulated by its norms and regulations.

Another factor may have been that South Korea experienced a financial meltdown in the late 1990s. Between 1996 and 1998, the unemployment rate increased from 2.0 to 6.8%, and the crude divorce rate increased from 1.8 to 2.5 per 1,000 population. Many companies became insolvent, and many middle-aged employees were forced to retire during this period of economic crisis. The suicide rate rose from 12.9 per 100,000 in 1996, 1 year prior to the economic crisis, to 18.4 in 1998, the peak year of the crisis. That was the biggest increase in suicide rates during any 2-year interval in South Korea's history.

Age

As in most developed countries, the suicide death rate of the elderly in South Korea is much higher than those of younger age groups. In 2014, the suicide rates of the 10–19, 20–29, 30–39, 40–49, 50–59, 60–69, 70–79, and 80+ age groups were 4.5, 17.8, 27.9, 32.4, 36.4, 37.5, 57.6, and 78.6 per 100,000 population, respectively. Between 2004 and 2014, the under-50 age group showed an increase in suicide rates, while the 50-and-older group experienced a decrease. Suicide was the leading cause of death for the 20–29 and 30–39 age groups, while it was the second leading cause of death for the 10–19, 40–49, and 50–59 age groups.

Gender

The suicide death rate for South Korean males in 2014 was 38.4 per 100,000, while the rate for females was 16.1. The male suicide rate was about 2.4 times higher than that of females. Suicide was the fourth leading cause of death for males, and the sixth leading cause of death for females. The gender differential in suicide rate was substantially greater for older age groups than for younger age groups. Cheong et al. (2012, as cited by Shin, personal communication, November 12, 2015) reported that the age-standardized suicide rate in rural areas was significantly higher than in urban areas for both males and females in the 20–64 age group.

Socioeconomic Status

Previous studies (Kim et al., 2006, 2010, as cited by Shin, personal communication, November 12, 2015) have found that, after controls for age, marital status, and area of residence, the risk of suicide was higher for those at the lowest SES levels than for those at middle and upper levels. Cheong et al. indicated that such variables as educational attainment level, automobile ownership, and quality of housing environment showed a strong negative correlation with suicide risk for both males and females.

Methods of Suicide

Lim et al. (2014, as cited by Shin, personal communication, November 12, 2015) analyzed 5,388 South Korean cases of completed suicide and found that hanging was the most common method (52.2%), followed by jumping (17.7%) and pesticide or herbicide poisoning (13.8%). Due to the fact that the government has strict control over firearms, there were very limited cases of completed suicides involving guns. Females tended to use poisoning and jumping more than males. The proportion of suicides involving pesticide or herbicide poisoning has declined because of stricter guidelines for selling those chemicals in recent years, whereas the proportion of hanging as a method of suicide has increased.

The Werther Effect

There have been quite a few celebrity suicides in recent years in South Korea. For instance, top actress Choi Jin-sil committed suicide in 2008, and in May 2009 former President Roh Moo-hyun committed suicide by jumping off a cliff near his retirement home amid a bribery investigation of his family members. Suicide cases of well-known film stars, popular music singers, fashion models, athletes, and business and political figures receive extensive media coverage. In fact, the mean number of suicides during the 2-month periods following five selected celebrity suicide cases in 2005–2008—which included the just-mentioned Choi Jin-sil, as well as Lee Eun-ju (also an actress), U;Nee (an actress/singer), Chung Da-bin (another actress), and Ahn Jae-hwan (an actor)—was 2,632, while the mean number of suicides for the same 2-month periods of the years preceding these cases was 1,947.

The South Korean government has implemented a series of suicide prevention programs in recent years. For example, it has expanded education programs to increase public awareness of suicide risk factors, increased screening and treatment of individuals at high risk, developed guidelines for responsible reporting on suicide by the media, and reduced access to poisoning agents. President Park Geun-hye's administration (2013–2017) enacted various social welfare programs that aimed to expand the social safety net for the poor and the elderly. It is hoped that these social welfare programs will help reduce South Korea's suicide rate. It is a promising sign that the suicide death rate declined from a record high of 31.7 per 100,000 in 2011 to 27.3 in 2014. However, it rose again to 28.9 in 2015 (see Table 8.1).

Australia

Australia's suicide rate is considered moderate at 10.6 per 100,000; its world ranking in Table 8.1 is 63rd. Australian suicides tend to be similar to U.S. suicides: Male rates are about three times higher than female rates, and alcohol abuse and depression are major risk factors.

Particularly noteworthy is the suicide problem among Australia's Aboriginal youth. For example, an Australian Broadcasting Corporation (ABC) News report (June 14, 2015) claimed that in far north Queensland, the Aboriginals make up just

4% of the population, but more than 50% of the suicides. This Aboriginal suicide epidemic mainly affects young people, especially in the 25–29 age group, in which Aboriginal suicide rates are about 5.1 times those of non-Aboriginals. Factors in Aboriginal suicides include disempowerment, acute poverty, racism (much like that against Native Americans), and the abuse of alcohol and drugs. Some researchers point out that before the arrival of Europeans in Australia in the late 1700s, Aboriginal suicide was virtually unheard of.

Elevated suicide rates among indigenous peoples (especially among young persons) also tend to occur outside Australia. Examples include various First Nations groups in Canada, various Native American tribes and nations in the United States (see Chapter 5 and Figure 5.1), and Inuit and other indigenous groups in Alaska and far northern Canada.

Countries with Low Suicide Rates

At the low end of the suicide rate continuum shown in Table 8.1 are countries like Mexico, the Philippines, Haiti, Bahamas, Libya, Egypt, Iraq, Jamaica, Syria, and Saudi Arabia. Whereas Guyana had a suicide rate of 44.2 per 100,000, Saudi Arabia and Syria, for example, had rates of only 0.4 per 100,000. What accounts for these vast differences in suicide rates, and what (if any) implications do they have for suicide prevention?

Although cultures are very diverse and one needs to be cautious about making categorical assumptions about human nature or suicide, I suspect that the countries with low suicide rates countries just listed tend to have the following characteristics: (1) religious convictions, beliefs, norms, or customs that strongly discourage or even forbid suicide, except in extraordinary circumstances (e.g., those of the Muslim and Roman Catholic faiths); (2) much younger populations, in which suicide is usually more uncommon and suicidal careers are less developed or advanced; (3) lower rates of depressive disorder and other mood disorders; (4) lower rates of alcohol and other substance use or abuse (especially among Muslims); and (5) more beneficial climatic conditions, diurnal rhythms, and lifestyles, in which food is more abundant and survival is comparatively easier (e.g., Jamaica vs. Finland). However, many climatic theories of suicide have been discredited, and climatic conditions or diurnal rhythms at best are only minor risk factors.

Now I consider two low-suicide countries. One is Egypt, a Muslim country, and the other is Mexico, a Catholic country. I visited Cairo in 2004 to investigate a suicide case involving Egypt Air, and I traveled repeatedly to Mexico while teaching at Arizona State University. The backdrop to this discussion is whether or not there could be places, cultures, or climates in which a properly socialized citizen would be less likely to commit suicide or even in rare cases be immune to suicide. If so, could these conditions be simulated elsewhere, and at what costs? (See Huxley, 1932, for his mordant answers to these questions.) Of course, life and suicide are not simple. An individual with a particular trait (like being male) or mental disorder could still be suicidal, even in utopia.

Egypt

The 2015 WHO data for Egypt (Table 8.1) indicate a male suicide rate of 2.4 per 100,000 and a 1.2 rate for females. Egypt's overall suicide rate was ranked 163rd (tied with Iraq) out of 171 countries. Ninety-five percent of Egyptians are Muslims, and many of them live very densely (about 3,820 people per square mile) along the Nile River, especially in Cairo and Alexandria. When I visited Cairo, people were everywhere; it was difficult just to cross a street, given the traffic. Cars did not stop for red lights; I had to pay a policeman to stop traffic for me. About 75% of Egyptians are under age 25. Since Egypt's suicide rates are so low, one could doubt their veracity. They could be artifacts of the Egyptian death certification process, or could reflect partial fabrication or distortion due to religious or political ideology

Interestingly, in ancient Egypt the afterlife was seen as a continuation of existence before death; that is, there was no dramatic break between life and death (Silverman, 1997; Spencer, 1988). Thus death for ancient Egyptians was not viewed so much an escape from life, and, as such, it was not seen as a solution to life's problems. In countries with high suicide rates, death is often seen as dramatically different from life (such as heaven vs. hell on earth).

Mexico

From 1970 to 1994, the Mexican suicide rate increased from 1.13 to 2.89 per 100,000. Some articles expressed concern about rise in the Mexican rates (Borges et al., 1996). The greatest increase was among males age 65 or older. Men had a suicide rate of 6.1 per 100,000, versus 1.3 in women. The highest rate was in men over age 65, at 13.6. Hanging was the most frequent method for both men and women. Interestingly, increased per capita alcohol consumption among Mexicans did not seem to be correlated with higher suicide rates. Nevertheless, the WHO (1999) commented that "Mexico has one of the lowest suicide rates in the world." However, Mexico's suicide rates are still slowly but consistently increasing, especially among males. In 2015 the WHO reported that Mexico had a suicide rate of 4.2 and a 137th world ranking out of 172 countries (see Table 8.1).

Mexicans have several suicide protective factors. For example, the median age is 24.6 years, and 50% of the population is under age 25. Only 5.5% of Mexicans are age 55 or older. Thus, demographically speaking, Mexicans tend to be in low-suicide-risk groups. Furthermore, about 89% of the Mexican population is Roman Catholic, and Catholicism has a strong proscription against suicide. Suicide is still considered a mortal sin that could result in eternal damnation and a non-Catholic burial, although views in this area have become somewhat more lenient in recent years. Catholics strongly oppose abortion and euthanasia, as well as suicide.

Chapter 9 is the concluding chapter of Part III on sociodemographic issues. It addresses who makes suicide attempts, how (i.e., what methods are used), how many suicide attempts are made by which people, what kinds of attempts are made (e.g., lethal or not), and what attempters have to say about them (e.g., in suicide notes).

Who Makes Suicide Attempts, How, and What Do Suicide Notes Say about Them?

Suicide notes are cryptic maps of ill-advised journeys.
—EDWIN S. SHNEIDMAN

Earlier in this text, I have talked about a "continuum of suicidality" (see Chapter 1, Figure 1.1). One estimate in the United States for 2015 was that there were (1) 1,024,000 suicide ideators, (2) 1,194,825 nonfatal suicide attempters (ideators can make more than one attempt), and (3) only 44,193 suicide completers. Klonsky and May (2014, 2015) and Joiner (2005) point out that the risk factors for suicide ideation, suicide attempting, and suicide completion are not the same (see also Qiu et al., 2017; Chesin et al., 2017; cf. O'Connor, 2018), and that many of our suicide risk factors are mainly for suicide ideas or nonfatal suicide attempts, not for completed suicides. So the question is this: How do we get from many suicide ideas and nonfatal suicide attempts to very few (1 in 10,000 per year) completed suicides?

One obvious answer has been provided in previous chapters: If a person is male and uses a firearm to attempt suicide, then he is much more likely to complete the suicide attempt and die (see also Table 9.2, below). Men can be almost twice as likely as women in the United States to use lethal firearm methods; women are about four to five times more likely to utilize less lethal drugs and poisons to attempt suicide than men are.

The current chapter examines who attempts suicide; how they do it; and what the suicides themselves say (if anything) about their suicide attempts in notes, diaries, journals, computer searches, patient interviews, and so on. Most research shows that only about 10–25% of suicide attempters go on to complete suicide. Interestingly, this means that 75–90% of attempters never complete suicide. The vast majority of people making a suicide attempt never die by it (*www.griefspeaks. com/id121.html*; cf. Maris et al., 2000).

155

As I have said before, the majority of suicide completers make relatively few suicide attempts before dying. Thus, even though suicide attempts are significantly correlated with suicides, it is often too late to use attempts to prevent suicide. For example, in my Chicago surveys (1969; 1981), almost 90% of males age 45 or older who suicided made only one suicide attempt before dying (see Tables 9.2 and 9.3, below).

There are many factors (some public health or population based) influencing the choice of suicide attempt methods (Maris et al., 2000). They include availability (e.g., a gun in the house or car; see Anestis & Houtsma, 2018; Anestis, 2017), lethal means restrictions (e.g., guns locked in a safe without bullets; Lester, 2012), knowledge (e.g., most women's more limited familiarity with guns), occupation (e.g., the military or police), suggestion (especially for young people; see Chapter 7), and state of mind (e.g., impulsivity or a mood disorder).

There are also many ways people can try to kill themselves. The most common and most lethal (Card, 1974) are, in order, (1) firearms, (2) hanging, and (3) carbon monoxide poisoning (often the second and third methods are reversed, depending on the attempters' gender and ethnicity). Table 9.1 lists 17 possible methods of suicide, although many of them are rare and exotic, even bizarre. For example, I had a case of a young man who taped a Hefty bag filled with dry ice around his head and neck. Below I elaborate on methods, such as firearms, hanging, carbon monoxide, and jumping.

Suicide Attempts and Methods

Data on Fatal Methods

Table 9.2 presents data on fatal suicide attempt methods in the United States from 1970 to 2015 by gender. Some of the methods categories overlap or are vague, but clearly firearms are the most common method for both men and women (about 60% and 30%, respectively). For one year (2002), J. L. McIntosh (personal communication) found that firearms and poisons (including drugs) were virtually tied for women (at 33% each).

Drugs, medications, and poisons combined usually constitute the second leading attempt method for women, and hanging is for men (especially in institutions like jails, prisons, and hospitals). Carbon monoxide poisoning is normally the third most common suicide attempt method for both men and women. Although McIntosh's 2002 data do not separate out poisons and drugs or control for gender, the 2015 data for firearms, hanging, and drugs were 51.5%, 24.5%, and 16.1%, respectively. In 2012 (not shown in Table 9.2), firearms accounted for 51% of suicides, hanging for 25%, and poisons and drugs for 16.1%.

Clearly, gun control could result in better suicide prevention. When I interned at the Los Angeles Suicide Prevention Center, I was advised by Bob Litman and Mickey Heilig to have a suicide hotline caller carry his or gun outside and put it down the nearest sewer drain. They emphasized the need for great care and discretion in giving a caller such an instruction. My mentor, Edwin Shneidman, used to collect guns in his office desk drawer (this is *not* a recommendation). Should a

TABLE 9.1. A Partial List of Possible Suicide Methods

- Firearms (the most common method in the United States, especially pistol shots to the head, temple, and mouth; sometimes rifles and shotguns are used).

- Hanging (the most common method in confinement in the United States, such as jails, prisons, and hospitals; also the most common method in Asia and much of Europe). The body is usually not above the floor. Blood flow is cut off in carotid arteries in the neck, to cause anoxia in a few minutes and death in about 4–5 minutes.

- Carbon monoxide poisoning (usually from car or truck exhaust in a confined space with windows up and engine running; it can also occur from burning charcoal in a confined space). The body turns cherry red or orange.

- Medication and other drug overdoses (this method is more likely to be used by females). Possible drugs include over-the-counter pills like Tylenol; pain medications such as opiates; barbiturates, especially where assisted suicide is legal; tranquilizers; antidepressants; or whatever is in the bathroom medicine cabinet. Overdoses are typically not rapidly fatal (cf. Benson et al., 2018).

- Poisons (solids and liquids, like pesticides in rural China and India, cleaners like Drano or Clorox, antifreeze, and other toxins such as rat and insect poisons).

- Jumping from heights (particularly in large cities like New York City, where 40% of suicides are jumpers; also used are bridges like the Golden Gate Bridge, or the steep gorges in Ithaca, New York). Sylvia Plath (1963/2005) estimated the necessary building height for suicide to be about six to seven stories.

- Bleeding, cutting, stabbing, or piercing (e.g., *seppuku* or *hara-kiri* in Japan; stabbing in several of Shakespeare's plays; self-cutting as described in the book *Skin Game* [Kettlewell, 1999], which is very common in people with borderline personality).

- Suffocation or asphyxiation (most commonly with a plastic bag over one's head and a rubber band around the neck, often accompanied by barbiturate or alcohol use; dry ice may be put in the bag over the head; less commonly, autoerotic asphyxiation).

- Drowning (walking or swimming into an ocean, lake, or river, as the novelist Virginia Woolf did).

- Vehicular blunt force trauma (some single-driver car wrecks; lying or jumping in front of trains or subways, as Anna does with a train in *Anna Karenina* [Tolstoy, 1877/2000]; intentional plane crashes).

- Explosions (blowing oneself up, like *jihadist* suicide bombers).

- Immolation (setting oneself on fire, like Buddhist martyrs, political protesters, Indian *sati* or *suttee* victims).

- Electrocution (putting an electrical device in bathtub water; touching high-voltage wires).

- Hypothermia (intentional self-freezing).

- Opocarteresis (starving oneself, like some political prisoners or hospital patients).

- Dehydration (refusing to drink liquids or water).

- Helium (asphyxiation with a helium hood, tubing, and helium gas).

Note. None of these methods are endorsed or recommended.
Source: Original table by Maris.

TABLE 9.2. Percentage of Completed Suicides by Method, Sex, and Year

Method of attempt	1970 M	1970 F	1980 M	1980 F	1990 M	1990 F	2002 M	2002 F	2011 M	2011 F	2015 M + F
Firearms	58.5	30.1	63.5	38.7	64.0	39.8	59.2	33.0	51.8	38.3	51.5
Medications and other drugs					5.2	25.0			6.9	22.0	
Hanging	14.3	11.9	14.1	10.5	13.5	9.4	21.1	17.7	23.1	15.6	24.5
Carbon monoxide	11.2	11.8	8.7	12.4	9.6	12.6	4.5	5.0	5.6	6.4	
Jumping from high place					1.8	3.0			5.2	5.7	
Drowning					1.1	2.8					1.0
Suffocation by plastic bag					0.4	1.8			2.1	5.0	
Cutting, piercing					1.3	1.4					1.9
Poisons	9.2	36.8	6.6	27.3	0.6	1.0	7.6	33.2	6.9	22.0	16.1
Other	6.8	9.4	7.1	11.1	2.5	3.2	7.6	11.1	5.4	7.1	5.0
Total	100	100	100	100	100	100	100	100	100	100	100

Note. M, male; F, female. Some method categories are unclear and overlapping, such as "poisons" and "drugs and medications" (e.g., in 1990, where "poisons" are separated from "drugs and medications").

Sources: 1970, 1980, 1990 data from the National Center for Health Statistics; 2002 data from J. L. McIntosh (personal communication); 2011 data from Callanan and Davis (2011); 2015 data from *www.suicidology.org/resources/facts-statistics*. All U.S. data. Government statistics are in public domain.

therapist collect guns or pills? Usually not. But this issue is related to lethal means restrictions. If a patient has suicide ideas, a clinician should always ask about the intended suicide method and the specific plan in detail.

Completed Suicides versus Nonfatal Suicide Attempts

Tables 9.3 and 9.4 show that 70–75% of all completed suicides make only one fatal suicide attempt. Again, in my Chicago data, the figure rose to 88 or 90% if the suicide attempter was male and age 45 or older. Forty-nine percent of suicide completers die in less than 1 hour of attempting (Table 9.5).

TABLE 9.3. Number of Suicide Attempts Made by Completers

Number of attempts	Percentage
1	70.0
2	13.8
3	4.8
4	3.9
5	3.5
6	0.0
7	1.1
8+	0.7
Don't know	2.2
Total	100.0

Note. N = 246 in Chicago. Percentage making one fatal attempt was 88%, if decedent was white, male, and age 45 or older.

Source: Maris, Ronald W. with Bernard Lazerwitz. *Pathways to Suicide: A Survey of Self-Destructive Behaviors.* Copyright © 1981 The Johns Hopkins University Press. Reprinted with permission of Johns Hopkins University Press.

TABLE 9.4. Number of Suicide Attempts Made by Completers, by Sex and Age

Number of attempts	Male (%)		Female (%)		Total (%)
	< 45 years (*n* = 55)	> 45 years (*n* = 90)	< 45 years (*n* = 44)	>45 years (*n* = 77)	(*N* = 266)
1	79	88	50	71	75
2–4	19	10	34	26	20
5+	0	0	16	3	3
Don't know	2	2	0	0	2
Total	100	100	100	100	100

Source: Adapted from Maris, Ronald W. with Bernard Lazerwitz. *Pathways to Suicide: A Survey of Self-Destructive Behaviors.* Copyright © 1981 The Johns Hopkins University Press. Adapted with permission of Johns Hopkins University Press.

TABLE 9.5. Time Interval between Suicide Attempt and Completion (Death)

Time interval between attempt and death	Completed suicides (%)
1 week or more	7
4–6 days	3
2–3 days	2
4–24 hours	3
2–3 hours	6
1 hour or less	15
Instantaneous death	34
Don't know	30
Total	100

Note. N = 266 in Chicago. Note that about 50% of attempters died within an hour or less.

Source: Maris, Ronald W. with Bernard Lazerwitz. *Pathways to Suicide: A Survey of Self-Destructive Behaviors.* Copyright © 1981 The Johns Hopkins University Press. Reprinted with permission of Johns Hopkins University Press.

Multiple Suicide Attempts

The other side of the suicide attempt coin is that multiple attempts among eventual completers are relatively rare. Most multiple attempts are by women. Eighty-four percent of my completed suicides in Chicago made no more than two attempts. The only age and gender group making two to four attempts before dying were younger women (34%) under age 45 (see Table 9.4).

Lethal Means Restrictions

Kreitman (1976; cf. Lester, 2012) reported that in Great Britain when lethal home gas was detoxified, the suicide rate went down and stayed down. People did not suddenly shift to other methods (Anestis et al., 2017; Lubin et al., 2010). We have also seen earlier (Chapter 8, Figure 8.1) that when alcohol was controlled in Russia during *perestroika,* the suicide rate dropped 40% and only went back up after the alcohol control policy was reversed. Since 40% of New York City suicides are jumpers (Maltsberger, 1998), imagine what might happen to the urban suicide rate if all buildings there and in other major cities were only two stories high. Although difficult, gun control is extremely important for suicide prevention.

Perturbation, Constriction, and Lethality

Shneidman (1985) argued that suicide methods are more likely to be lethal (i.e., to have a high probability of death) if one is highly agitated or perturbed, and if one's thinking about how to reduce that perturbation is rigid and constricted—for example, if suicide is seen as the only alternative resolution to one's problems. Shneidman liked to say that *only* was the four-letter word in suicidology (as in "It was the only thing I could do"). What determines the perceived *only*-ness of suicide—failure of previous adaptations, depression, or a correct assessment (rational suicide)?

Role of Age

One reason why almost 90% of older white males in the United States die on their first attempt is that they shoot themselves in the head (not something you can usually do twice). The older an attempter is, the more likely the person is to choose a lethal method (like a gun) for attempting suicide.

Nonsuicidal Self Injury

A history of nonsuicidal self-injury (NSSI) indicates significantly greater risk of a suicide attempt throughout adulthood (Chesin et al., 2017; note that Chesin's sample was 68% female).

Triggering and Chronicity

An important question is whether suicide attempts are triggered by exceptional circumstances or events in an otherwise nonsuicidal individual, or whether a fatal suicide attempt is more like tipping the suicidal scale or slowly breaching the adaptive threshold of the chronically suicidal person (see Chapter 2, Figure 2.1, for the general model of suicide). Both Joiner (2005) and I (Maris, 1981, 2015) have argued that most suicides are usually not triggered merely by immediate situational precursors. In general, a completed suicide is a multifactorial product of lifelong repetition of problems that gradually breaches an adaptive threshold in a vulnerable individual, who is often in repeated physical and/or psychic pain, and who has accumulated many years of experience with prior self-destructive behaviors. One reason why suicide attempts are completed is that over time (normally about 40–50 years), the alternatives to suicide in one's adaptive repertoire are gradually depleted. This process is usually catabolic, a slow entropy, rather than an acute crisis.

Thus, when suicide methods and lethality are assessed, it is wise to differentiate between acute and chronic lethality. Some methods are highly lethal but slow-acting, such as alcoholism. Roy and Linnoila (1986) claim that 18% (Murphy, 1992, claims it is more like 10%) of alcoholics eventually commit slow suicides (after about 25 years), and by not taking life-saving medications, accumulating stress, overeating the wrong foods, or even overworking. However, most methods are lethal and short-acting (Table 9.5), such as a bullet to the brain, hanging (which normally results in anoxic brain damage or death in about 4–5 minutes), or jumping from a heights.

Meanings of Suicide Methods

The lethality of suicide methods varies considerably by sex, age, race, ethnicity, culture, and even geographic region. Almost all suicides are ambivalent about the act; that is, they want both to die and to live. Most suicides with minimal ambivalence, such as those motivated by the desire to escape, tend to use more lethal methods (like guns in the United States) to attempt suicide; suicides whose motivation is to change inter-personal relationships are more likely to use less lethal methods, such as overdoses or cutting, perhaps because they want at some level to stay around and see the effects.

Culture, geography, or both often determine suicide methods, as we have seen in Chapter 8 for pesticide use by rural females in China and India. Why are guns preferred by suicides in the United States, but in Europe the preferred method is hanging? Guns are much more accessible in the United States. Why do so many suicides jump to their deaths in large cities and only 3–5% elsewhere? Well, that's where the tall buildings are.

In the United States, women have a suicide rate about four times lower than men do, but make three to four times more suicide attempts than men do (see Chapter 1). Why? One reason is that women are more likely than men to use rela-tively low-lethality suicide attempt methods like drug overdoses or cutting, while men typically shoot themselves.

This still begs the question of why women tend to overdose and not shoot them-selves (as much as men do). There is no simple, single answer. Women tend to own fewer guns and have less access to and familiarity with them. They are more likely than men to get treated and be prescribed psychiatric medications. Even when women do shoot themselves, they are less likely to do so in their heads (i.e., they tend to choose less lethal sites; see Eisele et al., 1981).

In Chapter 6, I have argued that women are also more aware than men of the con-sequences of their suicides for their families, especially for their dependent children. This might tend to act as a deterrent for choosing a lethal method to attempt suicide.

Distinguishing Characteristics of Suicide Methods

A medical examiner or coroner certifies the manner of death on the death certifi-cate as natural, accidental, suicidal, or homicidal (NASH). The manner of death is different from the cause of death. The coroner often relies on the distinguishing physical characteristics of suicide methods. For example, contact gunshot wounds (abbreviated as GSWs on death certificates) to the head (especially to the temple) are usually suicides, as are most hangings (unless there is autoerotic asphyxia). Fatal car wrecks are normally thought to be accidents. Cutting, piercing, or stab-bing deaths are often presumed to be homicides. Most medical examiners classify Russian roulette deaths as suicide (not accidents), since the probability of death would have been zero if Russian roulette had not been played.

Some manners of deaths are unclear or cannot be determined from the physi-cal evidence alone. In such cases in Baltimore, I was deputized by the medical exam-iner to do psychological autopsies to supplement the physical autopsies. You will recall from Chapter 3 that a psychological autopsy is a procedure for reconstructing an individual's psychological condition after the fact of death. For example, did the decedent (DCD, on the death certificate) leave a suicide note, make plans to die, talk to family and friends about suicide, make any prior nonfatal suicide attempts, or suffer from depression or chronic pain?

Four suicide methods are common and worth examining in detail. These include death by firearms, hanging, drug overdoses, and jumping from heights.

Firearms

As shown in Table 9.2, 50–60% of all U.S. suicides utilize guns (more than homicides do). This is especially true if the DCD is male. The United States is the only country in the world whose residents use guns so frequently for suicide. Some of the distinguishing characteristics of firearm suicides include these:

- Where the wound was located.
- The proximity of the weapon to the wound (e.g., was it a contact wound?).
- How accessible the wound location was (e.g., was the shot to the side, front, or back of the head?).
- The ipsilaterality of the wound (was it where right- or left-handed persons would normally shoot themselves?).
- Whether there was barium, antimony, or lead residue (gunshot residue, or GSR) on the DCD's hands or wound.
- Whether there was one or many wounds.

Figure 9.1 and Table 9.6 show that most suicides shoot themselves in the right temple, if they are right-handed. Eighty-two percent of suicides using handguns shoot themselves in the head, and 98% either in the head or chest. (For an excellent reference on this topic, see DiMaio, 1999.) Interestingly, in Figure 9.1, only 4.2 of 175 suicidal head wounds (2%) were to the eyes. Why is that?

Most suicidal GSWs are proximate or contact wounds to the head. The wounds leave GSR, tattooing, stippling, or muzzle or barrel patterns on the skin (DiMaio, 1999). Most accidents or homicides are normally not contact wounds, except for some executions.

The typical suicide is not a contortionist. Suicides usually choose the most accessible or convenient head site (see Figure 9.1), most often the right temple. Sites are determined in part by the length of the victim's arms (about 28 inches on average), although I have seen cases in which suicides shot themselves in the midline of the back of their heads.

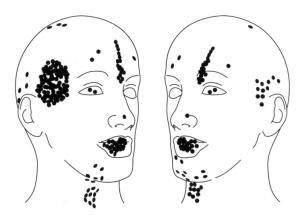

FIGURE 9.1. Location of 175 head and neck suicidal gunshot wounds. *Source:* Eisele et al. (1981). Reprinted, with permission, from the *Journal of Forensic Sciences,* Volume 26, No.3, copyright ASTM International, 100 Barr Harbor Drive, West Conshohocken, PA 19428.

TABLE 9.6. Suicidal Gunshot Wound Location by Type of Weapon

Site	Handgun		Rifle		Shotgun	
	n	%	*n*	%	*n*	%
Head	116	82	38	67	11	47
Temporoparietal	88	62	16	28	4	17
Frontal	10	7	9	16	2	9
Mouth	10	7	6	11	4	17
Submental	3	2	3	5	1	4
Other head	5	4	4	7	0	0
Neck	1	1	8	14	1	1
Chest	23	16	8	14	8	35
Presternum	20	14	6	10	6	26
Precordium						
Other chest	3	2	2	4	2	9
Abdomen	2	2	3	5	3	13
Epigastrum	1	1	2	3	2	9
Other abdomen	1	1	1	2	1	4
Total *n*	142		57		23	

Source: Eisele et al. (1981). Reprinted, with permission, from the *Journal of Forensic Sciences,* Volume 26, No.3. Copyright © ASTM International, 100 Barr Harbor Drive, West Conshohocken, PA 19428.

Ipsilaterality refers to wounds that are on the same side of the body as the DCD's dominant hand. So, usually, right-handed suicides would shoot themselves in the right temple (see Figure 9.1). Eisele et al. (1981) estimated that only about 8% of right-handed suicides shoot themselves in the contralateral side.

As noted above, GSR consists of barium, antimony, and lead deposited on the wound and hands of the individual firing the gun (usually a handgun). Often the DCD's hands are bagged, then tested for GSR. However, one study showed that GSR tests were positive only 38% of the time, even when it was 100% clear that the DCD had in fact fired the gun (Reed et al., 1990).

Unless the suicide is committed with a low-caliber gun (like a .22), the vast majority (99%) of suicidal GSWs involve only a single shot. I have had a case in which a .22 GSW ricocheted off the deceased's skull, only to be followed by a second fatal shot. Anecdotally, I have even heard of a GSW resulting in a crude lobotomy, allegedly curing the would-be suicide.

Hanging

Hanging is the second leading suicide method in the United States, but is much more common worldwide. In some European countries, about 90% of all suicides are by hanging (e.g., in Lithuania, 91.7%; in Poland, 91.2%; and in Romania, 87.3%). In other countries, about two-thirds of all suicides are by hanging (in Mexico, 68.8%; in Japan, 68.7%; and in Hungary, 70.3%; Adacic-Gross et al., 2008).

When a person is hanged, there is constriction of the blood flow of the carotid arteries in the neck; the windpipe is blocked (thus depriving the brain of oxygen);

and/or there is cardiac arrest. The brain and the body need to utilize oxygen and eliminate carbon dioxide. If it does not, then in 4–5 minutes there can be anoxic brain damage and/or death. Fifteen-minute checks for suicide watches are often ineffective. Hanging victims lose consciousness almost instantaneously. Contrary to popular opinion, most hanging suicides are not suspended off the ground (as in executions). The tension of a rope, cord, shoestring, belt, or torn cloth only needs to have 7–8 pounds of pressure to block the carotid arteries in the neck.

Hanging is common in U.S. jails, prisons, and hospitals (see Chapter 22). A patient or inmate just needs to take off a t-shirt, put the shirt over the neck, put an armhole over a doorknob, and then lean forward (this is not a recommendation!). Alternatively, materials can be tied to a shower head, cabinet, door, toilet paper holder, or the like. Normally, the hanging victim's feet (or other parts of the body) are touching the floor. Virtually any item of clothing can be used to make a noose or constriction, although thick, untearable comforters or "antisuicide blankets," gowns, or smocks can be provided to patients or inmates.

Drug Overdoses

As noted earlier in this chapter and in Table 9.2, drug overdoses are the second leading suicide attempt method in the United States for women, at about 25% of female suicides. Among the drugs that can be used to assist in or commit suicide (this is not a complete list) are these:

- Alcohol (ethanol).
- Prescription medications, especially antidepressants or anxiolytics (some other types fall into other categories in this listing; see Benson et al., 2018), as well as over-the-counter medications.
- Illegal or street drugs (like heroin).
- Opiates and other painkillers, including gabapentin (Neurontin).
- Barbiturates.
- Stimulants (including ADHD medications and methamphetamine) and cocaine.
- Hallucinogens.
- Household chemicals (e.g., cleaners, bleaches, poisons, pesticides, antifreeze).

Alcohol

Alcohol is probably the most dangerous drug there is. We have seen in Chapter 8 how powerful a risk factor it is in Russian suicides. Murphy (1992) and Roy and Linnoila (1986) estimate that 10–20% of those with alcoholism will eventually suicide. Alcoholism was considered a slow form of suicide by Menninger (1938). Alcohol use in the long run reduces brain serotonin and causes or worsens depressive disorder.

Prescription and Over-the-Counter Medications

Women are more likely than men to get treated psychiatrically and to receive antidepressant and anxiolytic prescriptions. When women are depressed, they often swallow a handful or a bottle of their psychiatric medications (Benson et al., 2018). All major antidepressants now carry an FDA-mandated black-box suicide warning (the strongest available) for antidepressant users up to age 24. Interestingly, actor-comedian Robin Williams was taking Remeron and Seroquel when he suicided. Sylvia Plath was on an antidepressant (probably a tricyclic) at the time of her death. Over-the-counter drugs, like Tylenol, can also be fatal in small overdoses (Tylenol can cause liver failure and is very dangerous in overdose).

Opiates and Other Painkillers

Many suicides are on prescription opiates or other painkillers (like gabapentin) for chronic pain. Illegal opiates like heroin are also widely used (there has been a resurgence in heroin use recently). Opiates are dangerous in part because their effective recreational dose is very close to their lethal dose (think of the cases of Philip Seymour Hoffman and John Belushi). Opiates worsen depression, cause nausea, and disturb sleep, all of which in turn increase suicide risk. Most pain medications increase brain GABA. GABA depletes brain serotonin and norepinephrine, which worsens depression. The most striking biological marker for depression and suicide is low brain serotonin (5-HT) in the prefrontal cortex of the brain (Maris, 2015; Mann & Currier, 2012; see Chapter 16).

Barbiturates

Barbiturates are recommended by Humphry (1991/1996, 2015; Maris, 2015) for assisted suicide in U.S. jurisdictions where assisted suicide is legal (at this writing, Oregon, Washington, Vermont, Montana, Hawaii, Colorado, California, and the District of Columbia; this list is in flux). Veterinarians still use barbiturates to euthanize dogs and cats, followed by another drug to stop their heartbeat.

Stimulants and Cocaine

Many celebrities use themselves up prematurely like Fourth of July sparklers (such as John Belushi, Kurt Cobain, Judy Garland, Marilyn Monroe, John Candy, Chris Farley, and Heath Ledger), and stimulants and cocaine are often factors in these deaths. For example, Belushi snorted cocaine on *Saturday Night Live,* and died probably accidentally of a "speedball" (a stimulant and opiate combination) overdose. Nor is the problem confined to celebrities. In one study in New York City, 29% of all suicides ages 21–30 had cocaine in their bodies at death (Marzuk et al., 1992). Less glamorous but equally dangerous is the methamphetamine epidemic currently ravaging the United States, especially in rural areas. People often do not realize how much caffeinated coffee or soft drinks they are ingesting. There is also nicotine: 90% of schizophrenics smoke cigarettes.

Most ADHD medications are stimulants as well. Adderall is an amphetamine combination (others include Strattera and Concerta) used for the treatment of ADHD; this disorder often includes trouble concentrating and sleeping, which Adderall helps. Adderall is frequently used as a "study drug" (to stay awake) by students without ADHD. Males with ADHD (depending on their age) also tend to be diagnosed with conduct disorder, oppositional defiant disorder, and later antisocial personality disorder. All of these diagnoses are risk factors for suicide.

Hallucinogens

Hallucinogens include LSD, Ecstasy, PCP, and psilocybin (in mushrooms). They can induce psychotic symptoms and confusion. For example, someone taking them may try to fly home from a party in a high-rise apartment and fall to their death. PCP is also related to bizarre acts of violence in emergency rooms. Any hallucinogenic drug can increase suicide risk (Maris, 2015).

Household Chemicals

Some agitated suicides impulsively drink whatever they find in their cupboards, such as Drano, Clorox, bleach, or vermin/insect poison. If death results, it is usually slow and painful. A notable example of such suicides is farm pesticides ingested in rural China and India, especially by younger females (see Chapter 8, particularly Box 8.1).

Jumping

Suicide by jumping is relatively rare (2–6%), except in large cities. Most jumpers are males jumping from their apartments. A jump of over six stories has about a 90% chance of death. Suicides tend to jump from celebrated sites like the Golden Gate Bridge in San Francisco (which has a 2% survival rate), the Empire State Building in New York City, the Eiffel Tower in Paris, the gorges at Cornell University, and Mount Mishara in Japan.

Jumpers raise puzzling questions about suicide prevention. Why not just "suicide-proof" bridges with protective railing or mesh? Why not just close the sides of the observation deck at the Empire State Building? I had a case of a young male jumper who put on a life jacket before jumping off a bridge, but drowned anyway. Sometimes accidents resulting in falls are difficult to distinguish from suicide jumpers. But suicide jumpers often leave evidence of their intent at the site. For example, they have no other reason to be there, they fold their clothes neatly before jumping, they jump feet first, may leave a cell phone, and so on.

Suicide Notes

Suicide notes might seem like windows to the suicidal mind (Shneidman, 1973). Are they the proverbial "last words," straight from the horse's mouth? If the deceased does not know why he or she is suiciding, who does? Medical examiners and the police often assume that a suicide note clearly indicates that the manner of death was suicide. Indeed, some medical examiners may only certify a death as a suicide if a suicide note is found; this is rare.

But are suicide note writers reliable sources of data? Suicides tend to be depressed, and one prominent feature of depression is not seeing alternatives or having insight. They are also often intoxicated by alcohol and/or other drugs, which can make them temporarily more impulsive and confused. They are often desperate and agitated, perhaps angry, seeking revenge, hopeless, and not rational. In short, suicide note writers may have limited insight into their own condition and may not be their usual selves at the time of death.

Some suicide notes are threats and manipulations of significant others, designed to change life, not end it—for example, "If you don't do *XYZ*, then I will kill myself, and it will be on your conscience." Some people write multiple notes with very different contents to various people. However, the biggest problem with suicide notes is that the vast majority of suicides do not leave suicide notes at all (Maris et al., 2000).

Who Leaves Suicide Notes?

The scientific study of suicide notes probably began with Shneidman and Farberow's work (in 1949–1957), after they found a trove of suicide notes stored in boxes in the basement of the Los Angeles County Medical Examiner's offices (Shneidman & Farberow, 1957).

These suicide notes were written from 1944 to 1953. During these years, only about 15% of all Los Angeles suicides left a suicide note; the other 85% did not. Worldwide, about 15 to 25–30% of suicides leave notes. In my 5-year Chicago survey (Maris, 1981), 23% of suicides and nonfatal attempters left notes. When I took a sabbatical in Calgary, Alberta, I discovered that 18% of suicides there left notes. Leenaars (1988), a disciple of Shneidman, concluded that 12–15% of all suicides are note leavers (see also Maris et al., 2000, p. 260).

Certainly, given these data, not finding a suicide note is not *prima facie* evidence of a nonsuicidal death. In fact, the most typical U.S. suicides (viz., older white males) seldom leave suicide notes. They may not have anyone to write to. Of course, this does not mean that older white male suicides do not leave clues to suicide; these clues are just not usually suicide notes.

Some (Tuckman et al., 1959) have argued that suicide note leavers are more likely to be younger females, to be separated or divorced, and to be white (whites are about three times more likely to leave a note than blacks are). Note, too, that if suicide methods are more slow-acting and less lethal (which is true for many younger females), then suicide attempters actually have more time to write notes.

Characteristics of Genuine Suicide Notes

In a systematic review of genuine and simulated suicide notes, Leenaars (1988) found the following characteristics to be statistically more common in genuine notes, roughly in descending order of significance:

1. Ambivalent feelings (e.g., having both death and life wishes).
2. A crucial significant other who "dooms" the individual to suicide (as in "Go ahead and do it! Here are the pills and a glass of water").

3. Figurative intoxication or constriction of thought (confusion or "It was the only thing I could do").
4. Active withdrawal of a significant other (such as through death, separation, or divorce).
5. An adult trauma (e.g., poor health, chronic pain, or loss of spouse).
6. Calamitous relationships (fighting, arguing, getting fired at work, etc.).
7. Love and hate expressed together ("Dear Bob, I hate you. Love, Mary").
8. A sense of total rejection (being all alone with no one to turn to).
9. Unconscious psychodynamics (e.g., identification with lost or rejecting person, depression, high perturbation, unfilled desire, a need to escape).
10. Feelings of helplessness.

Note the many interpersonal themes in the genuine notes, such as rejection, divorce, loss, or abandonment. Often such notes are written by younger females. However, it is also true that an older married person or long-time partner can be devastated by divorce/separation or by the death of the other spouse or partner, and just cannot imagine starting over without him or her. Note, too, that if older males did write notes, then themes might be different (e.g., more about their chronic pain or failing health).

Examples of Suicide Notes

What follows are two genuine suicide notes of typical middle-aged suicides. Sample notes of younger females also can be found in Maris et al. (2000). The suicide note in Case 9.1 is by Samuel Gardner (not his real name; as in most other cases in this book not involving celebrities, other facts have been changed to ensure privacy). He was a 41-year-old mathematician with a long history of severe headaches, and he had gone to a neurologist for relief. His doctor prescribed Inderal, prednisone, and Meclomen, and referred him for biofeedback therapy. He was also taking Serax. Gardner was married and had two young daughters, ages 8 and 13 at the time. He had no previous suicide attempts. He had lost his job and had been out of work for 2 months, however. His doctor did not advise him about any possible drug interaction effects with the Inderal and his diabetes medication. In fact, when Gardner came back to see his doctor about possible drug reactions he was experiencing, he was told: "It's your diabetes, not the medications."

On March 4, 1998, Gardner awoke with a severe headache and stayed home in the morning. On the evening of March 5, he passed out (syncope) in his kitchen after coming inside from working in his garden in an unusually hot temperature. Earlier that same day, Gardner had become confused and disoriented while out at lunchtime and was literally lost for over an hour. On March 6, he got up, made love to his wife, went to a biofeedback appointment, bought his wife a ring, then went home and shot himself in the chest (an atypical wound site) with a .38 revolver he had had since 1979. He put garbage bags under his body before shooting himself, and held a Bible and a picture of his wife and daughters in his free hand. He left the suicide note in Case 9.1 to his wife.

CASE 9.1. Suicide Note of Samuel Gardner

My dearest _____,

    I love you very much and I need to talk with you this one last time. You will not understand what I did and there were no signals from me that could have enabled you to prevent me from doing what I did.

    I am, unlike you, a very weak person. I have had more pain in my head these last several weeks than you can ever know. The medications that I was on and the diabetes being out of control has done more to me and my mind than I could tolerate, and I see no other solution.

    I did not want to be a burden to you and I know that under the circumstances of my death things will be very difficult for you for a while. But I hope that your strong character and the love of your daughters and trusting in God will carry you through these troublesome times.

    I have left a list of what I know to be my assets. You know what's in the various savings and money market accounts. You also have various IRAs and mutual funds that were in my name that will also need to be withdrawn. At this time knowing that your parents are headed in this direction, they will be here soon and can comfort you through these times.

    I know that my mind has been confused these last several weeks and cannot understand what might be coming in the future. My lack of concentration has gotten worse and there have been a couple of times that I had complete loss of memory. There may be a solution to my problem and with God's help maybe I can find it. I have prayed and know it's wrong to do what I am doing, but I have not seen the final answer. I have made a tape for our daughters.

    I love you with all my heart. Take care of yourself. Goodbye. Pray for me for maybe God will take me into his world and I won't go to hell.

Source: Maris. The identifying data have been altered and facts changed to protect confidentiality.

Gardner's note says that his suicide was not his wife's fault, and that he had intolerable pain in his head. However, he demonstrated rigid thinking (he saw his suicide as the only way to solve his problems); he demonstrated obsessive–compulsive traits (he took care to make sure that his wife's parents would be coming soon); he was clearly depressed and hopeless; and he had what Joiner (2005) calls "perceived burdensomeness." Finally, he took comfort from his religion (but note that his fear of going to hell did not stop him from suiciding).

The second suicide note, in Case 9.2, is by John Parsons (again, his name and other case facts have been altered to ensure confidentiality). He was a 49-year-old white male who overdosed on oxycodone in a recreational area in the West. He had earned a BA degree in history, worked in military intelligence (he spoke German), and collected military memorabilia. He had made one prior failed suicide attempt with a gun, which had failed (the gun misfired). Parsons's note is addressed to his dad and mom. In his note, Parsons described his suicide as transformation, not death, and he concludes with "See you soon" (i.e., he did not see suicide as the end).

CASE 9.2. Suicide Note of John Parsons

Dear Dad (and Mom),

    First my sincere apologies for making this letter necessary. I know you have both have been there before, though, and will understand that sometimes a person just despairs too much.

That sometimes we have to have the courage to take control of our lives and say, "I am not going to take it anymore." And that's where I am.

Before either of you leap to conclusions know that nobody is to blame. I have a wonderful marriage, perfect children, and perfect parents. I have a lot of understanding friends and don't owe thousands of dollars to anyone. My problem is simply that my brain chemistry is not working right and hasn't been for some time. I've tried to get help, but cannot get anything done soon. And even then, it will be listening to somebody respond. "Yeah" and "Uh Huh." Then give me another drug to try.

What none of it will do is solve the problems that I have and that make every day a living hell for me. My head and chest feel like they are on fire from 11 o'clock every day. I am driving _____ mad with my incurable moping, and I am yelling at the dogs for being dogs.

I love you both very much and have enjoyed being able to honestly tell people that my childhood was perfect. Because it was. But having to live with constant physical and emotional pain has driven me to my extreme limit and I am just not happy with anything anymore. My greatest desire is to fall asleep and wake up in Heaven, where we will all be together, young, happy and healthy again.

Please, take care of _____. She is so very precious to me and has always been the perfect companion. I love her so. As for my stuff, I've left instructions for Dad to get whatever militaria he wants. Family stuff at some point should go to _____, unless somebody else seems worthy, but only after _____ is ready to part with it. That goes for the piano and everything else. It's hers for as long as she wants it. I've sent _____ instructions for dealing with the militaria. Her phone number is _____.

I love you both and will see you soon. When you get to heaven, dinner will be waiting for you, along with the cat of your choice to warm up your lap.

Source: Maris. Again, the identifying data have been changed.

Motivations for Suicide

By definition, suicides intend to die, but why? What are their motivations? According to Shneidman (1993), suicide indicates psychic pain (which he called "psych-ache"), constricted or rigid thinking ("It was the only thing I could do"), and denial. Often suicide notes suggest the motivations of individuals for suiciding. Leenaars (1988) claims that suicide notes, although limited, can give us some insight into the suicidal mind and the unconscious (*à la* Freud; see Maris et al., 2000).

Based on my Chicago research (Maris, 1981), I claim that the core motives for most completed suicides are the following:

1. Escape (maybe 75% of suicides, especially for older white males).
2. Revenge (maybe 20% of suicides, especially for younger females).
3. Self-sacrifice or self-transformation (taken together, this motive and the next one account for about 5% of suicides).
4. Risk taking.

Escape

Most suicides (correctly or incorrectly) see death as the only real resolution to their life problems—as both Samuel Gardner and John Parsons did, although the motives in Parsons's case also included self-transformation (see Cases 9.1 and 9.2). Becker

(1973) points out that the human condition is finite, fragile, and often painful (cf. DeSpelder & Strickland, 2015). If there is no afterlife or vengeful God, suicide stops all feeling, suffering, and cognition, albeit at a high price. If the person is older, chronically in pain or ill, alone, hopeless, depressed, and angry, then suicide may seem to solve all problems as nothing else really can.

In a passage I have quoted more briefly in Chapter 2, Ishmael makes this comment on the suicidal motivation of escape or fugue in the opening paragraph of *Moby Dick* (Melville, 1851/1981, p. 2): "Whenever I find myself growing grim about the mouth; whenever it is a damp, drizzly November in my soul; whenever I find myself involuntarily pausing before coffin warehouses, and bringing up the rear of every funeral I meet . . . then, I account it high time to get out to sea as soon as I can. This is my substitute for pistol and ball."

Revenge

Many younger people see suicide as a way of getting even or revenge (as in the Biblical story of Samson)—a kind of desperate interpersonal communication, a last gesture to punish or win back estranged loved ones, or even an oblique statement that there is no interpersonal support system for them.

Self-Sacrifice or Self-Transformation

A minority of people see their suicides as a sacrifice for a higher good or cause (i.e., altruistic suicide as described by Durkheim, 1897/1951). Examples include the World War II Japanese *kamikaze* pilots. In the novel *Sophie's Choice* (Styron, 1979), later made into a film starring Meryl Streep, Sophie offers her own life to try to save the lives of her two children in a Nazi concentration camp. But she is forced to pick (her "choice") the one who will die; that is, her offer does not work. As John Parsons's note in Case 9.2 indicates, he believed his suicide would transform him, change his life, not end it, that he would be pain-free, and reunited with his family in heaven.

Risk Taking

A minority of suicides know that their behavior could kill them and accept this possible outcome, but their underlying motivation is to enhance or embellish their lives, to live life to its fullest, even if it kills them (Klausner, 1968). Risk taking is seen in those who die pursuing dangerous sports (e.g., mountain climbing, race car driving, hang gliding, whitewater rafting), as well as in those who play Russian roulette.

This completes our examination and consideration of sociodemographic issues in Part III. Part IV turns to what many suicidologists think are the key suicide risk factors, (viz., mental disorder and the biology and neurobiology of suicide).

PART IV

MAJOR MENTAL DISORDERS, BIOLOGY, NEUROBIOLOGY

CHAPTER 10

Mental Disorder

The Most Important Suicide Risk Factor?

> The best evidence to date indicates that around 95 percent of those who die
> by suicide have a diagnosable mental disorder at the time of their death.
> —THOMAS JOINER

If over 90% (or more; see Joiner, 2005 and the epigraph above) of all suicides have a diagnosable mental disorder, then obviously we need to look closely at mental disorders (www.nami.org). Most suicides never see a mental health professional, nor ever actually get diagnosed with mental disorder. One caveat: This percentage (viz., 90–95%) ignores the widespread prevalence of mental disorders, especially anxiety and mood disorders, in nonsuicidal populations. Kessler (2005: cf. Maris, 2015, p. 8) claims that fully 50% of all Americans will have at least one mental disorder during their lifetime, and yet only 1 in 10,000 Americans commit suicide each year. Clearly, there are other factors in suicide outcome than mental disorders. For example, 85–90% of depressed individuals die natural deaths.

Murphy and Robins (1967) argued that in their St. Louis research, fully 47% of all suicides had a primary depressive disorder. The next most prevalent suicide risk factor was alcohol abuse at 25% (cf. Maris et al., 2000, p. 80). I found the same prevalence (47%) in Chicago for at least *mild* depressive disorder on the original Beck Depression Inventory (BDI) among suicides (Maris, 1981).

We need to be careful here. To say that many suicides have mental disorders is not the same as saying that they are "crazy," psychotic, confused, or intoxicated (Joiner, 2010). For example, only about 5–10% of suicides (1% of the general population) have schizophrenia (Maris, 2015, p. 121), and roughly a third of suicides are intoxicated when they eventually suicide. Put differently, the majority (90–95%) of suicides are not psychotic, and at least 67% are not intoxicated. Most mentally disordered suicides are still capable of forming suicidal intent. They are usually not acting under some irresistible impulse as a result of their mental disorder. Certainly, most suicides are not "crazy." For the most part, they know what they are doing, are basically rational, and, rightly or wrongly, see suicide as problem solving.

Remember, suicidal behavior or ideation itself is not a mental disorder; it is just a diagnostic criterion for two of the mental disorders in DSM-5, major depressive disorder (MDD) and borderline personality disorder (BPD). Indeed, it is somewhat disconcerting that suicidal behavior (mainly, making a suicide attempt) is currently being considered for inclusion in the next edition of DSM as a mental disorder (see American Psychiatric Association, 2013, Section III, pp. 801 ff.). Why would making a suicide attempt mean that a person is mentally disordered? The people behind DSM always seem to want to create more new mental disorders, which perhaps justifies the use of new psychiatric drugs for treating them.

Furthermore, not all mental disorders are equally related to suicide risk and outcome. As shown in Table 10.1, Baldessarini et al. (2012) have found that bipolar disorder, severe depression, and substance use disorders are more highly related to suicide risk than are other mental disorders. Tanney (2000) claims that some mental disorders are not especially related to suicide risk at all.

Usually diagnosis and assessment of mental disorder determine the treatment of suicidal patients, and most of this treatment consists of medication management. To oversimplify, the wrong mental disorder diagnosis likely means the wrong treatment. Let us look at Case 10.1, a hypothetical example of a complete mental diagnosis for a suicidal patient, using the DSM-5 and ICD-10 codes.

CASE 10.1. A Hypothetical Mental Diagnosis

Major depressive disorder, single episode, no psychosis

Alcohol use disorder, moderate

Dependent personality disorder (rule out BPD)

Unspecified cirrhosis of the liver

Homelessness

Low income

Personal history of self-harm

Source: Fictitious case diagnosis compiled by Maris.

In Case 10.1, to minimize suicide risk, the clinician has to consider the following:

• Treatment for a first mild to moderate episode of MDD seems the most likely. This is probably best treated with a selective serotonin reuptake inhibitor (SSRI) like Lexapro, or a serotonin–norepinephrine reuptake inhibitor (SNRI) like Cymbalta or Pristiq (newer medications are marketed constantly). Dosage usually starts low and goes up slowly; for example, treatment with Prozac often begins with 10 mg/day and is increased to 20 mg or more later if necessary. If the MDD is severe, the clinician may need to hospitalize the patient. Depression severity has differing DSM-5 codes and can be confirmed with the BDI-II or the Hamilton Rating Scale

TABLE 10.1. Risk of Suicide in Patients with Specific Mental Disorders versus Controls

Mental disorder	Relative risk (SMR)	Suicide rate (%/year)	Lifetime risk (%)
Bipolar disorder	25	0.39	23.4
Severe depression	21	0.29	17.4
Mixed substance abuse	20	0.28	16.8
Severe anxiety disorder	11	0.15	9.0
Moderate depression	9	0.13	7.8
Schizophrenia	9	0.12	7.2
Personality disorder	7	0.10	6.0
Cancer	2	0.03	1.8
General population	1	0.014	0.8

Note. SMR, standardized mortality ratio to risk in the general population, adjusted for age and sex. Lifetime risk is based on the annual suicide rate multiplied by 60 years of potential risk.
Source: Baldessarini et al. (2012, p. 161). Reprinted with permission from *The American Psychiatric Publishing Textbook of Suicide Assessment and Management,* Second Edition. Copyright © 2012 American Psychiatric Association. All Rights Reserved.

for Depression (HAM-D), or clarified with a treatment team meeting with pooled clinical judgment.

• Since 65% of patients with MDD have at least moderate anxiety (Fawcett, 2012), the clinician may need to treat the anxiety with a long-acting benzodiazepine like Klonopin. Antidepressants usually take 6–8 weeks to work, and even then their efficacy is only 60–70%. Kirsch (2010) claims that 75% of the effect is placebo effect. So the patient's anxiety needs to be treated in the intervening 6–8 weeks at least. The clinician may need to give a major tranquilizer—perhaps a second-generation antipsychotic like Risperdal or Zyprexa.

• Since the patient also has a comorbid alcohol use disorder, the clinician may need to offer detoxification treatment with titrated doses of the benzodiazepine Librium or the antiepileptic drug Neurontin. Psychotherapy will also be needed. Alcohol abuse reduces serotonin levels in the brain and increases impulsivity and suicide risk.

• Dependent personality disorder along with MDD raises additional questions about using psychotherapy. Personality disorders are very hard to treat with just medication and are deeply ingrained. Most therapists use Beck's cognitive–behavioral therapy.

• How does the clinician deal with homelessness, low income, and a history of self-harm? Maybe patient improvement would reduce the threat of recurring self-harm to which the alcohol use disorder and depression contribute?

• What is missing here? Well, a suicide assessment should include consideration of the patient's age, sex, marital status, and SES (viz., demographic factors, including occupation and education); a mental status exam; a psychiatric history; support at home (obtaining contact information for a best friend or parents/family members is advised); a list of other medications; the primary care doctor's name and contact information; prior medical records; a social history; a treatment plan; consultations; maybe some psychological testing; and (of course) listing of the chief complaint. Ask about firearms at home, suicide ideas, specific plans to suicide, and so forth.

• Do not forget the importance of building rapport and creating a therapeutic alliance between patient and therapist. Convey that "I can [I am competent] and will help you [I care]." Do not just write a prescription for psychiatric medicine (think of all the things pills cannot do). Get involved with the patient—and do not take on too many suicidal patients.

Next, let us look at Case 10.2 for Bill Norris, and consider how mental disorder and psychiatric treatment of it affected his suicide risk.

CASE 10.2. Bill Norris

Bill Norris was a curious, sensitive man. He loved Sartre, Sophocles, and Mozart, but was able with equal enthusiasm to champion the virtues of Yeats, Shaw, and Beethoven. By trade, he was a pediatrician, and a good one. Mothers recall how he elicited giggles when he told children he could feel Popsicles and hamburgers in their stomachs as he was examining them, while children knew intuitively that he was someone they could trust with their small bodies and identities. When he died at age 45 by suicide, many in the community wept at his funeral. No one seemed to understand how it could have happened.

Well, how did it happen? Bill had problems with depression off and on for many years. The first episode occurred during his junior year at Harvard. Psychotherapy provided very little help. It seemed to clear up spontaneously after about 6 months. During Bill's senior year in medical school, his father died, and he plunged into terrible despondency. He saw a psychiatrist and was placed on medication. However, the episode lasted another 6 months, and the promotions committee decided that he should not graduate on time.

Because Bill had been held back, he had difficulty finding an internship and residency, even though he graduated *magna cum laude*. When he finished his residency, he went into private practice. Bill married a woman he had known since undergraduate days and had two daughters with her. During this time, he had another episode of depression and was again medicated; the depression cleared in about 1 month.

Things remained relatively quiet until Bill turned 35. But then his wife was diagnosed with inoperable cancer of the liver. She died within a year. Their daughters were 2 and 4 years old. Eventually he remarried; his second wife was a nurse 10 years younger than he was (she had been divorced). Unlike his first wife, Mary, Joann was unintellectual, light-hearted, and fun-loving. But when Joann turned 30, she said that she felt confined by their marriage and wanted to date other men and have an open marriage. Bill never had an affair, but watched his wife go out at 7 P.M. and return at 1 or 2 A.M., while he attended to the kids. Bill then insisted on monogamy, and Joann decided she wanted a divorce instead.

So, for the second time, Bill lost a wife. Since Joann still lived nearby, one night Bill drank 4 ounces of scotch, got inebriated, went to Joann's apartment, and started banging on the door. She called the police, and Bill was arrested for public intoxication and saw his name in a headline in the local newspaper. He was mortified.

Bill's fellow physicians in the community knew that he was having problems, but none of them offered to help. Bill had few close friends. Bill reentered the hospital for his recurring depression. He did not improve on psychiatric medication, and so was given ECT; this helped a great deal. However, the state medical examiners decided to suspend his license because of his recent arrest and hospitalization. His kids asked Bill what he had done wrong. Two weeks after his medical license was reinstated, he took his life. He left no suicide note.

Source: Adapted from *The Broken Brain: The Biological Revolution in Psychiatry* by Nancy C. Andreasen. Copyright © 1984 by Nancy C. Andreasen. Adapted by permission of HarperCollins Publishers.

What can we learn from Bill's case? For one, note the 25-year history of episodic MDD. Bill had what I call a "suicidal career," not just one acute triggering event. As we have seen in earlier chapters, Joiner (2005) calls this "the acquired ability to inflict lethal self-injury." After 25 years of mental illness, one can become hopeless and unable to cope with yet another hospitalization. As we will see below and in Chapter 11, hopelessness is usually more suicidogenic than depression is (Hawton et al., 2005).

The treatment of Bill's depression with psychiatric medication was relatively ineffective. Some people need not only to find an antidepressant (or combination of antidepressants) that works, but to stay on it for life. Bill had what Kramer (1993) calls "kindled depression." It was smoldering and could easily burst into another major depressive episode. Moreover, Bill had lost two wives and lacked a crucial significant other. A person who has at least one other person for support may be able to keep on trying. Bill also lacked close friends, quality of friendships is important too; as I have said in Chapter 7, almost 50% of my Chicago suicides had no close friends. Bill must have felt all alone. Furthermore, Bill's illness was made public, and it stained his reputation; it stigmatized him. He lost his medical license and perhaps the public's trust. If he were hospitalized again, he would probably lose his license permanently. Then what? How could he provide for his daughters? Perhaps the disease of depression alone did not kill Bill, so much as the lack of support and understanding of mental disorder from key people around him. In part because he had a mental disorder, people shunned, avoided, and even disdained him.

Definitions of Mental Disorder

Psychiatry is "the branch of medicine that focuses on the diagnosis and treatment of mental disorders" (Black & Andreasen, 2011, p. xi; also see newer 2014 edition). Psychiatry's primary organ of focus is the brain. Historically, scholars like Freud and Shneidman have countered that the focus should be on the mind. Neuroscience is a big part of modern psychiatry. In this text, I talk a lot about neurotransmitters (serotonin, norepinephrine, GABA, dopamine, acetylcholine, glutamate, etc.), neuroimaging (magnetic resonance imaging [MRI], positron emission tomography [PET], computed tomography [CT], single-photon emission computed tomography [SPECT], etc.), the anatomy of the brain (e.g., the Brodmann areas), psychopharmacology, lab tests (e.g., the dexamethasone suppression test [DST]), and molecular genetics.

There is no one standard nomenclature for either suicidology or mental disorders (O'Carroll et al., 1996; Mundt et al., 2013). At this writing, most mental health professionals rely on either the American Psychiatric Association's DSM-5 or the WHO's ICD-10 (p. 20). In DSM-5, *mental disorder* is defined as "a syndrome characterized by clinically significant disturbance in an individual's cognition, emotion regulation, or behavior that reflects a dysfunction in the psychological, biological, or developmental processes underlying mental functioning" (American Psychiatric Association, 2013, p. 20).

In ICD-10, suicidal acts are assigned E codes to describe their external causes ("due to . . ."). As noted above, they are included in DSM-5 only as symptoms in two mental disorders, MDD and BPD. ICD classifies many physical disorders, conditions, or injuries that are not mental; only one ICD chapter is devoted to mental disorders. Suicide per se is not a mental disorder (although, again as noted earlier, DSM-5 includes suicidal behavior disorder as a "condition for further study" in its Section III). DSM-5 uses ICD-10 diagnostic codes for mental disorders.

In the DSM system, "symptoms and/or signs cluster into clinically recognizable syndromes that when they impair normal functioning are disorders (dysfunctions) and when causative (etiology) mechanisms and natural history are known become diseases, or illnesses" (Tanney, 2000).

DSM-5 recognizes about 22 main types and roughly 478 specific types of mental disorders, depending on how they are counted. In DSM-5, all of the specific mental disorders have symptom checklists, conditions, severity indices, and specifiers. For example, a diagnosis of MDD with an ICD-10 code of F32.2 indicates MDD, single episode, severe, without psychosis. Patients can have *comorbid* mental disorders (more than one mental disorder), and mental disorders can overlap (they are not completely discrete entities).

Most mental disorders are diagnosed by the clinical judgment of qualified mental health professionals using the DSM or ICD disorder symptoms and conditions. But there are psychological, biological, and neurological tests for mental disorders, such as those displayed in Table 10.2.

Models of Mental Disorder

Mental disorders involve eccentric, aberrant, abnormal, dysfunctional mental behaviors and thoughts. The question remains: Why do such behaviors and thoughts occur? Psychiatrists, psychologists, sociologists, and other disciplines have developed models or theories to explain the facts, research results, behaviors, and thoughts characteristic of mental disorders.

For our purposes, there are six major models (of course, there could be others, and the six overlap to some extent):

1. The medical model (Kraepelin, 1906; Sacks, 1973, 1985).
2. The psychoanalytic model (Freud, 1917/1957; Campbell, 1971).

3. The behaviorist (learning and exchange) model (Skinner, 1953; Homans, 1974).
4. Antipsychiatric (conflict and labeling) models (Szasz, 1977).
5. The stress–diathesis model (Holmes & Rahe, 1967).
6. The structural model (Blau, 1977).

The Medical Model

The medical model views mental disorder as a disease (Sacks, 1973, 1985) that is biologically generated and treated (Mann & Currier, 2012; Mann & Rudd, 2018). In other words, mental illness is a little like having the flu, heart disease, or cancer. Note, however, that for most mental disorders, there is not yet clear scientific evidence of a (single or complex) biological etiology; when that is known, the disorder can be called a disease. The argument is that mental disorder is partially genetic and certainly neurobiological. For example, an identical (monozygotic) twin of a person with schizophrenia has about a 50% chance of also being schizophrenic (Haberlandt, 1967). In another study of Amish families, those with a defective gene (viz., a narrow portion of chromosome 11) had about an 85% chance of contracting

TABLE 10.2. Selected Tests for Mental Disorder and Suicidality

Mental disorder or condition	Measurement, test, assessment tool
DSM clinical syndromes	MMPI-2, SCID-5, DIS, MCMI-IV
Mood and depression	HAM-D, BDI-II, SADS
Suicide, suicidality	Cull & Gill SPS, risk factor scales
Psychological autopsy	Shneidman, Maris, et al. autopsy scales
IQ	WAIS-IV
Personality disorders	TAT, Rorschach
Mental disorder for children	House–Tree–Person, observation of play
Brain function and structure	MRI, CT, PET, SPECT, DST
Mental status	Mini-Mental State Exam (30 questions), various clinical interviews
Neurocognitive disorders	Imaging and psychological tests for cognitive function, memory, attention, language, executive function–dysfunction
Personality disorders	CPI

Note. This is just a partial list. Many tests have different versions for different age groups and situations. MMPI-2, Minnesota Multiphasic Personality Inventory–2; SCID-5, Structured Clinical Interview for DSM-5; DIS, Diagnostic Interview Schedule; MCMI-IV, Millon Clinical Multiaxial Inventory–IV; HAM-D, Hamilton Rating Scale for Depression; BDI-II, Beck Depression Inventory–II; SADS, Schedule for Affective Disorders and Schizophrenia; SPS, Suicide Probability Scale; WAIS-IV, Wechsler Adult Intelligence Scale—Fourth Edition; TAT, Thematic Apperception Test; CPI, California Personality Inventory. For "Brain function and structure" tests, see text of this chapter.
Source: All tests selected by Maris; original table.

bipolar disorder at some time in their lives (Egeland et al., 1987). With Huntington's chorea, each child of an affected parent has a 50% chance of getting the disease, too.

The medical model tends to explain mental disorders in terms of system abnormalities in brain neurotransmitters and systems; such as serotonin, dopamine, epinephrine, GABA, acetylcholine, and glutamate. To oversimplify, people with depressive disorders tend to have low serotonin or serotonergic dysfunction, especially in their prefrontal cortex (compared to nondepressed, healthy controls), and people with schizophrenia have overactive dopamine and/or overactive dopamine synapses. The D_2 dopamine receptors are often targeted to be blocked by antipsychotics. Those with Parkinson's disease have brains and CSF low in dopamine. Patients with panic disorder and other anxiety disorders tend to have GABA irregularities, and patients with Alzheimer's disease tend to have acetylcholine irregularities.

SSRIs like Prozac or Lexapro, and SNRIs like Cymbalta or Prestiq, are normally the first line of treatment for depressive disorders. There are also *atypical* antidepressants that act on dopamine (like Wellbutrin) or multiple neurotransmitters, and other newer antidepressants that are used as augmenting drugs; even ketamine (Nemeroff, 2018). The serotonergic system in the brain is related to abnormalities in sleep, aggression (including suicide and homicide), impulse control, pain proneness, headaches, mood volatility, and poor peer relationships. Antidepressants like Prozac are also *neurotropic;* that is, they grow neurons in rat brains (Reynolds, 2012). In neuroanatomy, the concentrations of neurotransmitters in various sites in the brain—such as the frontal cortex, hypothalamus, cerebellum, temporal lobe, parietal cortex, raphe nuclei, limbic system, and hippocampus—are studied. There are also dopaminergic, GABAergic, and other neurosystems.

Of course, mental disorders are much more complicated than mere chemical imbalances. For example, patients with schizophrenia tend to have larger ventricles than nondisordered patients (i.e., they have structural brain differences from healthy controls). Mental disorder is often related to neuroanatomy, and certain brain injuries or diseases can (such as head trauma or tumors) can produce or be associated with mental disorder. Note that the brain is also an electrical system, and some treatments of mental disorder are electrical, such as ECT for mood disorders (Maris, 2015). PET, SPECT, MRI, and CT can show changes in the brains of those with mental disorders (Black & Andreasen, 2014).

Most treatments of mental disorder in the medical model are psychopharmacological (i.e., drug treatments). However there are some other technical procedures, such as transcranial magnetic stimulation, or TMS (see the inside cover of the May 2018 *American Journal of Psychiatry*), and bilateral cingulotomy. Contemporary psychiatrists are mainly psychiatric medication managers, not psychotherapists. For example, SSRIs like Lexapro raise brain serotonin levels, and Thorazine blocks overactive dopamine brain synaptic activity, especially at the D_2 receptors.

The Psychoanalytic Model

The psychoanalytic model was originally developed in the late 1800s; the leading figure in the psychoanalytic movement was Sigmund Freud, a physician in Vienna (Gay, 1988). This model overlaps with the medical model, but its focus is more on the mind than on the brain (see Yakeley, 2018). Although a physician Freud concentrated on early traumas that were repressed into what he called the "unconscious." Freud felt that these early repressed conflicts later caused mental disorder in adults. He treated mainly phobias and neuroses, not psychoses. For example, Freud thought that the disorder of hysteria (which is no longer in DSM) arose from early trauma that led to sexual repression. The treatment consisted of making the unconscious conscious through hypnosis, free association, and dream analysis. Once the repressed childhood traumas were made conscious in adulthood, the mental disorder symptoms tended to abate.

Carl Jung (a younger contemporary of Freud) dealt primarily with hospitalized psychotic patients in Basel, Switzerland. Jung believed in what he called the "collective unconscious," and thought that getting in touch with it could produce psychosis. Jung was much more of a mystic than Freud was. For the most part, psychoanalysis plays a very small part in modern psychiatry. In my own university's psychology department, not one single course is offered today on Sigmund Freud.

The Behaviorist (Learning and Exchange) Model

The learning and exchange model focuses on actual face-to-face interaction. The model asserts that if mental disorders exist, then they have been reinforced, rewarded, and made valuable/profitable in actual social interaction. George Homans (a sociologist at Harvard), a developer of the exchange model, suggested that the mentally disordered learn to act crazy. Both B. F. Skinner (1953), also at Harvard, and Homans (1974) contended that originally random behaviors get differentially rewarded or punished (as pigeons in a so-called "Skinner box" do). Those behaviors that are rewarded tend to get repeated, even institutionalized.

What are some of the possible rewards of being mentally disordered? In Ken Kesey's (1962) novel *One Flew Over the Cuckoo's Nest,* "Chief" Bromden is allowed to be left alone on the ward because he feigns autism. Sociologists talk about the "sick role," in which mentally or physically disordered people are given a temporary reprieve from social responsibilities. Goffman (1961) said that mental hospital patients are rewarded if they accept their diagnoses, take their prescribed drugs, and in general conform to the hospital's expectations. If they try to act "normal," then they are punished. This has been called "iatrogenesis" (i.e., illness caused by health care).

Sensitivity and creativity are often thought to be associated with bipolar disorder. Some poets or artists with bipolar disorder might be considered rewarded for being mentally disordered. If artists could be cured of this disorder, would they still produce art?

Antipsychiatric (Conflict and Labeling) Models

Antipsychiatric (conflict and labeling) models of mental disorder (Szasz, 1961; Singer, 2013) tend to conceive of mental disorder as products of culture or value differences, not as diseases. For example, a more sociocultural model may define mental disorder simply as "behavior that exceeds the tolerance of others" and that tends to get the person locked up involuntarily (Eitzen with Zinn, 1989) for "breaking residual rules" (Scheff, 1974). To put this another way, some rules or norms are considered so fundamental that not observing them suggests mental disorder; an example might be coming to a college class naked, which has happened at the University of California, Berkeley.

Unlike persons with physical illness, people can become mental patients just because others (especially people in positions of power, such as police officers, judges, or physicians) label them crazy or dangerous, perhaps through an arrest or commitment procedure. And these labels stick (Lemert, 1951). Applying psychiatric labels or diagnoses can be a power move by those in authority to control difficult, annoying, eccentric people who are not in fact crazy but just oppositional or eccentric. For example, Mary Baker Eddy, the founder of the Christian Science religion, was committed to the Massachusetts State Hospital.

Psychiatrist Thomas Szasz (1961) said that psychiatry is for controlling people who have a religion or belief that most of us do not like. He said that a city hospital's psychiatry department ought to be housed in City Hall, next to the police station. Szasz thought that mental disorder was something one *does*, not something that one has. He talked about the "myth of mental illness." Szasz said that after death you cannot do an autopsy and determine if the formerly living patient were mentally disordered, which you should be able to do if the medical model were correct that mental disorder is a disease. I had an interesting debate with Szasz in Washington, D.C., on February 1, 1985 (which was broadcast on C-SPAN), in which he argued against suicide prevention.

The conflict model says that we lock people up in mental hospitals in part because of their low social status, rather than their mental disorder. One study (Szasz, 1961) found that about 30–42% of mental patients were involuntarily committed.

The Stress–Diathesis Model

As discussed in Chapter 7, Holmes and Rahe (1967) argued that when people with certain vulnerabilities (diathesis) have an excess of especially negative life events (stressors), they will tend to become mentally (and physically) disordered (cf. Kees van Heeringen, cited in Dwivedi, 2012). For example, anxiety, panic, and migraines can all result from repeated stress. Think of the stress associated with concentration camps in World War II, natural disasters (like Hurricanes Katrina, Hugo, Matthew, Harvey, Irma, or Maria), or returning from combat with PTSD. In one study, a significant life event or life change was related to a relapse of schizophrenia. On the Holmes and Rahe stress test (see Table 7.1), other things being equal, a life events score of 150–200 in a year can put an individual at risk for a health disorder.

The Structural Model

Social structure is important because it affects our opportunities for social interaction, and interaction tends to increase liking (see Ginn, 2011). The structural model focuses on the size and proximity of the mentally disordered population. One of the key concepts in Blau's (1977) structural theory is *heterogeneity*. Heterogeneity is the probability that any two people selected at random will come from different groups, such as a mentally disordered group and a nondisordered group. Heterogeneity equals 1 minus the sum of the proportions of (here) two groups squared ($H = 1 - \Sigma p_i^2$). For example, if 3% of the population is treated for mental disorder each year, heterogeneity would equal $1 - (.03)^2 + (.97)^2$ or .06. Thus any two people selected at random in the United States would have a 6% chance of one coming from a mentally disordered population and one from a nondisordered population (all other things being equal). This is important, because opportunities for social interaction affect our attitudes toward mental disorder (Maris, 1988). That is, the more we interact with others, the more we tend to like them.

Types of Mental Disorders

Given the DSM definition of mental disorder, what are the basic types of disorders, how many are there, and how are they differentiated? As noted earlier, DSM-5 has about 22 basic types of mental disorders and 478 specific diagnoses. As shown in Table 10.3, in every edition of DSM since it was first published, the number of mental disorder diagnoses has increased.

Table 10.4 lists the 22 basic types of mental disorders and a few examples of each type. Of course, these examples are neither exhaustive nor especially representative. I always wonder why there are 22 and not (say) 17 or 25. Each category seems to have a distinctive, coherent, and relatively consistent subject matter, although there is some overlap among them. The types of disorders are decided by a committee vote; the choice is not based on just scientific evidence, such as biological evidence from clinical trials (Carlat, 2010).

The 22 types of mental disorders are differentiated by subject matter and also by patients' age, sex, gender, and mood; the presence–absence of psychosis, personality problems, impulse control problems, stress, dissociation, and related bodily dysfunctions; whether or not they are related to the use of a substance or medication; severity; and number of episodes. In addition, there are the conditions that used to be called the *V codes* and are now the *Z codes*—conditions that are not mental

TABLE 10.3. Numbers of Psychiatric Diagnoses in Successive Editions of DSM

Year published	Edition number	Approximate number of psychiatric diagnoses
1952	I	128
1968	II	182
1980	III	265
1994	IV	300
2000	IV-TR	312
2013	5	478

Source: Numbers of psychiatric diagnoses counted and compiled by Maris.

TABLE 10.4. Basic Types of Mental Disorders

Type	Examples
1. Neurodevelopmental	ADHD, autism spectrum, intellectual disability
2. Schizophrenia spectrum, other psychotic	Schizophrenia, schizotypal, schizophreniform
3. Bipolar	Bipolar I and II
4. Depressive	MDD
5. Anxiety	Specific phobia, panic
6. Obsessive–compulsive	Body dysmorphic, trichotillomania
7. Trauma- and stressor-related	PTSD
8. Dissociative	Dissociative identity, depersonalization
9. Somatic symptoms	Conversion
10. Feeding and eating	Anorexia, bulimia nervosa
11. Elimination	Enuresis
12. Sleep–wake	Narcolepsy
13. Sexual dysfunctions	Delayed ejaculation, erectile, orgasmic
14. Gender dysphoria	Gender dysphoria
15. Disruptive, impulse-control, conduct	Oppositional defiant, conduct
16. Substance-related, addictive	[Name of substance] use disorder
17. Neurocognitive	Delirium, major neurocognitive due to Alzheimer's
18. Personality	Three clusters
19. Paraphilia	Voyeurism, frotteurism, sadism, fetishism
20. Other mental	Due to another medical condition
21. Medication-induced	Neuromalignant syndrome, tardive dyskinesia
22. Other conditions	Abuse, neglect, economic problems, academic or educational problems

Note. The disorders in the "Examples" column do not constitute a complete list of disorders.
Source: Table compiled and examples chosen by Maris.

disorders per se, but that "may be a focus of clinical attention." Of course, not all disorders are related to suicide, as we have seen above. However, major depression, bipolar disorder, and schizophrenia are more highly related to suicidal behaviors than other mental disorders, except perhaps for BPD.

In the initial paragraphs for the chapter on each basic type of mental disorder in DSM-5, there is an attempt to categorize and differentiate that group. The medical model of psychiatry might suggest that there are distinctive biological, genetic, and/or neurobiological characteristics and etiologies for each type of mental disorder—for example, serotonin dysfunctions for major depression, dopamine irregularities for schizophrenia, acetylcholine dysfunctions for Alzheimer's, GABA irregularities for anxiety, and so on. Unfortunately, the science is not quite there yet, and thus the DSM remains a work-in-progress.

Diagnosis of Mental Disorder

How are the roughly 478 specific mental disorders diagnosed? There are checklists of symptoms, signs, and other criteria for each of the mental disorders; conditions that must be met (e.g., how many and which symptoms must be present); specifiers of various sorts (e.g., rapid cycling in bipolar disorders); and severity indices (e.g., mild, moderate, or severe depression). The specific mental disorder needs to differ from an individual's normal baseline functioning and to impair typical functioning to a clinically significant degree for various lengths of time.

Armed with mental disorder symptoms and criteria, a qualified mental health professional does a thorough initial assessment (often lasting 1–1½ hours; Rudd, 2012). The types of questions asked in a psychiatric evaluation of an adult are listed in Table 10.5. Unfortunately, there can be a lot of disagreement on which diagnoses are appropriate for a particular patient.

Let me give one example of psychiatric diagnosis here. More detailed information is given for diagnosis of specific types of disorders in Chapters 11, 12, 13, and 14. Given its prominent association with suicide, I focus here on MDD. For a diagnosis of MDD in DSM-5, a patient has to meet at least five of the nine criteria (including at least criterion 1 or 2) listed under A below for at least 2 weeks, and the condition must be a change from the individual's normal functioning (the list below is elaborated as my own, not just the DSM's). Criteria A–C constitute the criteria for a major depressive episode or MDE; criteria D and E must be met for a diagnosis of MDD to be made.

A. Five (or more) of the following symptoms have been present during the same 2-week period and represent a change from previous functioning; at least one of the symptoms is either (1) depressed mood or (2) loss of interest or pleasure.
1. Depressed mood most of the day, nearly every day, as indicated by either subjective report (e.g., feels sad, empty, hopeless) or observation made by others (e.g., appears tearful). (Note: In children and adolescents, can be irritable mood.)
2. Markedly diminished interest or pleasure in all, or almost all, activities

TABLE 10.5. Sample Adult Psychiatric Evaluation

I. Identifying information
II. Chief complaint
III. History of present illness
IV. Substance abuse history
V. Past psychiatric history
VI. Past medical history
VII. Family, social history
VIII. Mental status exam
IX. Diagnoses and codes
X. Treatment plan, including psychiatric medications

Source: Hypothetical mental health form by Maris.

most of the day, nearly every day (as indicated by either subjective account or observation.)

3. Significant weight loss when not dieting or weight gain (e.g., a change of more than 5% of body weight in a month), or decrease or increase in appetite nearly every day. (Note: In children, consider failure to make expected weight gain.)

4. Insomnia or hypersomnia nearly every day.

5. Psychomotor agitation or retardation nearly every day (observable by others, not merely subjective feelings of restlessness or being slowed down).

6. Fatigue or loss of energy nearly every day.

7. Feelings of worthlessness or excessive or inappropriate guilt (which may be delusional) nearly every day (not merely self-reproach or guilt about being sick).

8. Diminished ability to think or concentrate, or indecisiveness, nearly every day (either by subjective account or as observed by others).

9. Recurrent thoughts of death (not just fear of dying), recurrent suicidal ideation without a specific plan, or a suicide attempt or a specific plan for committing suicide.

B. The symptoms cause clinically significant distress or impairment in social, occupational, or other important areas of functioning.

C. The episode is not attributable to the physiological effects of a substance or to another medical condition.

D. The occurrence of the major depressive episode is not better explained by schizoaffective disorder, schizophrenia, schizophreniform disorder, delusional disorder, or other specified and unspecified schizophrenia spectrum and other psychotic disorders.

E. There has never been a manic episode or a hypomanic episode.[1]

I, and most medical students, remember the nine symptoms listed under A by the following mnemonic: <u>D</u>epression <u>I</u>s <u>W</u>orth <u>S</u>tudiously <u>M</u>emorizing <u>E</u>xtremely <u>G</u>rueling <u>C</u>riteria, <u>S</u>orry (DIWSMEGCS). The underscored letters of this mnemonic stand for criteria 1–9 under A above, in order.

For a case of MDD, the diagnostic code stands for either a single or a recurrent episode that can be characterized as mild, moderate, or severe; with psychotic features; in partial or full remission; or unspecified. (Other specifiers may also be applied, but these do not affect the code number.) Let us apply the MDD criteria to the fictional individual in Case 10.3.

CASE 10.3. A 30-Year-Old Man with Depression

A 30-year-old man was transferred to a long-term facility for long-standing feelings of depression. History revealed that he first experienced a depressive episode at age 23. At that time he

---

was dysphoric and hopeless, lost considerable weight due to lack of appetite, withdrew from all social contacts, and heard voices (which he believed came from God) telling him he was being punished for past sins. He was hospitalized for 2 months, was tried on various antidepressants with little success, and was eventually given a course of ECT. He showed some partial improvement for 6 months or so, and his psychotic symptoms remitted. However, he became depressed again and has been depressed off and on ever since. Currently, he has been depressed for at least 3 years, without any periods of remission of his symptoms. He has severe depressed mood, insomnia, poor appetite, fatigue, and feelings of worthlessness nearly every day. He feels hopeless, has recurrent suicide ideation (although he has no specific plan to act on his ideation), has little interest in anything, and has no energy.

He has not worked since age 23 and is receiving Social Security Disability benefits. Apparently, the man has never really been happy. History reveals that he felt dysphoric throughout high school, long before he experienced severe depression in adulthood. He has never had much energy, has always suffered from insomnia, and has chronic feelings of low self-esteem. As a result, his functioning was always somewhat marginal. He had few friends, rarely dated, and never established a career. There is no history of elevated or irritable mood or a history of substance abuse. He has no significant medical problems.

Source: June Sprock, *www.indstate.edu/cas/psychology/faculty-and-staff/clinical-faculty/june-sprock-phd* (personal communication). Used with permission.

The diagnoses for Case 10.3 would be as follows:

- MDD, recurrent episode, severe.
- Persistent depressive disorder (dysthymia), early onset, with persistent MDE, severe.

This combination of diagnoses means that criteria for MDD have been met throughout the past 2 years (hence "persistent"); the patient has had at least one period of remission in the past, but has MDD now (hence "recurrent"); and the number and intensity of the symptoms have gone far beyond what is needed to make either diagnosis (hence "severe").

Prevalence of Mental Disorder

Let me reflect a little more on the prevalence of mental disorder and its relationship to suicide. I have begun this chapter saying that over 90% of all suicides could be diagnosed as mentally disordered. This seems to suggest that if we could just diagnose and control mental disorder (especially depression), then the suicide rate would drop precipitously.

One estimate for 2013 was that 43.8 million people in the United States had one of the DSM mental disorders (*www.nimh.nih.gov/health/statistics*); I have estimated the prevalence to be 46 million (see Maris, 2015). This would have amounted to 14.6–15.3% of all U.S. adults (out of a total of 300 million at that time) having a mental disorder. By 2015, the U.S. population was 321 million and the world population was 7.2 billion.

About 17% of all Americans will get a depressive disorder at some time in their lives. The rate is about twice as high for women. The WHO calls depressive disorder the single most disabling illness in the world, including physical illnesses (see Chapter 11). About 10% of Americans over age 6 take an antidepressant.

Generally, we would expect that the larger the population and the more mental disorder diagnoses there are, the higher the suicide rate (Whitaker, 2010). So how has the mentally disordered population changed over time? Table 10.6 might suggest that the number of those with mental disorders has actually gone down. In the United States, there were 512,501 patients (mainly with schizophrenia) in state and county mental hospitals in 1950, but only 54,015 in 1997 (an 89–90% decline). This phenomenon is often referred to as "deinstitutionalization."

But the Table 10.6 data are misleading. We do know that phenothiazine drugs like Thorazine were introduced in the 1950s, and thereafter persons with schizophrenia or psychotics could function better outside the mental hospitals. So, in a sense, the mentally disordered population was not reduced; it was just moved. A lot of former mental patients also ended up in jails and prisons or returned later (recidivism) to the state and county hospitals. Note that most depressed and anxious patients are in private hospitals or seeing their family doctors. Thus, to get a true count of the number of the mentally disordered, one would need to take the censuses of (1) state and county hospitals, (2) private psychiatric hospitals, (3) Department of Veterans Affairs hospitals (which take in a lot of patients with alcoholism), (4) psychiatric wards in local hospitals, and (5) family practice

TABLE 10.6. Number of Resident Patients, Total Admissions, Net Releases, and Deaths: State and County Mental Hospitals, United States, 1950–1997

Year	Number of hospitals	Resident patients	Admissions that year	Net releases	Deaths
1950	322	512,501	152,286	99,659	41,280
1955	275	558,922	178,003	126,498	44,384
1956[a]	278	551,390	185,597	145,313	48,236[a]
1960	280	535,540	234,791	192,818	49,748
1965	290	475,202	316,664	288,397	43,964
1970	315	337,619	384,511	386,937	30,804
1975	313	193,436	376,156	384,520	13,401
1980	276	132,164	370,344	366,766	6,800
1985	286	109,839	335,940	NA	NA
1990	281	92,059	277,813	NA	2,321
1992	275	83,320	254,932	NA	NA
1994	260	72,258	231,089	NA	NA
1997	234	54,015	190,183	NA	NA

Note. NA, not available.
[a]First year of widespread use of pharmaceuticals in state and county hospitals.
Source: National Institute of Mental Health, data over various years. Data in public domain.

patients being treated for mental disorders. However, most modern research methods resolve these issues (e.g., see Kessler, 2005; Kessler et al., 2015).

From other data (Whitaker, 2010, Ch. 6), we know that in 1955, 1 in 468 people were hospitalized (a rate, not just a frequency) for any mental disorder. By 1987, that number had risen to 1 in 184. By 2007, 1 in 76 suffered from any mental disorder. Overall, from 1955 to 2007, the mental disorder rate had increased sixfold (Angell, 2011a, 2011b). Whitaker (2010) calls this a virtual "epidemic" of mental disorder. By 2007, the United States had a 22–23% total rate of any mental disorder (i.e., about 44 million people). Angell claims that in 2003, 46% of the U.S. population met DSM criteria for mental disorder.

There were 76 million Americans in 1900, but 315 million by 2015. We also know (see Table 10.3) that the number of mental disorders (i.e., specific diagnoses) increased from 128 in 1952 to 478 in 2013. It only seems reasonable that the number of mentally disordered Americans increased from 1950 to 2015, but the exact size of the increase is unknown.

Yet the U.S. suicide rate over that same time has stayed almost constant (viz., 11–1213.2 per 100,000, with a few peaks and troughs). If mental disorder causes suicide, then it makes no sense that the mental disorder rate should have increased so dramatically, while the suicide rates have stayed virtually the same. Let us take a closer look at the prevalence of suicide over time (i.e., from about 1900 to 2015). As the U.S. population grew, the absolute number of suicides also grew. For example, there were 32,533 suicides in 2005, 38,364 in 2010, 41,148 in 2013, and 44,193 in 2015 (the latest available data). But we must convert absolute numbers of suicide to rates to control for population growth or change. When we do that, we see that overall U.S. suicide rates have stayed about the same for the last 115 years (again, 11–13.2 per 100,000). However, see Tavernese, 2016.

There have been small peaks and troughs in the suicide rate in times of economic depression (e.g., 1929 and 1987) and during World Wars I and II, but overall from 1900 to 2015 the U.S. suicide rate has been very constant—virtually a flat line. For example, the rate in 1985 was exactly the same as it was in 2013. Even though rates of mental disorder have increased over time, the suicide rate has stayed about the same, with a slight but steady increase recently. Suicide rates among hospital patients with major depression (lifetime) has stayed about 10–15 out of 100. The suicide rate in the general population is about 1 in 10,000 per year. It seems as if mental disorder is highly related to the suicide rate, but is it? The general population has roughly a 50% lifetime chance of becoming mentally disordered, but only a 1 in 10,000 chance of suiciding in a given year.

Clearly, a lot of depressed or mentally disordered patients never commit suicide. Again, about 85–90% of depressed patients die natural deaths. In sum, although mental disorder is a very important risk factor for suicide outcome, the etiology of suicide is multifactorial (i.e., suicide is not just a result of mental disorder). There are many different interacting causes of suicide and many different types of suicide. In Chapters 11–13, I now turn to three specific groups of mental disorders closely related to suicide and examine them in much more detail.

CHAPTER 11

Major Depression
Undiagnosed and Untreated

Depression is a disorder of mood, so mysteriously painful and elusive . . . as to verge close
to being beyond description. It thus remains nearly incomprehensible to those who have
not experienced it . . . a veritable howling tempest in the brain . . . a brainstorm.
—WILLIAM STYRON

Depression is a terrible illness. People with depression would rather be asleep
than awake, dead than asleep. Vizzini (2006) writes, "It was almost like a reverse
nightmare, I woke up into a nightmare." The smallest challenges, like getting out
of bed and dressing, seem Herculean, and life is devoid of pleasure or interest. You
cannot sleep or eat. People who are depressed have a sad, despairing mood or profound dejection most of the day, almost every day; a loss of spontaneity, decrease in
mental productivity, reduction of libido and sex drive (which antidepressants often
finish off), and inability to accept responsibility; motor retardation (usually) or excitation; diminished ability to give or receive gratification or love; loss of self-esteem;
self-contempt and increased guilt; disintegration of ego; and pathological, narcissistic aspirations, if any (Maris, 1981, 2015; Maris et al., 2000; Black & Andreasen,
2014).

As Muncie (1963) said long ago, "Depressed patients are those people who find
themselves essentially bankrupt in self-esteem, once they can no longer produce
the effort necessary to gain contingent approval." However, this does not really capture the private, subjective feelings of the depressed individual. For example, David
Foster Wallace (1998), a novelist who hanged himself in 2008, wrote:

> The so-called psychotically depressed person who tries to kill herself, doesn't do
> so out of "hopelessness" or of any abstract conviction that life's assets and debits
> do not square. The person in whom its [depression's] agony reaches a certain
> unendurable level [psychache] will kill herself the same way a trapped person will
> eventually jump from a burning high-rise.

Although about 15% of the American population each year could get a DSM diagnosis of some form of depression, only about 3% ever get treated. Most depressed people are never diagnosed or treated (especially men). That is, "People who die by suicide are often experiencing undiagnosed or untreated depression" (*https://suicideprevention.ca/the-relationship-between-suicide-and-mental-health*). This is especially true for the typical U.S. suicide, an older white male. Older men are very likely not to get diagnosed or treated for depression; even if they do, the antidepressant dosage may be too low, or they may have the wrong combination of psychiatric medications (Sher, 2015; Benson et al., 2018). Also, can pills alone get the job done?

I recently had a methicillin-resistant Staphyloccus aureaus (MRSA) infection in my knee, which was treated surgically and then with intravenous (IV) vancomycin and oral cephalexin, which caused nausea (1,500–2,000 mg/day for 15 months, which seemed like forever). After surgery, in an opiate haze, psychotic, nauseous, and in chronic pain, I felt acutely suicidal for the first time in my life. As Wallace wrote, I did not know if I could endure this situation. My "house" was on fire and it felt like I was burning alive. When the pain subsided and the hydrocodone was stopped, my suicide ideation slowly abated too, and life seemed possible once again. Everyone (even suicidologists) has a pain threshold (both physical and psychic) beyond which life may be impossible. That is, death is sometimes not really a choice.

Epidemiology of Depression

Depression in all of its types accounts for about 10% of all costs for biomedical illness worldwide, including physical illness. In its Global Burden of Disease project, the WHO (1996, 2008, 2012a) has reported depressive disorders to be the number one source of disability (as measured in *disability-adjusted life years,* or *DALYs*). *Prevalence* refers to the total existing cases, and *incidence* indicates the number of new cases in a given time period, usually within a year. The 12-month prevalence (Kessler, 2005) for MDD is about 6.7% of all adults, and its lifetime prevalence is about 17% (Black & Andreasen, 2014). About 30% of depressive disorders are severe. The lifetime prevalence of bipolar disorder (see Chapter 12) is about 2%.

Females on average have rates of depression roughly twice those of males (e.g., 8.3 vs. 4.6 in 2008 in the United States). Depression rates for black females are about four times higher than those of black males, but their suicide rate is still very low. Why? Females are 70% more likely than males to experience lifetime depression, but have lower suicide rates than males do. For youth ages 12–17 in 2008, depression was about three times higher in girls than in boys. Blacks (before researchers control for gender) are 40% less likely than whites to experience lifetime depression. Obviously, for women especially, some factors other than depression cause suicide (see the data on China and India in Chapter 8; see also Maris et al., 2000).

Generally, the lifetime prevalence of depression decreases with increasing age (which seems counterintuitive). For example, in 2008 the prevalence of depression in people ages 18–25 was 8.7% percent, but in ages 50 and over it was 4.5%; it was higher in midlife. The median duration of MDD is about 3 months, but about 20% are not recovered after 24 months (Spuker et al., 2002). Surprisingly, there is evidence (Pasternick et al., 2006) that MDD may have a shorter duration when untreated (13 weeks) than when treated (23 weeks). The median onset age for major depression is 32 years, and for bipolar disorder is 25 years.

In a 2009–2010 survey (*N* = 5,639) of drug use and health, Mojtabai (2013) found that only 38.4% of participants with clinician-identified depression met the DSM criteria for MDD. Mojtabai concluded that depression was overdiagnosed and overtreated pharmacologically on a remarkable scale (I realize that this finding is at odds with the main thesis of this chapter). The study also found that 10% of Americans took antidepressants, including 25% of women ages 40–50. Elderly patients were most likely to be misdiagnosed with depression.

My Chicago suicide surveys (Maris, 1969, 1981) revealed that depressive disorders were the number one single risk factor for suicide outcomes (see also Maris et al., 2000; Green et al., 2015). About 47% of the completed suicides in Chicago had moderate to severe depression, as measured by the original BDI (Maris, 1981). Guze and Robins (1970) found that about 15% of patients hospitalized for primary affective (mood) disorders later killed themselves. Bostwick and Pankratz (2000) later revised that figure downward to about 10%.

Depression and Suicide

What does it mean to say that suicide is related to depressive disorders, bipolar disorder, or major depression (Hawton, 2005)? It means that in appropriately drawn (random, the proper size, etc.) samples of suicides and controls, rates of depressive disorders are statistically significantly higher in suicides than in the controls. For example, Fawcett (2006, 2012) claims that 60% of all U.S. suicides have MDD, versus only 6.7% of all adults (see Box 11.1). Jamison (1993) further points out that writers and artists not only have higher suicide rates than the general population (see Figure 11.1), but have significantly more MDD and bipolar disorder than nonsuicidal controls do.

These findings do not mean that depression necessarily or by itself *causes* suicide, for which there are very stringent criteria (Maris, 2015, pp. 36–37). The vast majority of depressed individuals never suicide. But of all suicide risk factors, MDD and bipolar disorder are the most highly related single suicide risk factors.

What if there were a causal relationship between suicide and depressive disorder? What might the neurobiological etiology be? As noted in earlier chapters, the main biological hypothesis is that the brains and CSF of suicides show lower serotonin levels than do healthy nondepressed controls, especially in the prefrontal cortex of the brain (i.e., too little serotonin in the wrong place) (Äsberg et al., 1976; Mann & Currier, 2012; Dwivedi, 2012; see also Chapter 23). Most antidepressants (such as the SSRIs and SNRIs) try to correct this chemical imbalance by increasing CSF serotonin and boosting the serotonergic system (among other things). Of course, this theory of depression and suicide (and there are several competing theories) is far more complex than stated here.

Following the medical model of mental disorder (see Chapter 10), modern psychiatry tends to assume that depressive disorders result from or are characterized

BOX 11.1. Key Points about Depressive Disorders and Suicide

- About 60% of all suicides in the United States occur in people with MDD.
- In spite of depression treatment advances, there has been no significant decrease in suicide ideation.
- A Finland study of completed suicides showed that only 3% had received adequate doses of any antidepressant.
- Suicide is not predictable in an individual patient. Clinicians can only assess chronic or acute risk.
- It is important to assess the severity of psychic pain and the patient's ability to tolerate it.
- Chronic high suicide risk is indicated by past history, prior suicide attempts, plans, hospital admissions, and DSM Cluster B personality disorders.
- Factors associated with acute high suicide risk are agitation, panic attacks, global insomnia, and severe anxiety.
- Sixty-five percent of patients with MDD have at least moderate anxiety.
- Assiduously monitoring and aggressively treating anxiety in depression are recommended.
- A previous history of suicidal tendencies may be a better predictor than current state.
- Fifty-six percent of suicides in Finland died on their first attempt.
- Fewer than 20% of suicides had communicated suicidal thoughts to a physician or helper.
- Symptoms of anxiety or agitation should be treated with a benzodiazepine like clonazepam.
- Protective factors for children under age 18 include spiritual interests and religious beliefs.
- It is important to offer realistic hope for relief from pain and suffering.
- When a therapist feels hopeless about a suicidal patient, it may be time for the patient to get another therapist.
- It is important to assess both high and low, chronic and acute suicide risk, and to treat the different types differently.
- About 50% of patients are at chronic high suicide risk.
- Lithium treatment produces an eightfold reduction in suicide.
- Cognitive therapy reduces suicide ideation better than other therapies.
- There are no data demonstrating that 8 weeks of an antidepressant alone prevents suicide better than a placebo.
- A major goal of medicine is the battle against an untimely death.

Source: Excerpted and rewritten by Maris from Fawcett (2006).

by various dysfunctions in the brain's neurochemical systems. These dysfunctions involve neurotransmitters like dopamine, serotonin, epinephrine, norepinephrine, cholinergics (like acetylcholine in dementia), GABA (the "brake" in the brain), glutamate (an excitatory amino acid), and so forth. As of 2015, a total of about 30–100 neurotransmitters had been identified, but about 10 do most of the work.

The whole theory of depressive disorders, brain neurotransmitters, and neurosystems is not well understood or categorically convincing. It was first proposed by Bowers in 1969 (see Whitaker, 2010, p. 71). Whitaker (2010, p. 263) refers to it as "the dogma of biological psychiatry." It is just that: a theory, not a cogent, scientific

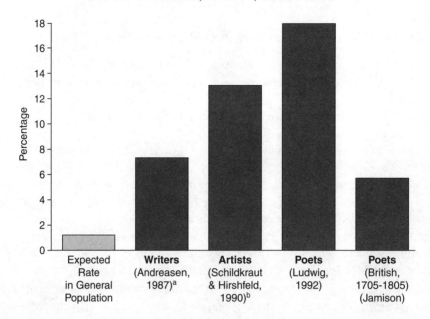

FIGURE 11.1. Suicide rates in writers and artists. References for the studies cited may be found in Jamison (1993). [a]Suicide rate at time of study completion. [b]Two other artists died individually in single-car accidents. *Source:* From *Touched with Fire: Manic–Depressive Illness and the Artistic Temperament* by Kay Redfield Jamison. Copyright © 1993 by Kay Redfield Jamison. Reprinted with the permission of The Free Press, a division of Simon & Schuster, Inc. All rights reserved.

fact (Carlat, 2010; Kramer, 1993; Mann & Currier, 2012). Angell (2011a, 2011b) says that the neurobiological explanation of mental disorder is a little like arguing that too little aspirin causes headaches. In spite of the simplistic claims and the ads of drug companies, the human brain is extremely complex. We have just begun to understand it. For example, there are about 14 times more neurons in a single human brain than there are people on our planet. When Pfizer (for example) talks about "cell A" communicating with "cell B" in its Zoloft television commercials, it is describing nothing more than a crude, oversimplified theory. Note, too, that a healthy, normal person cannot be made depressed simply by lowering his or her CSF serotonin level.

Diagnosis and Classification of Disorders Involving Depression

The specific criteria for MDD have been discussed in Chapter 10; I am not going to repeat these criteria here, except to refer readers to section 1 of Table 11.1. I do, however, comment more here on a few select details about the diagnosis of the principal disorders that involve depression. The anhedonia criterion is not intuitively obvious. *Anhedonia* has the same root as the word *hedonism,* or "pleasure seeking." Depressed patients are _anhedonic;_ that is, they tend to be unable to experience pleasure from ordinary life activities that most nondepressed people find gratifying.

TABLE 11.1. Selected Disorders Involving Depression

1. Major depressive disorder (MDD)
   a. Mnemonic is DIWSMEGCS (see Chapter 10); includes at least five of nine "A" criteria (including either criterion 1 or 2, plus any four others) for a minimum of 2 weeks, and a change from baseline functioning.
   b. Codes depend on episode and severity specifiers. For example, F32 (not codable by itself) = single or first episode (mild = F32.0, moderate = F32.1, severe = F32.2, and with psychotic features = F32.3); F33 (not codable by itself) = two or more episodes (mild, moderate, severe, and severe with psychotic features = F33.0, F33.1, F33.2, and F33.3, respectively). HAM-D or BDI-II can also be used to measure severity.
   c. Treat for 4–5 months, or for the patient's lifetime if kindled depression is present (see Kramer, 1993).
   d. First-line treatment: SSRIs (like Lexapro), or SNRIs (like Pristiq), for 4–8 weeks. If no change (or serious adverse effects), then change the antidepressant or the dosage or augment it with other antidepressants (e.g., lithium or Abilify). Start anxiolytics earlier (like Klonopin). Use antipsychotics, benzodiazepines, and ECT as needed.
   e. There is a 17% lifetime prevalence of MDD; females have rates twice as high as male rates.
2. Persistent depressive disorder (dysthymia) (code = F34.1) The essential feature of dysthymia is a depressed mood that occurs for most of the day, for more days than not, for at least 2 years (1 year for children and adolescents).
3. Bipolar I (BP I) or bipolar II (BP II) disorder
   a. A mnemonic for mania is GSTIDAP (the first letters of the seven "B" criteria in DSM-5 for a manic episode—grandiosity, sleep disorder, excessive talking, etc.). A patient must have at least three of the seven criteria, for a minimum of one week, and a change from baseline function.
   b. BP I is the classic bipolar disorder; it requires at least one manic episode, accompanied by at least one major depressive episode and possibly by hypomanic or unspecified episodes.
   c. BP I codes depend on current or most recent types of episodes and specifiers. For example, current or most recent episode manic (codes are different if most recent episode was depressed): F31.11 = BP I mild, F 31.12 = moderate, F 31.13 = severe, and F 31.14 = severe with psychotic features (there are other specifiers, such as rapid cycling, etc.).
   d. BP II involves at least one hypomanic episode plus a depressive episode. A hypomanic episode is similar to a manic episode, but less intense. The BP II code is F31.81.
   e. Treatment: lithium, Depakote, Tegretol, Lamictal, Gabapentin, Trileptal, Gabitril, Topamax, Latuda, and other psychiatric drugs as needed.
   f. The BP disorders have a 4% lifetime prevalence.
4. Cyclothymia (code = F34.0)
   a. In cyclothymia, a patient meets both some depressive episode criteria and some hypomanic episode criteria for at least 2 years, but the symptoms are not of sufficient number or dysfunction to merit a MDD or BP diagnosis.
   b. Cyclothymia is like dysthymia, in that it is a low-grade form of BP: The mood dysfunctions do not reach BP diagnostic levels.

Note. Not all possible disorders, codes, or specifiers are listed here.
Source: Original table by Maris, referring in part to DSM-5 (American Psychiatric Association, 2013) and in part to Black and Andreasen (2011, Ch. 6).

Let us also consider the sleep disturbance criterion (insomnia or hypersomnia). In my survey of Chicago suicides (Maris, 1981; cf. Peterson, 2016a), using the original BDI, I found that *terminal* insomnia (early morning waking and the inability to fall back to sleep) was one of the distinctive depressive traits of suicides, even distinguishing them from nonfatal suicide attempters. Note, that depression is often worse early in the morning, and that, ironically, many antidepressants disrupt sleep or cause nightmares. Difficulty falling asleep in the first third of the sleep cycle (*initial* insomnia) was more characteristic of anxious patients.

How do we measure *severity* of depression? Generally, the more depression (e.g., DSM-5) criteria the patient has, the more severe the depression is considered to be. There is a severity specifier that the clinician judges: For example, DSM code F32.0 indicates mild, F32.1 indicates moderate, and F32.2 indicates severe MDD, single episode. However, in clinical trials, severity of depression is usually measured with a depression scale like the BDI-II or the HAM-D. The BDI-II and most other versions of the BDI comprise 21 Likert scale items, scored from low (0) to high (3) of four fixed choices.

There are different versions of the depression scales with different high scores. For example, the 17-item HAM-D has a high score of 50, but the 21-item scale has a high of 62. The BDI-II has a high score of 63. No (or minimal), mild, moderate, and severe depression are often measured on the HAM-D and BDI-II as follows:

HAM-D	BDI-II
25+ = severe depression	29–63 = severe depression
18–24 = moderate depression	20–28 = moderate depression
7–17 = mild depression	14–19 = mild depression
> 7 = not depressed or recovered	0–13 = minimal depression

Drug companies often claim that a HAM-D score of less than 7 indicates that their antidepressant is effective (cf. Green et al., 2015). In my study in Chicago using the original BDI, I found that 30% of the completed suicides scored 26+ (the range for severe depression in that version), compared to only 11% of the natural death controls ($t = -5.6$, $p < .001$). That is, suicides were statistically significantly more depressed that a control sample of natural deaths.

However, once again, the sterile, objective DSM criteria do not seem to fully capture the subjective, private feelings of depressed individuals. Subjectively, depressed people often:

- Do not feel like doing anything, and become anxious about that feeling.
- Seem as if they are moving and thinking in slow motion.
- Feel totally alone in the world, as if enclosed in an airless glass cage (like the metaphorical bell jar in Sylvia Plath's [1963/2005] novel) over them.
- Find themselves crying or even sobbing for no apparent reason.
- Find that getting up in the morning and getting dressed requires tremendous effort.
- Feel that suicide would be a relief (i.e., a solution to their problems).
- Find that food has no taste and flowers do not smell sweet.
- Feel that things just seem "off."
- Find that maintaining conversations and social propriety is a struggle.
- Feel that their family and friends *really* irritate them.

Author William Styron was asked what depression felt like. In response, he wrote in his book *Darkness Visible* (1990):

It was not really alarming at first, but I did notice that my surroundings took on a different tone at certain times: the shadows of nightfall seemed more sober, my mornings were less buoyant, walks in the woods became less zestful, and there was a moment during my working hours in the late afternoon when a kind of panic and anxiety overtook me.

Are there biological markers for depressive disorder or suicide that could help us diagnose it or measure severity? As mentioned earlier, the most significant marker is a low CSF serotonin level. However, this measure is not very practical, since it involves doing spinal taps (Äsberg et al., 1986; Maris, 1986). One psychiatric test for depression that has been used widely (Mann & Currier, 2012) is the dexamethasone suppression test (DST). Dexamethasone suppresses cortisol in non-depressed normal patients. The patient is given 1 mg of the steroid dexamethasone at about 11 P.M. the night before discharge is intended. When measured the next morning, the patient may hypersecrete the hormone cortisol, if depressed. However, dexamethasone does not suppress cortisol in some depressed patients. Some research has utilized the DST in suicidal patients (see Black & Andreasen, 2014, p. 392; Mann & Currier, 2012).

As noted in Table 11.1 and in Chapter 12, there are other mood disorders besides MDD. They also have elevated associations with suicide outcomes. For example, DSM-5 presents criteria for manic and hypomanic episodes and for disorders like bipolar I and II, cyclothymia (a low-grade bipolar disorder), and dysthymia (a low-grade, chronic depression, requiring fewer than the nine A criterion symptoms for major depression, over a longer period of time). Bipolar and related disorders are considered in Chapter 12.

One could also talk about the older concept of *reactive* depression (which is often correlated with stress), versus more *endogenous* (literally, "in the genes" or "growing from within") depression and its vegetative symptoms (see below). Other types that have been described include *atypical* depression, *agitated* depression, and *double* depression (MDD on top of dysthymia), as well as schizoaffective disorder, which combines mood and psychotic symptoms. Some of these disorders are not official DSM categories.

Dysthymia is a chronic, low-grade depressive neurosis, although the concept of *neurosis* is not used much any more. Patients need only have three of the nine "A" criteria for a major depressive episode. To be diagnosed with dysthymia (also called persistent depressive disorder in DSM-5), the patient must have the condition for at least 2 years.

Endogenous depression is sometimes still called by an older name, *melancholia* (Black & Andreasen, 2011, p. 154). Prominent features of endogenous depression are *vegetative* symptoms, which are reflected in the patient's vital or biological signs. These symptoms can be tracked in various ways:

- Sleep charts.
- Eating logs.
- Weight gain or loss charts.
- Records of bowel and urine movements.

- Notes on libido fluctuations.
- Pulse, blood pressure, respiration, and temperature readings.
- Activity therapy notes.
- Observations of diurnal rhythms.

Patients with endogenous depression are often thought to be more responsive to biological treatments like monoamine oxidase inhibitors (MAOIs) and other specific types of antidepressants, or to ECT.

One reason we pay special attention to a patient's vital signs is that changes in them often occur *before* mood lifts or suicide ideation diminishes. For example, weight, sleep, motor activity, energy, and libido may improve before the sad mood, anhedonia, thoughts of death, guilt feelings, and trouble concentrating do. The theory is that continuing depressed mood, coupled with increased physical energy and arousal, may give the patient a sufficient catalyst and window of opportunity for suicide. Psychiatric improvement is not uniform across all dimensions or symptoms of depression. Many suicides occur when the patients are actually getting better physically; they may appear less suicidal, since they now (or had one in reserve earlier, per Joiner, 2010) have a planned resolution (dying) to their life problems and are more able to act on it.

Finally, when classifying disorders that involve depression, remember that some bad feelings actually may be good for you (Kramer, 1993). See the discussion in Chapter 12 of Kay Jamison's own bipolar I disorder. We have to be careful not to eliminate or stifle art when we treat depression or manic–depressive disorder. It is astounding how many poets, novelist, musicians, sculptors, and painters have mood disorders and comorbid substance abuse.

Humor and Depression

Sometimes it is instructive to consider the opposites of depression, such as happiness, humor, and laughing, rather than somberness (Riley, 2003). Let me be clear, suicide itself is not funny. It is a tragic waste of life, and it devastates survivors. But could humor help us understand and prevent suicide?

The reader is invited to look at the data in Figure 11.2 and then reflect on the following questions. There may not be definitive answers to these questions, but they need to be raised anyway.

- If laughter protects against suicide, or suicide attempts, then why did it not protect the comedians Robin Williams and John Belushi from committing suicide, or Owen Wilson from attempting it? Perhaps their substance abuse and mental disorder overpowered their humor?
- Could depressed patients benefit from induced laughter? If so, how many times a day should they laugh? The former editor of the *Saturday Review,* Norman Cousins (1979), said that watching 10 minutes of Marx Brothers or *Candid Camera* comedy routines was better for his severe cancer pain than opiates were.

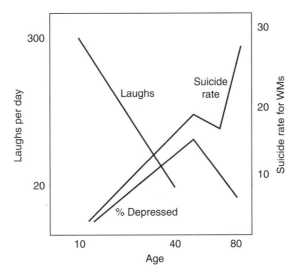

FIGURE 11.2. Laughs per day, percentage depressed, and suicide rates of white males (WMs) by age (however, see *www.laughteronlineuniversity.com/children*). *Source:* "Daily Occurrence of Laughter," R. A. Martin and N. A. Kuiper, *International Journal of Humor Research, 12*(4), 1999, pp. 335–384.

- What are the purposes of jokes, psychiatrically speaking? Perhaps jokes provide a window to our unconscious or to our repressed traumatizing thoughts and feelings, as our dreams do (see the work of Freud as described in Gay, 1988). If so, are there advantages to getting or keeping in touch with repressed experiences and feelings? What does humor get in touch with, and how might it be related to suicide prevention?
- Humor often involves unexpected juxtapositions, like a suicide "helpline" ("No, no! Turn off the safety, then pull the trigger"), or a fish jumping out of the water and onto a bridge to commit suicide, while a person standing on the bridge is contemplating jumping into the water. Maybe juxtaposition offers an alternative to suicidal solutions?
- Is happiness the opposite of depression? There are a lot of perpetually happy people who are not especially admired. The philosopher Aristotle said in his *Nicomachean Ethics* (2002) that happiness entailed moderation, not extremity.
- Humor and suicide can both be escapes. Perhaps humor is more diversion or distraction than it is true escape. Can humor be a true alternative to suicide? Even though we can laugh at death, we still have to die.
- Humor is often a psychological defense mechanism. It can make an intolerable situation possible or more tolerable.

Both laughter/humor and antidepressants are needed (and many other things, such as psychotherapy) to treat depression effectively. Clinicians could encourage conditions conducive to happiness and humor, as well as alter the biology and neurobiology of depression.

Treatment of Depression

This section focuses on specific treatments for MDD, especially the antidepressants. I follow a similar procedure in Chapters 12 and 13 for bipolar and schizophrenic spectrum disorders, respectively. Later, in Chapter 23, I talk about the generic treatment of suicide and mental disorder according to the medical model (Salin et al., 2013). Thus some redundancy will be inevitable.

Psychopharmacology

In treating mental disorders like MDD, psychiatry currently uses the medical model (rather than psychotherapy) most of the time. This model assumes that one's neurochemistry or neurobiology is out of balance when one has a depressive disorder, compared to that of healthy, nondepressed controls. What exactly needs titrating to restore balance? As discussed above, most psychiatrists and pharmaceutical companies target neurotransmitters, like serotonin (or the serotonergic system), or epinephrine, norepinephrine, dopamine, and their respective neurosystems. Thus most psychiatric treatment of depression is medication management. Modern psychiatrists actually do very little psychotherapy themselves. A word of caution here: Treating depression and other mood disorders involves far more than just titrating neurotransmitters (see Chapter 24).

The types of antidepressants include the following: tricyclics, MAOIs, SSRIs, SNRIs, atypicals, and augmenters (often antipsychotics like Abilify or Latuda, even ketamine [an anesthetic; see Grunebaum et al., 2018)], etc.).

Tricyclics

One of the first antidepressants was imipramine (Tofranil), a tricyclic introduced in 1957–1958 (Maris, 2015). It and similar drugs were called *tricyclics* because of the three cycles in their molecular structure (or *tetracyclics* if they have four cycles, like Ascendin). They are not used that much any more, due to their anticholinergic side effects and the fact that they are often fatal in overdose.

Monoamine Oxidase Inhibitors

MAOIs came out in 1959. MAO is an enzyme that degrades serotonin, tyramine, and norepinephrine. If MAO is inhibited, then theoretically monoamines (like serotonin) are increased, and depression is reduced. One major problem with MAOIs is that they interact with tyramines and can cause orthostatic hypotension, stroke, and even death. People on MAOIs have to monitor their diets closely, because a number of foods contain tyramines. Consequently, MAOIs are not used very much today, either. Common MAOIs include Parnate, Nardil, and Marplan.

Selective Serotonin Reuptake Inhibitors

The first SSRI, fluoxetine (Prozac), was marketed in 1987. These medications took the psychiatric world by storm (Maris, 2015, p. 42). In theory, SSRIs like Prozac, Paxil,

Zoloft, Celexa, and Lexapro block the reabsorption of serotonin presynaptically in the cleft between brain neurons, and thus make more serotonin available in the CSF of depressed patients. SSRIs are also *neurotropic*; that is, antidepressants like Prozac actually increase the neurons in the brain (at least in rats). A common side effect of SSRIs is sexual dysfunction, such as failure to get an erection, have an orgasm, or take an interest in sex. Some 40–60% of patients taking SSRIs report sexual dysfunctions (Black & Andreasen, 2011, p. 518), but drug companies have argued that the proportion is much less (maybe 1–5%). The sexual and other side effects of Prozac, as experienced by the writer Lauren Slater, are reported in Case 11.1.

CASE 11.1. Lauren Slater

The list below outlines Lauren Slater's experience with taking Prozac, as described in her 1998 book *Prozac Diary* (and excerpted in a 2010 anthology titled *Voices from the Inside*).

- Slater was told at the beginning, "We will start with 20 mg of Prozac." (*Start low, go slow* is the usual prescribing procedure.)
- At first, Slater "didn't think much of the stuff."
- Slater likens her Prozac changes to having a piano tuner fine-tune her brain.
- Prozac has been the single most stunning experience of her life.
- Slater has lived with chronic depression before, and she used to cut herself.
- She says that Prozac empties her, leaving a void that needs to be filled.
- For a year, she never wrote a short story or a poem (she was a writer).
- She concluded that Prozac "posits God as a matter of molecules": "Behind every crooked thought . . . lies a crooked molecule."
- Slater decided to write her thesis in Kentucky; then 2 weeks after she went to Kentucky, the Prozac just stopped working (the medical term for this phenomenon is *tachyphylaxis*).
- Her doctor reacted by doubling her Prozac dose to 80 mg each morning.
- The 80 mg helped, but she never felt as well as before.
- Slater concluded that Prozac is a feminist tablet that makes previously hungry women less interested in "corporeal platters" (like sex) laid out by the patriarchy.
- Given Prozac's sexual dysfunction side effects, Slater felt freed from the shackles of heterosexual sex.
- Ten years have gone by since Slater started taking Prozac. Her hands shake sometimes, and she thinks maybe she should stop taking Prozac.
- When Slater has tried to stop taking Prozac, however, eventually a big "kaboom" and "wreckage" ensue. She has concluded that she cannot get off it for very long.
- Slater worries about Prozac's making her complacent and compromising, causing her to give up the search for what she calls the "gem."

Source: Excerpted and rewritten by Maris from Slater (2010). Direct quotes are Slater's own words.

Today the first line of treatment for depression consists of SSRIs or SNRIs (see below). There is controversy (Kirsch, 2010) about whether much of the effect of SSRIs is *placebo* and not neurochemical. Antidepressants are only about 60–70% effective even when they do work. We now know that for young people up to age 24, SSRIs double suicidality (not suicide) risk. The FDA now requires black-box suicidality warnings on most antidepressants (Maris, 2015, p. 63). In my opinion, antidepressants are often ineffective and sometimes may not be worth the risk of side effects if a person is only mildly depressed. However, some patients really do need their antidepressants.

Serotonin–Norepinephrine Reuptake Inhibitors

The first SNRI, venlafaxine (Effexor), was introduced in the early 1990s. Dulox-etine (Cymbalta) came out in 2004 and was later also approved for pain control. Pristiq was marketed in 2008 and Fetzima in 2013. SNRIs boost both serotonin and norepinephrine (and their neurosystems). Thus SNRIs combine the serotonin and catecholamine theories of depression. In the latter theory, depression is associated with a deficiency of the catecholamine neurotransmitters norepinephrine or dopa-mine in the synaptic cleft. Like SSRIs, SNRIs can cause sexual dysfunction.

Atypical and Augmenter Antidepressants

Atypical antidepressants include the important and popular bupropion (Well-butrin). Unlike the SSRIs and SNRIs, Wellbutrin does not cause sexual dysfunc-tion. (In fact, it is even used to treat sexual dysfunction.) Unlike SSRIs, Wellbutrin works on dopamine and norepinephrine. Another atypical is Trazadone (Desyrel), which is a sedating antihistamine/antidepressant (given at bedtime). It has hyp-notic effects. Augmenting or facilitating medications, such as aripiprazole (Abilify) or lurasidone (Latuda), may also be used. Most depressed patients are on psycho-tropic "cocktails," consisting often of five to six different psychiatric medications.

Effectiveness, Administration, and Combinations of Antidepressants

For a list of the top 10 most effective (i.e., they work) and acceptable (i.e., patients like them and keep taking them) antidepressants, see Table 11.2. Most patients con-tinue taking antidepressants for about 4–5 months after their depressive symptoms resolve, usually as determined by clinical judgment or by a score below 7 on the HAM-D (Black & Andreasen, 2014). However, if patients have repeated depressive episodes (called "kindled" depression by Kramer, 1993), they may have to remain on antidepressants for the rest of their lives. They may need to take other psycho-tropic drugs as well. Antidepressants take up to 4–8 weeks to become effective. In the meantime the patient may need a concomitant long-acting benzodiazepine anx-iolytic, like clonazepam (Klonopin) (Fawcett, 2012), to relieve their anxiety. What causes people to suicide is often not their depression, but rather their acute, severe anxiety (see Shneidman, 1993, on "psychache").

 If the initial antidepressant does not work, then often the dosage is increased (e.g., up to 40 or 80 mg of Prozac), changed, or augmented. Often patients take multiple antidepressants at the same time. If the patient is having serious side effects or drug interactions, then he or she may have to stop or change medica-tions. For a small, vulnerable minority of younger patients (up to age 24), antide-pressants actually may increase their suicidality. One needs to know the half-life of

TABLE 11.2. Efficacy and Acceptability of Antidepressants

Most efficacious	Most acceptable
1. Remeron	1. Zoloft
2. Lexapro	2. Lexapro
3. Effexor	3. Wellbutrin
4. Zoloft	4. Celexa
5. Celexa	5. Prozac (esp. for children)
6. Wellbutrin	6. Savella[a]
7. Paxil	7. Remeron
8. Savella[a]	8. Effexor
9. Prozac	9. Paxil
10. Cymbalta	10. Cymbalta

[a]Savella (milnacipran) is an SNRI approved for depression in 45 countries, but approved only for fibromyalgia treatment in the United States.

Source: Reprinted from *The Lancet, 373,* A. Cipriani et al., "Comparative Efficacy and Acceptability of New-Generation Antidepressants," pp. 736–758, Copyright © 2009, with permission from Elsevier.

antidepressants, since that helps determine withdrawal time. Prozac can be stopped "cold turkey" due to its long half-life, but Paxil has to be titrated slowly downwards and is hard to get off of. If the patient is acutely suicidal or antidepressants have not worked, then ECT is the gold standard for treatment of depression (Carlat, 2010, Ch. 8). ECT is more effective (about 80%) than antidepressants and works more quickly, but there are reasons not to consider it a first-line treatment (see below).

Recently (Grohol, 2017), pharmacogenetic tests have been developed to estimate the likelihood of a favorable response to specific antidepressants. For example, Duke ranks a list of antidepressants in order of their likely effectiveness for a specific patient. These tests costs about $100, and insurance normally will not pay for them. It is estimated that only about 20% of first antidepressant trials are positive, so avoiding a long trial (such as 6–8 weeks of several different types of medications) is important and perhaps cost effective to prompt depression treatment.

Ketamine

One recent promising off-label treatment for MDD (i.e., it is not approved by the FDA for this use) is the anesthetic ketamine (Andrade, 2017; Oaklander, 2017; Grunebaum et al., 2018; Nemeroff, 2018). In addition to its human medical and veterinary uses, it was ingested as a hallucinogenic party drug ("Special K") on the street. In 2017 ketamine was thought to be rapidly effective in reducing depression and suicide ideation, but its effects are transient (days or weeks). The patient gets subanesthetic infusions or uses nasal sprays at ketamine clinics. Infusions last about 40–60 minutes, require constant monitoring, and can cost $400 to $2,000 per infusion (insurance will not pay for them). Ketamine is thought to work on the neurotransmitter glutamate, but there are few clinical trials to date. Patients are cautioned that ketamine itself is not a sufficient treatment for depressive disorders and that adverse effects can be problematic.

ECT and Related Procedures

If pharmacotherapy fails to produce an antidepressant response, or a patient's suicidal crisis is acute and severe, then the patient may receive ECT every other day for up to 2 weeks (Manning, 1995; Behrman, 2002; Gambino, 2018).

ECT is like a minor outpatient surgical procedure. The patient can have nothing to eat after midnight the day before. An IV line is started, and electroencephalographic (EEG) sensors are attached to the head. Other sensors are put on the patient's chest, and a blood pressure cuff is attached to the arm. A rubber guard is inserted over the teeth to keep the patient from biting the tongue or cracking teeth. A medication (like thiopental or the barbiturate methohexital) is then injected through the IV, causing the patient to sleep for about 5–10 minutes. Once the patient is asleep, another medication is given to relax the muscles and prevent injury during the seizure. Since the medication also inhibits breathing, patients are given oxygen through a mask until they resume breathing on their own.

The treatment itself consists of a brief (a few seconds) intermittent electrical charge (about enough electricity to light a 20-watt bulb) through electrodes that have been placed on one or both of the patient's temples. Some claim that the right temporal location causes less confusion afterwards. The ECT machine lets out a loud "*beeeep*" when discharging (Carlat, 2010). The electrical charge stimulates the brain and produces a grand mal seizure that lasts for about a minute.

Modern ECT does not cause patients' bodies to convulse, and they do not feel any pain. There will be an elevated heart rate (*tachycardia*), followed by a slow heart rate (*bradycardia*). The patient's toes can twitch, fists clench, and chest heave. After the treatment, the patient is taken to a recovery area and usually wakes up 10–15 minutes later. Upon awakening, the patient may have a headache, confusion, nausea, and muscle stiffness. If present, these symptoms normally last about 20–60 minutes (cf. Anderson, 2018). Memory loss for events immediately preceding the procedure (*retrograde amnesia*) often occurs. The patient can go home within about 30–60 minutes, although some hospitals require an overnight stay. ECT probably affects the serotonergic system and is about 80% effective, versus 60–70% for antidepressants; it is also more quickly effective (1–2 weeks vs. 4–8 weeks for antidepressants).

In addition to ECT, there are other technical procedures to treat depression, including vagus nerve stimulation, transcranial magnetic stimulation (Weisman et al., 2018), bi- and unilateral cingulotomy, and various imaging procedures that are mainly diagnostic (see Chapter 24). Of course, psychotherapy (Beck's cognitive therapy or Linehan's dialectical behavior therapy; see Maris, 2015) is often used conjointly with antidepressants and ECT (see Chapter 23).

Hopelessness versus Depression as a Suicide Risk Factor

Although no single suicide risk factor predicts suicide, there is some evidence that hopelessness is a better predictor than depression is (however, see Qiu et al., 2017). Beck and his colleagues pioneered the research on depression and suicide. Beck created the original 21-item BDI in the 1960s; scores on both it and the BDI-II (Beck et al., 1996) range from a low of 0 to a high of 63. Beck determined that patients with a score of 26 or higher on the original BDI had severe depression and a higher suicide risk than normal controls. In research such as this, one needs to be careful that both the suicides and controls are dead (e.g., not living suicide attempters).

When I surveyed Chicago suicides, I tested Beck's depression hypothesis (Maris, 1981). I found that 30% of the completed suicides scored 26 or higher on the original BDI, compared to just 11% of the natural death controls. This difference was statistically significant ($t = -0.56$, $p < .001$). Beck et al. (1974a) went on to create a Hopelessness Scale (see Table 11.3). They concluded that a hopelessness score of 15+ (the maximum was 20) indicated severe hopelessness and a definite suicide risk.

However, Beck and colleagues did not stop here. They developed a correlation matrix (Kovacs et al., 1975; see Table 11.4) that examined the comparative relationships of depression and hopelessness scales to current suicidal intent (or the wish-to-live). Table 11.4 shows that (1) hopelessness has a higher correlation with current suicidal intent (+.68) than depression does (+.57); (2) hopelessness has a higher negative correlation with the wish-to-live (–.74) than depression does (–.57); and (3)

TABLE 11.3. Beck's Hopelessness Scale

True	False
2. I might as well give up because I can't make things better for myself.	1. I look forward to the future with hope and enthusiasm.
4. I cannot imagine what my life would be like in 10 years.	3. When things are going badly, I am helped by knowing that they cannot stay that way forever.
7. My future seems dark to me.	
9. I just don't get the breaks, and there's no reason to believe I will in the future.	5. I have enough time to accomplish things I most want to do.
11. All I can see ahead of me is unpleasantness rather than pleasantness.	6. In the future, I expect to succeed in what concerns most.
12. I don't expect to get what I really want.	8. I expect to get more of the good things in life than the average person.
14. Things just don't work out the way I want them to.	10. My past experiences have prepared me well for my future.
16. I never get what I want, so it's foolish to want anything.	13. When I look ahead to the future, I expect that I will be happier than I am now.
17. It is very unlikely that I will get any real satisfaction in the future.	15. I have great faith in the future.
18. The future seems vague and uncertain to me.	19. I can look forward to more good times than bad times.
20. There's not use in really trying to get something I want because I probably won't get it.	

Note. Hopelessness scores (each item is worth 1 point): 0–3, none or minimal; 4–8, mild; 9–14, moderate (not immediate danger, but requires frequent monitoring); 15+, severe (definite suicide risk).
Source: Beck, Weissman, Lester, and Trexler (1974). Copyright © 1974 American Psychological Association. Reprinted with permission.

TABLE 11.4. Correlations of Beck et al.'s Depression, Hopelessness, Current Suicidal Intent, and Wish-to-Live Scores

	Hopelessness	Depression	Wish-to-live
Depression	+.68	–	–
Wish-to-live	–.74	–.57	–
Current suicidal intent	+.68	–.57	–.76

Source: "Hopelessness: An Indicator of Suicide Risk" by M. Kovacs, A. T. Beck, and A. Weissman, *Suicide, 5,* 98–103. Copyright © 1975 by the American Association of Suicidology. Reproduced with permission of John Wiley & Sons, Inc.

the relationship between depression and current suicidal intent is likely due to a common source of variance (viz., hopelessness).

Thus, hopelessness is a better predictor of suicide than depression is. This makes common sense as well: After having repeated depressive episodes (perhaps some with hospitalization), it makes sense that patients might become hopeless and more suicidal. Partly for this reason, I made hopelessness a separate predictor in my own list of 15 suicide risk factors (see Chapters 3 and 4).

Beck et al. (1985) tested the relationship of hopelessness to suicide. They did a 10-year follow-up of 165 patients hospitalized for suicide ideation. Of the 11 patients who eventually suicided, 10 (91%) had hopelessness scores greater than 9, and only 1 had a hopelessness core below 9. Ideally, a longer follow-up period would have been preferable to test this hypothesis, since suicidal careers are normally much longer than 10 years, and we cannot know the outcome until all 165 patients have died.

Chapter 12 examines another major mood disorder category, bipolar disorder, and its relation to suicide. Bipolar disorder includes manic/hypomanic as well as depressive episodes.

Bipolar Disorder

A Suicidogenic Cycle of Despair

For no reason I started to feel very good. Suddenly I knew how to enter into the life of everything around me. I knew how it felt to be a tree, a blade of grass, even a rabbit. I didn't sleep much. I just walked around with this wonderful feeling.

—THEODORE ROETHKE

Unlike major depression, the two major bipolar disorders in DSM-5 require having at least one manic or one hypomanic episode in addition to a major depressive episode (MDE). *Mania* can be defined as "a distinct period of abnormality and persistently elevated, expansive, or irritable mood and abnormally and persistently increased goal-directed activity or energy, lasting at least 1 week" and meeting at least three of seven symptom criteria during that time (American Psychiatric Association, 2013, p. 124). In bipolar I disorder (BP I), there must be at least one MDE and one manic episode. DSM codes depend upon whether or not the current or most recent episode was manic, hypomanic, or depressed.

In bipolar II disorder (BP II), there must be at least one MDE and one hypomanic episode. A hypomanic episode consists of at least three of the seven manic criteria or symptoms over at least 4 consecutive days. *Hypomania* is a less elevated mood state than mania, but it is still more elevated than normal mood (i.e., it is still manic). Below, in the section on classification and diagnosis, I also define cyclothymia, medication-induced bipolar disorder, medical-condition-related bipolar disorder, and various specifiers for the bipolar disorders.

BP I, severe, would be coded as F31.13, and BP II as F31.81 (with severity specified in writing rather than coded). BP II is not milder than BP I; there is just hypomania, not mania, but it is still elevated mood.

Both MDD and bipolar disorder (which I use in the singular as an overall term for this group of disorders) are related to elevated rates of suicide (see Table 10.1). Unfortunately, much of the literature on bipolar disorder and suicide is related to prevalence, risk factors, and treatment issues, and does not consider why this disorder category might cause or contribute to elevated rates of suicide (however, see Hawton, 2005; Gilbert et al., 2011). I address this issue in the next section, but I suspect that it has to do with the impulsivity, poor judgment, faulty cognition, increased risk taking, and unstable mood involved in mania, plus poor treatment, pharmacological effects, and neurobiological factors (Maris, 2015). Al Alvarez (with whom Sylvia Plath had an affair) comments in his book *The Savage God* (1971) that when he was manic, he felt his life was out of control. And, of course, depression is associated with bipolar disorder as well.

Bipolar disorder and suicide also concern psychopharmacological issues, especially the neurotransmitter GABA. In 2008, the FDA (Maris, 2015, p. 90) said that users of antiepileptic drugs or mood stabilizers had a relative risk (odds) ratio for suicide ranging between 1.8 and 2.92. This range is two to three times as high as the range for those not on these drugs. The FDA required drug manufacturers to add a warning to their product description.

Jean-Pierre Falret identified what he called *folie circulaire* in 1843, and mood disorders as early as 1859. By 1875 the disorder was often called *manic–depressive psychosis*. In 1913 Emil Kraepelin was probably the first to systematically describe manic–depressive disorder. Australian John Cade was the first to use lithium, a naturally occurring salt, to treat mania in 1949. After 1980, the term *bipolar disorder* began to replace *manic-depressive disorder*. One of the first major textbooks on manic–depressive disorder (still using the older term) was published by Goodwin and Jamison (1990).

Jamison herself suffers from bipolar disorder (see Case 12.1, below) and attempted suicide, as did many other historical and contemporary artists and celebrities. A partial list of those with bipolar disorder includes Robert Schumann, Vincent van Gogh, Ludwig van Beethoven, Edgar Allan Poe, Ernest Hemingway, Virginia Woolf, Frank Sinatra, Catherine Zeta-Jones. Dick Cavett, Robert Downey, Jr., Mel Gibson, and Robin Williams. For example, Vincent van Gogh had his greatest artistic productivity when he was manic, according to Jamison (1993), and was least productive when he was depressed. As in the Hemingway family (see Chapter 1, Figure 1.3), several of van Gogh's family members suffered from psychiatric disorders and were suicidal (see Figure 12.1). Cases like van Gogh's suggest that there is a likely genetic component to both bipolar disorder and suicide (Simon & Hales, 2012).

Epidemiology of Bipolar Disorder

MDD (unipolar depression) has a 17% lifetime prevalence and is twice as common in women as in men. Bipolar disorder has a lifetime prevalence of about 2% and affects males and females about equally (Black & Andreasen, 2014). No one seems to know why. The WHO (1996, 2008, 2012) rates bipolar disorder as the sixth leading cause of disability (including physical disorders).

The median age of onset for bipolar disorder is about 25 years. In children and adolescents, any bipolar disorder diagnosis is controversial (see DSM-5; American

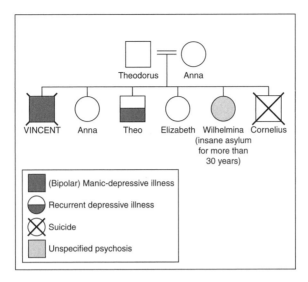

FIGURE 12.1. Partial family history of Vincent van Gogh. *Source:* From *Touched with Fire: Manic–Depressive Illness and the Artistic Temperament* by Kay Redfield Jamison. Copyright © 1993 Kay Redfield Jamison. Reprinted with the permission of The Free Press, a division of Simon & Schuster, Inc. All rights reserved.

Psychiatric Association, 2013, p. 123 and Section III), and apparent bipolarity in younger patients is thought to overlap with ADHD (Black & Andreasen, 2014). In fact, some of the criteria for any diagnosis of bipolar disorder occur only *after* puberty or in adulthood, such as sexual inappropriateness or reckless spending. So how could young children have bipolar disorder?

As with van Gogh (Figure 12.1), bipolar disorder tends to run in families. This is especially the case with BP II. There is a clear genetic component to bipolarity. For example, the concordance rate (i.e., the rate that if one twin has the disorder, so will the other twin) for bipolar disorder is 72% in monozygotic twins (Simon & Hales, 2012, p. 163), but in dizygotic twins the rate is just 14% (Black & Andreasen, 2014).

There is a high comorbidity rate for bipolar disorder and alcohol/other substance abuse in general—about 45% for patients with BP I and 31% for patients with BP II. The rate of suicide is probably slightly higher in patients with BP II (Baldessarini et al., 2012), although the suicide rate is also elevated in MDD.

Bipolar Disorder and Suicide

Those with bipolar disorder whose current mood episode is an MDE suffer the same suicidogenic symptoms of MDD discussed in Chapter 11. These include perpetual sadness, anhedonia, fatigue, apathy/listlessness, and thoughts of death and/or suicide. To these, a manic or hypomanic episode of bipolar disorder adds its own suicidogenic factors (Hawton, 2005). These include high rates of alcohol and other substance abuse, anxiety, impulsivity, lack of insight, and poor treatment compliance.

Part of the problem is that bipolar patients enjoy their manic or hypomanic highs (see similar reactions in patients taking Adderall, as described by Schwartz, 2016), but usually not the full-blown mania of BP I. One bipolar patient wrote, "To me being hypomanic has to be better than any drug one could ever market" (quoted in Maris, 2015, p. 83). Even when bipolar patients realize that their manic behavior is self-destructive, it is hard for them to give up the euphoric highs. This was Kay Jamison's experience, as described in Case 12.1. She managed to write a 938-page tome on manic–depression. Staying up for days and having unbounded energy can have their rewards. She did not want to take lithium, because it slowed her down.

CASE 12.1. Kay Redfield Jamison

Kay Redfield Jamison is a psychologist and a professor of psychiatry and behavioral sciences at Johns Hopkins Medical School. She has described her coping with bipolar disorder, and has emphasized how the disorder has been both good and bad for her. Since she was often manic, she was able to work hard. But eventually she had a neuronal pileup on the highways of her brain. Mania can make a person impulsive and reckless. She had suicidal ideas about jumping off a bridge. She became financially irresponsible and accumulated $30,000 in debt after two manic episodes. With mania, her life went at a frightening pace. Sounds and music were intense; colors were very vivid. She resisted treatment and liked her highs. After separating from her husband, she dated another man, a doctor, who encouraged her to take lithium.

She then saw a psychiatrist at UCLA who asked her about her sleep, ability to concentrate, and talkativeness, as well as her being overly energetic, undertaking overly ambitious projects (e.g., writing a 938-page book), behaving impulsively, and spending money irresponsibly. Jamison concluded that her mind was beholden to her brain and that she would likely have to stay on lithium indefinitely. Only lithium could slow her down to the pace of normal people.

How does one solve the dilemma between creativity and self-destructiveness (see also Jamison, 1993)?

Source: Excerpted and rewritten by Maris from Jamison (1995).

Jamison (1993) argues that not only did her mania make her feel good and more able to work, but also that the work of bipolar writers, artists, and poets (see Figure 11.1) actually benefits from mania. She points out that creative thinking, feeling, and hypomania share traits of enhanced fluency, rapidity of thought, flexibility, and the ability to combine ideas to form new connections. She worries that effective treatment of bipolar disorder might destroy art and turn former artists into bland, uninteresting people.

Jamison (in Ann, 2016) claimed that van Gogh had his greatest artistic productivity when he was manic (also Jamison, 1993, Figure 4.6), and that he was least productive when he was depressed. As noted above, several van Gogh family members (like several Hemingway family members) suffered from psychiatric disorders and were suicidal. Vincent himself lacked self-control, slept very little, smoked and drank too much, ate poorly, and had little money in his lifetime—ironic, given what his paintings are worth now. He also had headaches and abused substances. van Gogh once came after his fellow artist Paul Gauguin with a razor, but ended up cutting off his own ear. He painted a self-portrait of his head after the incident. In April,1890, Vincent was living in the village of Auvers-sur-Oise north of Paris with a medical doctor, Gachet. He went out into the countryside, shot himself in the stomach, and died at age 37.

Consider also the much more recent case of comedian Robin Williams (Case 12.2). Williams suicided in August 2014. For much of his life, his mania sustained his creativity. He was like a Fourth of July sparkler, except that he somehow managed to live until age 63, unlike John Belushi, Janis Joplin, Heath Ledger, Judy Garland, Marilyn Monroe, and many others, who died much younger.

CASE 12.2. Robin Williams

Robin Williams died August 11, 2014 at age 65. He committed suicide by hanging himself with his belt. At the time, he was taking Seroquel (an antipsychotic) and Remeron (an SNRI antidepressant) for severe depression and bipolar disorder. He also suffered from mild dementia, Parkinson's disease, and paranoia. He had been married three times and had three children.

Williams's mother was a model from Mississippi, and his father was a senior executive at Ford Motor Company. He was born in Chicago, but moved to Detroit due to his father's job. He studied at Julliard in New York City, where his roommate said that Robin "talked a mile a minute" and was "caroming off walls." His comedy routines were so intense that it sometimes seemed he would have a complete meltdown on stage.

At times Williams was psychologically dependent on cocaine, and he often abused alcohol to the point of needing detoxification. He said that cycling (i.e., riding a bike) saved his life. His comedic idols were Peter Sellers and Jonathan Winters. His films included *Good Morning, Vietnam* (1987); *Dead Poets Society* (1989); *Awakenings* (1990), in which he played the psychiatrist Oliver Sacks; and *Good Will Hunting* (1997), for which he won an Academy Award. He also won several Emmy and Grammy Awards.

Source: Original case description by Maris, compiled from various news accounts.

Eventually, after mania, there is an inevitable major depressive crash. There is a limit to how many nights in a row a person can stay awake. Sooner or later, the suicidogenic effects of mania catch up with the person. For example, as described in Case 12.1, Kay Jamison eventually thought about jumping off a bridge. She stated that only lithium saved her (Jamison, 1995). But Robin Williams suicided even though at the time of his death he was taking Seroquel and Remeron (i.e., these psychiatric medications did not save him).

The suicide rate of bipolar patients is 28 times that of the population without bipolarity (Baldessarini et al., 2012). When patients fail to take appropriate psychiatric medications and stay on them, the resulting substance abuse, anxiety, impulsivity, lack of self-control, busted marriages, poor relationships, and constant ups and downs often eventually do them in. Box 12.1 outlines various key points about bipolar disorder.

BOX 12.1. Key Points about Bipolar Disorder and Suicide

- According to Goodwin and Jamison (2007), the prevalence of bipolar disorder is about 5%. Other estimates say 2–5%.
- Patients with bipolar disorder have a slightly higher suicide risk than patients with MDD.
- The bipolar disorder suicide risk of 329 per 100,000 is 28 times the risk of suicide in the general population.
- About 15–19% of patients with bipolar disorder complete suicide.
- The suicide risk (not the prevalence) of bipolar disorder is several times higher in men than women.
- Suicide risk is especially high early in the course of bipolar disorder.
- BP II has an especially high suicide risk.
- Additional suicide risk factors include prior suicide attempts, current depression, previous severe depression, hopelessness, impulsivity, and substance abuse.
- It is not clear that rapid cycling increases suicide risk.
- Predisposing and precipitating factors interact.
- To assess suicide risk, consider intensity of suicide ideation, details of suicidal plans, access to lethal means, presence of a major psychiatric illness besides bipolar disorder, past suicide attempts, and social support. Also, do an adequate mental status exam.
- Do not be too reliant on objective risk factors alone in assessing the suicide risk of patients with bipolar disorder.
- Antidepressant treatment for both MDD and bipolar disorder is a plausible intervention.
- Treatment with lithium provides the strongest evidence for reducing suicide risk.
- Long-term lithium treatment results in a sixfold reduction in the suicide rate.
- Lithium may reduce impulsivity or aggression by enhancing serotonin.
- The antipsychotic clozapine (Clozaril) was the first FDA-approved drug for reducing suicide risk.
- ECT is the treatment of choice for patients with acute suicide risk.
- Bipolar disorder is associated with high rates of substance abuse, anxiety disorder, impulsivity, lack of insight, and poor treatment compliance.

Source: Excerpted and rewritten by Maris from Baldessarini et al. (2012).

Diagnosis and Classification of Bipolar Disorders

The diagnostic criteria for BP I and BP II have already been outlined in Table 11.1 and mentioned briefly at the beginning of this chapter. Here I elaborate on the diagnostic features and criteria, specifiers, and modifiers for BP I, BP II, and cyclothymia. More precisely, a manic episode consists of elevated or irritable mood, with increased activity or energy to achieve goals, lasting at least 1 week. At least three of the following seven symptoms are clearly evident most of every day for at least 1 week:

- Grandiosity or inflated self-esteem.
- Sleep is decreased (often to no more than 3 hours a night for several days in a row).

* Talkativeness and pressure to speak.
* Ideas are flighty or racing.
* Distractibility to irrelevant external stimuli.
* Actions or projects with unrealistic goals.
* Pleasure-seeking acts (including sexuality and spending)

As with the symptom criteria for an MDE (see Chapter 10), one can take the first letter of each symptom and come up with a mnemonic (GSTIDAP) that uses these seven letters in a sentence, like Great Sex Through Impulsivity Denies Appropriate Planning. Other diagnostic criteria are that the manic behavior must be a definite change from normal or usual baseline functioning, and it must be dysfunctional. It also needs to be specified if the mania is the result of drug abuse or a medical condition; if so, a diagnosis of BP I is not given.

There are many specifiers and modifiers for BP I (and other bipolar disorders), such as mild, moderate, or severe; severe with psychotic features; in full or partial remission; and so forth. One also needs to specify whether the current or most recent episode is depressed, manic, hypomanic, or unspecified. A condition with mixed features will have, for example, depressive symptoms during hypomania. In addition, are anxious distress, rapid cycling (at least four or more mood episodes in the previous 12 months), melancholic features, atypical or psychotic features, catatonia, peripartum onset, or seasonal features present?

Moreover, any bipolar disorder needs to be distinguished from schizoaffective disorder (which has mixed schizophrenia and depressive disorder symptoms) and schizophreniform disorder (which is prodromal to and shorter than schizophrenia). Finally, clinicians need to consider and correct for gender and cultural variations.

One of the pertinent diagnostic features of bipolar patients is that often they are not even aware that they are ill. During their manic or hypomanic phases, they tend to be euphoric (not dysphoric), excessively cheerful and talkative, high, and feeling on top of the world (see the epigraph to this chapter). They have haphazard enthusiasm for interpersonal, sexual, or occupational interactions. Often their mood is irritable (not just elevated) and *labile* (i.e., they have rapid mood shifts). When they are manic, they tend to take on multiple, overlapping, excessively ambitious projects.

Bipolar patients have inflated, unjustified self-esteem and a decreased need for sleep. Their speech can be pressured, loud, and hard to interrupt. It can be hard to talk with them, since they do all the talking and do not listen well. They tend not to be able to censor or shut out external, irrelevant stimuli. As mentioned earlier, the differential diagnosis for any bipolar disorder in children is difficult and controversial, in part because the criteria for these disorders are mainly for adults (Whitaker, 2010).

BP II must include an MDE for a minimum of 2 weeks and hypomania for at least 4 days. Cyclothymia is chronic (at least 2 years), with mood fluctuation between hypomanic symptoms (but not full hypomania) and less severe depression (but not an MDE) more days than not and for most of the day. In BP II, criteria for a manic episode have never been met.

Treatment of Mania or Hypomania in Bipolar Disorder

Treatment of mania or hypomania in bipolar disorder is problematic and tricky, since mood stabilizers do not work for depression (except perhaps for Lamictal). In fact, like antidepressants, they may even induce or worsen depression. For example, gabapentin (Neurontin) and carbamazepine (Tegretol) may reduce monoamines (like serotonin and norepinephrine), which are related to increased risk for depression. Thus, it is common for a bipolar patient to be on an antidepressant in addition to a mood stabilizer. However, even this treatment is tricky, since antidepressants can make a bipolar patient have an induced or worsened manic or hypomanic episode.

Mania is the polar opposite of depression, and so the treatment of mania is different from that of an MDE. Psychiatric medications used to treat mania are variously called *mood stabilizers, anticonvulsants, antiepileptics, antiseizure drugs,* or *antimanic drugs* (see Baldessarini, 2002). Although the mechanisms of mood stabilizers are not well understood (especially for lithium), most of them seem to affect (to enhance or be agonists of) GABA (and sometimes glutamate, acetylcholine, and serotonin).

GABAergic mood stabilizers increase the neurotransmitter GABA and stimulate its brain system. But there are possible suicidogenic implications (for a dissenting view, see Rothschild, 2017). Neurontin is a GABA agonist; it raises brain GABA (Trimble, 2007; Cooper et al., 2003). Increases in brain GABA can lead to negative effects on mood and behavior (according to Trimble, 2007). Glutamate is the brain's main excitatory neurotransmitter. Gabapentin reduces glutamate at cortical synapses. Depletion of monoamines leads to significant increased risk for depression (or can make existing depression worse), dysphoria, depersonalization, agitation, aggression, suicidal behaviors, and possibly even completed suicide (Brown et al., 1992). As discussed earlier, depleting serotonin or norepinephrine in the CSF of the brain is related to higher rates of both suicide and depressive disorders (Äsberg et al., 1976).

Mood stabilizers are similar to antianxiety and antipsychotic medications. In fact second-generation antipsychotics (e.g., Zyprexa, Respirdal, Abilify, Seroquel, and Latuda) are also often used to treat mania (sometimes conjointly with a mood stabilizer and/or antidepressant). Lilly manufactures a drug that combines Prozac and Zyprexa into one medication called Symbyax.

The leading antimanic drugs (this is not a complete list) include these:

- Lithium carbonate: a salt with many generic brands; it can be toxic and requires blood tests.
- Valproic acid (Depakote).
- Carbamazepine (Tegretol).
- Lamotrigine (Lamictal): one of the most popular medications for bipolar disorder, especially for BP II.
- Gabapentin (Neurontin): used for off-label indications like pain control.
- Topiramate (Topamax).
- Oxcarbazepine (Trileptal).
- Omega-3 fatty acids.

Other drug treatments for bipolar disorder include the following:

- Pregabalin (Lyrica).
- Tiagabine (Gabitril).
- Vigabatrin (Sabril).
- Levetiracetam (Keppra).
- Zonisamide (Zonegran).
- Clobazam (Onfi).
- Lurasidone (Latuda): an atypical antipsychotic often used as an augmenter.

Treatment of bipolar disorder often consists of a combination of therapy with lithium, anticonvulsants, antidepressants, and sometimes minor tranquilizers (like the benzodiazepines) and/or a major (antipsychotic) tranquilizer (like Risperdal or Zyprexa). Of course, concomitant psychotherapies may be advised as well (Maris, 2015, pp. 84ff.). Treatment of mania in BP I is difficult, since mood stabilizers do not work for depression. They may even induce or worsen depression. For example, as noted above, Neurontin reduces serotonin and norepinephrine (monoamine neurotransmitters), but these neurotransmitters help prevent depression. Thus it is common for bipolar patients to be on an antidepressant, in addition to a mood stabilizer. However, even this is problematic, since antidepressants can make a bipolar patient manic or hypomanic or worsen mania. The bottom line is that bipolar patients are difficult to treat and need to be monitored closely. Below, I consider lithium, Tegretol, Depakote, Lamictal, and Neurontin.

Lithium Carbonate

Since lithium is the only bipolar treatment with clinical trial data supporting a significant reduction in suicide risk and attempts (Simon & Hales, 2012; Baldessarini et al., 2012; Ishii et al., 2015), I discuss it here at greater length than I discuss other treatments. Recall that Jamison (1995) described lithium as her most effective drug. All psychiatric medications can have (1) main intended effects (like reducing mania), (2) minor adverse effects (often transitory), (3) serious adverse effects (discussed for mood-stabilizers and suicide risk at the end of this chapter; see Hawton et al., 2005), (4) interaction, and (5) withdrawal effects.

Although we do not understand the mechanisms of lithium very well (Black & Andreasen, 2011, p. 532; 2014), it seems to block acetylcholine and may be related to decreased cellular response to neurotransmitters. Some have argued that in mania there is an increase in protein kinase C (PKC), and that lithium may inhibit PKC (see below). Lithium, like Latuda, can be used as an augmenting drug with antidepressants for major depression (see "Lithium: Patient Drug Information," 2013).

Lithium is a naturally occurring salt. Bottled lithium water, called Lithia, is produced in Ridgeway, Colorado; there are even lithium health spas, such as Lithia Springs, Georgia, 12 miles outside Atlanta. Lithium may be the drug of choice for the initial stabilization of mania, although many patients will not take it (Maris et al., 2000). It has been used medicinally at least since 1843 (as a bladder stone solvent) and since 1859 for gout, rheumatism, headaches, and mood disorders.

Some patients cannot tolerate lithium, in which case they are usually put on various anticonvulsants (Goldsmith et al., 2002). Lithium can result in intoxication and in rare cases even death. One has to monitor blood plasma levels carefully to achieve a therapeutic lithium level (initially 0.9–1.4 mEq/L and a maintenance level of 0.5–0.7 mEq/L). The typical patient is started on 300 mg of lithium twice a day, and the dosage is then titrated upward until a therapeutic plasma level is achieved. There is a slow-release form of lithium to reduce gastric irritation (see "Lithium: Patient Drug Information," 2013).

There can be side effects of polyuria or thirst, weight gain, edema, diarrhea, and tremors. As many as 15% of patients taking lithium get hypothyroidism, which can be treated with Synthroid (although concerns have recently been raised about the effectiveness of Synthroid). Lithium (like Prozac) can be stopped without tapered doses. The reduction of suicide risk with lithium is most pronounced after a minimum of about 2 years of treatment.

Given the clinical trial data, bipolar patients with serious suicide risk probably should be put on lithium treatment as soon as possible. Unfortunately, almost 50% of patients who are prescribed lithium are nonadherent with their treatment and will not take the drug as prescribed. As noted earlier, often the manic highs are so pleasurable that bipolar patients are reluctant to control them.

Carbamazepine (Tegretol)

Carbamazepine was first synthesized in 1960 and then later marketed as an anticonvulsant. Tegretol has a molecular structure similar to that of the tricyclic antidepressants (see Chapter 11). Many patients take 200 mg three times a day; the maximum dose is about 1,600/day. It has dampening effects on kindling—depression that smolders and can easily burst into full-blown depression (Kramer, 1993). Like Lamictal, Tegretol can cause rashes or skin disorders. It may result in drowsiness, dizziness, ataxia (muscle incoordination), and possible fetal malformations. Tegretol can also have rare hematological effects, like infection, anemia, and petechiae.

Valproic Acid (Depakote)

Valproic acid is found naturally in valerian and was first synthesized in 1882. Like gabapentin, Depakote enhances the neurotransmitter GABA. It was first approved only for epilepsy, and then later as a mood stabilizer. Many patients receive 1,250–2,500 mg each day. It needs to be taken with food and may cause gastrointestinal problems. Many patients will not take Depakote, since it causes weight gain (no improvement here over lithium). Patients can also feel sedated or get tremors, and pregnant women can develop birth defects. Finally, Depakote can cause a rare hepatotoxic (toxic to the liver) reaction, possibly leading to death.

Lamotrigine (Lamictal)

Lamictal was marketed as an anticonvulsant by Glaxo-Smith-Kline in 1994, and it is one of the more popular mood stabilizers. Its target dose is 200 mg/day, through a slow titration in 25-mg increments. Lamictal blocks calcium channels and delays the occurrence of depressive episodes in bipolar patients. Many patients not on lithium take Lamictal. Although Lamictal has relatively few adverse effects, it does have a black-box FDA warning for rashes and skin disorders—including the rare but dreaded Stevens–Johnson syndrome, in which the skin can become necrotic (and be shed like a snake's skin), and the throat can swell and impair breathing. Other adverse effects of the syndrome can include damage to vital organs, such as liver failure.

Gabapentin (Neurontin)

Neurontin was first marketed in 1994 by Parke-Davis and was later manufactured by Pfizer. It was approved for treatment of refractory epilepsy and later for shingles. However, about 90% of Neurontin's use has been off-label, especially for pain control (it is often preferred to opiates) and bipolar disorder. Neurontin is a GABA agonist (Trimble, 2007). Many have argued (Trimble, 2007) that increase in brain GABA leads to negative effects on mood and behavior. Glutamate is the brain's main excitatory neurotransmitter. Neurontin reduces glutamate release at cortical synapses, says Trimble (2007, p. 15). As discussed above, depletion of monoamines (serotonin and norepinephrine) can lead to significantly increased risk of depression (or can make an existing depression worse) and of suicidal behaviors (Trimble, 2007; Brown et al., 1992).

Neurobiology of Mania

Up to this point, I have considered the neurobiology of depression and the treatment for mania/hypomania. What I have not examined is how people become manic (or hypomanic) in the first place. The neurobiology of mania is far more complex, subtle, and interactive than can be discussed in this text (see Manji et al., 2003). Furthermore, the neurobiology of bipolar disorder is not fully understood. Consideration of the pathophysiology of mania requires answers on the genetic, molecular, cellular, and behavioral levels. I review only briefly genetics, PKC, and neurotransmitter systems.

Genetics

It is well known that mania tends to run in families far more frequently than by chance alone (Black & Andreasen, 2014). For example, 65% of monozygotic twins develop mania, but only 14% of dizygotic twins do; that is, the stronger the genetic bond, the greater the chance of developing mania. For other examples, see the presence of bipolarity and major depression in the genealogies of Virginia Woolf, Ernest Hemingway and Vincent van Gogh (Figures 1.3 and 12.1, respectively).

Candidates for bipolar genes include (1) G72 (the D-amino acid oxidase gene), (2) BDNF (the gene for brain-derived neurotrophic factor), (3) NRG1 (the neuregulin gene) (4) DTNBP1 (the dysbindin gene), and (5) circadian rhythm genes (the Clock, Timeless, and Period 3 genes). A serotonin transporter gene polymorphism is also a candidate for developing depression. The serum BDNF gene level is reduced in bipolar patients. BNDF promotes survival of nerve cells. Remember that Prozac is neurotropic; it actually increases brain neurons (in rats). The BDNF gene is located in the region of chromosome 11.

Protein Kinase C

In mania there is an increase in PKC, and lithium (for one) inhibits it. Although the mode of action of acetylcholine is still unknown, it could be that lithium reduces mania by blocking acetylcholine (Trimble & George, 2010). Other inhibitors are the drugs riluzole (Rilutek) and valproate (Depakote). Mania is associated with overactive PKC intracellular signaling or abnormalities in the regulation of signal transduction cascades. Genomewide studies have isolated an enzyme that reduces activation of PKC. Overactive PKC signaling occurs in the prefrontal cortex.

Imaging studies show reduced activity in the right prefrontal cortex during manic episodes. Disinhibition of the right prefrontal cortex leads to a disinhibited profile (e.g., poor impulse control, risk taking, distractibility and delusion). There is also loss of prefrontal volume in untreated bipolar patients. Mania is related to prefrontal functioning from abnormal signaling cascades, especially of PKC signaling. Sustained elevation of PKC signaling may result in loss of grey matter in the prefrontal cortex.

Neurotransmitters

As already discussed, amine neurotransmitter systems, such as the serotonergic system, are dysfunctional in bipolar disorder. When depressed, there is lower serotonin (5-HT) and its chief metabolite, 5-HIAA, in the prefrontal cortex. Other neurosystems are also involved in bipolar disorder, including the dopamine, GABA, glutamate, norepinephrine, and acetylcholine/cholinergic systems (Black & Andreasen, 2011, pp. 66 ff.). For example, dopamine and its chief metabolite, homovanillic acid, is reduced in depression or depressive episodes. Glutamate is the main excitatory neurotransmitter. GABA reduces glutamate, as does lithium. Antidepressants that increase glutamate can trigger a manic episode. Finally, note that there are probably some intercycle dynamics in bipolar disorder. For example, if a person is manic for long he or she will become exhausted, deprived of sleep, and thus more vulnerable to switching to a depressive episode.

Suicidogenic Effects of Bipolar Disorder Treatment

Bipolar disorder is mainly treated with psychiatric medications, like those just discussed since manic and depressive episodes themselves increase suicide risk. Baldessarini et al. (2012) claim that patients with bipolar disorder have a suicide mortality risk 25 times that of the general population (see Chapter 10, Table 10.1; Baldessarini, 2002). Suicide prevention is one of the main intended effects of taking a mood stabilizer or an antidepressant. Other therapeutic effects include issues related to quality (not length) of life, such as reducing depression, anhedonia, weight loss, sleep disorders, and low energy/libido; improving concentration, control, decision making, and ability to work; and preventing disorganized thought and self-destructive sexual or financial acting out.

But what if the treatment of mania itself were suicidogenic? Can antidepressants or mood stabilizers increase suicidality, induce or worsen depression, or result in other serious adverse effects that make life intolerable? If so, then the treatment of bipolar disorder is paradoxical, since it may contribute to the very thing it is supposed to prevent. In this last section of this chapter, I consider some of the possible serious adverse effects of the treatments of both mania and depression. It is my argument that antiepileptic or mood-stabilizing drugs can contribute substantially, directly, and proximately to suicidality outcomes. In other words, they can be suicidogenic, although the effects may be rare, small, and worth the risk.

The FDA issued a warning about antiepileptics and suicide risk on July 10, 2008, based on an advisory committee vote (see more below). However, the FDA has issued an even stronger (black-box) warning for antidepressants. The summary risk for suicidality (up to age 24) for patients treated with any of nine antidepressants was 2.19 overall (roughly two times the suicidality risk of controls not taking antidepressants). The FDA then issued two black-box warnings (the strongest possible) for young people (on September 14, 2004) and young adults (on October 13, 2006) taking any of the nine antidepressants (namely Prozac, Luvox, Effexor, Celexa, Paxil, Zoloft, Wellbutrin, Serzone, and Remeron).

Among the antiepileptic adverse effects most often claimed to be related to suicidality (i.e., suicide ideation, nonfatal suicide attempts, and completed suicides) are these (cf. Hawton, 2005):

- Increased suicidality.
- *De novo* or worsened depression.
- Ego-dystonia, or feeling and acting out of character.
- Emergent hopelessness.
- Chronic pain.
- Behavioral changes.
- Akathisia.

The emphasis in what follows is mainly on gabapentin (Neurontin).

Increased Suicide Ideation or Behavior

In the July 10, 2008 FDA alert, patients receiving antiepileptic medications were described as having approximately twice the relative risk for suicide ideation or suicide behavior (0.43) as patients receiving placebo (0.22). Note that even though the difference was statistically significant, it was still under 1%. These results were based on 199 placebo-controlled studies of 11 antiepileptic drugs ($N = 43,892$, of whom 27,863 received antiepileptic medications).

There were 4 completed suicides in this population, equaling a suicide rate of 14.4 per 100,000. Since the suicide rate in the general population is rare (about 12 per 100,000), the FDA studied suicidality (as broadly defined above). For psychiatric patients, the relative risk difference for suicidality equaled 3.1 times that of the placebo group.

The 11 antiepileptics studied by the FDA for suicidality were Tegretol, Depakote, Felbatol, Neurontin, Lamictal, Keppra, Trileptal, Lyrica, Gabitril, Topomax, and Zonegran. On December 16, 2008, the FDA ordered the manufacturers of all 11 of these drugs to include a warning for increased suicide ideation or suicidal behavior with their product information (in each product's package insert). The elevated suicidality risk was consistent across all 11 antiepileptics, although there was individual drug variation in risk levels.

Russell Katz, MD, of the FDA (in the July 10, 2008 FDA alert) added: "Patients being treated with AEDs [antiepileptic drugs] for any indication should be monitored for the emergence or worsening of depression, suicide ideation, suicidal behaviors, or for any unusual changes in mood or behavior." Moreover, suicide ideation and/or suicidal behavior among users of antiepileptic drugs did not vary by the patients' ages, as they did among users of antidepressant medications.

De Novo or Worsened Depression

As discussed above, any medication that lowers monoamine (serotonin or epinephrine) tends to generate depression or make existing depression worse (Trimble, 2007; Trimble & George, 2010; Maris, 1986); drug company manufacturers of AEDs often contest this. Since Neurontin and Tegretol deplete monoamines, they tend to induce or worsen depression. Depleting these neurotransmitters leads to more depression and less excitation or pleasure. For example, Neurontin shifts the balance of neurotransmitters from excitatory to inhibiting. The *Physicians' Desk Reference* (2013) says that the relative risk of depression in patients taking Neurontin is 1.6 times higher than that in patients receiving a placebo.

Also, patients taking Neurontin have a 3.3 times greater risk for anxiety and restlessness than the placebo group (McCormick, 1992). McCormick adds that two psychobiological adverse events that are "frequent" are depression and anxiety. We have seen that anxiety increases suicide risk (Fawcett, 2012).

Ego-Dystonia

Antiepileptics can make changes in a person's sense of ego, as antidepressants can. Patients are often not their usual, predrug selves after ingesting Neurontin, for example. All of us have psychic and physical pain thresholds beyond which it is difficult to keep living. People are not infinitely flexible; they have coping boundaries. When a medication changes people's perceptions of who they are (i.e., causes ego-dystonia) and what they can tolerate, life and coping may become untenable, if not impossible.

Emergent Hopelessness

As a result of adverse events resulting from antiepileptic drugs (such as depression or suicide ideation), some patients may lose hope that they can maintain or sustain a life of sufficient quality. These patients may conclude that they have to escape from a future they perceive as intolerable (Tandon et al., 2013). As I have noted in Chapter 11, Beck et al. (1985) claimed that hopelessness is more suicidogenic than depression. When patients are depressed, they cannot consider their best alternatives (Brandt, 1975). Depression generates dichotomous, rigid thinking and hopelessness—for example, "I must be either miserable or dead by suicide."

Chronic Pain

Since many patients are taking antiepileptic drugs (such as Neurontin) and even antidepressant drugs for chronic pain, manufacturers often claim that the patient's chronic pain (not the drugs) caused the patient's suicide. For example, Ilgen et al. (2008) found that chronic pain makes some sufferers contemplate suicide to relieve their pain. Note that the vast majority of people in pain are not suicidal. It usually takes more than just physical pain to result in a suicide.

One aspect of Neurontin treatment pain may be what Shneidman (1993) called "psychache" (cf. Motto, 1992, pp. 625–639; Ducasse et al., 2018). When a patient says, for example, "The pain pills are not working," this patient may be reflecting antiepileptic-induced depression, hopelessness, and heightened suicidality, not primarily physical pain.

Behavioral Changes

Some of the adverse effects in which patients taking antiepileptics exceed patients taking a placebo (see the 2007 package insert for Neurontin) are dizziness, somnolence, ataxia, abnormal thoughts, fatigue, back pain, hostility, and emotional lability. Although none of these effects are particularly life-threatening, they can raise suicide risk. Notice particularly the sedating and disorienting effects of Neurontin. One patient I spoke with recently said that this drug made him feel like a "zombie." If not being manic is a problem, then so is being severely depressed and lethargic.

Serious adverse effects are often not separated out from other adverse effects in clinical trials. *Serious* in this context usually means "leading to death, a suicide attempt, or hospitalization." Adverse effects in clinical trials are not psychiatric diagnoses, but rather what are called "coding symbols for a thesaurus of adverse reaction terms" (COSTARTs). For example, *emotional lability* or *depression* may not be defined the way most clinicians understand them.

Akathisia

Akathisia is a diffuse psychomotor restlessness, which affects both a patient's body and mind (Van Putten, 1975; Healy et al., 2006). Typically the akathisic patient cannot sit still, constantly paces, shifts weight from one foot to another while standing, has restless legs while sitting or sleeping, and can walk miles each day (American Psychiatric Association, 2013). Akathisia has both outer (behavioral) and inner (mental and emotional) aspects. DSM-5 refers to medication-induced acute akathisia (code G25.71). The condition is caused by a psychiatric drug, such as antipsychotic medications.

Chapter 13 considers suicide and psychotic disorders, especially the schizophrenias. There is often something bizarre or distinctive about psychotic suicides.

CHAPTER 13

Schizophrenia
Bizarre and Psychotic Suicides

My good fortune is not that I have recovered from mental illness. I have not,
nor will I ever. My good fortune lies in having found my life.

—ELYN SAKS

Schizophrenia is among the most devastating and debilitating of all mental disorders. It tends to strike patients in their late teens to early 20s (on average, at age 21 for males and 27 for females). Most people with schizophrenia, but not all, have a poor prognosis (Black & Andreasen, 2014). Once symptoms emerge, people are often unable to return to (or even commence) normal adult lives, such as going to school, working, marrying, or having children. Schizophrenia is in the top 10 causes of disability worldwide for people ages 15–44 (WHO, 1996, 2008, 2012a).

Although schizophrenia is the most important of the psychotic disorders, there are other psychotic disorders on the schizophrenia spectrum (see the discussion of differential diagnosis and "rule-outs," below). These include medical-condition-induced psychosis (e.g., resulting from a brain tumor); substance-related psychosis (e.g., caused by a hallucinogen such as LSD or PCP), brief psychotic disorder; delusional disorder; schizoaffective disorder (a mix of schizophrenic and mood symptoms); schizophreniform disorder (which is prodromal to and briefer than schizophrenia); schizotypal personality disorder (a pervasive pattern of social and interpersonal deficits marked by acute discomfort with and reduced capacity for close relationships, as well as by cognitive or perceptual distortions and eccentricities of behavior; American Psychological Association, 2013); and what DSM-5 labels *other specified* or *unspecified* schizophrenia spectrum and other psychotic disorders. By definition, schizophrenia is a psychotic disorder.

Schizophrenia is a multidetermined disorder combining many different causes, such as (1) genetics (e.g., a person has about a 46% chance of getting schizophrenia if both parents are schizophrenic); (2) stress–diathesis factors; (3) development (it is age-related, it can result from brain injury, and it may be influenced by hormones); (4) neuroanatomy (schizophrenic patients tend to have hypofrontality and so-called negative symptoms, ventricular enlargement and more CSF than is normal); and (5) neurotransmitter abnormalities (see the later discussion of the dopamine hypothesis).

Schizophrenia and Suicide

Originally schizophrenia was called *dementia praecox* or "precocious dementia" by French psychiatrist Benedict Morel in 1856, since it presented early in the life cycle. He described the dementia-like symptoms of a 14-year-old boy. This adolescent had been bright and active but gradually became silent and withdrawn, in what Morel thought was a kind of precocious senility.

In 1896, Emil Kraepelin combined several previously distinct psychotic disorders. For example, in 1868 Kalbaum spoke of *catatonia* (marked by abnormal motor behavior and either excited or stuporous states, such as waxy inflexibility); in 1868 Sander identified *paranoia* (characterized by delusions of persecution or grandeur); and in 1870 Hecker coined the term *hebephrenia*—that is, silliness, inappropriate smiling/grimaces, disorganization, and primitive behavior, such as Lisa's behavior in the movie *David and Lisa* (Perry, 1962). Kraepelin subsumed all these concepts under the rubric of *dementia praecox*. Kraepelin also felt that (unlike most of those with manic–depressive disorders), patients with dementia praecox deteriorated and never improved.

In 1911 Eugen Bleuler formed the basis for the modern concept of schizophrenia around four primary symptoms, the so-called "four A's": Affective disorder (usually flat affect), loose Associations, Autism (withdrawnness or self-centeredness), and Ambivalence (having two opposite feelings toward the same object or person at the same time). The terms *schizophreniform* (1939), *schizoaffective* (1943), and *atypical schizophrenia* (1960) were added by Langfeld, Cobb, and Leonard, respectively.

Bleuler felt that other schizophrenic symptoms (like hypersensitivity, hallucinations, delusions, loss of ego boundaries, and verbal disorders) were all secondary symptoms. Bleuler, unlike Kraepelin, did not view terminal deterioration as a necessary feature of schizophrenia. Those with schizophrenia have two more of the following characteristics over most of one month: (1) delusions, (2) hallucinations (which can be auditory, visual, olfactory, or somatic/tactile), (3) disorganized speech (such as derailment of thought or incoherence), (4) catatonic or grossly disorganized behavior, and (5) so-called "negative symptoms" (such as flat affect, alogia, and avolition). These five sets of symptoms are grouped together in DSM-5 as criterion A for a diagnosis of schizophrenia; a person must exhibit symptoms in three of these groups, including at least one from the first three (see "Classification and Diagnosis," below).

Antipsychotic medications were discovered in 1952–1953 by French physicians Delay and Deniker, who used chlorpromazine (Thorazine) as an anesthetic at first. They later discovered that it calmed agitated patients and reduced their hallucinations and delusions (Black & Andreasen, 2011, p. 501). Some of the first antipsychotic drugs were the phenothiazine medications introduced in the 1950s, like Thorazine, Stelazine, Haldol, and Mellaril. Phenothiazines were crucial in lowering the census of state and county mental hospitals. Clozaril, the first of the second-generation antipsychotics, appeared in 1989 and has proven effective for suicide prevention.

Schizophrenic patients exhibit a lot of movement disorders; these may be related to their disease or to treatment with antipsychotics (often first-generation antipsychotics). Medications in second category, such as Cogentin or Artane, are often given to control these movement disorders. A few of the more important and common movement disorders are these:

- Parkinsonism—flattening of facial expression, stiffness of gait, muscular rigidity in trunk and extremities, so-called "pill-rolling" tremors of fingers, and excessive salivation.
- Catatonia—withdrawal, muteness, bizarre posturing, rigidity or immobility, and waxy flexibility.
- Akathisia—a subjective sense of inner and outer motor restlessness, impatience, nervousness, restless legs, fidgeting, pacing or compulsive walkingrocking back and forth, and foot shifting.
- Tremor—rhythmic alternating movements of opposing muscle groups, most often in the fingers.
- Tardive dyskinesia—sometimes stereotyped, involuntary movements of the nose, tongue, mouth, face, and extremities; the movements are writhing and purposeless. (*Tardive* means "slow" or "tardy"; in this context, it refers to symptoms that develop slowly or appear long after inception.)

What are some of the symptoms of schizophrenia that might raise suicide risk? Since the onset of schizophrenia tends to be in the late teens or early 20s and the prognosis is usually poor, it seems reasonable to assume that people with schizophrenia would also have higher rates of hopelessness and depression, which in turn can increase suicide risk.

Since schizophrenia by definition is a psychotic disorder, one has to pay particular attention to voices, especially command hallucinations and what they are telling a patient to do (Tandon et al., 2013: see the description of Elyn Saks in Case 13.1).

CASE 13.1. Elyn Saks

Elyn Saks is a very bright person with schizophrenia who graduated first in her undergraduate class at Vanderbilt, received a master's of letters from Oxford University, graduated from Yale Law School, and then became a well-known professor. She underwent deep talk therapy with Melanie Klein, a famous 20th-century psychoanalyst in England; Saks described Klein as making "blank" observations and as being detached and distant. Saks's dreams were very strange (e.g., "I made golf balls out of fetuses"). The closer Saks got to her therapist, the more terrified she became of her ("I must kill her," she thought).

Saks describes psychosis as like an infection that leaves some facilities intact. She would stay in her room for days, withdrawn and isolated. She became a hypochondriac. Saks had great trouble discontinuing treatment with her therapist when she had to leave England for New Haven, Connecticut.

One wonders why no antipsychotic medications are mentioned in the treatment of Saks. Thorazine was first introduced in 1952, and Saks was born in 1955. How much talk therapy can one do with a psychotic patient? Notice, too, that although Saks was totally psychotic at times, she still managed to excel at Oxford and at Yale Law School.

Source: Excerpted and rewritten by Maris from Saks (2010).

The presence of psychosis raises the interesting question of whether schizo-phrenic patients know what they are doing when they suicide. Suicides have to be able to form the *intent* to die by suicide. But can those experiencing psychosis enact intentional behavior? For example, if a psychotic person is at a party in a high-rise and decides to fly home, jumps out of a window, and falls, is this an accident or a suicide? Schizophrenic suicides often behave strangely and utilize unusual, bizarre methods. Remember Silvia Suarez (see Chapter 4, Case 4.1): She was a 30-year-old woman taking an SSRI whose behavior and speech were becoming increasingly psy-chotic. At her death, she cut herself in multiple locations, in a way that seemed more like self-mutilation than a clear-cut suicide attempt. Before she exsanguinated, she collected her own blood in bowls and then set them neatly on a kitchen table. What was she thinking?

Another bizarre suicide case was that of Franklyn Thornwell (Case 13.2), a 28-year-old African American male. Sometimes hallucinations can include com-mands to suicide. For example, Franklyn was told by his voices: "You are evil and you should cut your heart out."

CASE 13.2. Franklyn Thornwell

Franklyn Thornwell was a 28-year-old black male from a U.S. coastal city. He heard voices that told him to kill himself: "You are evil and you should cut your heart out." He tried to do that, but failed. After stabilization in an emergency room, he was committed to the state mental hospital for stabbing himself and was diagnosed with schizophrenia, paranoid type (according to the typology then used in DSM). Franklyn was put on the antipsychotic Haldol.

In the summer of 1981, Franklyn stopped taking his medications and ran away from home. He was arrested while hitchhiking. He assaulted the arresting officer, behaved "bizarrely," and was put in a local jail over the weekend (on a Friday).

His mother was notified of his arrest, and she told the jailer, "Franklyn ain't right. He has mental problems. Go to the ER and start Haldol for him." Nothing was done. Franklyn calmed down for a while, but then again became very agitated. First he ran back and forth in his jail cell, and then he began hitting his head on the bars.

About this time, Franklyn told the jailer, "Everything is evil and should be destroyed," and "I am tired of being in this world." He then started speaking in tongues (*glossolalia*), which sounded like gibberish to the other inmates who heard him, but it was perhaps just the typical free association of thoughts and words that is common in schizophrenia. As a result, Franklyn was supposed to be put on constant watch for the weekend.

About 8:00 A.M. on Monday, Franklyn could still be heard talking, and the jailer took a 5-minute phone call. At the 8:15 A.M. check, Franklyn was found naked and dead in his cell. He had taken off his jogging pants, forced one leg of the pants down his throat, and then drowned himself in the toilet in his cell.

Source: Even though this case was heard in public court, most identifying information (names, dates, places, etc.) has been changed to maintain the confidentiality of the family.

Going in and out of psychosis itself would seem to be suicidogenic, as in "I don't think I can tolerate yet another psychotic episode." The brother of a famous South Carolina novelist, Pat Conroy (author of *The Prince of Tides,* etc.) was schizophrenic and jumped to his death from his eighth-floor apartment after emerging from yet another psychotic episode.

Both suicide and schizophrenia have genetic components. In my survey of Chicago suicides (Maris, 1981), 11–12% of the first-degree relatives (mother, father, and siblings) had also committed suicide, but none of the healthy control relatives had. Genetics are even more powerful in schizophrenia, as I discuss in the next section.

Comorbid substance use and sleep disorders occur at high rates in people with schizophrenia, in those who suicide, and in depressed patients, although sleep can also be affected by antipsychotic drug treatment. Alcohol and drug abuse are common in schizophrenic patients (Black & Andreasen, 2011). Those who suicide tend to have disturbed rapid-eye-movement (REM) sleep (which occurs during dreaming) and terminal insomnia (early morning awakening and the inability to fall back to sleep) (Maris, 1981, 2015; Maris et al., 2000). Severe insomnia may be a prodromal clue to an incipient psychotic episode. Schizophrenic patients also have decreased non-REM sleep early in the sleep cycle. People with schizophrenia tend to sleep during the day and less at night (Black & Andreasen, 2014). For a recent review of schizophrenia see Hor and Taylor (2010).

Epidemiology of Schizophrenia

About 1% of the American population has schizophrenia, but not all of them have been diagnosed or treated. About one-third of these persons will attempt suicide, and about 5–10% will complete suicide at some time during their lives. Many people are surprised by the prevalence of this serious mental disorder. For example, in 2013 the U.S. population was 316 million, and 1% were schizophrenic (3,160,000). Five percent of the schizophrenic population equals 158,000, which is the estimated number of those who will eventually suicide. One could calculate similar rates for world estimated lifetime schizophrenic suicide rates, starting with a figure of 7 billion people in the world. The WHO (2015c) claims that there are about 800,000 to 1 million total suicides in the world each year (see Chapter 8).

Males have earlier onset of schizophrenia than females do (about 5–6 years earlier) and higher rates of suicide as well. The first psychotic episode in males tends to occur between the ages of 18 and 25, but in women it is between ages 21 and 30. Maleness in general is related to higher mortality, including that from schizophrenia. Even the *in utero* death rate of male fetuses is higher than that of females. In the United States at least, schizophrenic suicide risk factors include being male, being African American (see Table 13.1), and being under age 30 (see Table 13.1), as well

TABLE 13.1. Prevalence Rates for Schizophrenia in Monroe County, New York, by Age, Sex, and Race

| | Males | | | | Females | | | | | |
| | White | | Nonwhite | | White | | Nonwhite | | Total | |
Age	No.	Rate	No.	Rate	No.	Rate	No.	Rate	No.	Rate
0–14	44	0.47	7	0.64	18	0.20	4	0.37	73	0.35
15–24	357	6.69	36	8.60	240	4.11	16	3.00	649	5.35
25–34	362	8.74	46	12.46	338	9.13	44	10.09	840	9.13
35–44	339	9.30	47	17.11	432	11.44	43	14.75	861	10.78
45–54	231	2.75	8	8.37	141	4.45	7	6.80	596	7.25
55–64	78	2.75	8	8.37	141	4.45	7	6.80	234	3.77
65+	17	0.63	2	3.03	46	1.13	1	1.27	66	0.96
Total	1428	4.49	172	6.91	1575	4.61	144	5.32	3319	4.65

Note. Rates per 1,000 population. Observe the higher rates for nonwhites, especially males.

Source: H. M. Babigian, "Schizophrenia Epidemiology," in A. M. Freedman et al., eds., *Comprehensive Textbook of Psychiatry* (2nd ed., Vol. 2), 1975. Copyright 1975 by Williams & Wilkins. Reprinted with permission of Lippincott Williams & Wilkins.

as prior depression, a chronic course of the illness with an early start, substance abuse, recent mental hospital discharge, and unemployment (Yoon & Carter, 2012). It is likely that the male XY chromosomal combination is more highly associated with death in general (regardless of the cause) than the female XX is. In a sense (as noted in an earlier chapter), we all begin our development as females, and then about half of us develop as male.

Throughout this textbook, I have alluded to the role of genetics in suicide. Generally, the closer the biological tie (such as being twins from the same egg), the more likely it is that if one twin becomes schizophrenic, so will the other twin. This is called *concordance*. For example, if both parents are schizophrenic, their child has about a 46% probability of becoming schizophrenic. The probability is 17% if only one parent is schizophrenic. Twins who share the same egg (monozygotic) have a roughly sixfold greater concordance rate for schizophrenia. As shown in Table 13.2, several studies of twins with schizophrenia indicate that the concordance rate for schizophrenia in monozygotic twins (*heritability*) is about 0.54 on average. Although the authors of the studies listed in Table 13.2 did not calculate the heritability scores for fraternal (dizygotic) twins, they are much lower for the dizygotic twins (e.g., about 0.10 for the Rosanoff study and about 0.02 for the Kallman study). See Hilker et al. (2010) for a more recent study, though the results are about the same.

Some young people with prodromal/incipient schizophrenia may be especially suicidal, since they realize that something is terribly wrong with their brains and they may never recover from it. They may realize that they perhaps cannot return to college, have a career, get married, or have children. From this perspective, it is no wonder that schizophrenic individuals have elevated suicide rates.

Classic research in New Haven, Connecticut by Hollingshead and Redlich (1958), a sociologist and a psychiatrist, respectively, found that persons with schizophrenia tended to have lower SES and that about 60% of the population

TABLE 13.2. Concordance Rates in Monozygotic (MZ) and Dizygotic (DZ) Co-Twins of Schizophrenic Twins

Investigator(s), country, year	Zygosity	No. of pairs	Concordance	Heritability
Rosanoff, United States, 1934	MZ	41	67	0.63
	DZ	101	10	
Essen-Moller, Sweden, 1941	MZ	7	71	0.65
	DZ	24	17	
Kallman, United States, 1953	MZ	268	86	0.84
	DZ	685	15	
Inouye, Japan, 1961	MZ	55	76	0.69
	DZ	17	22	
Harvald and Hauge, Denmark, 1965	MZ	7	29	0.25
	DZ	59	5	
Cohen et al., United States, 1972	MZ	81	23	0.19
	DZ	113	5	

Note. If you average the six heritability scores above, the mean is 0.54. Although the authors of these studies (references for these studies can be found in Leo, 2003) did not calculate the DZ twin heritability scores in this table, they are much lower for the DZ twins—for example, about 0.10 for the Rosanoff study and 0.02 for the Kallman study.

in state and county hospitals were schizophrenic. In New Haven, 86.8% of those with schizophrenia were in the lower two SES classes (classes IV and V), versus only 65% of the general population. Although the Hollingshead and Redlich data are old, they call attention to an important aspect of schizophrenia: Lower-SES schizophrenic patients may be more likely to be in state hospitals, in part because they cannot afford treatment "on the outside." Even when they do get antipsychotics, they are more likely to get older phenothiazine medications with more side effects than to be prescribed the more expensive second-generation antipsychotics.

It would be negligent here not to mention what happened to the state and county mental hospital census from about 1955 to 1997. Essentially, the populations of such hospitals were drastically reduced with the advent of phenothiazine drugs (like Thorazine). You can turn back to Chapter 10, Table 10.6, to see this for yourself. In 1955 state and county mental hospital censuses went from 558,922 inpatients to only 54,015 in 1997, roughly a 90% drop.

Classification and Diagnosis

Schizophrenia is conceptualized as one of many psychotic disorders on a spectrum. Through a process of *differential diagnosis,* a clinician sorts through and rules out the competing psychotic (and other) disorders that are possibilities for a given patient, until the clinician arrives at the most appropriate psychotic disorder (if any).

Differential diagnosis involves giving a series of yes-or-no answers in a decision tree to a series of questions such as these: (1) Are two or more groups of symptoms present (delusions, hallucinations, disorganized speech or thought, catatonic behavior, or negative symptoms—see below), including at least one from the first three? If yes, then: (2) Are the symptoms due to a medical condition? If no, then: (3) Are they due to a substance or medication? If no, then: (4) Have the symptoms lasted at least 1 month? If yes, then: (5) Is there a concurrent major depressive or manic episode? If no, then: (6) Is the total duration at least 6 months? If yes, then the diagnosis is schizophrenia. There are many specifiers, such as for a first episode versus multiple episodes, for catatonia, and for severity. Clinicians also need to rule out other psychotic disorders.

Today schizophrenia is thought to consist of five major factors determined by the statistical procedure of factor analysis. These factors are the five groups of symptoms included in DSM-5's criterion A, as noted earlier: (1) delusions, (2) hallucinations, (3) disorganized speech, (4) disorganized or catatonic behavior, and (5) negative symptoms. First and second, hallucinations and/or delusions (the so-called "positive symptoms") are excessive and pathological activities of the five senses (*Hopkins Brain Wise*, 2015). Delusions are fixed beliefs held despite contradictory evidence; paranoia is a common delusion. Hearing voices is the most common hallucination, with about 75% of schizophrenic patients experiencing these. Visual hallucinations tend to be second, experienced by about 45% of patients. Positive symptoms are usually treated with second-generation antipsychotics like Clozaril, Abilify, Zyprexa, Risperdal, Geodon, or Saphris (Maris, 2015). The third major factor is disorganized speech, such as derailment of thought, loose association, neologisms, and incoherence (Black & Andreasen, 2014). Fourth, grossly disorganized or catatonic behavior can include motoric immobility, stupor, excessive motor activity, stereotypic behaviors, echolalia, hygiene and grooming deficiencies, and so on. Fifth, the so-called "negative symptoms" include being withdrawn, mute, catatonic, alogic, or anhedonic. Negative symptoms often also require treatment with second-generation antipsychotics (see Table 13.3 for an overview of positive and negative symptoms). These factors must represent a change from the patient's normal, baseline functioning and meet several other conditions (length of disturbance, current severity from 0 to 4, etc.) specified below.

Here is an example of schizophrenic speech and thought. A schizophrenic college professor was asked by his psychiatrist what his chief complaint was. He replied:

> "It should be extrusively notated that my imago has been ensnared in the viscosity of time. That is why my transcendent self has been importuned (but not without resisting) despite the hydraulic pressure I have succinctly initiated in an attempt to laminate and delineate those teotons whose essential god-like characteristics have been laminated into an irreducible minisculate, atomized, and indeed lionized canister. Such is the enraptured entrapment of my condition."

TABLE 13.3. Percentages of 111 Schizophrenic Patients with Positive and Negative Symptoms

Negative symptoms	Positive symptoms
Affective flattening (unchanging facial expression, 96%) (paucity of expressive gestures, 81%)	Hallucinations (auditory, 75%) (voices, 58%)
Alogia (poverty of speech, 53%) (poverty of speech content, 51%)	Delusions (persecutory, 81%) (delusions of reference, 49%)
Avolition/apathy (lack of persistence at schoolwork, 95%) (impaired grooming and hygiene, 87%)	Bizarre behavior (social/sexual behavior, 33%) (aggressive/agitated, 27%)
Anhedonia/asociality (few recreational interests, 95 %) (impaired intimacy/closeness, 84%)	Positive thought disorder (tangentiality, 50%) (derailment, 45%)
Attention (social inattentiveness, 78 %) (testing inattentiveness, 64 %)	

Note. Only two examples per symptom are given, even though there are usually more.
Source: Excerpted and adapted by Maris from Black and Andreasen (2011).

Most of the words sound real, and the syntax seems to be correct (although verbose). Note, however, that there are several neologisms or made-up words, such as *extrusively, teotons.* and *minisculate.*

To summarize, the diagnosis of schizophrenia involves examining and making decisions on at least six criteria:

A. The presence of (1) delusions, (2) hallucinations, (3) disorganized speech, (4) disorganized or catatonic behavior, and (5) negative symptoms; the schizophrenic patient must have symptoms for much of a 1-month period in at least two of these five groupings, including at least one of the first three.

B. The behavior (such as in work, personal relationships, or self-care) must be dysfunctional and/or leading to disability compared to baseline functioning (such as in occupation or school).

C. The symptoms must be present more or less continuously for at least 6 consecutive months (including at least 1 month of continuous A symptoms).

D. Other disorders (schizoaffective and bipolar disorders, etc.) must be ruled out.

E. The symptoms are not physically induced (such as by substance abuse or a medical condition).

F. There must be clarifications for autism spectrum disorder or childhood communication disorders.

Again, specifications must be made for the episode, severity of the disorder, presence of catatonia, and so forth.

Treatment of Schizophrenia

With psychotic disorders, antipsychotic medication treatments are usually necessary (Lehman, 1980). It can be nearly impossible to do psychotherapy with a floridly psychotic patient. Most psychotic patients start out with one of the second-generation atypical antipsychotics. Three of the most common second-generation antipsychotics (see Table 13.4) are Clozaril, Risperdal, and Zyprexa. Given their serious adverse effects, the first-generation antipsychotics tend not to be used as much any more, although for agitated episodes in emergency rooms or jails, a patient may receive an intramuscular injection of 5–10 mg of the high-potency antipsychotic Haldol. Clinical trials have shown that Clozaril is especially effective in lowering suicide risk, but it can induce agranulocytosis (lowered white blood cell counts and increased risk of infection) in about 1% of all patients taking it. Two of the newer antipsychotics are Rexulti (brexpirazole) and Abilify (ariprazole); see Chapter 23, Table 23.6.

Some of the most common adverse effects of antipsychotics are akathisia, headache, dizziness, parkinsonism and other movement disorders, fatigue, weight increase, and dry mouth (see the last section of this chapter for a discussion of the serious adverse effects that are specifically related to suicide risk). In discontinuation of antipsychotic treatment, there can be depression, agitation, anxiety, and akathisia, all of which can be suicidogenic. The second-generation antipsychotics tend to work better for negative symptoms (the absence of something that should be present); the first-generation antipsychotics (like Thorazine and Haldol) work well on positive symptoms (like hallucinations and delusions), but can also have long-term, adverse effects like tardive dyskinesia.

When I was a professor at Dartmouth, I tried to interview schizophrenic patients at the Concord State Hospital. Most of them were mute (a negative symptom) and would stare at me or just repeat my questions back verbatim (*echolalia*). Most of them were also taking first-generation antipsychotics, so it was difficult to sort out the effects of their psychosis from the effects of the medications.

Another important thing to note is that psychotic patients may be taking antipsychotics, antidepressants, and anxiolytics all at the same time. That is, many psychotic patients get a cocktail of psychiatric medications. In a study of antipsychotic medications, Tiihonen et al. (2006) compared the risk of re-hospitalization (as a measure of antipsychotic medication effectiveness) after a mean time of 3.6 years. The drug of reference was haloperidol (Haldol). The lowest risks for re-hospitalization after various drug treatments, in order, were as follows:

- 59% for perphenazine (Trialfon) depot (just 31% for the tablet alone).
- 41% for olanzapine (Zyprexa).
- 39% for clozapine (Clozaril).
- 23% for risperidone (Risperdal).

The effectiveness of Trialfon, a first-generation phenothiazine medication, is related to the form of administration. A *depot* is an injectable medication; its use improves compliance, and it normally stays effective in the body for about 30 days. Decanoic acid is a saturated fatty acid from which one may develop a long-acting

TABLE 13.4. Antipsychotic Medications

Generic name/Brand name (drug type)	Dosage in mg/day (half-life in hours)	Company (year first manufactured)	Adverse events/other characteristics	
			Generic	Specific[a]
First-generation antipsychotics				
Chlorpromazine/Thorazine (phenothiazine/aliphatic)	100–400 (16–30)	SmithKline (1952)[b]	EPS, weight gain, akathisia, anticholinergic, sexual dysfunction, muscle stiffness and tremors, sedation, heart	Revolutionary first antipsychotic; led to reduction of psychiatric inpatients
Thioridazine/Mellaril (phenothiazine/piperidine)	30–800 (7–13)	Novartis (1959)		Tardive dyskinesia, anorgasmia
Trifluopromazine/Stelazine (phenothiazene/aliphatic)	5–40 (10–20)	SmithKline (1958)		Lower seizure threshold, tardive dyskinesia
Thiothixene/Navane (thioxanthene)	5–60 (10–20)	Pfizer (1967)		Somnolence
Fluphenazine/Prolixin (phenothiazine/piperazine)[d]	0.5–20 (15–30)	App Pharma (1960s)		Tx for BP off-label; "rabbit syndrome"; injectable
Haloperidol/Haldol (butyrophenone)[e]	3–50 (10–30)	Janssen (1958)		Used for ER agitation via IM injection; depression
Second-generation (atypical) antipsychotics[c]				
Clozapine/Clozaril	200–600[d] (6–26)	Novartis (1971)	Fewer EPS; weight gain, sexual dysfunction, type II diabetes	Agranulocytosis in 1%; sedation

Generic/Brand	Dose range	Manufacturer (year)	Characteristics/adverse events
Risperidone/Risperdal	2–6 (3–20)	Janssen (1994)	Blood pressure effects, muscle stiffness, neuroleptic malignant syndrome
Olanzapine/Zyprexa	15–30 (21–54)	Eli Lilly (1996)	Orthostatic hypotension, auditory hallucinations
Quetiapine/Seroquel	300–500 (6)	Astra-Zeneca (1997)	Somnolence; augmenter for MDD[e]
Ziprasidone/Geodon	40–160 (7)	Pfizer (2001)	Akathisia, sexual dysfunction, mortality in elderly patients; IM adm.
Aripiprazole/Abilify[f]	10–15 (75)	Otsuka (2002)	Augmenter, AΨ/AD enhancer; weight gain, type II diabetes
Asenapine/Saphris	10–20 (24)	Schering Plough (2007)	Severe akathisia, sedation, extreme weight gain

Note. This table is not a complete list; no foreign brand names are given; sometimes drug manufacturers change. Abbreviations in table: EPS, extrapyramidal symptoms or movement disorders; Tx, treatment; BP, bipolar disorder; ER, emergency room; IM, intramuscular; MDD, major depressive disorder; AΨ/AD, antipsychotic/antidepressant.

[a]Specific does not mean that an adverse event or other characteristic occurs only in a specific drug (e.g., tardive dyskinesia occurs in other antipsychotics), just that the adverse event or characteristic is highlighted for the particular medication cited.

[b]Synthesized in December 1950; antipsychotic properties observed by Delay and Deniker in 1952.

[c]Relatively new second-generation (atypical) antipsychotics are iloperidone/Fanapt (2009, Vanda) and lurasidone/Latuda (2010, Dainippon Sumitomo). Others include amisulpride/Solian, adasuve/Loxapine (inhaled) (2013), and paliperidone/Invega. Latuda is also marketed in the United States for depressive episodes in bipolar disorder.

[d]Clozapine starts with low doses (e.g., 12.5 mg two times a day) and is increased in small increments (with monitoring for agranucytosis) until a therapeutic level is achieved.

[e]Sometimes used as a date-rape drug.

[f]Sometimes called a "third-generation antipsychotic."

Source: Adapted from Maris (2015). Copyright © 2015 by the University of South Carolina. Adapted with permission.

injectable drug (depot injection). Compliance is important; presumably most patients get better if they keep taking their medication. Tiihonen et al. (2006) also rated the various antipsychotics by rates of discontinuation; those with the lowest risks of discontinuation, in order, were (1) Clozapine, (2) Trilafon, and (3) Zyprexa.

A Note on Clozaril

As noted above, a striking research finding is that Clozaril is extremely effective in lowering suicide risk, compared to other antipsychotics. One clinical trial (Goldsmith et al., 2002, p. 236) reported an 80–85% decline in suicide risk with Clozaril. This seems to be a beneficent effect, although about 1–2% of patients taking Clozaril do get a serious white blood cell disorder called "agranulocytosis" (again, as noted above). Some psychiatrists have argued that Clozaril reduces suicide risk by lowering impulsive aggression.

This raises the interesting question of what price should be paid for suicide prevention. For example, we could probably drastically reduce the suicide rate by giving all agitated psychotics an antipsychotic like Clozaril. We often do just that by giving Haldol in jails, hospitals, and emergency rooms. But antipsychotic medication can also be a kind of psychic castration. There is even the absurd argument that acutely suicidal individuals should be given a general anesthesia (i.e., be put in an induced coma for a while). I am not talking about reasonable anesthetic treatment like ketamine here (see Chapter 11). The dilemma is a little like that of a police officer who shoots a would-be bridge jumper to prevent his suicide.

Neurobiology of Schizophrenia

One of the classic (but flawed) theories of what causes schizophrenia was the dopamine hypothesis (Black & Andreasen, 2011; Whitaker, 2010). Most antipsychotic drugs are dopamine blockers or *antagonists;* that is, they block excess dopamine. An *agonist* is a substance that promotes a receptor-mediated biological response. To oversimplify, schizophrenia was thought to be caused by an excess of dopamine in the brain and CSF (and dopaminergic dysfunction in general). The older phenothiazine drugs (Table 13.4) were thought to block mainly dopamine (D_2) receptors postsynaptically, whereas second-generation antipsychotics (like Clozaril) were thought to block both D_2 and serotonin (5-HT) receptors. Notice that if 5-HT receptors are blocked by antipsychotics, then schizophrenia cannot be explained just by the dopamine hypothesis. For example, Zyprexa blocks $5\text{-}HT_2$, D_1, D_2, D_3, D_4, and other receptors. Geodon is a D_2, D_3, $5\text{-}HT_{1A}$, and $5\text{-}HT_{2A}$ antagonist.

One function of neurotransmitters is to move chemicals across the synaptic cleft into the postsynaptic neurons via chemical charges and/or neurochemicals (or they can also be reabsorbed back into presynaptic vesicles). The dopamine hypothesis assumes that schizophrenic individuals tend to have excess dopamine in their brains. By blocking dopamine receptors, antipsychotics inhibit the transmission of dopamine into the postsynaptic neurons, thereby reducing excessive neuronal dopamine (at least that is the crude theory).

Again, however, the dopamine hypothesis is obviously overly simplistic, because antipsychotics also affect serotonin receptors and dopamine receptors other than D_2. Mental disorder is in fact the result of complex interactions of many different neurotransmitters in many different combinations in different parts of the brain (neuroanatomy), as well as of different factors like psychotropism (neuronal growth) or neuronal changes (both growth and depletion) and other organic considerations. For example, patients with schizophrenia exhibit hypofrontality (declining frontal lobe size, functioning, and metabolism) and enlarged ventricles (and a reduced ratio of CSF to ventricle area), compared to healthy controls (Black & Andreasen, 2014). The hypofrontality can be seen on a functional MRI that looks at regional blood flow, or on a PET scan. The relative size of the temporal region is also decreased in schizophrenia.

There are four main types of adverse events or effects from antipsychotics: (1) oversedation; (2) orthostatic hypotension (low blood pressure when changing positions); (3) anticholinergic effects (dry mouth, etc.); and (4) extrapyramidal symptoms (tremors, slurred speech, akathisia, etc.) One of the most serious of these adverse effects of antipsychotics is a movement disorder called *tardive dyskinesia*—an irreversible writhing of the mouth, tongue, and face, often seen in patients with chronic schizophrenia who have been taking Thorazine for a long time.

Other movement disorders related to antipsychotics include *parkinsonism* (flattening of facial expression, stiffness of gait, rolling tremors of the fingers, excessive salivation); *acute dystonic reaction* (tightening of the facial, neck and jaw muscles, difficulty opening the mouth); catatonia (bizarre posturing, rigidity or immobility, withdrawal); *akathisia* (restless legs, fidgeting, pacing, rocking, and inner restlessness); *akinesia* (depressed motor movements); so-called *"rabbit syndrome"* (fine, rapid tremors of the lips); rhythmic alternating movements, mostly of the fingers; and *atheotis*, which is writhing, purposeless movements.

Patients taking antipsychotics can also have anticholinergic adverse effects, which reduce the effects mediated by acetycholine in the central and peripheral nervous systems. Some of these symptoms include dry mouth, urinary retention, constipation, ataxia, increased body temperature, double vision, tachycardia, shaking, lack of perspiration, and respiratory depression. As we saw above, about 1–2% of patients taking Clozaril get *agranulocytosis,* an inhibition of white blood cell production that can lead to infection and even death.

Because of all the adverse effects of many antipsychotics, patients may need to take antiparkinsonian agents along with their antipsychotic medications. Some of these agents are Cogentin (1–2 mg), Artane (1–15 mg), over-the-counter Benadryl (25–200 mg), various beta-blockers (like Corgard or Tenormin), and vitamin E.

Suicidogenic Adverse Effects of Psychosis and Its Treatment

There are several adverse suicidogenic effects of psychosis and its treatment. Some of these serious adverse effects should be familiar from the discussion of antidepressants in Chapter 11; thus the consideration of such effects is briefer here. These adverse effects include the following:

- The development of akathisia and other movement disorders.
- Increased sedation and worsened depression.
- The effects of dopamine transmission and its blockage.
- Intolerable physical consequences.
- Sexual dysfunction.

Some of these effects were listed by Howanitz et al. (1999), who compared Clozaril and Risperdal. Patients taking Clozaril exceeded those taking Risperdal in drowsiness, somnolence, salivation, and nausea. One profile of patients taking antipsychotics is that of highly sedated, drooling, nauseous, overweight patients with trouble sleeping.

Akathisia

Akathisia was first noticed as a side effect of taking early antipsychotic drugs like Thorazine. The term *akathisia* refers to a series of neuroleptically induced adverse effects. However, some second-generation antipsychotics (like Saphris) can also cause akathisia. Patients tend to find that akathisia makes them very uncomfortable, and often they will do anything (including suicide) to try to stop its intolerable sensations. I had a case in Wisconsin in which a nurse (a patient) with akathisia requested a straitjacket to help keep her from hurting herself. Nevertheless, she managed to climb on a bookcase, jump off head first, break her neck, and die.

Increased Sedation and Induced or Worsened Depression

Several antipsychotics have the side effect of excessive sedation. This can make preexisting depression worse or even cause a *de novo* depression. For example, see the side effects of Haldol in Table 13.4. Some antipsychotics are actually combined with antidepressants. One example is Symbyax, which combines Zyprexa and Prozac. Since antidepressants can paradoxically increase depression and suicide risk, schizophrenic patients who are given antipsychotics and antidepressants could experience a compounding depressive effect of both drug types.

Dopamine Transmission and Its Blockage

As noted above, most antipsychotics are dopamine antagonists; theoretically they work in part through reducing dopamine transmission by blocking dopamine (especially D_2) receptors, thus leaving more dopamine in the synapse and CSF. The antidepressant Wellbutrin is a dopamine agonist. Dopamine is involved with pleasure and reward functions. For example, taking cocaine increases dopamine, is extremely reinforcing, and difficult to control. About one-third of New York City suicides had cocaine in their body when they suicided. When I was at Johns Hopkins, there was a primate laboratory in which chimps in so-called "Skinner boxes" would self-administer cocaine until they starved to death. Extroverts tend to have higher dopamine levels than do introverts. Dopamine is important in allowing us to acquire new behavior, such as in psychotherapy. Given these associations of suicide with dopamine, titrating dopamine could have self-destructive consequences.

Intolerable Physical Consequences

Both psychosis itself and its treatment with antipsychotics can produce a number of intolerable physical consequences, such that suicide may be the only perceived way to resolve them, As noted above, some antipsychotics can cause tardive dyskinesia (permanent writhing of mouth and tongue) and other movement disorders. With parkinsonism there can be stiffness of gait, pill-rolling finger tremors, a flattened facial expression, and excessive salivation; again, such symptoms are tough to live with. There is an acute dystonic reaction to antipsychotics called *oculogyric crisis,* in which the patient's eyes rotate and may become fixed or locked, usually in the backs of their sockets. Disfigurement, especially of the face, is a stigma that some people cannot ignore, accept, or live with. Even psychotic-induced weight gain can be a problem, and suicide can be seen as solving the problem.

Sexual Dysfunction

Antipsychotics, like antidepressants, can cause sexual dysfunctions such as anorgasmia. Although most people do not commit suicide because of sexual dysfunction, sexuality is still an important aspect of life, enjoyment, and having a family. In fact, Sigmund Freud said that all energy is either sexual energy or sexual energy that has been sublimated, repressed, or projected. In a sense, if there is no sexual energy, then there is no life energy. One way people know they are recovering from a life-threatening injury or illness is that their libido returns.

In the next chapter, I turn to personality disorders (long-term, deeply ingrained character disorders, such as borderline and antisocial personality disorders) and their relationship to suicidality.

CHAPTER 14

Personality Disorders
Borderline, Antisocial,
and Obsessive–Compulsive Personalities

There was an honors student who had only received A grades his entire
life. In university he received a B+ and went home and shot himself. He
said that not getting an A was like an India ink stain on his character.
—HONORS STUDENT

Personality disorders are maladaptive sets of character traits or long-term developmental disorders that are deeply ingrained, stable, enduring, and inflexible patterns of relating, perceiving, and thinking, and so they are difficult to treat. By definition, they are of sufficient severity to cause at least moderate distress or impairment in functioning. Freud thought that personality disorders (he did not call them that) were rooted in repressed unconscious conflicts resulting from traumatizing infant or childhood experiences like physical or sexual abuse. The result was believed to be developmental fixation at an early psychosexual life cycle stage (such as the *anal* stage, from about age 18 months to 3 years). Personality disorders are usually neurotic, not psychotic disorders. Although they are bothersome to self and others, most of these disorders are not as incapacitating as other clinical disorders like schizophrenia or MDD.

Some of the traits associated with personality disorders can be suicidogenic (Szanto et al., 2018). For example, people with antisocial personality disorder (ASPD) tend to have the suicidal personality traits of impulsivity, disinhibition, risk taking, and hostility. Borderline personality disorder (BPD) includes as a diagnostic criterion recurring suicidal behaviors, especially self-cutting. Those with obsessive–compulsive personality disorder (OCPD) tend to be rigidly perfectionistic, like the young college student described in the epigraph to this chapter; such perfectionism also increases suicide risk.

240

In editions of DSM prior to DSM-5, personality disorders used to be coded on a separate diagnostic axis (Axis II) from Axis I clinical disorders like MDD, bipolar disorders, schizophrenia, panic disorder, and so on. One of the main ways Axis I disorders were distinguished from Axis II disorders was chronicity. To qualify for diagnoses of MDD, BP I (current episode manic), schizophrenia, or panic disorder, the symptoms must last at least for a minimum of 2 weeks, 1 week, 1 month, and 10–30 minutes (respectively); that is, the criteria are relatively acute (most of the time) for a shorter time.

Personality disorders, on the other hand, must be present for years in order to meet the criteria for diagnosis. For example, for a diagnosis of ASPD, a person has to be at least 18 years old. Before then, the person might be diagnosed with oppositional defiant disorder, ADHD, or conduct disorder. Normally personality disorders are recognized and diagnosed in late adolescence or early adulthood.

DSM-5 recognizes 10 personality disorders, grouped into three clusters (see Table 14.1), plus a few other personality diagnoses that do not fall into these clusters. Individuals with Cluster A personality disorders tend to be eccentric; those with Cluster B personality disorders tend to be dramatic; and those with Cluster C disorders tend to be anxious.

Although I could focus on the suicidogenic implications of all 10 personality disorders, I choose instead to single out 3 of these disorders (see Table 14.1): ASPD, BPD, and OCPD. I have chosen these disorders because BPD includes suicide attempts as a diagnostic criterion (as noted above), and because in my experience males with ASPD and persons with OCPD have many suicidogenic traits.

Another justification for this reduced focus is the need for emphasis on the important work of Marsha Linehan on dialectical behavior therapy (DBT) and BPD, and the work of Aaron Beck and colleagues on cognitive-behavioral therapy (CBT), suicide, and depression. Thus far, the FDA has approved no drugs or medications for the treatment of personality disorders, although SSRIs, valproic acid (Depakote), and flupenthixol decanoate (Fluanxol) are used off-label (Black & Andreasen, 2014). So, later in this chapter, I discuss the important psychotherapies for suicidal behaviors often used with these three personality disorders.

Epidemiology and Etiology of Personality Disorders

Epidemiology

Estimates of any personality disorder in the general U.S. population range from 9 to 16% (Black & Andreasen, 2014; Carballo et al., 2012; Lenzenweger et al., 2007). However, in self-destructive populations the prevalence of personality disorders is much higher:

- Those who die by suicide = 57% (Carballo et al., 2012).
- Psychiatric hospital patients = 91% (Carballo et al., 2012).
- People who make suicide attempts = 84% (Carballo et al., 2012).
- Completed suicides = 31–57% (Maris et al., 2000).

TABLE 14.1. List of Personality Disorders

Definitions of Personality Disorders

DSM-IV-TR (2000): Personality disorders are deeply ingrained, inflexible, maladaptive patterns of relating, perceiving, and thinking, of sufficient severity to cause impairment in functioning or distress. They are generally recognizable by adolescence or early adulthood, and continue through adulthood; some (borderline and antisocial) become less obvious in middle or old age.

DSM-5 (2013), Alternative DSM-5 Model for Personality Disorders: Personality disorders are characterized by (1) moderate or severe impairments in self and interpersonal functioning (criterion A), in two or more of four areas (identity, self-direction, empathy, and intimacy); and (2) pathological personality traits (criterion B), including one or more of negative affectivity, detachment, antagonism, disinhibition, and psychoticism (measured on a scale of 0–3 for each). These dysfunctions and pathological traits tend to be pervasive (criterion C) and stable, appearing by adolescence or early adulthood (criterion D). They are not better attributed to another mental disorder (criterion E), to substance use or a medical condition (criterion F), or to normal developmental or sociocultural processes (criterion G).

Cluster A (eccentric)

(1) **Paranoid** (DSM-5 codes 301.0, F60.0): Pervasive and long-standing suspiciousness and mistrust of others; hypersensitivity and scanning of the environment for clues that selectively validate prejudices, attitudes, or biases. Stable psychotic features such as delusions and hallucinations are absent.

(2) **Schizoid** (301.20, F60.1): Manifested by shyness, oversensitivity, social withdrawal, frequent daydreaming, avoidance of close or competitive relationships, and eccentricity. These persons often react to disturbing experiences with apparent detachment and are unable to express hostility and ordinary aggressive feelings.

(3) **Schizotypal** (301.22, F21): The essential features are various oddities of thinking, perception, and behavior not severe enough to meet the criteria for schizophrenia. No single feature is invariably present. The disturbance in thinking may be expressed as magical thinking, ideas of reference, or paranoid ideation. Perceptual disturbances may include recurrent illusions, depersonalization, or derealization. Often there are marked peculiarities in communication; concepts may be expressed unclearly or oddly, using words deviantly, but never to the point or loosening of association or incoherence. Frequently the behavioral manifestations include social isolation and constricted or inappropriate affect that interferes with rapport in face-to-face interaction.

Cluster B (dramatic)

(4) **Antisocial** (301.7, F60.2): A lack of socialization, along with behavior patterns that bring a person repeatedly into conflict with society; incapacity for significant loyalty, to others or to social values; callousness; irresponsibility; impulsiveness; and inability to feel guilt or learn from experience of punishment. Frustration tolerance is low, and such people tend to blame others or give plausible rationalizations for their behavior. Characteristic behavior is classifiable as antisocial at age 18 or older, although the diagnosis may not be apparent until adulthood.

(5) **Borderline** (301.83, F60.3): A disorder that includes instability in interpersonal relationships, inappropriate, intense, uncontrolled anger, identity disturbance, instability of affect, intolerance of being alone, physically self-damaging acts (especially self-cutting), and feelings of emptiness.

(6) **Histrionic** (301.50, F60.7): Excitability, emotional instability, overreactivity, and attention seeking; often seductive self-dramatization, whether or not the person is aware of its purpose. People with this disorder are immature, self-centered, vain, and unusually dependent. Sometimes referred to (especially in the older literature) as *hysterical personality*.

(continued)

TABLE 14.1. *(continued)*

---

(7) **Narcissistic** (301.81, F60.81): Grandiose sense of self-importance or uniqueness; preoccupation with fantasies of limitless success; need for attention and admiration; and disturbances in interpersonal relationships, such as lack of empathy, exploitativeness, and relationships that vacillate between the extremes of overidealization and devaluation.

Cluster C (anxious)

(8) **Avoidant** (301.82, F60.2): Inhibited, introverted, anxious, inadequate, reluctant to take risks, not involved with other people.

(9) **Dependent** (301.6, F60.7): Inducing others to assume responsibility for major areas of one's life; subordinating one's own needs to those of others on whom one is dependent to avoid any possibility of independence; lack of self-confidence.

(10) **Obsessive–compulsive** (301.4, F60.5): Restricted ability to express warm and tender emotions; preoccupation with rules, order, organization, efficiency, and detail; excessive devotion to work and productively to the exclusion of pleasure; indecisiveness.

Source: Adapted with permission from the *Diagnostic and Statistical Manual of Mental Disorders,* Fourth Edition, Text Revision, and Fifth Edition. Copyright © 2000 and 2013 American Psychiatric Association. All Rights Reserved.

- People with suicide ideation = 16.8% (Maris et al., 2000).
- People who have comorbid MDD = 51% (Black & Andreasen, 2014).

Self-destructive behaviors are especially high in people with ASPD (mainly males) and those with BPD (mainly females). As noted above, personality disorders tend to occur by adolescence or early adulthood. In general, there is a greater prevalence of personality disorders in people with comorbid MDD, bipolar disorders, ADHD, and substance abuse. Thus, we can conclude that self-destructive populations have a much higher prevalence of personality disorders than do the general population.

Etiology

Personality disorders are complex and multifaceted, and there is no one simple answer to the question of what causes them (Black & Andreasen, 2014). We suspect that their etiology includes genetics, neurobiology, childhood trauma (especially abuse), parenting and socialization, culture, and even high reactivity such as to light, noise, texture, and other stimuli. As mentioned above, psychoanalysts like Freud argued that personality disorders are rooted in developmental fixation in one of the psychosexual stages of development, such as the oral, anal, or phallic stages; developmental psychologists like Erik Erikson have made similar arguments (Black & Andreasen, 2014).

Studies of monozygotic (identical) twins suggest strong genetic influences, especially for ASPD and BPD. Other researchers have identified a gene related to OCPD (Huff, 2004). Aberrant serotonin neurotransmission has been related to impulsive and aggressive behaviors (Black & Andreasen, 2014). Also, altered metabolism in the prefrontal regions of the brain has been linked by PET scans to ASPD and BPD. Mann and Currier (2012) claimed that early childhood abuse leads to altered adult brain development and contributes to mental disorder. Even cultural factors play a role in the etiology of personality disorders. For example, we find very low rates of ASPD in China, Japan, and Taiwan.

Personality Disorders and Suicide Risk

An important question in this chapter is this: How do personality disorders affect suicide risk? Are people with personality disorders at greater or lesser risk for suicide, and why is that? Superficially, it appears that personality disorders increase, augment, or potentiate suicide risk. Just consider the comparisons made above. Only 9–16% of the general nonsuicidal population has a personality disorder, but 84% of suicide attempters and 57% of completed suicides do.

Consider this selection of personality disorder criteria:

- Impulsivity (which can affect the transition from suicide ideation to completion).
- Aggression (suicide is an aggressive act against the self).
- Disinhibition (personality-disordered patients are more likely to consider radical solutions to life problems, like suicide).
- Unstable interpersonal relationships (especially lack of a sustaining, crucial significant other).
- Rigidity and stubbornness (failure to see alternatives; Beck et al., 1985).
- Exclusion of play and leisure activities (can work alone sustain us?).
- Reluctance to confide in others (affects therapy and lack of social support).
- Distrust of others (including therapists and others who would be supportive).
- Suggestibility (contagion can increase suicide).
- Inappropriate sexual behaviors (cf. bipolar disorder).
- Unwillingness to get involved with other people (social isolation increases suicide risk).
- Discomfort when alone (more dependent and vulnerable to isolation).

What strikes you about this list of personality disorder criteria? For one thing, many of them are also suicide risk factors (see Chapters 4 and 10). This is especially true for BPD (Berk et al., 2009; Blasco-Fortecilla et al., 2010). Some of the known suicide risk factors that are more common in those with BPD include a history of prior suicide attempts, impulsivity, greater depression and hopelessness, poor problem-solving skills, a history of physical abuse, comorbid ASPD, more substance abuse, and more Cluster B traits like aggression. No wonder people with BPD are at greater suicide risk.

For purposes of suicide prevention, remember also that personality disorders are deeply ingrained and hard to treat. Thus the presence of a personality disorder complicates efforts at suicide prevention. With many of the major clinical disorders (such as MDD or bipolar disorder), psychiatrists use mainly medication management. Psychopharmacological treatment alone just does not work as well with personality disorders.

Borderline Personality Disorder

BPD and Suicide Risk

BPD is one of the single most important psychiatric disorders related to suicide (Simon & Hales, 2012). As emphasized here and in Chapters 10 and 11, BPD, like MDD, actually has recurrent self-destructive behavior as a diagnostic criterion. BPD is characterized by unstable relationships, affect, self-image, and impulsivity. It begins in early adulthood and includes five or more of the following: efforts to avoid abandonment; unstable relationships; identity disturbance; impulsivity (e.g., in use of money, sex, substances, driving, eating); suicidal behavior (especially self-cutting); unstable affect; chronic empty feelings; inappropriate anger; and paranoia or dissociation.

BPD is often comorbid with other personality disorders, as well as bipolar disorder, substance abuse, and MDD (Simon & Hales, 2012). The case of Juanita Delgado (Case 14.1) illustrates comorbidity with a possible bipolar disorder.

CASE 14.1. Juanita Delgado

Juanita Delgado, a single, unemployed Hispanic woman, sought therapy at age 35 for treatment of depressed mood, chronic suicidal thoughts, social isolation, and poor personal hygiene. She had spent the prior 6 months isolated in her apartment, lying in bed, eating junk food, watching television, and doing more online shopping than she could afford. Multiple treatments had had little effect.

Ms. Delgado was the middle of three children in an upper-middle-class immigrant family in which the father reportedly valued professional achievement above all else. She felt isolated throughout her school years and experienced recurring periods of depressed mood. Within her family, she was known for angry outbursts.

She had done well academically in high school, but had dropped out of college because of frustrations with a roommate and a professor. She attempted a series of internships and entry-level jobs with the expectation that she would return to college, but she kept quitting because "Bosses are idiots." She had dated men when she was younger, but never got close physically, because she became too anxious when any intimacy began to develop.

Ms. Delgado's history included cutting herself superficially on a number of occasions, along with persistent thoughts that she would be better off dead. She said that she had dozens of 1- to 2-day "manias" in which she was energized and pulled all-nighters. She tended to "crash" the next day and sleep for 12 hours.

She had been in psychiatric treatment since age 17 and had been psychiatrically hospitalized three times after overdoses. Treatments had consisted primarily of medications—mood stabilizers, low-dose neuroleptics, and antidepressants that had been prescribed in various combinations in the context of supportive psychotherapy.

During the interview, she was causally groomed, coherent, and goal-directed. She was generally dysphoric with a constricted affect, but did smile appropriately several times. She described shame at her poor performance, but also believed she was "on earth to do something great." She described her father as a spectacular success, but also as a "Machiavellian loser who was always trying to manipulate people." She described quitting jobs because people were disrespectful. Toward the end of the initial session, she became angry with the interviewer after he glanced at the clock: She said, "Are you bored already?"

Source: Yeomans and Kernberg, in Barnhill (2014, Case 18.5, p. 311). Reprinted with permission from *DSM-5 Clinical Cases.* Copyright © 2014 American Psychiatric Association. All Rights Reserved.

As many as 84% of patients with BPD report at least one prior nonfatal suicide attempt (Simon & Hales, 2012). About three-fourths of such patients engage in deliberate self-harm (like self-cutting, burning, and overdosing), and as many as 10% actually commit suicide. In the general population, as noted throughout this book, the corresponding number of completed suicides is 1 in 10,000 (Simon & Hales, 2012). BPD first appeared as a psychiatric disorder in DSM-III (American Psychiatric Association, 1980).

Dialectical Behavior Therapy

One of the pioneers in the nonpharmacological treatment of BPD has been Marsha Linehan, who developed DBT (Linehan, 1997; Maris et al., 2000; Brown et al., 2012; Miller et al., 2007). DBT can be especially effective in treating female suicidal patients with BPD. It differs from CBT in that it is based on making behavioral (not just ideational) techniques more compatible with psychodynamic models. DBT is intended to treat (among others) the chronic suicidal patient who lives what I call a "suicidal career" (Maris, 1981; Joiner, 2005)—that is, a life high in suicide ideation, in talk about or threats of suiciding, and in repetitive nonfatal suicidal attempts/ self-mutilating behavior (such as repeated self-cutting).

DBT assumes that chronically suicidal individuals lack and must acquire skills for self-regulation of their behavior, emotions, and stress tolerance, and must be motivated to strengthen these skills outside therapy situations. DBT uses a problem-solving strategy, addressing the patient's behaviors. Possible changes or behavioral solutions are then generated to be tested. DBT can range from an intensive year-long program to a 20-week treatment called STEPPS (Black & Andreasen, 2014).

The word *dialectic* probably first occurred in Plato's *Dialogues* (Jowett, 1950), in which two or more philosophers argued about a subject (e.g., "What is justice?") from different points of view to try to arrive at the truth. Later, the philosopher Hegel (1874) spoke of *thesis, antithesis,* and *synthesis* as a dialectical process. Dialectical strategies balance and attempt to synthesize coexisting opposites and tensions.

For example, Linehan et al. (1983) created a 72-item Reasons for Living Inventory, in which patients rate their reasons for not suiciding. A patient rates each of the 72 items on a 1–6 scale, where 6 equals the most important. The therapist then tries to validate the patient's views of life and death while implementing alternative problem-solving analyses and responses. Detailed analyses of environmental and behavioral situations linked to suicidal behavior are then conducted to elicit patterns and to identify alternative (nonsuicidal) resolutions. A commitment to learning nonsuicidal behavioral responses while tolerating negative affect is a major goal of DBT.

At age 17 in 1961, Linehan herself was committed to an inpatient psychiatric institute for 26 months with a diagnosis of schizophrenia and put on lithium and

Thorazine (Carey, 2011). She later claimed that her correct (or at least comorbid) diagnosis was BPD. She still has burn and cut scars on her body. Linehan claims that ideas and theories by themselves are not very useful for treatment; she says that patients with BPD need to change their behavior and develop day-to-day skills. DBT focuses on getting patients back in control of their own lives through learning skills in what Linehan calls *mindfulness, distress tolerance, emotion regulation,* and *interpersonal effectiveness* (Linehan, 2015; Pickert, 2014).

Linehan and her colleagues have argued (with cogent data and analyses) that DBT can significantly reduce suicidal behaviors and precursors to deliberate self-harm, such as depression, hopelessness, anger, eating disorders, substance use disorders, and impulsiveness. A pill alone certainly cannot do that. Linehan often reminds us and her patients that "you cannot do therapy with a cadaver." Probably patients in DBT do not "feel better off dead," even though they often think that they would (*www.borderlinepersonalitytreatment.com/dbt-marsha-linehan.html*). Dead people most likely do not feel anything at all, which is what many patients with BPD want, unfortunately.

Antisocial Personality Disorder

ASPD is to suicidal males, especially younger males, what BPD is to suicidal females. As many as 72% of those with ASPD attempt suicide (Pompili et al., 2014). Suicide attempts are about 3.7 times more likely in persons with ASPD than in normal controls, and 9 times more likely if the persons are under age 30 (Beautrais et al., 1996; Carballo et al., 2012).

ASPD is a strong pattern of disregarding and violating the rights of others that begins in childhood or in early adolescence and continues into adulthood. In childhood, the behavior pattern may be called conduct disorder, ADHD, or oppositional defiant disorder. An individual must be at least 18 years old to qualify for a diagnosis of ASPD, but the pattern of disregard for others will have started by least age 15.

Individuals with ASPD fail to conform to lawful behavior and perform acts that are often grounds for arrest. They tend to deny the rights and feelings of others. For a chilling example of this behavior, see the HBO documentary *The Iceman and the Psychiatrist* (Ginsberg, 2003), in which psychiatrist Park Dietz interviews mob contract killer Richard Kuklinski (see also *www.liveleak.com/view?i=d93_1178139940*). Those with ASPD often fail to plan ahead and repeatedly get into physical fights (including with their spouses/partners and children). Their drinking behavior is reckless and excessive. They tend to drive while intoxicated, speed, and have multiple accidents.

Individuals with ASPD are often extremely irresponsible, have many jobs, or are unemployed. They are frequently absent from work or school. They tend to default on debts and other financial responsibilities, including child support. Like the "Iceman," Richard Kuklinski, they seem to feel no remorse for their actions. The case of a 24-year-old white male, Charles Patterson (a pseudonym), illustrates typical ASPD traits. See Case 14.2 for his story.

CASE 14.2. Charles Patterson

Charles Patterson was a 24-year-old white male living in a major city. He had been a college football player at a well-known university. His psychiatric diagnosis was ASPD. He had been in jail twice for writing bad checks. His work history was erratic; he had been AWOL from the army, and he had a history of alcohol and drug abuse. A male cousin had suicided 6 months before Charles did. Charles had an aggressive, violent relationship with his father, who was a local football coach. His mother had left his father and her four sons several years ago, and Charles had been raised mainly by his grandmother. A few weeks before dying, Charles broke up with his girlfriend. He was on parole at the time and was scheduled to go to court for a hearing the day after he suicided. He told his grandmother and his girlfriend that he was thinking of killing himself.

The chronology of events leading up to his suicide was as follows. A few weeks before his death, Patterson went to a family practice physician for trouble sleeping and was prescribed a single bottle of 25 flurazepam (Dalmane) capsules (this case occurred in the mid-1980s). Just before his suicide, he took an overdose of about 20 of the Dalmane capsules. His grandmother found him sleeping deeply. She was so upset that after calling 911, she took the rest of the Dalmane and passed out herself.

The police took Charles to a local emergency room, where the incident was classified as "suicide attempt by overdose." The ER personnel stabilized Charles and then transferred him to a VA hospital (since he was a veteran), and later to a large regional hospital. His doctor at the regional hospital discharged Charles the next day, stated in his progress notes that Charles was neither suicidal nor depressed, and referred him to outpatient follow-up therapy in 2 weeks. Charles's father objected to the release, but agreed to drive him back to his own apartment (not the father's house), where he lived alone.

After arriving home, Charles drove his car into the side of a school bus; he was arrested and sent to jail. While in jail, he told other inmates that he wanted razor blades to kill himself with. After being released from jail, Charles went to his father's house, got his father's pistol, and stuck it in the back of his belt under his shirt. Later that same day, he was arrested a second time for driving his motorcycle erratically. He was not searched by the police at the jail, since he had been searched earlier that day. As soon as the police put Charles in his cell, he took out the pistol and shot himself in the head, dying instantly.

Source: A court case in which Maris testified. Although this was a court case and the information was public, all personal identifying information (the name, where the death happened, the day of death, etc.) has been changed or removed.

Prevalence and Etiology

The 12-month prevalence for ASPD is about 0.2–0.3%. Two to four percent of men and 0.5% of women have ASPD. Of males abusing alcohol, over 70% have ASPD. Having comorbid BPD increases the risk of suicidal behavior (Carballo et al., 2012, p. 194). Genetically, ASPD is more common in first-degree relatives of those with the disorder than in the general population. ASPD is chronic, but tends to remit or be less evident in adulthood. Adoption studies suggest that biology (nature) and environment (nurture) both contribute to ASPD risk, but adopted children are more like their biological parents than their adoptive parents with regard to ASPD.

ASPD seems to be associated with low SES and urban settings. Again, it is much more common in men than it is in women. ASPD was first diagnosed as *manie sans délire* ("mania without delirium") or *moral insanity;* both these terms indicated immoral or guiltless behavior in the absence of impaired reasoning. In the first half of the 20th century, it was called *sociopathic personality*. It was first termed *antisocial personality* in the first edition of DSM (American Psychiatric Association, 1952).

Differential Diagnosis and Classification

For the current diagnostic criteria for ASPD, see American Psychiatric Association (2013, p. 659). Here I consider differential diagnosis—that is, the process of excluding or ruling out competing alternative diagnoses. Unless ASPD was present in childhood and has continued into adulthood, we call a substance use disorder by its own name (not ASPD). If both ASPD and substance use disorder begin in childhood, then two separate diagnoses are required. If antisocial behavior occurs only during bipolar or schizophrenic disorders, it is not ASPD.

Sometimes other personality disorders are confused with ASPD and need to be differentiated from it. For example, narcissistic personality disorder does not include characteristics of impulsivity, aggression, or deceit. Individuals with histrionic personality disorder tend to be more exaggerated in their emotions. Antisocial behavior in paranoid personality disorder is more attributable to a desire for revenge. Finally, ASPD must be distinguished from criminal behavior without ASPD traits. A word of caution: One cannot always rule out other diagnoses and be left with only one correct diagnosis. A patient can have multiple comorbid psychiatric disorders.

ASPD and Suicide Risk

Many of the ASPD criteria are also suicide risk factors (Tanney, 2000). These characteristics include impulsivity, aggressiveness, disregard for safety (as in "Sure, let's play Russian roulette!"), and unemployment. Remember that about a third of suicides are unemployed.

Treatment of ASPD

No medications target the full ASPD syndrome. Think about it: If it takes 15–18 years to develop a personality disorder, the person is not going to be cured with a few pills in a few weeks. Often, in effect, those with ASPD need to be resocialized and reparented to correct damage that was a long time in the making. The damage related to ASPD comes more from pathological interpersonal relationships than from pharmacology or neurochemistry.

Lithium has been effective in reducing anger and aggression in prisoners. Mood stabilizers, including carbamazepine (Tegretol) and valproic acid (Depakote), are used as well. Benzodiazepines should not be used routinely, due to their abuse potential and encouragement of behavioral dyscontrol.

If patients with ASPD have distorted beliefs, attitudes, or reasoning, then CBT may be most effective (see the discussion of CBT later in this chapter). These patients are often challenging in therapy, since they tend to have low tolerance for frustration and tend to blame others, not themselves, for their problems.

Obsessive–Compulsive Personality Disorder

Like the honors student described in the epigraph to this chapter who had to have all A's, people with OCPD display a lifelong pattern of perfectionism and inflexibility. They are preoccupied with orderliness; prefer work over play; are obsessed with details, lists, and rules; tend to be overly conscientious; are reluctant to delegate to others; cannot throw things away; and are miserly (Black & Andreasen, 2014). Patients with obsessive–compulsive disorder (OCD) sometimes overlap with those patients with OCPD. One can have both OCD and OCPD, but there are also important differences.

Most patients with OCPD are not characterized by intrusive thoughts, images, or urges (obsessions), or by repetitive behaviors that must be performed in relation to these intrusions (compulsions). Instead, those with OCPD have an enduring pattern of excessive perfectionism and rigid control, as the honors student did. Individuals with OCD are more willing to identify their symptoms as pathological (Black & Andreasen, 2014; American Psychiatric Association, 2013). The "essential feature of OCPD is a preoccupation with orderliness, perfectionism, and mental and interpersonal control, at the expense of flexibility, openness, and efficiency" (American Psychiatric Association, 2013, p. 679).

To help clarify the differences between OCD and OCPD, Case 14.3 describes a patient with OCD who was first described by Judith Rapoport (2010). Eventually, with 100 mg/day of imipramine (Tofranil), the man's obsessive–compulsive symptoms had been under control for 2 years at the time Rapport described this case. That is, the man said he could defer obsessive–compulsive thoughts and behaviors, but they were still there. Can psychiatric medications like Tofranil alone treat OCD or personality disorders? If we remove the symptoms of obsessive anxiety with drugs like the benzodiazepines, is the illness still there, but just dormant and hidden?

CASE 14.3. The Auto Accident That Never Was

A young man with OCD was driving down a highway to take a final exam. He was doing 55 mph when, out of nowhere, an OCD attack occurred. A heinous thought intruded that he had hit someone, although the highway was deserted and he had no memory of an accident. He had to go back and check, and so he returned to the spot where *it* might have occurred. Nothing was there. He thought that maybe he should have checked the roadside brush. He arrived late at school for the exam.

He was 36 years old, but had had obsessions since he was 22. He had hidden the disorder from others. Valium had been only marginally helpful. His doctor then prescribed imipramine

(Tofranil). In the man's fifth month on the Tofranil, the OCD symptoms stopped, and he was then placed on a maintenance dose of Tofranil.

Source: Excerpted and rewritten by Maris from Rapoport (2010).

Notice how crippling and time-consuming obsessive–compulsive symptoms can be. Many of us have obsessions or compulsions, but they do not usually interfere with our daily functioning. Rapport wrote (2010) another case account of a boy who could not stop washing his hands. While it is good to take some things seriously and do a thorough job, it is another matter to obsess when a person knows intellectually that excessive concern is unnecessary and irrational, even dysfunctional. The problem is that obsessive–compulsive behavior and thoughts are irrational and cannot be easily controlled. In this respect, at least, OCD is like OCPD.

The features of OCPD (as opposed to OCD) include self-imposed high standards of performance, excessive devotion to work and productivity, and not wasting time. Even play is turned into a structured, nonspontaneous task. When it comes to morality, those with OCPD are often excessively conscientious, scrupulous, and inflexible (e.g., "One must always tell the truth," or "There should be no sex before marriage").

Individuals with OCPD can be rigidly deferential to authority, unable to discard worn-out or worthless objects, and prone to giving others very detailed instructions for simple tasks (e.g., how to mow the grass or make a bed). They often have trouble deciding which tasks to perform and are preoccupied with logic and intellect (see American Psychiatric Association, 2013, pp. 678 ff.).

Prevalence

According to DSM-5, the estimated prevalence of OCPD is 2.1–7.9% of the U.S. population. Others (Black & Andreasen, 2011) say that the prevalence is lower (viz., 1–2% of the general population). The Epidemiologic Catchment Area study (see Tanney, 2000) found that 5.9% of the population had a diagnosis of OCPD. Psychoanalysts often claim that OCPD results from fixation at an oral stage of development. In the first DSM (American Psychiatric Association, 1952), OCPD was called *compulsive personality*. Comorbidity of OCPD with anxiety disorders is common.

Differential Diagnosis and Classification

Those with OCPD are preoccupied with order, perfection, and control at the expense of flexibility, openness, and efficiency. OCPD begins in early adulthood. It is indicated by four or more of the following; concern with details, rules, lists, and schedules; paralyzing perfectionism; overconcern with work and being productive; overconscientiousness and inflexibility; keeping worthless objects; unwillingness to delegate tasks; miserly spending habits; and rigidity and stubbornness.

Since I have considered the diagnostic features of OCPD above, I have little more to add here. However, it should be noted that several other disorders are related to obsessive–compulsive behaviors but have their own distinct DSM codes.

These include body dysmorphia, hoarding, trichotillomania (compulsive hair-pulling), excoriation (skin picking), and some disorders related to use of a substance/medication or to a medical condition.

OCPD, Perfectionism, and Suicide Risk

As for suicide risk and personality disorders, Brent et al. (1994) found a higher prevalence of Cluster C personality disorders (which include OCPD) among completed suicides. In Finland (Isometsa et al., 1996), 10% of suicides met the criteria for Cluster C personality disorders. Some (Johnson et al., 1999) have claimed that Cluster C disorders had an increased risk for suicide attempts and suicide ideation, even after affective (mood) disorders were controlled for.

As a university professor, I have seen a lot of self-destructive students who exhibit signs of OCPD, especially in my honors classes. Virtually all of my prepro-fessional students (especially honors medical school aspirants) believe they have to get all A's in order to be sure of even getting into a medical school (and they are right).

Perfectionism is hard to define, but usually it refers to one's own unrealistically and rigid high standards, not some objective, external standard. Thus one could do "perfectly" on an exam, get all the answers correct, and still not be satisfied with the performance.

Dean et al. (1996) did an empirical study of perfectionism and suicide ideations (see Table 14.2). They obtained the following correlations:

1. Perfectionism and suicide ideation: .55.
2. Perfectionism and depression: .53.
3. Perfectionism and hopelessness: .48.
4. Reasons for living (Linehan et al., 1983) and suicide ideation: −.64.

TABLE 14.2. Correlations of Negative Life Events, Perfectionism, Depression, Hopelessness, and Reasons for Living with Suicide Ideas

	NLE	PERF	DEP	HOPE	RFL	SI
NLE						
PERF	0.32					
DEP	0.48	0.53				
HOPE	0.25	0.48	0.67			
RFL	−0.15	−0.26	−0.38	−0.63		
SI	0.30	0.55	0.59	0.83	−0.64	
Mean score	12.90	51.45	36.40	2.41	219.88	2.31
SD	10.63	17.52	10.44	3.94	37.63	6.57

Source: "An Escape Theory of Suicide in College Students: Testing a Model That Includes Perfectionism" by P. J. Dean, L. M. Range, and W. C. Goggin, *Suicide and Life-Threatening Behavior, 26,* 181–186. Copyright © 1996 by the American Association of Suicidology. Reproduced with permission of John Wiley & Sons, Inc.

That is, (1) the more perfectionism, the greater the suicide ideation; (2) the more perfectionism, the more depression; (3) the greater the perfectionism, the more hopelessness; and (4) the more reasons for living, the lower the suicide ideation (among other associations). All of these associations were statistically significant (i.e., not likely to occur by chance alone).

Psychotherapy and CBT

Since suicide is a multidimensional malaise, its treatment should usually be complex, and varied, yet specific to the individual. However, most treatment of suicidal patients is merely neurobiological titration of the patients' neurotransmitters (serotonin, norepinephrine, dopamine, GABA, acetylcholine, etc.) and neurosystems. Shneidman (1993) insisted that instead we should focus on suicidal patients' minds (not just their brains) through psychotherapy. Most people take many years to develop mental disorders, especially personality disorders. They are not going to be fixed in a few weeks by neurochemistry.

Nevertheless, today psychiatric treatment is usually medication management of a suicidal person in an outpatient setting (Maltsberger & Stoklosa, 2012). Inpatient treatment for about 1 week is also fairly common for more acute and severe self-destructive behavior. To oversimplify, if Hx = history, Sx = symptoms, Ax = assessment, Dx = diagnosis, Tx = treatment, and Rx = medication, then:

$$(Hx + Sx + Ax) \rightarrow Dx \rightarrow Tx \text{ (usually Rx only)}$$

Treatment of suicidal individuals can include (1) pharmacology (most often with antidepressants and anxiolytics for depression or other mood disorder); (2) psychotherapeutic approaches (especially Linehan's DBT and Beck's CBT), (3) treatment of concomitant biological problems (pain, physical illness, sleep disorders, problems with diet and appetite, sexual difficulties, etc.); (4) various modes of crisis intervention (suicide prevention centers, online sites, or emergency rooms); (5) behavioral modification schedules (like those of Linehan); (6) group or family psychotherapy; and, rarely, (7) technical procedures like partial laser lobotomies, transcranial magnetic stimulation, and vagus nerve stimulation.

Most suicidal patients will be started on one psychotropic medication or a cocktail of two to six drugs (Carlat, 2010; Maris, 2015). The medications can include antidepressants, mood stabilizers, antipsychotics, anxiolytics, and sleep aids. But what if one does not want to use just psychiatric medications, or they are not very effective (such as with personality disorders)? What other treatment options exist (see Chapter 24)? I have already discussed DBT above in connection with BPD. CBT or a related approach, cognitive therapy for suicide prevention (CT-SP; Brown et al., 2012), involves training in problem-solving skills. Suicidal persons tend to have faulty cognitions, including dichotomous thinking, catastrophic thinking, and rigid tunnel vision. They tend to see suicide as the one and only way to resolve their life problems. Suicide is irrational when something short of suicide would have the same effect. Such self-destructive individuals need to be persuaded or educated to avoid fallacious reasoning—to be able to see and believe that there are alternatives to suicide.

CBT for suicide ideations and behaviors should start with a complete assessment of the patient's perceived problems and a suicide risk assessment linked to these problems (Rudd, 2012). According to Beck et al. (1985), hopelessness is more highly associated with a suicidal outcome than depression alone. Hopelessness, deficits in problem solving, perfectionism, dysfunctional attitudes and irrational beliefs (e.g., "I'm a loser and would be better off dead") are all characteristic of self-destructive individuals and can often be successfully treated with CBT, often conjointly with psychiatric medications.

Medications may make a person feel more euphoric, calm, less depressed, and so on, but feelings do not necessarily change behavior. To eliminate or lessen the chances of suicide, individuals need to change their catabolic lifestyles and avoid boxing themselves into an increasingly self-destructive corner or career. Sometimes a qualified mental health professional is needed to look such a person squarely in the eye and say, "I care about you, I am competent to help you, and I will stick with you until you get better." Can a pill alone do that?

Remember, too, that suicide is not itself a mental illness or a DSM diagnostic category. (Not yet, anyway—although suicide ideation and/or attempts do appear in DSM-5 as a criterion for MDD and BPD, and although suicidal behavior disorder now appears in Section III of the manual as a proposed separate mental disorder.) Suicides may be agitated, impulsive, or perturbed, but they are not usually crazy (Maris, 1982). The next chapter considers what is perhaps the second most important suicide risk factor: substance abuse, especially alcoholism.

CHAPTER 15

Alcoholism and Other Substance Abuse
The Second Most Important Suicide Risk Factor

> Beverage alcohol is fecal matter. Alcohol is not made of grapes or grain. It is those which are devoured by the ferment germ and the germ then evacuates alcohol as its waste product. The thought of swallowing the excrement of living organism is not an esthetic idea, but people will do such things.
>
> —OAKLEY RAY

After mood disorders, alcohol intoxication and/or abuse is the second leading single risk factor for a suicide outcome. Murphy and Robins (1967; see also Murphy, 1998) found that the second most common single suicide risk factor in their 5-year St. Louis suicide sample was alcohol abuse or intoxication at 27%. In my Chicago sample, the corresponding percentage of alcohol-related suicides was 33%. Forty-seven percent of their St. Louis suicide sample had one of the depressive disorders. I found exactly the same percentage (i.e., 47% for at least mild depression) in my own 5-year Chicago (Cook County) suicide sample (Maris, 1981).

What is important to note here is that no other single suicide risk factor was present in more than 5% of all suicides (see Maris et al., 2000, p. 80). Thus mood disorders and alcohol intoxication or alcoholism at the time of death (see Bagge & Borges, 2017, who found that drinking alcohol within 24 hours before a suicide attempt increased the odds of an attempt by a factor of 4.4) are far and away the most important single suicide risk factors (however, see Joiner, 2010, pp. 91–97). *Caveat emptor,* suicides are not just the product of acute or situational depression and alcohol abuse; rather, they are key components (albeit very significant ones) in a complex, interactive causal model for suicide outcome that unfolds over a long suicidal career.

In DSM-5 (American Psychiatric Association, 2013), alcohol is just one of 10 classes of substances associated with substance-related disorder diagnoses. The 9 others are caffeine, cannabis, hallucinogens (including phencyclidine [PCP]),

255

inhalants, opioids, sedatives (including hypnotics and anxiolytics), stimulants (including amphetamine and cocaine), tobacco, and other or unknown substances. "Polysubstance abuse" was a category in the DSM-IV but is no longer.

Alcohol-related disorders in DSM-5 include the following diagnoses: alcohol use disorder (code F10.10 [mild = 2–3 symptoms] or 10.20 [moderate = 4–5 symptoms] or severe [6+]; see American Psychiatric Association, 2013, p. 491, for definitions of *tolerance* and *withdrawal*); alcohol intoxication, a reversible syndrome due to recent ingestion (F10.129, F10.229, F10.929); and alcohol withdrawal (F10.239, 10.232). Specifier codes vary by mild, moderate, or severe and by other specifier categories, such as remission. Most substance abuse is polysubstance abuse (i.e., abuse of multiple substances), as in the case of comedian John Belushi (see Case 15.2, below). Withdrawal from alcohol often involves tapered doses of chlordiazepoxide (Librium) or gabapentin (Neurontin; Black & Andreasen, 2011, p. 255).

For our purposes, a *drug* is any substance (usually other than food) that by its chemical nature alters the structure or functioning of a living organism. I focus on *psychotropic* drugs (ones that alter mood, perception, consciousness, and/or behavior), especially those used in psychiatry to treat mental disorders (see Table 15.1). Psychiatric medications are also discussed in Chapters 16 and 23.

Psychiatric patients who take overdoses or attempt suicide often ingest large quantities of one or more of their psychiatric medications. As described earlier for depressive disorders, physicians may prescribe one or more of the SSRIs, SNRIs (Cipriani et al., 2018), atypicals, older tricyclics, or tetracyclics. They may also prescribe *stereoisomers* of earlier drugs (right- or left-hand versions of the same molecular structure). Antidepressant treatment may further include augmentation with an atypical antipsychotic, like lurasidone (Latuda) or aripiprazole (Abilify) (Maris, 2015).

TABLE 15.1. Psychiatric Medications among the Top 50 Prescribed Drugs in the United States, 2008

1. Hydrocodone/Lortab, Vicodin, etc. (pain), 121.3 million prescriptions, $1.78 billion retail cost[a]

9. Alprazolam/Xanax (anxiety), 43.6, $468 million

15. Sertraline/Zoloft (anxiety and depression), 29.5, $648 million

19. Escitalopram/Lexapro (depression), 26.3, $2.4 billion

25. Fluoxetine/Prozac (depression), 23.3, $349 million

29. Lorazepam/Ativan (anxiety), 22.0, $340 million

30. Clonazepam/Klonopin (anxiety), 21.8, $287 million

31. Citalopram/Celexa (depression), 21.6, $260 million

33. Gabapentin/Neurontin (pain, epilepsy, bipolar disorder), 20.7, $809 million

42. Venlafaxine/Effexor, Effexor XR (depression), 16.9, $140 million

47. Paroxetine/Paxil (depression), 15.6, $359 million

Source: Excerpted and rewritten from Towner (2009).

[a]Hydrocodone is not really a psychiatric medication, but a lot of psychiatric patients take it occasionally. (Also, what does it mean that the number one prescribed drug is a pain control drug? The pain being controlled may be psychic as much as physical.) Note, too, that almost all of the unarguably psychiatric medications on this list are for anxiety and/or depression.

In this chapter, I also focus on the following suicidogenic substances, in addition to psychiatric medications: alcohol, opiates, barbiturates, stimulants (including cocaine and methamphetamines), and hallucinogens. Some aspects of suicide related to disorders involving these substances are summarized in Box 15.1.

Alcohol/Ethanol

The vast majority of the scientific literature and research on suicide and substance abuse concerns alcohol (Joiner, 2010, pp. 90–97). The mere fact that about one-third of all suicides are alcohol-intoxicated (see below for definition) at the time of their death means that we need to examine alcohol use and abuse carefully. Ethanol is one of the most problematic drugs. Although I focus on alcohol and suicide,

---

BOX 15.1. Substance-Related Disorders and Suicidal Behavior

- Substance-induced contributors to suicidality include (1) disinhibition, (2) agitation, (3) psychosis, (4) impulsivity, (5) irritability, (6) depression, (7) violence, (8) overdose, (9) withdrawal effects, and (10) hopelessness.

- A substance-associated factor contributing to suicide risk is central nervous system injury, especially to the frontal lobes.

- The WHO says that substance-related disorders are involved in 17% of completed suicides.

- Conwell found in New York City that alcohol misuse was present in 56% of elderly suicides.

- Factors associated with alcohol-dependent suicide completers, according to Murphy, are (1) heavy drinking just prior to suicide, (2) poor social support, (3) living alone, (4) having talked to others about suicide, (5) suffering serious medical complications of alcohol abuse, and (6) unemployment.

- Marzuk et al. found that 29% of suicides in New York City aged 21–30 tested positive at death for cocaine.

- Barraclough found that marijuana users had a suicide risk four times greater than that of nonusers.

- For individuals in correctional settings (i.e., jails or prisons), the following confluence of factors related to arrest while intoxicated that increase suicide risk were found: impulsivity, antisocial personality, shame, disinhibition, and agitated withdrawal.

- There is an unmistakable dose-dependent association between nicotine use and suicide (Malone).

- The increase in adolescent suicide risk is related to the increase in adolescent substance abuse.

- For completed suicides, DSM-IV alcohol dependence or abuse was present in 43% of cases and was twice as common in men as in women.

- For bipolar patients who are alcohol abusers, lithium is not well accepted, particularly if the patients are also rapid cyclers.

Source: Box by Maris, excerpting and rewriting some factual materials from Mack and Lightdale (2006). For the specific references cited above, see the Mack and Lightdale chapter's references.

some general background information is necessary first. Ethanol (its molecular structure is CH_3CH_2OH) is a volatile colorless liquid used not only for intoxication, but as a fuel, solvent, anesthetic, and antiseptic, among others. It has been used since at least since 6000 to 4000 B.C. and is derived from the fermentation of plant products. To oversimplify, yeast eats sugar and makes alcohol and carbon dioxide. Alcohol is a central nervous system depressant or tranquilizer, similar in structure and function to benzodiazepines like Valium and Xanax. For example, ethanol is an agonist of GABA receptors.

Alcohol has both positive and negative short- and long-term effects, as listed in Table 15.2. The effects of alcohol seem to turn on whether or not usage is moderate and occasional. In 2010, according to the Centers for Disease Control and Prevention (CDC; 2010), about 90% of the American population had ever had a drink of alcohol. Of those who drank, about two-thirds (66%) were occasional users, and 10–12% were heavy drinkers. This compares with 63% who had ever smoked cigarettes and 40–50% who had used marijuana. Men were about two to three times more likely to drink alcohol than were women and also made up the bulk of alcoholic suicides. Perhaps 50–60% of psychiatric patients have comorbid diagnoses of alcohol use disorder.

An alcoholic is more than just a heavy drinker. For our purposes, an *alcoholic* can be defined as follows:

> An excessive drinker who has lost control of his/her drinking and whose dependence on alcohol is so extreme that there is a noticeable mental disturbance or interference with bodily health, interpersonal relations, and social and economic functioning. An alcoholic is unable to refrain from drinking or to stop drinking before getting intoxicated. Treatment is required. (Maris, 1988)

TABLE 15.2. Effects of Alcohol

Effects	Positive	Negative
Short-term	Relaxing, calming, disinhibiting, socializing	Decreases judgment and decision making; increases impulsivity; slows reaction time, contains little nourishment but makes one feel full; depresses immune system; decreases sleep quality; irritates GI tract
Long-term	Moderate alcohol decreases heart disease, reduces arterial calcification (esp. red wine), reduces stroke through anticlotting properties, increases good cholesterol (HDL), reduces type II diabetes, stimulates economy (e.g., $13.50 federal tax per "proof gallon" for hard liquor; federal government alcohol tax revenue totaled $9.6 billion in fiscal year 2015)	Causes fatty liver/cirrhosis, brain atrophy; increases breast cancer, cognitive impairment, sexual impotence/erectile dysfunction, testicular atrophy; raises blood pressure; causes vitamin B deficiency, acne rosacea (nose); drunk driving is leading cause of death at ages 16–21; alcohol is linked to crime and accidents (80% of violent crime involves alcohol, 41% of all motor vehicle accidents are related to alcohol); alcohol abuse increases suicide rates.

Sources: Original table by Maris, with data from Maris (1988), CDC (2010), and Tax Policy Center (2016).

Alcohol intoxication is legally defined as a specific *blood alcohol level* (BAL), or blood alcohol content measured by a blood or breath test. The BALs defining drunkenness vary among states and jurisdictions. For example, in South Carolina an individual is considered legally intoxicated at a minimum BAL of 80 milligrams of alcohol per deciliter of blood (or 80 mg/dL), usually expressed as a percentage (0.08%). The BAL drunkenness criteria across the 50 states range from about 0.05 to 0.20% (not 20%!). One's BAL metabolizes (decreases) at about .016% per hour.

Assuming that no tolerance for alcohol has developed, BALs are associated with specific mental and physical conditions as noted below. Other conditions that are relevant to BAL are body weight and whether or not the individual has been eating. Beer is generally 3–6% alcohol, wine 9–14%, and whiskey 35-50%. The term *100 proof* means 50% alcohol content. Some conditions and behaviors related to specific BALs (Black & Andreasen, 2014; Maris, 1988) are as follows:

BAL	Behaviors/conditions
0–100 mg/dL	Sedation, tranquility, sense of well-being
100–150	Incoordination, irritability
150–250	Slurred speech, ataxia
> 250	Unconsciousness
> 350	Coma or death

One of my first forensic suicides (which I discussed in Chapter 1) was a Las Vegas case in which the individual had a BAL of 0.50% and was still able to play Russian roulette. Given his BAL, the question arose as to whether he could even form the intent to suicide (i.e., whether his death was an accident). He had taken five of six bullets out of his revolver and then spun the cylinder. He had an 83% probability of surviving each spin and shot. Of course, if all of the bullets had been taken out or if he had not played Russian roulette, the probability of dying would have been zero.

Alcoholic Suicides

As noted at the start of this chapter, Murphy and Robins (1967) reported that 27% of St. Louis suicides had some type of alcohol involvement. As shown in Box 15.1, the WHO has said that substance-related disorders are involved in 17% of all suicides (Mack & Lightdale, 2006, p. 352; see also Leamon & Bostwick, 2012; Bagge & Borges, 2017).[1] Alcohol and other substance abuse may be especially relevant to adolescent suicides (Mack & Lightdale, 2006) and to females, who tend to utilize medications or other drugs (not especially alcohol) as their number one suicide method.

In one of the best books on alcohol and suicide, George Murphy (1992) argued that alcohol-dependent suicides tend to have years of heavy drinking (what I call a "suicidal career" [Maris, 1981], and what Joiner [2005] refers to as "the acquired

---

[1]Joiner (2010) emphasizes that most suicides cannot be described as alcoholics or substance abusers.

ability to inflict lethal self-injury"), to have poor social support, to live alone, to have talked to others about suiciding, to have serious medical complications of alcoholism, and to be unemployed. Mack and Lightdale (2006; see also Leamon & Bostwick, 2012) say that substance abuse increases suicidality through disinhibition, agitation, psychosis, impulsivity, irritability, depression (remember that alcohol is a depressant itself), violence, overdose, withdrawal effects, and hopelessness.

In 1986, I asked Alec Roy and a colleague to review the literature on alcohol and suicide (see Roy & Linnoila, 1986). One of the results from their synopsis of the scientific literature was astounding: They found that almost one in five alcoholics eventually committed suicide (18% on average), and they were not talking about partial self-destruction or cirrhosis. They meant that these alcoholics were mainly putting guns to their heads and pulling the triggers. Later, George Murphy (1992) claimed that the eventual lifetime suicide rate among alcoholics was a little lower (about 10%), but it was still a major risk factor. Roy and Linnoila (1986) went on to say that alcoholic suicides were mainly men (87%) and older; their mean age was 47. At the time of their suicides, the men had been alcoholic for about 25 years on average. Thus alcoholic suicide was a chronic, slow-developing condition, not normally the result of an acute episode (although drinking consumption tends to increase just before suicide; Maris, 1981, pp. 172–180)). Most of the male alcoholics had ASPD (if they had a secondary diagnosis), while the female alcoholics tended to have an affective (mood) disorder (Roy & Linnoila, 1986, p. 271). Notice that the male-to-female ratios of suicide rates and alcoholism rates are both about 4:1 to 5:1.

Karl Menninger, in his classic book *Man against Himself* (1938), called alcoholism "partial suicide." This suggests that early on alcoholism may be a slow substitute for suicide, or initially may even be self-medication. Ballenger et al. (1979) argued that alcoholics have preexisting low brain serotonin and serotonin dysfunction that is transiently raised by initial alcohol consumption, but that in the long run alcoholism leads to the depletion of serotonin. And, as we have seen above, lowered serotonin and serotonin dysfunction are associated with suicide, especially with violent suicides. Brown and Goodwin (1986) reported that depressed patients with a positive history of alcoholism had significantly lower CSF levels of the chief metabolite of serotonin (5-HIAA).

Alcoholic Suicides in Chicago

In my Chicago survey, I studied alcoholic suicides (Maris, 1981). Using a 0.10% BAL as the standard for drunkenness, I found that about 10% of completed suicides drank to the point of intoxication, when they drank. This compared with about 5% of the natural death control population. Thus drunkenness was roughly twice as common in suicides.

Suicide completers were also more likely than nonfatal suicide attempters to engage in repeated excessive drinking. Seventy-two percent of the suicide completers had six or more alcoholic drinks and had them every day, whereas only 50% of the attempters drank that much every day. When I asked survivors about changes in the deceased's drinking habits in the last 5 years of life before the suicide or death, 31% of the suicides had changed their drinking, and 67% of those had increased their drinking. Completed suicides age 45 or older drank more if they were both depressed (as measured by the original BDI) and relatively socially isolated. All differences reported from the Chicago study were statistically significant.

Murphy (1992) and Roy and Linnoila (1986) found that suicides tended to be both alcoholic and depressed (Bagge & Borges, 2017). In four different studies, 57% of alcoholic suicides were also depressed. Interpersonal loss was a significant factor in alcoholic suicides. Roy and Linnoila (1986) found that 48% of suicides had a loss of some kind (e.g., death, separation, divorce) in the year just before their suicide. One-third of suicides suffering from alcoholism had experienced the loss of a close personal relationship within 1 year of their suicides. Finally, alcoholic suicides showed more aggressiveness and violent behaviors than did other suicides.

A few words are in order about overdoses and their relationship to alcohol use in suicides. In 2002–2004 (see Chapter 9, Table 9.2), the number one method for attempting suicide for females was medication and other drug overdose (it was virtually tied with use of firearms). In the Chicago survey, suicide completers did not overdose on drugs much. Only 21% of suicide completers also had at least one overdose (Maris, 1981). Seventy-five percent of suicide completers had no (zero) overdoses. Also, only 8% of suicides consumed both high levels of alcohol and non-alcoholic drugs. Do not forget, too, that male suicides tend to shoot themselves (about 60% do) rather than to overdose.

Finally, one should not minimize or misrepresent the role of alcohol or other substance abuse in suicide. Joiner (2010) has pointed out that in one study, 67% of 2,000 intentional overdoses had no alcohol in their bodies. This means, however, that 33% did have alcohol present. Overdoses and alcohol tend to be mutually exclusive in male suicides, who have the highest rates. Joiner concludes that the majority of people are not drinking at the time of their suicide or suicide attempt. The majority of suicides are not depressed, either, but about 47% are. Do these figures mean that depression and alcohol abuse are not suicide risks? Hardly. Even when suicide can be described as rational or sensible, intoxication may still be an important factor in suicide outcome (Maris, 1982).

Since Joiner (2010) wants to argue that most suicides know what they are doing and that their suicides make sense to them, he emphasizes that most of them are not drunk or intoxicated by a substance when they attempt suicide (which is true). He goes on to point out that the BAL of most suicides is below 0.08%, the legal limit for drunkenness in South Carolina and elsewhere. He claims that if a person drinks regularly, and has some tolerance, then even a 0.10% BAL is not much different from a BAL of 0. Joiner (2010, p. 94) argues that suicides tend not to be all that impulsive, since their suicide plan is "in reserve" and the intoxication only facilitates rather than causes the suicide. However, Joiner's arguments do not mean that alcohol and other substance abuse are not important pieces in the puzzle of why people suicide.

Opiates and Narcotics

Opiates are often used for pain control and have suicide risk associated with overdose, addiction, and withdrawal (Benson et al., 2018). Physicians and dentists have easy opiate access and can sometimes abuse their availability and overdose on these drugs; this is especially true of females (Maris, 2010). One problem with opiates is that their effective dose is very close to their lethal dose. With illegal street opiates, doses are not standardized, and quality is uncontrolled and uncertain; accidental overdose is fairly common. Gabapentin (Neurontin) is used off-label for pain control, but as a GABA agonist it can contribute to depression and suicide (see below).

Surprisingly little research has been done on the relationship of opiates to suicide, especially given the current wave of opiate deaths in the United States (Mack & Lightdale, 2006, p. 355; Sarasohn, 2017). However, a lot of suicides (mostly older white males) are in physical pain, especially musculoskeletal or orthopedic pain, and many of them take opiates for pain control (see Table 15.1). In 2009 I had a case of a 79-year-old white male who was taking hydrocodone (Lortab), 500 mg up to eight times a day; rofecoxib (Vioxx), 50 mg as needed; and Neurontin, 500 mg three times a day. He was also receiving epidural steroid injections and physical therapy. He had had a laminectomy and a knee replacement. This poor man had been in chronic pain for some time. When he shot himself, it was argued by his estate that the Neurontin and opiates had either induced or worsened his clinical depression, which in turn contributed to his suicide. Both Neurontin and opiates are GABAergic (i.e., GABA agonists), and the theory is that they lower serotonin and norepinephrine, thereby increasing the risk of depression and suicide (Trimble, 2007; Trimble & George, 2010; however, see Rothschild, 2017).

Opioid drugs are natural, synthetic, or semisynthetic analgesics or narcotics that reduce pain. The opium poppy naturally produces two alkaloids: morphine and codeine. Although there are some 120 species of poppies, only 2 of them produce morphine. Heroin (morphine diacetate) was first synthesized in 1874, and it was sold in New York City in over-the-counter bottles in 1898 along with aspirin by Bayer. Poppies have been harvested for opiate effects since about 3400 B.C. in Mesopotamia.

Other synthetic opioids and pain control medications are methadone (which, given its long half-life of 22–56 hours, is used for opiate withdrawal treatment) and tramadol (Ultram) (which is actually an SNRI antidepressant and pain control medication, with fewer adverse side effects than most opiates). Semisynthetic opioids include hydrocodone (Lortab, Vicodin, etc.) and oxycodone (Oxycontin). There are many other opioids than the ones mentioned here. Interestingly, the human body also produces endogenous morphine (*endorphins*). There is actually a neurological disorder related to a gene (SCN9A), in which children cannot feel pain, but are normal otherwise. Being able to feel pain is important; it signals a need for treatment that otherwise might be neglected.

If one is in moderate to severe pain, opiates reduce pain and produce euphoria (a sense of well-being, in the short run), as well as drowsiness and relative inactivity. Since the passage of the Harrison Narcotics Tax Act in 1914 in the United States, opioids have been controlled substances (Schedule I). They have been illegal for nonmedical use since 1924. Given the euphoria that opiates produce and the limited legal access to them, much opiate use in the United States is illegal and big business. Many people do not realize that only six countries consume about 77% of the world's morphine supply. About 87% of opiates worldwide come from Afghanistan, and the second most from Mexico. The current drug wars in Mexico (see Harris, 2017) are essentially fights for control over the enormously profitable illegal trade in narcotics, as well as marijuana and cocaine.

Pharmacologically, opiates work by binding to opioid receptors, such as mu, kappa, and delta. There are about 17 different opioid receptors; for example, at least 3 mu receptors have now been identified (μ_1, μ_2, and μ_3). The exact pharmacological response depends upon the receptor to which the opiate binds. It is important for suicidology that opioids affect GABAergic neurotransmission, which is related to mood; as noted above, they tend to worsen or induce depression.

Opiates, of course, can have several adverse effects. In the short run, they can cause nausea and vomiting, loss of appetite, constipation, drowsiness, depression, hallucinations (transient psychosis), and disrupted sleep/dreams. In the longer run, they are associated with hepatitis from intravenous use, pneumonia, collapsed veins, heart problems, addiction, withdrawal, and death in overdose. Opiates interact with alcohol, benzodiazepines, and other substances (see the description of Philip Seymour Hoffman's "mixed drug intoxication" in Case 15.1). Note that several of the adverse effects of opiates also relate to depressed mood, and that depression elevates suicide risk (see the description of Nirvana's Kurt Cobain in Chapter 26, Case 26.3).

CASE 15.1. Philip Seymour Hoffman

One famous accidental heroin overdose was that of actor Philip Seymour Hoffman on February 2, 2014. He died in his Manhattan apartment early that Sunday morning of "acute mixed drug intoxication"; the drugs included heroin, cocaine, benzodiazepines, and amphetamines. That morning he was supposed to pick up his three children (a son and two daughters) from his estranged girlfriend, Mimi O'Donnell, but he was a no-show. Hoffman and O'Donnell were together from 1999 to 2013. He left his entire estate of $35 million to her. Hoffman was found dead by a friend, David Bar Katz, with a syringe still stuck in his arm and with 5 empty bags and 65 full bags of heroin in his apartment. He was 46 years old.

Hoffman was born on July 23, 1967 in Fairport, New York. His mother was a lawyer and family court judge, and his father worked for Xerox. He had one brother. All of the Hoffmans were Roman Catholics. His parents divorced (which tends to increase suicide risk) when Philip was 9 years old. Little is known about his family. Hoffman commented that he would "rather not [talk about them] because my family doesn't have any choice [about my disclosures]."

Hoffman liked sports until he injured his neck at age 14, at which time he turned to acting. After high school, Hoffman went to the Tisch School of Arts at New York University and graduated in 1989 with a bachelor's degree in drama. Even back then, he abused alcohol and drugs. He was in a drug rehabilitation program at age 22, but then mostly remained sober for 23 years. However, in May 2013, Hoffman relapsed and again went to drug rehab for 10 days. He commented during a *60 Minutes* interview with Steve Kroft in 2006 that he liked "anything [drugs] I could get my hands on."

Hoffman was pudgy and not especially good-looking. He tended to play creeps, misfits, sniveling wretches, insufferable prigs, braggarts, and outright bullies. He once said, "I didn't go out looking for negative characters; I went out looking for people who have a struggle and a fight to tackle." He may be best known for his performances in *Capote* (2005), for which he won the Best Actor Academy Award, and in Parts 1 and 2 of *The Hunger Games,* his last films. He died with two scenes of Part 2 left to film.

Sources: Wikipedia and various news accounts selected by Maris, with comments by Maris. Data in public domain.

Like all substance use disorders, the psychiatric diagnoses related to opiates are problematic drug patterns related to use or abuse. They include opioid use disorder (mild = F11.10, etc.), opioid intoxication (e.g., with use disorder, moderate or severe, F11.222), and opioid withdrawal (F11.23).

Treatment for opiate addiction primarily involves giving tapered doses of methadone (Black & Andreasen, 2014; Sonntage, 2013). Methadone centers are licensed federally. The detoxification process can take 7–10 days, or even 2–3 weeks. The first day the patient is given 5–20 mg (usually not more than 40 mg) of methadone, depending upon the symptoms. This dose is repeated (Black & Andreasen, 2014) after about 12 hours (there can be supplemental 5- to 10-mg doses, as needed). Once a reference 24-hour dosage is established (usually divided doses three times each day), the dose is tapered by about 20% each day for short-acting opiates and ten percent for long-acting opiates. Clonidine (Catapres) can also be used for opiate detoxification. On the first day, normally 0.3–0.5 mg is given twice a day, and then on subsequent days 0.9–1.5 mg is administered in divided doses three or four times a day.

Barbiturates

In Derek Humphry's (1991/1996) best-selling book *Final Exit,* barbiturates such as secobarbital (Seconal) or pentobarbital (Nembutal) are part of his recommended suicide scenario. Humphry has been heavily criticized in the media for ignoring treatment for depression.

Barbiturates are central nervous system depressants, similar to ethanol, that have been used as sedatives, hypnotics, or anxiolytics (Black & Andreasen, 2014). They have largely been replaced by benzodiazepines. Barbiturates today are mainly used as anticonvulsants. Veterinarians also still use them as anesthetics and (together with potassium chloride, a drug that stops the heart) in euthanasia for animals. Since 1970 barbiturates have been controlled substances (Schedule II) in the United States. Barbiturates are used for physician-assisted suicide or "self-deliverance" in Oregon, Washington, Vermont, Colorado, California, Hawaii, and Montana, and the District of Columbia—jurisdictions where physician-assisted suicide is legal.

The first barbiturates were created by Adolf von Baeyer in Munich, Germany, in 1862. He synthesized barbiturate acid in 1864 by combining urea and malonic acid. One rumor had it that Bayer called it a "barbiturate" because he made it from the urine of a local waitress named Barbara. The main barbiturates are secobarbital (Seconal), pentobarbital (Nembutal), phenobarbital (Luminal), and amobarbital (Amytal). Recreational barbiturate users often prefer short-acting barbiturates like Tuinal, which combines Amytal and Seconal.

Pharmacologically, barbiturates potentiate $GABA_A$ receptors, as the antiepileptics (such as Neurontin) do. Barbiturates also block the neurotransmitter glutamate, which is the principal excitatory neurotransmitter in the brain. Therefore, barbiturates should depress levels of serotonin and norepinephrine and worsen or cause depression and suicide ideation, especially in older adults. The adverse effects of barbiturates resemble those of alcohol intoxication (viz., sluggishness, incoordination, difficulty thinking, slowed speech, staggering, shallow breathing, and even coma and death). Both Marilyn Monroe and Judy Garland died from self-induced barbiturate overdoses in the 1960s.

In Oregon, after October 27, 1997 (and later in other states), a physician under highly specified conditions could write a patient a prescription for barbiturates to be used later by the patient for suiciding. This law was initially blocked, it was not ultimately enacted until 1997. Barbiturates were one of three drugs used initially by Jack Kevorkian (1991) when he assisted his early suicides. (He later switched to carbon monoxide gas.) Kevorkian (1991) built a machine that he called a "Mercitron" (as in mercy killing), which time-released the contents of three vials into a single IV line. The first vial contained sodium pentothal (a barbiturate); the second vial contained succinylcholine (a muscle relaxer like the curare used by pygmies to hunt monkeys; it is also used in the emergency room when a patient is put on a ventilator, so that the patient will not fight the ventilator); and the third vial contained potassium chloride, which stopped the heart. The IV liquids were driven by a motor from a toy truck that Kevorkian got at Toys'R'Us. Kevorkian put the IV in the patient's arm, but the would-be suicide flipped the switch on the motor (as a rule of thumb, Kevorkian never touched a patient if assisting a suicide). All this took place at first in the back of Kevorkian's old Volkswagen van.

Stimulants

Stimulants have been involved in the deaths of many celebrities. They burn brightly, then flame out and die, often before age 40. They include artists like John Belushi, Janis Joplin, Kurt Cobain, John Candy, Chris Farley, and Heath Ledger. For example, Belushi snorted cocaine during skits on *Saturday Night Live* and sometimes drank LSD-laced punch at parties after the show. He died from his recreational use of opiates and cocaine (see Case 15.2).

CASE 15.2. John Belushi

Comedian John Belushi, best known for his groundbreaking work on *Saturday Night Live* (*SNL*) and for the film *Animal House* (1978), died of a heroin and cocaine overdose (a "speedball") on March 5, 1982 at age 33. He had a long history of substance abuse and was on cocaine during skits for *SNL*. He was one of the entertainers who lived to excess with few boundaries except his own mortality, like the Bob Fosse character in *All That Jazz* (1979).

John's wife, Judy, was concerned that for John drugs and music were practically synonymous. Drugs were interfering with their marriage and sex life, which is fairly common for opiate abusers. (Opiates are often a substitute for sex.) Cocaine gave John a positiveness about himself; it made everything important and intense.

John's friend and trainer, Bill Wallace, drove to the Chateau Marmont where John and a female companion had gone to do drugs. When Wallace found John, he thought he was asleep in bed. "John, it's time to get up." There was no response, no movement, not a breath, a nerve, a moan. John was dead.

Sources: Factual materials from Maris (1988, p. 317) and Woodward (1984, pp. 402–403), with comments by Maris.

There is a vast panorama of stimulating drugs, which include cocaine, the amphetamines (including Adderall, methamphetamine, and Dexedrine), caffeine, and nicotine. Fifty-seven percent of Americans drink caffeine every day. There are about 80–150 mg of caffeine in a single 5-ounce cup of coffee. The half-life of caffeine is about 3 hours (Black & Andreasen, 2014). Of course, caffeine increases anxiety, and anxiety is a risk factor for suicide (however, in 2017 it was argued that coffee tended to extend life expectancy).

About two-thirds of Americans (63% in 2010) have smoked tobacco. Nicotine is another stimulant. Since the U.S. Surgeon General's (1964) report linking smoking with lung cancer, there has been a 25–35% decline in cigarette smoking. Today roughly 25% of adults in America smoke, but 90% of schizophrenic patients smoke (Black & Andreasen, 2014). Smokers are twice as likely to have a fatal heart attack as nonsmokers are. About 30% of the annual U.S. cancer deaths are tied directly to cigarette smoking, as are a large percentage of fatal motor vehicle accidents (especially in young males). One disturbing consequence of smoking is Berger's disease, progressive gangrene due to cigarette abuse and requiring amputation of the extremities:

If a patient with this condition continues to smoke, gangrene may eventually set in. First, a few toes may have to be amputated, then the foot at the ankle, the leg at the knee, and ultimately at the hip. . . . Patients are strongly advised that if they will only stop smoking, it is virtually certain that the inexorable march of gangrene will be curbed. (Maris, 1988, p, 340)

This sounds a lot like slow suicide.

Cocaine

Cocaine is the second most researched substance in relation to suicide (Lester, 2000; Simon & Hales, 2012, pp. 148–149). As mentioned in earlier chapters, Marzuk et al. (1992) found that 29% of suicides in New York City ages 21–30 tested positive for cocaine. Cocaine was isolated from the leaves of coca plants in South America by a German chemist, Albert Niemann, in 1860. In the early 1880s in Vienna, Freud experimented with the anesthetic and aphrodisiac properties of cocaine. In fact, he thought he would become famous for his research on cocaine, not for what later came to be called psychoanalysis.

In 1903, Coca-Cola (Coke) had 60 mg of cocaine in each bottle. In fact, the manufacturers of Coke were once sued because the product was thought to have *less* cocaine than advertised. About 7–10% of Americans have used cocaine (CDC, 2010). Crack is a form of cocaine; it got its name from the cracking sounds it makes when being smoked. About three-fourths of cocaine users cannot control their cocaine ingestion. Cocaine is not addicting, but it still produces a strong psychological dependence. Cocaine users tend to become preoccupied with getting and using cocaine, to the exclusion of other responsibilities like work, school, and family.

Pharmacologically cocaine increases brain dopamine by blocking the removal of dopamine from the synapse. In a sense, cocaine hijacks the brain reward system by flooding it with large amounts of dopamine (Black & Andreasen, 2011, pp. 66, 260). The brain reward system is a network for the experience of pleasure, including especially the ventral tegmental area and the nucleus accumbens (see National Institute of Drug Abuse, 2010).

Some of the beneficent effects of cocaine include short-term mood elevation, euphoria, decreased appetite, and sexual arousal. It has been used as a diet pill. Unfortunately, cocaine also has many adverse effects. These include paranoia, visual hallucinations, depression, violence (including suicide), impaired judgment, asocial behavior, and heart problems, among others. Withdrawal from cocaine can be related to depression, even suicide. Usually withdrawal is facilitated with a tapered benzodiazepine dose.

Adderall and Other ADHD Medications

A large number of young (adolescent) male suicides tend to have ADHD and to be on stimulating psychiatric medications like Ritalin, Adderall, or Strattera (see Schwartz, 2016). Interestingly, almost all of the 200–300% increase in the adolescent suicide rate from 1950 to 1977 was among males (Maris, 1985). From 1960 to 1977 the increase was 237%, and from 1950 to 1996 the increase was 317%. But, of course, these increases were obviously not necessarily because of ADHD or the medications used to treat it.

Adolescent males who suicide tend, early in their development, to get diagnoses of conduct disorder or oppositional defiant disorder. After age 18, they often have ASPD diagnoses (see Chapter 14). A number of very bright young male university students who later suicided used Adderall as a study drug because it focuses energy and increases concentration (Schwartz, 2016). Note the paradox of giving amphetamines to hyperactive young people.

Adderall is an amphetamine-salt-based medication introduced for the treatment of ADHD in 1996. Adderall increases dopamine and norepinephrine in the brain; that is, it is a dopamine and norepinephrine reuptake inhibitor. Adderall affects the mesolimbic reward pathway in the brain. It also decreases appetite. Patients with ADHD tend to have trouble sleeping and concentrating, which Adderall helps control.

The half-life for Adderall is 10 hours for adults (some patients with ADHD are adults) and 11 hours for adolescents. The dosage of Adderall usually is 10–25 mg twice a day, up to 120 mg per day. Twenty milligrams of extended-release Adderall (Adderall XR) is about the same as 10 mg of instant-release Adderall. Adderall has a high abuse potential; patients taking it can be medically noncompliant and try to get early refills from their doctors. Adderall interacts with serotonin-specific anti-depressants and Wellbutrin, and can result in excessive serotonin (the "serotonin syndrome") and suicide outcomes.

Methamphetamines

Ephedrine was first synthesized in Japan in 1893. In one study, 20% of Japanese female prisoners with methamphetamine addiction showed psychoses resembling those of schizophrenic patients. Methamphetamine has a high association with both depressive disorder and suicide and is highly addictive. It is a neurotoxin that forces dopamine molecules out of their storage vesicles and expels them into the synaptic cleft, thereby increasing CSF dopamine. This results in an intensely plea-surable rush from dopamine release. Methamphetamine is a controlled substance (Schedule II) in the United States. Lately there have been restrictions added to over-the-counter products containing pseudoephedrine, such as cold/allergy medica-tions and cough syrups. The pseudoephedrine in these products can be converted to methamphetamine in illegal methamphetamine labs. (See Box 15.2 about the popular television series *Breaking Bad*.)

Hallucinogens

Several, mainly recreational, hallucinogenic drugs can cause altered consciousness, perception, and sense of time (Simon & Hales, 2012, p. 147); euphoria and more intense emotions; a sense of intimacy or empathy with others (*entactogenesis* or ego death); psychedelic changes in perception, such as seeing radiant or sparking col-ors, surfaces that ripple or breathe, or tracers/trails of moving objects; and feelings of unreality and psychotic-like experiences. These sensations are normally short-acting (e.g., with LSD, they start within an hour of ingestion and last 6–12 hours).

BOX 15.2. *Breaking Bad*

Breaking Bad was an American crime drama television series created by Vince Gilligan. The show aired on the AMC network from January 20, 2008 to September 29, 2013. It told the story of Walter White (played by Bryan Cranston), a struggling high school chemistry teacher with inoperable lung cancer. Together with a former student, Jess Pinkman (Aaron Paul), White turns to a life of crime—producing and selling crystallized methamphetamine to secure his family's financial future before he dies. The title comes from a Southern colloquial-ism that means "raising hell." *Breaking Bad* was set and filmed in Albuquerque, New Mexico.

   Ironically for White, his family, and Pinkman, the methamphetamine business turns out to be self-destructive, even suicidal. Creator Gilligan said that *Breaking Bad* represents a human desire for wrongdoers to be punished. So it is not so much about the pharmacology of amphetamine use, but rather its self-destructive lifestyle and moral aspects. *Breaking Bad* is widely regarded as one of the best television series of all time. The show received numer-ous awards.

Source: Factual information from Wikipedia, with comments by Maris.

Hallucinogenic drugs include lysergic acid diethylamide (LSD), a synthetic; peyote and mescaline, both of botanical origin; Ecstasy or MDMA (technically an amphetamine, viz., methylenedioxymethamphetamine); PCP (phencyclidine); psilocybin (a hallucinogen found in some mushrooms); and various designer or synthetic drugs. As noted above, John Belushi was a recreational user of LSD, but his death was caused by a mixture of opiates and cocaine (see Case 15.2).

LSD

LSD was first synthesized on November 19, 1938 by Swiss chemist Albert Hoffman, who worked for Sandoz (now Novartis). Hoffman later experimented with psychedelic mushrooms (psilocybin) in the late 1950s. Hoffman ingested LSD on April 19, 1943, and Sandoz first marketed it as a psychedelic drug, Delysid, in 1947. A single dose of LSD, 250 micrograms, is roughly equivalent to 10% of the mass of a grain of sand. Several psychiatrists, including Joel Elkes at Johns Hopkins, experimented with the creative and conjoint psychotherapeutic uses of LSD. The British author Aldous Huxley (see his novel *Brave New World,* 1932) advocated consumption of LSD, as did Harvard professor Timothy Leary in the 1960s.

LSD affects all the dopamine receptors, and adrenoreceptors, as well as most serotonin receptors (but not 5-HT$_3$ or 5-HT$_4$). The psychedelic effects of LSD are attributed to its strong agonist effects at 5-HT$_{2A}$ receptors. A very small dose of LSD (100–500 micrograms or 1 mg/kg) can produce an effect lasting 6–12 hours, with a plasma half-life of 5.1 hours and a peak plasma level at 3 hours postdose. LSD does not lead to death in overdose, is not especially correlated with suicidal behaviors, and seems to have few long-lasting effects. Some people do reexperience the drug's effects (i.e., have "flashbacks") and can become anxious or paranoid. DSM-5 lists hallucinogen persisting perception disorder as a diagnosis. LSD may have the effects of temporarily compromising sensible judgment and the ability to understand common dangers. If death results, these are probably accidents, not suicides.

Sometimes LSD takers, especially those who are also on antidepressants or lithium, have dissociative fugue states in which they have an impulse to wander. These states can be dangerous, if time perception and consciousness are also altered. LSD can cause panic attacks, but does not produce schizophrenia or permanent psychosis in otherwise healthy individuals.

MDMA/Ecstasy

Methylenedioxymethamphetamine, called MDMA or Ecstasy, is another popular hallucinogenic drug. Several university student suicides have used the drug recreationally. Ecstasy produces altered consciousness; an extreme mood lift; feelings of compassion, empathy, and intimacy toward others (entactogenesis); mild psychedelia; and hyperactivity, such as an uncontrollable urge to dance (from which the dance events called "raves" originated). In 2013 a more concentrated derivative of Ecstasy called Molly led to several deaths at rock concerts.

MDMA was synthesized in 1912 by Merck chemist Anton Köllish. However, the first scientific article on MDMA did not appear until 1958 as part of research on antispasmodics. Shulgin and Nichols (1978) reported on MDMA's psychotropic effects.

The primary precursor to the manufacture of MDMA is the liquid Safrole, which is extracted from the root-bark of the sassafras plant. MDMA is a releasing agent of serotonin, norepinephrine, and dopamine. Its entactogenic effects might come from indirect oxytocin secretion via activation of the serotonin system. Peak plasma levels of MDMA occur in 1.5–3 hours, with a half-life of peak concentration in about 8 hours. After May 1985, MDMA was classified as a Schedule I drug in the U.S. MDMA is one of four widely used illicit drugs, along with cocaine, cannabis, and heroin.

In overdose, MDMA can result in serotonin syndrome and stimulant psychosis, both of which can be suicide risk factors. Long-term MDMA use causes reduction in the concentration of serotonin transporters in the brain, as well as clinical depression, which is related to suicide risk. Since MDMA is illegal like heroin, the purity of ecstasy sold is unknown. Paramethoxyamphetamine (PMA), sold as Ecstasy, has resulted in deaths. Benzodiazepines have been utilized for treatment of those having adverse MDMA effects (Black & Andreasen, 2014).

PCP/Angel Dust

A third drug with hallucinogenic properties is phencyclidine, called PCP or angel dust. PCP was synthesized in 1926, and eventually patented in 1952 by Parke-Davis as Serynl. After World War II PCP was tested as a surgical anesthetic, but it proved not to be very useful for this purpose, given its adverse effects of hallucinations, mania, delirium, and disorientation. In 1967 PCP began to be used recreationally in major U.S. cities. By 1978 Mike Wallace, on *60 Minutes,* was calling PCP the country's number one drug problem. In 1990, however, only about 3% of high school students had ever tried PCP, down from 13% in 1979.

PCP produces numbness in the extremities, analgesia, intoxication, staggering/unsteady gait, schizophrenia-like changes, and unpredictable alterations of mood. It lands many recreational users in big-city emergency rooms. Some bizarre acts of violence, both homicidal and suicidal, have been reported with PCP use. Since users feel diminished pain, they have been known to break handcuffs, pull their own teeth out, or otherwise self-mutilate. Emergency room treatment is mainly supportive, including benzodiazepines like lorazepam (Ativan) or diazepam (Valium).

PCP binds to different receptor sites. It acts most notably on glutamate receptors, such as N-methyl-D-aspartate (NDMA) receptor antagonists. Glutamate and NDMA receptors mediate excitation. Nitrous oxide is another NDMA receptor antagonist. PCP also acts as a D_2 receptor partial agonist, which may be related to its psychotic effects. D_2 antagonists like haloperidol (Haldol) can be used to treat PCP psychosis. The onset of PCP effects can occur in about 5 minutes and peak in 30 minutes (Black & Andreasen, 2011, p. 276). Effects last a few hours, but total elimination typically may require 8 days or more. PCP comes in both powder and liquid forms. The powder can be inhaled (insufflated). Typically PCP is sprayed onto leafy material (like cannabis). Cigarettes can be dipped in liquid PCP (sometimes called "embalming fluid" on the street) and then smoked. Of course, since PCP is illicit, it can contain a number of contaminants.

Psilocybin

Psilocybin is a naturally occurring psychedelic compound produced by over 200 species of mushrooms, mostly from Mexico. It has been used for thousands of years as an *entheogen* (a psychoactive drug used in religious or spiritual contexts). Users report feelings of euphoria, disorientation, giddiness, hallucinations, anxiety, paranoia, or even depression. Often psilocybin makes users feel as if time has slowed down. Panic attacks occur in about 25% of users. There can be violent, aggressive behavior, including homicide or suicide attempts. Albert Hoffman, the chemist for Sandoz (Novartis) who had earlier created LSD, purified psilocybin from *Psilocybe mexicana* in the late 1950s. Sandoz marketed psilocybin for use in psychedelic psychotherapy, such as the experiments in the early 1960s by Timothy Leary at Harvard and later by Griffiths et al. (2011) at Johns Hopkins.

The effects of psilocybin begin 10–40 minutes after ingestion and last two to six hours. A typical recreational dose is 10–50 mg of psilocybin or 10–50 g of fresh mushrooms. Psilocybin is a tryptamine compound and is structurally similar to the neurotransmitter serotonin. It is chemically related to the amino acid tryptophan. Psilocybin is a partial agonist of several serotonin receptors (especially 5-HT_{2A} receptors). The functions of serotonin receptors include regulation of mood and motivation. The psychotic-like effects of psilocybin can be blocked by 5-HT_{2A} antagonist drugs, like risperidone (Risperdal). Psilocybin has no affinity for dopamine receptors. It should be noted that any drug that heightens anxiety, panic attacks, depression, psychotic-like behavior, violence, and aggression can also increase suicide risk, *ceteris paribus*.

Other Chemical Substances

Other chemicals are used for suicide, especially household cleaning chemicals and farm pesticides. This residual drug category includes a multiplicity of suicidogenic substances. For example, some people may drink caustic cleaners like Clorox or Drano, or eat vermin and insect poisons. As noted in Chapter 8 (see especially Box 8.1), young women in rural China and India tend to overdose on farm pesticides. Chemicals like potassium cyanide will stop the heart (e.g., some Nazis carried cyanide suicide pills in the lapels of their coats; see the accounts of Hermann Goering's death). Even Tylenol (acetaminophen) is very fatal in relatively slight overdoses. Lately there also have been suicides by helium gas (see Chapter 9, Table 9.1).

In the concluding chapter of Part IV (Chapter 16), I examine the biology, genetics, and neurobiology of suicide. This area seems to be the wave of the future, given the prominence of the medical model in psychiatry and the pharmacological treatment of mental disorders.

CHAPTER 16

Biology, Genetics, and Neurobiology
Suicidal Biogenics of the Brain

> Although neurological factors are diverse, complex, and interactive;
> the primary biological marker for suicide is probably too little
> serotonin in the wrong place; viz., i.e., in the prefrontal cortex.
> —J. JOHN MANN

Modern psychiatry tends to assume that mental disorders result from or are characterized by various dysfunctions in the brain's (as opposed to the mind's) neurochemical systems (see Trimble & George, 2010; Mann & Currier, 2012; Cooper et al., 2003; Dwivedi, 2012; Oquendo et al., 2017). These alleged dysfunctions involve neurotransmitters and neurosystems, including small-molecule neurotransmitters like serotonin, dopamine, norepinephrine, and gamma-aminobutyric acid (GABA, the "brake" in the brain); cholinergic systems (such as acetylcholine in dementia); glutamate (an excitatory amino acid); neuropeptides like endorphins; and others like nitric oxide. There are about 30–100 different molecular types of neurotransmitters, but about 10 of them do 99% of the work (King, 2017).

Most psychiatric treatment of depressive disorders, for example, consists of adjusting these alleged neurochemical imbalances with one or more antidepressants (see Chapters 10 and 11, as well as Black & Andreasen, 2014). Carlat (2010) says that most of his psychiatric patients are taking about five or six medications at the same time—antidepressants, anxiolytics, antipsychotics, mood stabilizers, and even anesthetics (like ketamine; Grunebaum et al., 2018) and augmenting drugs (like Abilify, Latuda, Rexulti, or lithium). Of course, concomitant psychotherapies, as well as electroconvulsive therapy (ECT) and other technical procedures, can be used in addition to psychiatric medications. Two more exotic treatments for refractory depression include transcranial magnetic stimulation and vagus nerve stimulation (Black & Andreasen, 2014).

Neurotransmitters are chemicals that transmit signals from a neuron to a cell across a neuronal gap called a *synapse* or *synaptic cleft*. In addition to the neurotransmitters listed above, others include histamine, many other neuropeptides, and tyramine. The human brain has about 100 billion neurons (Black & Andreasen, 2014), far more than the total number of people on earth (see Joiner, 2005, Ch. 5; Mann & Currier, 2012; and Black & Andreasen, 2011, Ch. 3).

The key research results on the biology of suicide center on the serotonergic system in the brain. For example, early research in Sweden in the mid-1970s (Äsberg et al., 1976; Mann & Currier, 2012) discovered that the cerebrospinal fluid (CSF) of suicidal patients contained lower levels (below 92.5 nmol/liter) of serotonin (5-HT) and 5-hydroxyindoleacetic acid (5-HIAA, the chief metabolite of 5-HT) than the levels of normal controls, especially in the prefrontal cortex of the brain (see this chapter's epigraph by Mann). Of all the neurotransmitters, 5-HT is probably the most important for suicide risk (Joiner, 2005, p. 182). It affects sleep, impulsivity, and mood, and reduced levels of 5-HT have been linked to headaches, conduct problems, poor peer relationships, and suicidal behaviors (Brown & Goodwin, 1986; Brown et al., 1992; Joiner, 2005). A blunted response to a fenfluramine challenge suggests less 5-HT. Much of the research on serotonin and suicide has focused on the suicidogenic factor of impulsivity (Joiner, 2005).

The vast majority of the pharmacological treatments of suicide and depression concern titrating 5-HT levels and boosting the serotonergic system. Think back to Chapter 11 and the discussion of SSRIs, like Prozac, Paxil, Zoloft, Luvox, Lexapro, and Celexa. To oversimplify, SSRIs block the reuptake of 5-HT presynaptically in the synaptic cleft between brain neurons; this makes more CSF 5-HT available, and theoretically reduces depressive disorders. SSRIs are also *neurogenic;* that is, they create more neurons and synapses. This can be seen with an electron microscope in rat brains after treatment with megadoses of Prozac.

Serotonin is also enhanced by the over-the-counter herbal St. John's wort, as well as by other factors. For example, the dietary precursor to 5-HT is tryptophan. There are sociological studies of early American colonies in which the colonists' diets were low in tryptophan and entire communities tended to become depressed (Soh & Walter, 2011). Of course, the brain is also electrical (not just neurochemical), and one of the treatments for depression is also electric (viz., ECT). ECT is about 80% effective (vs. the 60–70% effectiveness of SSRIs), and it enhances serotonin.

More recent antidepressants focus on boosting both serotonin and norepinephrine, and thus are called SNRIs. These include Pristiq, Cymbalta, Fetzima, Brintellix, Rexulti, and Deplin. There are also atypical antidepressants like Wellbutrin that focus on dopamine (and can help with weight loss as well). Whereas SSRIs have about a 50% sexual dysfunction rate, Wellbutrin causes much lower rates of sexual dysfunction and may be preferred for treating sexually active young adults.

An *agonist* enhances a neurochemical reaction or response, and an *antagonist* inhibits a response. Most antidepressants are serotonin agonists, but, strangely, some are serotonin antagonists (such as tianephrine, used in France). Most biological treatments of suicidality also include antianxiety medications (like Klonopin or Xanax), antipsychotics (like Risperdal or Zyprexa), and/or some mood stabilizers (like lithium or Depakote), as well as antidepressants. It is common to give depressed patients more than one antidepressant (e.g., adding trazodone [Desyrel] at bedtime for sleep to an SSRI prescription).

An overview of the genetics and neurochemistry of suicide can be found in Box 16.1. Many biological markers have been considered, including those pointed out by Joiner and outlined in Box 16.2. I discuss details for many of these points in the rest of this chapter.

BOX 16.1. Selected Overview of the Genetics and Neurochemistry of Suicide

- Suicidal behaviors are too complex for there ever to be a single *suicide gene,* but genes can be related to suicide risk factors. Mapping the human genome for gene- and suicide-related behaviors is in its infancy and on the cutting edge of future suicide research (Mann & Currier, 2012).

- In a study in *Nature,* depressed Amish people were found to have a chromosome 11 defect (Egeland et al., 1987).

- For serotonin, a single gene on chromosome 17 affects control of the available 5-HT in brain synapses.

- The short/short (s/s) allele combination is related to a dysregulated serotonin system (Joiner, 2005). Joiner says that his father (who committed suicide) had an s/s genotype.

- The tryptophan hydroxylase (TPH) gene breaks down tryptophan and affects serotonin.

- The catechol-O-methyltransferase (COMT) gene breaks down dopamine and norepinephrine, which in turn are related to suicide.

- Kaminsky (see Minkove, 2016) has identified a protein (SKA_2) that appears to be a link in the stress response pathway. SKA_2 and epigenetic regulation of the gene that makes it are reduced in postmortem brains of suicide victims.

- Pain dysfunction in children (they do not feel pain) is related to the SCN9A gene.

- If both parents are schizophrenic (itself a risk factor for suicide), their child has about a 50% chance of becoming schizophrenic. (However, see Leo, 2003.)

- Monozygotic (MZ) twins have a six times greater suicide concordance than do dizygotic (DZ) twins (cf. Joiner, 2005, p. 175). Concordance rates for suicide in MZ twins is 13–19%, but for DZ twins it is only 1%.

- Fenfluramine stimulates 5-HT release; if you give fenfluramine to suicide attempters, they show a decreased release of 5-HT (a blunted response). A blunted response suggests less 5-HT activity, which in turn is related to increased depression and suicide risk.

- Completed suicides show decreased prefrontal cortex activity.

- The hypothalamic–pituitary–adrenocortical (HPA) axis under stress causes the cortical release of corticotropin-releasing hormone (CRH). Major depression is associated with hyperactivity of the HPA axis, the body's main stress reaction system.

- The dexamethasone suppression test (DST) should reduce cortisol. In depressed patients, however, it tends to fail to suppress cortisol.

- The 5-HT system probably relates to impulsivity, which in turn increases suicide risk.

Source: Excerpted and rewritten by Maris from Maris (1986) and Mann and Currier (2012).

BOX 16.2. Thomas Joiner (2005) on Neurobiology and Suicide

- Serotonin is key with regard to mood, sleep, and appetite (p. 172).
- The serotonin transporter gene codes for recycling 5-HT back up into the neurons after it is released into the synaptic cleft, and it codes for 5-HT receptors (p. 173).
- Another serotonin system gene is the tryptophan hydroxylase (TRH) gene (p. 178).
- The catechol-O-methyltransferase gene (COMT) gene is responsible for breaking down dopamine and norepinephrine. A gene on chromosome 22 codes for COMT activity.
- Fenfluramine stimulates serotonin release. In a fenfluramine challenge, suicide attempters show decreased release of 5-HT, indicating less serotonin activity despite the challenge (p. 180).
- Patients who attempt suicide by more lethal means show decreased activity in the prefrontal cortex (p. 180).
- A postmortem study of suicides found decreased serotonin transporter binding in the prefrontal cortex (p. 180).
- Serotonin plays an important role in sleep regulation (p. 181).
- Depressed patients with repetitive and frightening nightmares are more likely to be suicidal (p. 181).
- Joiner doubts that true spur-of-the-moment suicides exist (p. 185).
- Plasma levels of serotonin metabolites were lower in impulsive suicide attempters (p. 186).
- A blunted response to fenfluramine challenge suggests less 5-HT activity (p. 186).
- Joiner argues that impulsivity is related to suicidal behavior indirectly (p. 187).
- Impulsivity has the most clearly documented association with suicidal behavior (p. 188).
- 65% of suicides with BPD have made a prior suicide attempt, versus 33% of those with major depression. Those with BPD in effect "practice" suicide (p. 196).

Source: Excerpted and rewritten by Maris from Joiner (2005).

Chemical Synapses

Starting with the work of Bowers in 1969 (see Whitaker, 2010), the research of Sol Snyder at Johns Hopkins at about the same time (see Kramer, 1993), and especially the suicide research of Marie Äsberg (Äsberg et al., 1976, 1986) in Sweden, mental disorders in general and depressive disorders in particular came to be conceptualized as chemical imbalances. In the case of depressive disorders, serotonin deficiencies or dysfunctions were implicated. As described in Chapter 11, the basis for the simplistic serotonin (or monoamine) hypothesis of depression was that patients tended to have lower CSF brain serotonin, especially in the prefrontal cortex, compared to healthy controls. Carlat (2010) has jokingly called this the "dipstick" theory of neurotransmitters, like an auto mechanic checking under a car's hood for fluid levels: "Your serotonin is low, and we need to top that off with Prozac, but your dopamine level is fine." Other mental disorders (like schizophrenia, anxiety disorders, bipolar disorder, and dementia) were also seen as chemical imbalances of dopamine, GABA, acetylcholine, norepinephrine, and so on.

One obvious question that arose from the serotonin hypothesis was this: How do we adjust the brain's serotonin imbalance? At a chemical synapse, a neuron releases a neurotransmitter into a small space (or *cleft*) adjacent to another neuron (see Figure 16.1). The human brain has about 100–500 trillion synapses. The word *synapse* is from the Greek, meaning "to clasp together."

Synapses are functional connections between neurons or other cells. Most synapses connect axons to dendrites. You can actually see a synapse like the one depicted in Figure 16.1 with the naked eye through an electron microscope. Chemical synapses pass information from a presynaptic cell to receptors in a postsynaptic cell. The neurotransmission process begins with a wave of electrochemical excitation.

At a synapse, various neurotransmitters, like serotonin, norepinephrine, GABA, dopamine, and acetylcholine, pass information from a presynaptic cell to a postsynaptic cell. When neurotransmitters are released into a synaptic cleft, they (1) are transmitted to a postsynaptic receptor, (2) are reabsorbed presynaptically by a *reuptake pump*, (3) remain in the brain CSF, or (4) are broken down metabolically.

Having said all this, I must add that we really do not know what causes depression or other mental disorders; we just have theories or hypotheses backed by some clinical trials and not by others. To make the serotonin hypothesis more complex, certain antidepressant medications affect different neurotransmitters (not just serotonin or only some 5-HT receptors) at the same time in different concentrations in different anatomical sites in the brain.

Any one neurotransmitter theory of mental disorder oversimplifies what is in fact a very complex neurochemical process that we really do not understand well yet.

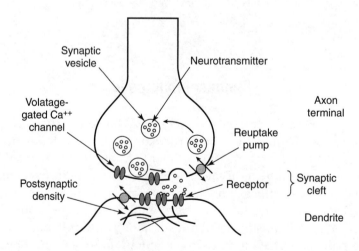

FIGURE 16.1. Structure of a typical chemical synapse. *Source:* Thomas Splettstoesser (*www.scistyle.com*), as posted on Wikipedia. Created July 3, 2015. Permission granted under Creative Commons Share Alike 4.0 Internations. (I know that Wikipedia tends not to have the scientific reliability and validity that original scientific studies do, but for various reasons I have decided to use Wikipedia here and in a few other places in my book. For a more professional depiction of a synapse, see Black & Andreasen, 2014, which portrays an actual synapse as seen through an electron microscope.)

Also, drugs like Prozac are *neurotropic* or *neurogenic;* that is, they increase or grow neurons and synapses (see the discussion of neurogenesis later in this chapter).

Antidepressants like Prozac, Paxil, and Zoloft (and, more recently, Luvox, Celexa, and Lexapro) are called *selective serotonin reuptake inhibitors* because when serotonin is released into the synaptic cleft and CSF, the SSRIs prevent their reuptake presynaptically, leading to higher levels of serotonin in the brain. Although the mechanism of mood elevation is not entirely clear, it is thought that keeping levels of neurotransmitters like serotonin higher may improve communication between the nerve cells, and that this can strengthen circuits in the brain which regulate mood. We still have a lot to learn.

Neurotransmitters

As noted above, *neurotransmitters* are chemical messengers that transmit signals across a chemical synapse (Black & Andreasen, 2014). As shown in Figure 16.1, neurotransmitters are released from synaptic vesicles into the synaptic cleft, where they are received by receptors on the target cells. A released neurotransmitter is typically available in the synaptic cleft for a short time before it is (1) metabolized by enzymes, (2) pulled back into the presynaptic neuron through reuptake, or (3) bound to a postsynaptic receptor. A neurotransmitter is released in response to a threshold action potential or graded electrical potential.

Psychiatry is especially interested in the neurochemical systems that are associated with major mental disorders, like dopamine, acetylcholine, serotonin, GABA, and glutamate—some of the 10 neurotransmitters that King (2017) describes as doing most of the work (cf. Mann & Currier, 2012, pp. 481 ff., and Black & Andreasen, 2011, Ch. 3). Some major types of neurotransmitters include the following:

- Amino acids, like glutamate and GABA.
- Monoamines, like dopamine (DA), norepinephrine (NE), serotonin (5-HT), histamine, and epinephrine (adrenaline).
- Gastrotransmitters, like nitric oxide (NO) and carbon monoxide (CO).
- Peptides, like cocaine- and amphetamine-regulated transcript, and opioid peptides.
- Purines, like adenosine.
- Others, like acetylcholine (ACh), and over 50 neuroactive peptides.

The most common neurotransmitter is glutamate, which is 90% excitatory. The next most prevalent is GABA, which is 90% inhibitory.

5-HT Receptors

Given the important relationship of depression to both serotonin and suicide, I have tended to focus on the serotonin system and the 5-HT receptor. Up to this point I have acted as if there were only one type of 5-HT receptor, and that titrating it (usually elevating its level or function) in the brain improves mood. In fact, the relationship of serotonin to depression or mood is far more complex than suggested up to now.

There are at least 13 types of 5-HT receptors (Glennon & Dukat, 1991). There are $5\text{-}HT_{1-7}$, and the subtype serotonin families: $5\text{-}HT_{1A, 1B, 1D, 1E,}$ and $_{1F}$, and $5\text{-}HT_{2A.}$ Most 5-HT receptors are excitatory, but a couple are inhibitory. The inhibitory 5-HT families include $5\text{-}HT_1$ and $5\text{-}HT_5$; excitatory 5-HT families include $5\text{-}HT_{2-4}$ and $5\text{-}HT_{6-7}$. Each receptor tends to affect different specific functions (mood, aggression, anxiety, sexual behavior, sociability, penile erection, memory, learning, sleep, and many more). Thus different antidepressants target specific types of 5-HT receptors. For example, the antidepressant Viibryd is a $5\text{-}HT_{1A}$ agonist.

Antipsychotic medications target specific dopamine (not just D_2) and serotonin combinations. For example, Zyprexa blocks D_1, D_2, and $5\text{-}HT_{2A.}$ Geodon is a D_2, D_3, $5\text{-}HT_{2A}$, and $5\text{-}HT_{1A}$ antagonist. Note that if antipsychotics affect both dopamine and serotonin, then on its face, the dopamine hypothesis of psychosis by itself is inadequate. The serotonin receptors also modulate the release of glutamate, GABA, dopamine, epinephrine, norepinephrine, acetylcholine, and many hormones.

Dopamine and GABAergic Receptors

Theories similar to the serotonin hypothesis have been developed for other mental disorders with their own unique or focal neurotransmitters. One example is the flawed dopamine hypothesis of schizophrenia, described in Chapter 13 (Black & Andreasen, 2014; Whitaker, 2010). The disorder was thought to be caused by an excess of the neurotransmitter dopamine in the brain and CSF, and dopaminergic system dysfunction in general. The older phenothiazine drugs (like Thorazine or Haldol) were thought to block mainly dopamine (D_2) receptors postsynaptically. Second-generation antipsychotics (like Clozaril) block D_1, D_2, D_3, and D_4 receptors and serotonin ($5\text{-}HT_2$) receptors. Again, if 5-HT receptors are also blocked or altered, then schizophrenia cannot just be explained by a dopamine hypothesis.

Another theory for titrating synaptic neurotransmitters can be given for anxiety disorders and the neurotransmitter GABA (a GABA hypothesis, if you will). For short-term use and acute or time-limited situational anxiety generally, the benzodiazepines are normally prescribed either alone or (more often) with an antidepressant. Unlike antidepressants, benzodiazepines act relatively quickly and are very effective. Acute, highly agitated patients in the emergency room or psychiatric inpatients may be given a drug cocktail, one of which can be referred to as "5–2–25" (i.e., 5 mg of Haldol + 2 mg of Ativan + 25 mg of Benadryl). The benzodiazepine clonazepam (Klonopin) has a long half-life and is often recommended for suicide prevention while a patient is waiting for an antidepressant effect to kick in (Fawcett, 2012).

According to Trimble and George (2010), however, GABA-enhancing drugs like the benzodiazepines or the antiepileptic gabapentin (Neurontin) tend to deplete central nervous system serotonin and norepinephrine, and lowered levels of monoamines are positively associated with depression (perhaps even with increased suicide risk; Maris, 2007). Thus, in theory, GABA-enhancing medications can be suicidogenic (however, see Rothschild, 2017).

Genetics of Suicide

The existence of discrete inheritable units was first suggested by the 19th-century Austrian monk Gregor Mendel. James Watson and Francis Crick (1953) first published the model of a double-stranded deoxyribonucleic acid (DNA) molecule (the *double helix*). A *gene* is the basic physical and functional unit of heredity. Each person has two copies of each gene, one inherited from each parent. Genes, which are made up of DNA, act as instructions to make molecules called *proteins* (see *https://ghr.nlm.nih.gov/primer#basics*). Genes also encode functional ribonucleic acid (RNA). RNA itself is a polymeric molecule implicated in various biological roles in coding, decoding, regulation, and expression of genes.

Genes can acquire mutations, leading to different variants known as *alleles*. Alleles encode slightly different variations of proteins, which cause different phenotype traits. The *phenotype* is the totality of an organism's visible traits, and the *genotype* is all of the organism's genetic material.

An increasingly important question for suicidology is this: Do genes determine or affect suicidal behaviors, and if so, how? Although the genetic process is complex and interactive, we are starting to identify specific genes related to both mental disorder and suicide. More than 50% of genes are expressed in the brain. We would like to be able to discover mechanisms of mental disorder and suicide at the molecular level. The Human Genome Project (*www.genome.gov*) has estimated that humans have about 20,000–25,000 genes.

Early genetic studies of suicide focused on (1) twin studies, (2) adoption studies, and (3) family history. More recent research has begun to examine possible specific genes related to mental disorder and suicide (Mann & Currier, 2012; Fiori et al., 2014). No single-gene defect has been identified that leads to suicide (Lester, 1988), unlike (say) Huntington's chorea, which is determined solely by a locus on chromosome 4 (Black & Andreasen, 2014). Most mental illnesses are due to the interactions of multiple genes, each having a small individual effect, with nongenetic factors.

Twin Studies

One of the key issues in the genetics of suicide is trying to tease out the effects of nature versus those of nurture. Is suicidal behavior genetically determined, or is it the result of socialization and nurturing, especially by one's parents? We know that twins from the same egg (monozygotic, or MZ) have higher rates of suicide concordance than do dizygotic (DZ) twins. *Suicide concordance* is the probability that if one twin is suicidal, the other also will be. This would suggest a genetic effect. For example, Roy et al. (1991) found that 11.3% of MZ twins were concordant for suicide, versus 1.8% of DZ twins. In a more recent study, Voracek and Loibl (2007) found the concordances to be 24.1% for MZ versus 2.8% for DZ twins. In general, suicide concordance in MZ twins is higher than that of DZ twins (Kallman, 1953; Black & Andreasen, 2011).

Mental illness concordance in general is greater in MZ than in DZ twins, and greater than concordance for physical illness is (Black & Andreasen, 2014). For example, see Table 16.1.

TABLE 16.1. Concordance of Monozygotic (MZ) and Dizygotic (DZ) Twins for Selected Mental Disorders and Heart Disease

Mental illness	% in MZ twins	% in DZ twins
Schizophrenia, bipolar disorder	60	5
Depression	50	15
Coronary heart disease	40	10

Source: Black and Andreasen (2014, p. 77). Reprinted with permission from the *Introductory Textbook of Psychiatry,* Sixth Edition. Copyright © 2014 American Psychiatric Association. All Rights Reserved.

Adoption Studies

One way to control for nurturance effects and separate out biological or genetic effects is to look at MZ and DZ twins separated at birth and raised apart from each other. Twins in these studies have the same genes, but were raised by different parents and hence have different nurturance. Adoption studies tend to show a higher concordance rate for MZ than for DZ twins than we would expect, given different socialization (Mann & Currier, 2012). A methodological problem is that it is very rare for twins to be adopted and raised apart from each other or from their own biological parents (Lester, 1988).

Family History Studies

A lot of studies seem to suggest that both mental disorders and suicidal behaviors tend to run in families. By itself, however, this does not prove genetic determination. Joiner (2005) claimed that having a family history of suicide raises a child's suicide risk by about 2:1, compared with controls with no family history of suicide. In my survey of Chicago suicides (Maris, 1981), I found that individuals with a first-degree relative who suicided had a suicide rate of 24 per 100,000, versus 12 per 100,000 for natural death controls. Thus, in the Chicago study there was a two-fold increase in suicide risk if a prior first-degree family member suicided. Note, however, that the association of mental disorder and suicide with next-generation mental disorder or suicides, does not explain why most people with mental disorder (about 85–90%) never commit suicide at all (Joiner, 2005).

Specific Genes and Suicide Outcomes

In recent years, scientists have started to hypothesize and run clinical trials on self-destructive behaviors and specific genes (cf. Sample, 2011). Here are some examples:

- A single gene on chromosome 17 is responsible for plans for the *serotonin transporter gene* (STG) (Mann & Currier, 2012; Rujescu et al., 2007). The STG has two alleles of that gene and three combinations of short and long alleles (viz., long/long, long/short, and short/short). There is evidence that the short/short genotype has more dysregulated 5-HT systems (cf. Joiner, 2005, p. 177).

- Mann and Currier (2012) have reported on the following:
  - The CD44 gene was correlated with the immune system in three suicide studies.
  - There are hypotheses of depression in which neurodegradation and reduced neurogenesis were thought to be caused by inflammation.
  - There is a possible link between suicide and allergic reactions.
- There is a higher frequency of the A218 allele in patients with suicidal behavior (Rujescu et al., 2007).
- There is a significant association of the short allele with suicidal behaviors as a whole. Such patients are more impulsive and aggressive.
- The tryptophan hydroxylase gene is another 5-HT gene.
- In studies of the hypothalamic–pituitary–adrenocortical (HPA) axis, genes related to CRH are promising candidates for predicting suicidal behaviors. (See below for further discussion of the HPA axis.)
- *Epigenetics* involves changes in an organism through the modulation of gene expression, rather than through altering the gene itself. It is biochemical modification of the function of the primary DNA sequence.
- The COMT gene is related to aggression and violence.
- Low-fat diets increase aggressive behavior; low serum cholesterol levels are associated with a higher risk of violent, aggressive behavior (cf. Rujescu et al., 2007).
- See below and Black and Andreasen (2014) for discussion of other hypothesis-driven candidate genes, like the brain-derived neurotropic factor (BDNF) gene.

Other Suicide-Related Biological Findings

The HPA Axis

The HPA axis is the body's main stress reaction system (Mann & Currier, 2012, p. 485). Prolonged stress stimulates release of a hormone from the hypothalamus, which in turn acts on the pituitary gland, causing release of another hormone, which causes the adrenal cortex to release cortisol, the stress hormone (Joiner, 2005). More specifically, with stress the HPA axis is activated by the release of CRH, which acts on the CRH_1 receptor in the pituitary to stimulate release of adrenocorticotropic hormone (ACTH). ACTH is responsible for the peripheral release of cortisol from the adrenal cortex (Mann & Currier, 2012, p. 489). The hyperactivity of the HPA axis in suicidal patients mediates some 5-HT abnormalities.

Earlier in this textbook, I have spoken of the stress–diathesis model (see especially Chapter 4). In the present context, *diathesis* refers to trait predisposition to suicide, and *stress* to current or acute stressful state circumstances. Early family life adversity, including sexual and physical abuse and severe family discord, has been associated with suicidal behavior. For example, lower levels of CSF 5-HIAA (the chief metabolite of serotonin) and lower SERT[1] binding on PET scans were seen in some rhesus macaques who experienced maternal deprivation (Mann & Currier, 2012). Also, adult women with BPD who reported a history of severe childhood adversity had a blunted response to a serotonin agonist. Suicide attempters who reported sexual abuse had significantly higher levels of CSF MHPG.[2] According to Mann and Currier (2012, p. 489), early adversity or abuse is associated with abnormal HPA axis function in adulthood; that is, early stress changes the adult brain. Finally, some women with a history of childhood abuse had lower basal cortical concentrations.

The Dexamethasone Suppression Test

One test of HPA axis function evaluates cortisol feedback inhibition using dexamethasone (Mann & Currier, 2012). As described in Chapter 10, the DST checks overnight changes in the level of the hormone cortisol in the blood. The patient's blood is drawn the night before at about 11 P.M. The patient then swallows a pill containing 1 mg of dexamethasone. At about 8 A.M. the next morning (and maybe also later in the day) another blood sample is drawn.

If depressed, the patient may hypersecrete the hormone cortisol when measured the next morning. Dexamethasone suppresses cortisol in nondepressed control groups. But dexamethasone does not suppress cortisol in some depressed patients (Maris, 2015). The DST has been studied in suicidal patients (Black & Andreasen, 2014).

Although ECT concerns treatment, there is evidence that ECT is more effective and quicker in boosting 5-HT levels in depressed patients than antidepressant medications are (Maris, 2015). (See Chapters 11 and 23 for more on ECT.)

Sociobiology

de Catanzaro (1986, 1992) has argued that suicide tends to occur in individuals experiencing severe coping impasses related to their sex, health, age, and social and reproductive potential. Sociobiology stresses biological fitness and reproductive capacity (cf. Joiner et al., 2017). As I have discussed briefly in Chapter 7, de Catanzaro created what he calls the "Ψ coefficient." Ψ is the residual capacity to promote inclusive fitness, or the capacity to act so as to promote your genes. A positive value for Ψ suggests more inclusive fitness and less suicide risk. A negative value for Ψ indicates less inclusive fitness and greater suicide risk. Consider these two examples:

- A polygynous male, age 25, with two wives but no nurturance behavior, would have a Ψ of 5.0.

---

[1] SERT or 5-HTT is known as the sodium-dependent 5-HT transporter. It removes serotonin from the synaptic cleft and enables its reuse by the presynaptic neuron.

[2] MHPG (3-methoxy-4-hydroxyphenylglycol) is a metabolite of norepinephrine degradation. Low levels of MHPG in the blood and CSF are associated with pathological gambling, for example.

- An infirm female, age 75, supported by her financially pressed daughter (who herself has to support three children), would have a Ψ of -0.5.

Ψ is calculated by $\Psi = P_i + \Sigma k \, b_k \, p_k \, r_k$, where p_i is the remaining reproductive potential of i; p_k is the remaining reproductive potential of each kinship member; b_k is a coefficient of benefit or cost to the reproduction of each k by the continued existence of i; and r_k is the genetic relatedness of k to i.

Neurogenesis

In the earlier discussion of the mechanisms of SSRIs, I have commented that medications like Prozac are *neurogenic* or *neurotropic* (Maris, 2015, p. 42). For example, if rat brains are examined with an electron microscope before and after administration of megadoses of Prozac, there are actually more neurons in the rat brains afterwards. BDNF and neurotropic growth factor (NGF) are both relevant in this discussion. BDNF is a candidate gene for several mental illnesses and for suicide (Black & Andreasen, 2014). For example, BDNF is a potentially vulnerable gene for schizophrenia. We know that progressive brain tissue loss occurs in some people with schizophrenia and shows an association with bipolar disorder (Black & Andreasen, 2011). Genes that regulate plasticity may also play a role in schizophrenia (Black & Andreasen, 2011). Neurogenesis is inhibited in mice under stress (Mann & Currier, 2012) and increases, if mice receive weeks of antidepressants like Prozac. BDNF may also be related to suicide outcomes (Mann & Currier, 2012, p. 491). There is evidence that exercise is related to neurogenesis (especially in the hippocampus) and can improve memory (van Praag et al., 2005).

Biotechnical Procedures

In addition to ECT, there are several less proven "seductions of technology," as Carlat (2010) calls them, in psychiatry. Some of these procedures include vagus nerve stimulation, transcranial magnetic stimulation, bilateral cingulotomy, and various imaging procedures. After reviewing these procedures, Carlat (2010) concluded that the primarily viable alternative (or cotreatment) to psychopharmacology is psychotherapy (described in Chapter 24), not the biotechnical treatments now described.

Vagus Nerve Stimulation

Vagus nerve stimulation is a procedure developed by Cyberonics for treatment of depression in which the vagus nerve (the 10th cranial nerve, in the neck) is connected to a wire and a battery (external or internal). The device gives a 30-second burst of electricity every 5 minutes; treatment times are adjusted by the therapist. The FDA approved this procedure in February 2005. Vagus nerve stimulation may alter norepinephrine and/or elevate GABA. However, vagus nerve stimulation has not been proven effective, and the device costs about $25,000.

Transcranial Magnetic Stimulation

On October 10, 2008, the FDA approved transcranial magnetic stimulation for depressed patients who had at least one prior failure of antidepressant treatment (Carlat, 2010; cf. Weisman et al., 2018). The patient sits in a chair like a dentist's chair, and the left frontal cortex is targeted by magnetic pulses for 30 minutes of treatment a day, for 10–20 total treatments over 4–6 weeks. The evidence of efficacy is unimpressive. At $300–400 per treatment, the out-of-pocket expense for the patient is about $10,000.

Bilateral Cingulotomy

The classical lobotomy severed frontal lobe nerve tracts to help calm agitated patients. In 1948 a new procedure was developed: severing supracallosal fibers of the cingulum bundle to target the anterior cingulate cortex. The treatment was intended for extreme, persistent OCD (e.g., constant hand washing), refractory depression, and chronic pain. After imaging studies, carefully positioned electrodes were put into the patient's brain thorough burr holes. Lesions were then made either by heating electrodes or by using lasers. The biggest problems with cingulotomies are permanent brain damage risk and undemonstrated effectiveness.

Imaging

It should be noted in passing that today there are several imaging techniques that can be used on the brain primarily for diagnostic purposes, but not so much for treatment. These include magnetic resonance imaging (MRI) and functional MRI (fMRI; e.g., for tracing blood flow), computed tomography (CT) scans, positron emission tomography (PET), and single-photon emission computerized tomography (SPECT).

Most imaging in psychiatry is used to rule out conditions like brain tumors, anatomical abnormalities, strokes, and regional blood flow problems. Some psychiatrists have claimed that they can diagnose psychiatric disorders by observing a patient's brain scans, but these claims are not convincing (Carlat, 2010). Nevertheless, the brains of psychiatrically disordered patients are often significantly different structurally from those of healthy controls, and may need to be examined unobtrusively. For example, the brains of patients with chronic schizophrenia may have ventricular enlargement, increase in the CSF in their ventricles, and decreased frontal lobe size (Black & Andreasen, 2014).

This chapter completes Part IV of this book. The chapters in Part V examine religion, culture, history, art, and ethics in relation to suicide.

RELIGION, CULTURE, HISTORY, ETHICS

CHAPTER 17

God, the Afterlife, Religion, and Culture

For those who have laid mad hands upon themselves, the darker regions of the netherworld receive their souls, and God, their father, visits upon the posterity the outrageous acts of the parents. With us it is ordained that the body of a suicide should be exposed unburied until sunset.

—JOSEPHUS

Religion can be defined as belief in and reverence for a supernatural power or powers as creator and governor of the universe, or as a set of beliefs, values, and practices based on the teachings of a divine being or spiritual leader, such as God, Jesus Christ, Adonai/Yahweh, Moses, Allah, Muhammad, Krishna, or Buddha (*American Heritage College Dictionary*, 2010). In some religions it is considered irreverent even to speak the name of God, and certainly one should never speak ill of God. Beliefs and practices are revealed in each religion's scriptures (e.g., the Bible for Christianity, the Torah for Judaism, the Qur'an for Islam, the Bhagavad-Gita for Hinduism, the Tripitaka for both Theravada and Mahayana Buddhism) and through prayer, meditation, or revelation.

For followers of most world religions, being religious protects one against suicide (Walker et al., 2018). Only God can give or take a life. Suicide is usually considered offensive to God, because it involves the "sin" of hubris or pride. God's wishes or plans for us can be inscrutable; they may even include suffering, as in the Judeo-Christian book of Job, and often are different from our own plans. You will recall from Chapter 8 (see Table 8.1) that predominantly Catholic (such as Mexico, Italy, and the Philippines), Jewish (Israel), and Muslim (Syria, Egypt, Libya, and Saudi Arabia) countries tend to have very low suicide rates. However, as we shall see, many religious cults in effect are death cults and do not protect one against suicide. Cults like Jonestown, Heaven's Gate, David Koresh's Branch Davidians, and the Solar Order are exceptions to the rule that religion is a protective factor against suicide.

Early in the history of Judaism and Christianity, suicide was not forbidden (van Hooff, 2000). For example, the Old Testament records the suicides of Samson (suicide as revenge) and Saul (defeat in battle), and the New Testament describes those of Judas (betrayal or shame) and perhaps even Christ himself (self-sacrifice for a higher good). Josephus records the mass suicides of 960 Jewish men, women, and children who killed themselves at Masada to avoid capture by the Romans (see below). It was not until St. Augustine's *The City of God* (completed by 426 A.D.,) and the Roman Catholic Councils of Arles (452 A.D.,) and Braga (563 A.D.,) that the commandment "Thou shalt not kill" or "Thou shalt do no murder" in the books of Exodus and Deuteronomy was interpreted to include self-murder. In fact even homicide was appropriate in very specific situations, such as if one was engaged in a holy war. Later in this chapter, I comment on the Muslim concept of *jihad*. Many people do not realize that in general, suicide is strongly condemned in the Muslim religion.

Most world religions contend that we are not alone here on earth, that we are not fully in charge of our own lives, and that God has plans or purposes for us. Religions typically teach that our 70–80 years on earth are not all there is. We may survive the death of our physical bodies and live on as souls, spirits, or disembodied minds, or we may even be reincarnated physically (however, Nietzsche claimed: "In heaven all the interesting people are missing"). Hindus assert that we may be reborn into this world (see their classical concept of transmigration of souls or *samsara*), and Buddhists argue that our physical bodies are not our true (*atman*) selves.

Religion as an institution typically concerns itself with death and the meaning and purpose of life. In many religions the goal of earthly life involves spiritual development, which transcends earthly flesh-and-blood existence. In a sense, then, part of the *false self* has to die or be transformed in order for a person to achieve or be granted spiritual maturity—for example, in heaven, the afterlife, *nirvana,* or *moksha* (i.e., in spiritual enlightenment and fulfillment). In most religions, suicide increases the prospect of going to a hell-like place, condition, or otherwise being punished. So for most of those who are religious, suicide does not resolve their problems, but rather makes them worse. If people are evil, selfish, deluded, lack faith, accumulate bad *karma*, or sin, then they cannot escape by suiciding; they may not enter into a good afterlife.

Although there are many world religions, here I mainly talk about Protestants, Catholics, Jews, Muslims, Hindus, and Buddhists. Typically Protestants tend to have higher suicide rates than Jews, followed by Catholics. Muslims have very low suicide rates. Martin Luther believed in the concept of a "priesthood of all believers." Thus Protestants typically assume greater individual responsibility for their own salvation and resolution of their daily problems than, say, Catholics do. Catholics are more communal and protected by ritual, such as the catechism, communion, saying the rosary, and going to mass frequently. They thus tend to find suicide, as well as abortion, euthanasia, and capital punishment, more abhorrent on average than Protestants do. Jews tend to be a little less protected against suicide than Catholics, but a little more protected than Protestants.

Unfortunately, there are few empirical studies of religion and suicide. One reason for this is that the U.S. Census Bureau and the Department of Vital Statistics are forbidden by the U.S. Constitution from asking about one's religious behaviors or opinions. However, my 5-year sample survey of Chicago suicides included questions about their religion (Maris, 1981). I now turn to some of the Chicago data on religion and suicide.

Empirical Findings on Religion and Suicide Rates

What do data about religion and suicide tell us? The short answer is that religion does tend to protect people from suicide, both individually and collectively; however, there is not a simple causal connection. There are variables, suicide risk and protective factors, other than religion involved and religious protection from suicide varies with the type of religion.

Much of the suicide and religion data are confounded by culture and ethnicity, such as the suicide rates (see Table 8.1) in countries that are predominantly Catholic, Protestant, Jewish, Muslim, Hindu, and Buddhist. Such data are inconclusive. For example, Hungary and Austria tend to have high suicide rates, but are predominantly Catholic (68% and 90%, respectively). However, the Philippines (ranked 150th out of 172 countries) and Mexico (ranked 137th out of 172) are also predominantly Catholic, but have low suicide rates (WHO, 2012, 2015c). How can Catholic countries have both high and low suicide rates? Clearly, the Catholic religion alone does not protect one against suicide. There must be other nonreligious risk factors or variables affecting suicide outcome.

We see a similar empirical pattern in predominantly Protestant countries. For example, Finland (ranked 33rd out of 170 countries) and Sweden (ranked 58th of 170 countries) are mainly Protestant, especially Lutheran, countries and have relatively high suicide rates as predicted. But Norway, which is also mainly Lutheran, has a relatively low suicide rate (ranked 81st out of 170).

The suicide rates of countries with a mainly Buddhist religious history include Japan (and Shinto), which has a high suicide rate (ranked 17th out of 170 countries), and South Korea (but 41% Christian), which has the second highest suicide rate in the world. China (which has the most Buddhists worldwide, even though Buddhism originated in India), however, has a modest suicide rate (ranked 94th out of 170). Only Muslim countries tend to have consistently low suicide rates (see Table 8.1). For comments on suicide and religion (Hinduism) in India, see Farberow (1975) on *sati, suttee, karma,* reincarnation, and so forth. India has a high suicide rate (11th of 170), especially among young females in rural areas. If we gloss over the subtleties and inconsistencies just described in the religious data, Protestants tend to have high suicide rates, followed by Jews and then by Catholics with lower rates. Muslims tend to have the very lowest rates.

As an aside, when I was a WHO Fellow in Berlin, Germany, I investigated Jewish suicides in Berlin during World War II (Maris, 1981). Table 17.1 shows data found in the Weissensee cemetery in Berlin (cf. MacRandle, 1965). There seems to be a strong correlation between increasing Jewish persecution by the Nazis and Jewish suicides during World War II. However, the data are not clear. One of my honors students did research on Jewish suicides in Nazi concentration camps, and she found that Jewish suicides there were relatively low, although other data sometimes

TABLE 17.1. Jewish Suicides in Berlin's Weissensee Cemetery, 1940–1945

Year	Number of Jewish suicides buried in the cemetery
1940	59
1941	254
1942	811
1943	214
1944	34
1945	2

Source: Maris, Ronald W. with Bernard Lazerwitz. *Pathways to Suicide: A Survey of Self-Destructive Behaviors.* Copyright © 1981 The Johns Hopkins University Press. Reprinted with permission of Johns Hopkins University Press.

show the opposite. She concluded that in the camps the main motivation was getting enough to eat. If you did not, then dying was easy.

In the sample survey of suicide in Chicago, I was able to get data on religion and suicide (Maris, 1981) and then compare it with similar data for New York City. Table 17.2 shows that overall in both Chicago and New York City, Protestants had the highest suicide rates, especially older white male Protestants. Protestant suicide rates were followed by those of Jews and Catholics, in that order. As Durkheim (1897/1951) predicted on the basis of his social integration theory of suicide, Protestants in general have the highest rates and Catholics the lowest rates of suicide,

TABLE 17.2. Suicide Rates (per 100,000) by Religion, Age, and Sex in Cook County (Chicago) and New York City (Controlled for Race)

Locality, religion, and race	≤ 24		25–44		45–64		≥ 65	
	M	F	M	F	M	F	M	F
Cook County								
White Protestants	25	12	16	10	28	13	40	14
White Jews	22	–	15	–	28	–	26	–
White Catholics	13	7	11	8	16	6	24	8
New York City								
White Protestants	47	19	46	17	42	22	62	20
White Jews	18	15	15	12	15	15	27	19
White Catholics	15	7	10	6	16	8	30	11

Note. Based on 1,056 white suicides in Cook County (Chicago, Illinois, 1966–1968) and 2,975 white suicides in New York City (1963–1967). Percentages rounded off to whole numbers.
Source: Maris, Ronald W. with Bernard Lazerwitz. *Pathways to Suicide: A Survey of Self-Destructive Behaviors.* Copyright © 1981 The Johns Hopkins University Press. Reprinted with permission of Johns Hopkins University Press.

while Jewish rates usually are somewhere in the middle. He did not study Muslims. In the data shown in Table 17.2, Protestant and Catholic males had suicide rates about twice those of females of the same age, but in the oldest age group (65+), male suicide rates exceeded those of females by a ratio of about 3:1. Jewish male suicide rates were about the same as those of females, except in the oldest (65+) age group.

In other Chicago data not presented here, Chicago Protestant and Catholic males preferred firearms for suicide; Protestant women preferred poisons and over-doses. Catholic women preferred hanging in Chicago, but poisoning in New York City. Suicide by jumping from heights was much more common in New York City across all religions and genders. Maltsberger (1998) says that jumping accounts for 20% to 40% of all suicides in New York City.

Of course, religious affiliation or preference is not the same as religious activity or behavior. In data not shown here, nonfatal suicide attempters and suicide completers were much less likely than those dying natural deaths to attend church every week. Table 17.3 further shows that all suicides, regardless of religious preference or gender, were less likely to attend Christmas services than was the general non-suicidal population. Also, the ratio of those attending services among Protestant and Catholic males was about 2.2:1 for the general population versus suicides (see boldface type in Table 17.3).

To conclude, there is some empirical evidence that religion does protect against suicide. Protestant males have the highest suicide rates and are the least involved in religion; Catholic females have the lowest suicide rates and are the most involved religiously. Data for African Americans, religion, and suicide show similar religious patterns to those of European Americans (Walker et al., 2018; Nisbet, 1996; Early, 1992).

Nevertheless, as I argue below, if the norms, values, or objectives of a religion are pro-suicide (such as in some cults), then obviously religion or social integration in the cults does **not** protect one from suicide—in fact, it does just the opposite.

TABLE 17.3. Church Attendance at Christmas by Sex and Religion for Suicide and Nonsuicidal (General) Samples in Cook County, Illinois (Percentages of Whites Only)

Church services last Christmas?	Protestant males[a]		Protestant females[b]		Catholic males[c]		Catholic females[d]	
	General	Suicide	General	Suicide	General	Suicide	General	Suicide
Did *not* attend	53	52	54	50	20	43	7	31
Did attend	**45**	**19**	44	46	**80**	**36**	93	45
Don't know	2	29	2	24	0	21	0	24
Total	100	100	100	100	100	100	100	100
	(n = 125)	(n = 57)	(n = 249)	(n = 69)	(n = 101)	(n = 72)	(n = 151)	(n = 51)

Note. For explanation of boldface, see chapter text.
[a]$z = 2.1, p < .05.$
[b]$z = 1.0,$ not significant.
[c]$z = 4.5, p < .001.$
[d]$z = 6.0, p < .001.$

Religious Cults and Mass Suicides

Religion does not always protect us against suicide. Mass suicides in religious cults are good examples of religion greatly *increasing* suicide risk. Here are a few examples of religious groups that were essentially death cults (Maris, 1997a):

- A mass suicide at Masada (a high plateau in Israel) in 72–73 A.D., was described by the Romano-Jewish historian Josephus. About 960 Jewish men, women, and children killed themselves to avoid capture by the Romans. Many, especially the children, were murdered by others in the group. John Mann, a physician and suicidologist at Columbia who is an Orthodox Jew, told me (personal communication) that the Talmud (a commentary on the Jewish scriptures) also records the mass suicides of approximately 200 young men and 200 young women in a similar incident. Suicide in order to avoid capture or after defeat in battle was fairly commonly mentioned in the Torah and Talmud.
- Perhaps the best-known mass suicide took place on November 18, 1978, when between 908 and 914 followers of evangelist Jim Jones drank cyanide and depressant-laced Kool-Aid. A few members of the cult were shot or shot themselves, including Jones himself. This event took place in a remote compound in the jungle of Guyana, South America, called Jonestown (see the data on the high suicide rate in general in Guyana in Chapter 8).
- Heaven's Gate was the mass suicide of 38 cult members in San Diego, California, on March 26, 1997. They were led by Marshall Applewhite.
- On April 19, 1993, 85 members of David Koresh's Branch Davidian cult killed themselves in Waco, Texas. The Waco deaths were a combination of suicides, homicides, and accidents. Most of the cult were burned to death, but up to 22 of them were shot (including Koresh), either by themselves or by agents of the FBI or the Bureau of Alcohol, Tobacco, and Firearms (*Fort Worth Star-Telegram*, May 12, 1993).
- On October 6, 1994, the Associated Press reported the suffocation, gunshot, and burning suicides of 48–53 members of the Order of the Solar Temple in Switzerland. There were 16 more immolation suicides by solar cult members in France on December 24, 1995.
- As a mass suicide aside (not a cult), about 200 of the 3,000 people who died on September 11, 2001 at the World Trade Center jumped or fell to their deaths. Interestingly, all of these deaths were classified as homicides, not suicides (Joiner, 2005).

Let us look in greater depth at two of the most famous of these mass suicides, Jonestown and Heaven's Gate, and then try to summarize what characteristics religious cults that encourage such suicides tend to have in common.

Jonestown

Jim Jones grew up in Indiana. His mother believed that he would eventually become the Messiah. Jones's father, on the other hand, was a bigot, racist, and Ku Klux

Klan member; this is noteworthy, since most of the cult members at Jonestown were African Americans. Jones went to Butler University in Indiana and originally was a Methodist minister. Later, Jones abandoned mainstream Christianity. He performed many faith-healing "miracles," which were actually cheap tricks, such as producing chicken entrails while supposedly purging ill people of their cancers. Jones founded his cult, called the People's Temple, in Indianapolis in the 1950s, but later moved it to San Francisco.

Many members of the People's Temple were poor, uneducated African Americans who signed over the deeds to their estates, homes, or life insurance policies to Jim Jones. Family members began to protest to Congressman Leo Ryan about losing their estates, property, money, and birthrights to Jones.

Partly to escape this ill will, Jones and his cult members fled to Guyana, in north central South America. As just noted, the country of Guyana has one of the highest suicide rates in the world; see Table 8.1. In Guyana, Jones and his cult were isolated, and the cult became even more extremist. For example, Jones came to believe that the world would be destroyed soon by nuclear war (the apocalypse or "end of days"). Jones grew increasingly paranoid, especially when one of his co-leaders, Grace Stoen, defected and exposed Jones for the charlatan he really was. Jones had fathered a son with her, and she later sued Jones for custody of their son.

The cult lived in crowded conditions, in temperatures often exceeding 100 degrees Fahrenheit with high humidity. There were physical beatings and promiscuity, particularly by Jones. Jones practiced a form of terrorism reminiscent of the novel *1984* (Orwell, 1949), in which children and spouses were encouraged to spy on other family members and then tell Jones. Jones chastised or severely beat transgressors. Spouses were often forbidden to have sex with each other, but Jones himself had sex with married females in the cult.

Jones thought that the end of the world was imminent. To prepare, Jones had drills called "white nights" in which cult members were asked to drink Kool-Aid, not knowing whether it was poisoned. Drinking it proved their faith in and loyalty to Jones and his cause. Jones decided that on November 18, 1978, over 900 (one estimate was 909) men, women, and children would commit mass suicide.

Heaven's Gate

A second suicidal religious cult was Marshall Herff Applewhite's and Bonnie Lu Nettles's Heaven's Gate. These two founders of the cult were originally from Houston, Texas. Applegate had been an opera singer, choir director, and college music teacher with an MA in music from the University of Colorado. He was the son of a Presbyterian minister. Bonnie Lu Nettles was a nurse and astrologist; she died of cancer in 1985. In the cult they were known as Bo (Marshall) and Peep (Bonnie).

Taking their scriptural foundations from the Christian Book of Revelations, Applewhite and Nettles believed in human metamorphosis. Their idea was that that the human being could "metamorph" (change into something or someone else) through ascetic discipline, hard work, and strict dieting and evolve to life in a higher kingdom. To prepare for this journey, the cult members had to give up alcohol, tobacco, sex (males were castrated), most material possessions, and regular jobs. In San Diego, they supported the cult financially by becoming webpage design-ers. They believed that spiritual salvation resulted from fasting and hard work.

Applewhite believed that if they prepared correctly, they could undergo what he called "chrysalis," being transformed like caterpillars into butterflies. During an interview, Applewhite said he could disappear and then reappear. When the interviewer said, "Show me," Applewhite strained, tensed up, and got red in the face—but, of course, did not disappear. The theory was that perfected cult members would become enlightened and able to alter their "vibration rates," allowing them to disappear from sight and then reappear at will.

Applewhite thought that he had come to earth in a spaceship (a UFO) and only woke up to his real-life mission in his 30s. Cult members contended that when they suicided, there would be bodily (not just spiritual) transformation. They believed that their perfected bodies would rise to a higher level and be transported to a spaceship hidden in the tail of the Hale–Bopp comet. They interpreted the appear-ance of the comet as a sign to them that it was time (the "apocalypse") to suicide.

The Heaven's Gate cult claimed that when we leave this world through ritual suicide, we are "harvested." Applewhite maintained that the world was nearing a cataclysmic crisis ("eschatology") and was about to be "recycled." Thorough ritual suicide, Heaven's Gate cult members felt they would escape this world (which was a sinking ship) just in time to be saved.

On March 26, 1997, 38 members of the cult committed mass suicide in San Diego (Rancho Sante Fe), California. Dressed all in black and wearing Nike sneak-ers, the cult members poisoned their bodies according to Humphry's (1991/1996) suicide method. Their elaborate death ritual included draping their bodies in shrouds, putting $5 in quarters in their pockets for "long-distance calls," and hop-ing to be transported to a spaceship.

Common Characteristics of Suicide Cults

Among the common characteristics of most of the mass suicides listed above (with a few exceptions, such as those who jumped to their deaths from the burning World Trade Center) are the following. First, the groups that encouraged these suicides were religious cults. More specifically, these suicidal societies tended to be *altruistic* (in Durkheim's sense). That is, being a member of the cult meant being willing to sacrifice oneself or die for the sake of a higher good. This is reminiscent of Japa-nese officers committing *seppuku* in front of their assembled troops, or of *kamikaze* pilots flying their planes into allied ships. Durkheim correctly observed that being socially integrated into some religious groups did *not* protect one against suicide, since the norms of these religious groups favored suicide in many circumstances. In Jonestown (contrary to Durkheim's theory), the more social integration, the higher (not lower) the suicide rate.

Second, in most suicide cults, the intentions of a charismatic leader are crucial (e.g., those of Jim Jones, David Koresh, and Marshall Applewhite). Most cult leaders have a diffuse concept of self. We know that both Jones and Koresh had sex with many of the women in their cults, sired many children in the cult, and often for-bade the women's own husbands to have sex with their wives. In a very literal sense,

Jim Jones was the *father* of his cult; he was in fact implanting his own genes in cult members. It follows that for either Jones or Koresh to kill himself, he probably felt he had to kill his extended family—that is, the entire cult. The cult leader, in effect, decides for everyone else that they will suicide. The leader's intentions or beliefs are paramount.

Third, there is usually a perceived danger to the cult or persecution from the outside. For example, Jones did not order the mass suicides at Jonestown until Congressman Leo Ryan of California came to Guyana with his entourage to investigate the People's Temple. In Masada the stimulus for mass suicide was the Roman soldiers, and in Waco it was the presence of the federal agents that seemed to trigger the suicides.

Fourth, the cults tend to become isolated from the rest of larger society. Jones and his followers left California for Guyana. This reminds us that suicide is a "transformation drive" (Hillman, 1977). That is, suicides do not want so much to die as to change or transform themselves, their lives, or their world. Routinely in death cults, the physical body is not held in very high regard. The soul or spirit is central, and often it is required that one must renounce the physical body in order to get into heaven, achieve *nirvana* or *moksha,* or achieve another religious transformation.

Finally, in almost all mass suicides there is coercion or even murder, especially of children or of cult members who try to escape rather than suicide, as was the case in Jonestown.

Jihad, Suicide, and the Muslim Religion

Muslim countries typically have very low suicide rates. For example, in Table 8.1 (WHO, 2015c), the female suicide rate in Syria was 0.2 (per 100,000) and the male rate was 0.7 (although given the civil war there, these data may be inaccurate). In Saudi Arabia, females had a rate of 0.2 and males a rate of 0.6 per 100,000. In Egypt the female suicide rate was 1.2, and that of males was 2.4. Are these extremely low suicide rates accurate, or are they reported low for political and religious reasons? If they are accurate, is that the result of cultural and religious forces? In this section I ask: What do the teachings of Islam say about suicide? If Islam usually forbids suicide, then how can *jihad* be allowed? Some of these issues are now examined with special reference to the main holy text of the Muslims, the Qur'an.[1]

Islam and Suicide

Many recent terrorist attacks around the world involving suicide bombers have been carried out by Muslims (cf. Lankford, 2009, 2013). Generally Muslims believe that out of all the bounties that Allah (the name of God for Muslims) has bestowed on human beings, the most precious is the gift of life. Since Allah has granted life to Muslims, it is not their own personal possession or property. Humans are no

---

[1] I wish to acknowledge the helpful assistance of Adnan Omar, a Muslim PhD student of mine from Malaysia, in the researching and writing of this section of the chapter.

more than trustees of life, and they must use their every living moment to worship and praise Allah.

Islam is unambiguous about its prohibition of suicide. In Islamic law there is a direct injunction against suicide. The Qur'an (all quotations from the Qur'an are from the Abdel Haleem [2004] translation) states:

> "And, do not kill yourself. Surely, Allah is the Most Merciful to you. Whoever does so in transgression and wrongfully, we shall roast him in the Fire, and that is an easy matter for Allah" (Qur'an 4:29–30).
> "And do not throw yourself in destruction" (Qur'an 2:195).

Similar prohibitions against suicide can be found in the Sahih al-Bukhari—the traditions (sayings, words, practices) of the Prophet Muhammad (all quotations from these are from Khan, 1995):

> "The Prophet said: 'and whoever commits suicide with a piece of iron, will be punished with the same piece of iron in the Hell-Fire'" (Sahih al-Bukhari, Vol. 2, Hadith 441).
> "The Prophet said: 'A man was inflicted with wounds and has committed suicide, and so Allah said: My slave has caused death on himself hurriedly, so I forbid Paradise for him'" (Sahih al-Bukhari, Vol. 2, Hadith 446).

Islam and *Jihad*

The primary meaning of *jihad* to the ancient Arabs is, surprisingly to many Westerners, not "fighting" or "killing" (the Arabic *qital* conveys that meaning). The word *jahada* (*jihad* being the associated noun) means "to toil, to become weary, to struggle, to strive after, or to exert effort." For example, the derivative *ijtihad* means "effort" or "diligence." A survey of the Qur'anic usage of the verb *jahada* shows its more general connotation:

> "And for those who strive hard [*jahada*] for Us, We shall certainly guide them in our ways, and Allah is surely with the doers of good" (Qur'an 29:69).
> "Then do not obey the unbelievers, and strive for a great striving [*jihadan*] against them [*jihadhum*] by it [the Qur'an]" (Qur'an 25:52).

This last verse occurs in a passage telling Muslims to make use of the Qur'an when they dispute with non-Muslims (cf. Taymiyyah, 2001).

In short, the concept of *jihad* embodies an action that a Muslim must take to struggle against evil as he or she lives life. Unfortunately, in the current political climate, the concept of *jihad* has wrongly become synonymous with "holy war" or "religious war." The meaning of *jihad* as "holy war" is foreign and not from Islam. Muslims are commanded to fight an inner spiritual struggle as well as to fight on the battlefield (such as for self-defense), because both struggles are considered doing *jihad* in the cause of Allah. The Qur'an states:

"And what is the matter with you that you do not fight in the cause of Allah and for those weak, ill-treated, and oppressed among men, women, and children whose only cry is: Our Lord, rescue us from this town whose people are oppressors and raise us from one who will protect and raise us from one who will help" (Qur'an 4:75).

The traditions of the Prophet Muhammad point to the fact that *jihad* is not just (or even mainly) fighting on the battlefield. It is generally believed that *jihad* can be done by at least three methods: with the heart (intentions or feelings), with the hands (such as with weapons), and with the tongue (speeches, writings, etc.):

"Narrated by Abu Hurairah the Prophet said: 'The best *jihad* is by the one who strives against his own self for Allah, the Mighty and Majestic'" (Sahih al-Bukhari, Vol. 4, 104).

This is an eloquent summary of the view that an individual's earthly life is an unremitting personal struggle.

Therefore, Muslims believe that since life is the most precious gift from Allah and since they are the trustees of life, they must perform *jihad* (internally as well as externally) as they live their daily lives. In the Muslim doctrine, *jihad* is the utmost respected action and the most rewarded act of worship. The reward is Paradise:

"Let those who fight in the cause of Allah who sell the life of the world for the Hereafter, and the one who fights in the cause of Allah, and then who is [either] slain or attains victory, we shall give him a mighty reward" (Qur'an 4:74).

The confusion exists when *jihad* is perceived to mean "holy war," "martyrdom," or "suicide bombing." Suicide, killing, or waging wars against innocents is strictly forbidden. The Qur'an states:

"If anyone killed a person not in retaliation for murder or to spread mischief in the land, it would be as if he had killed the entire humanity, And (likewise if anyone saved a life, it would be as if he saved the entire humanity" (Qur'an 5:32).

Qur'anic passages make it quite clear that fighting is allowed in self-defense or to help victims of tyranny or oppression who are too weak to defend themselves:

"Fight (*qatilu*) in Allah's Cause against those who fight against you (*yuqatilunakum*), but do not commit aggression, for truly, Allah does not love aggressors" (Qur'an 2:190).

"But if the enemy inclines toward peace, then you (too) incline towards peace, and trust in Allah, Truly He is All-Hearing, All-Knowing" (Qur'an 8:61).

It is significant that these passages occur in the second *surah* (chapter), which is believed by many Muslim scholars to be a recapitulation of the Qur'an's major themes. The Qur'an's attitude toward war is cautionary, circumspect, and yet realistic. One finds little Qur'anic support for the use of aggression to force non-Muslims to accept Islamic rules.

In summary, Islam completely prohibits suicide and waging warfare against innocents or most individuals. *Jihad* to Muslims encompasses the very essence of their living. Life must not only be preserved to the utmost, but also must be used to worship God through a continuous struggle at all levels of living. *Qital* (warfare) is allowed in some areas, but must be fought with religious, moral, and ethical caution.[2]

Religion, the Afterlife, and Concepts of Death

One of the basic functions of religion as an institution is to help individuals come to terms with death and dying. It is predicted here that how one conceives of death will be related to outcomes of suicide (completed and attempted) versus natural death. Do not forget that suicide is a form of problem solving, although it usually is not the best solution. Some tormented individuals in physical and emotional pain for many years could conclude that they might be better off dead. At least then their pain would stop (if there is no afterlife), albeit perhaps at the price of nothingness. This raises the question of what it means to die and how religion is related to death.

The topic of death is central to all world religions. Religions tend to assert that there is an afterlife of some sort, and that biological cessation does not imply cessation of the soul, spirit, or consciousness. To oversimplify, most religions claim that if individuals do good works, follow the religions' scriptures and God's commandments, and avoid selfishness and evil, then their souls at least are more likely to go to some type of heaven or positive afterlife. On the other hand, if people are not religiously compliant, do not follow God's expectations, are selfish, and so forth, then it is more likely that they will have a hellish afterlife.

If suicide is an anathema or sinful in God's eyes, then suicide is not problem solving. Suicide merely results in a kind of "out of the frying pan and into the fire" situation, perhaps one of eternal damnation and punishment. If there is an afterlife and the person goes to hell, then suicide geometrically compounds problems; it does not resolve them.

Although there are no data on concepts of death by religion, there are data from my Chicago research on how those who died natural deaths (from cancer, stroke, heart disease, etc.) conceived of death, compared to suicides and nonfatal suicide attempters (Maris, 1981). I hypothesized that that suicides would tend to conceive of death more favorably than nonsuicides would (cf. Joiner, 2005, p. 136, on "the desire for death"), since the suicides actually chose death over life.

---

[2]Obviously, I am not an Islamic scholar, and although Mr. Omar was the principal of a Muslim school in Malaysia, we would defer to those who are more qualified than we are for any unintended misinterpretations or citations of the Qur'an.

These Chicago data are presented in Table 17.4. Several differences among suicide completers, nonfatal suicide attempters, and natural death controls in relation to their concepts of death are worth noting.

First, suicide completers (89%) were much more likely than either attempters (51%) or natural death controls (68%) to conceive of death as "escape from pain and suffering." These differences were statistically significant (at the .001 level). This seems to suggest that the suicide completers saw death as more of a problem-solving method.

Second, both suicide completers (45%) and attempters (59%) were more likely than those dying natural deaths (34%) to conceive of death as "the end of it all" or nothingness. Thus, suicidal groups might tend not to fear punishment in the afterlife, if they died by suicide.

Third, both the completers (45%) and the attempters (41%) were much more likely than the natural death controls (12%) to dream about death, even though the controls in fact were closer to having to die. Death was probably more on the minds of the suicidal groups. In fact, people who suicide are more likely to have nightmares than nonsuicidal groups are (Joiner, 2005).

Fourth, the completers (14%) were about two times less frightened (see being "fearless" of death, per Joiner, 2005, p. 86) of death than the natural death controls (23%) were, and people who attempted but did not complete suicide were much more afraid of death (42%). Note that about 86% of the completers were not frightened about death. Thus completers were more likely to choose death, and nonfatal suicide attempters (who did not choose death) were three times more likely to be afraid of death. Perhaps this fear contributed to their avoidance of suicide.

Fifth, the completers were more likely to see suicide as "revenge on someone else" (25%) than either the natural death controls (2%) or the nonfatal suicide

TABLE 17.4. Concepts of Death by Suicide Completers, Nonfatal Suicide Attempters, and Natural Death Controls (Percentages Responding "Yes")

Concepts of death	Natural deaths	Attempted suicides	Completed suicides
Escape from pain or suffering	51	68	82
Punishment of self, damnation	5	23	9
Revenge on someone else	2	16	25
Nothingness, the end of it all	34	59	45
Is an afterlife, not the end of it all	63	54	59
Something talked about frequently	19	33	18
Something dreamed about	12	41	45
It is frightening	68	42	14
Other (not the eight concepts above)	68	67	22
Total number of cases	71	64	266

Note. Informants could respond "Yes" to more than one concept of death. Thus column entries do not total 100%.
Source: Maris, Ronald W. with Bernard Lazerwitz. *Pathways to Suicide: A Survey of Self-Destructive Behaviors.* Copyright © 1981 The Johns Hopkins University Press. Reprinted with permission of Johns Hopkins University Press.

attempters (16%). The motivation of revenge might thus have given the completers added incentive to die by suicide.

Sixth, the completers (9%) were much less likely than the attempters (23%) to see death as "damnation" or "punishment." Perhaps this contributed to the attempted suicides' being nonlethal.

Finally, the completers were much more likely (78%) to conceive of death in terms of one or more of the eight concepts listed in Table 17.4 than were the attempters (33%). That is, their views of death were more clearly characterized by these eight concepts than they were by other concepts.

Do concepts of death relate to suicide? Yes, the Chicago data seem to suggest that suicides are more likely to see death as an acceptable way out of their pain and suffering than nonsuicidal groups are. Of course, suicide outcomes are much more complicated (e.g., involve other variables) than what concepts of death alone might suggest.

Cultural Variations in Suicide

One serendipitous fact about suicide is that in some groups it is low to virtually non-existent, such as in the Muslim countries just discussed, among African American females (Walker et al., 2018, and Chapter 6 here), in the Tiv of Nigeria, and perhaps even among Irish Catholics (however, see Caollai, 2014). However, in other groups, it is so common that it is almost part of their national or group character, such as in Russia, South Korea, Hungary, Austria, Japan, and Finland, as well as among older white males in the United States. This empirical difference among groups, nations, or societies reminds us that suicide varies culturally.

That which is *social* usually refers to the reciprocal relations of interacting human beings. *Culture,* on the other hand, refers to patterns of behavior, thought, and feeling that are acquired or influenced through learning, and that are characteristic of groups rather than individuals. The emphasis in the cultural study of suicide is on shared products of social activity, especially on values and norms.

According to Marvin Harris (1971; Harris & Johnson, 2006), "A culture is the total socially-acquired life way or life style of particular groups of people." Language is a particularly important component of a group's life style, but culture includes much more than language. For example, Tylor (1871) claims: "Culture . . . is that complex whole which includes knowledge, belief, art, morals, law, custom, and any other capabilities and habits acquired by man as a member of society." Thus, religious beliefs and practices constitute an important part of a group's culture. Usually religion connotes the part of culture that deals with ultimate issues of life and death, the meaning or purpose of life, ethics and rituals related to the good life (as revealed in scriptures), magic and superstition, and the maintenance of hope and social order.

Most cultural or anthropological studies of suicide have focused on basic values or social types in societies, such as those reflected in French sociologist Emile Durkheim's (1897/1951) four main types of suicides: *egoistic, anomic, altruistic,* and *fatalistic* (see Chapter 7). *Egoistic* suicide has its origins in excessive individuation, social isolation, or lack of involvement with other people. *Anomic* suicide is thought to originate in a disruption (usually sudden, like a stock market crash) of the external and constraining power of social norms (*a-nomia* or "without norms"). *Altruistic* suicide is characterized by insufficient individuation. For example:

> Instead of apathy, we find energy and activity . . . the altruistic suicide tends to find the basis for existence beyond this life. Altruistic suicide was common among the North American Indians and Polynesians, Its primary attribute was duty (to a higher cause). A good example of altruistic suicide is the custom of "*suttee*" in India in which the wife was socially "obligated" to kill herself after her husband died. (Maris, 1969, p. 34)

Finally, *fatalistic* suicide refers to suicide stemming from excessive regulation, such as suicides among prisoners.

Most of the cultural studies of suicide refer to altruistic suicide types. The Japanese kamikaze pilots in World War II are an excellent example of altruistic suicide. In another example, the Gisu of Uganda are expected to suicide, if other means of alleviating problems are unsuccessful. I conclude this chapter with four examples of the role of culture in suicide.

* One famous case of suicide in the ethnographic literature is that of a 16-year-old Trobriand islander named K'ma'i (Malinowski, 1926). K'ma'i had broken the rules of exogamy by having sexual relations with the daughter of his mother's sister (his cousin). This behavior was tolerated until his cousin's rejected lover publicly accused K'ma'i of incest. Under these conditions, it was expected that the accused would suicide. Accordingly, the next morning K'ma'i dressed himself in festive attire and then climbed to the top of a 60-foot palm tree. There he bade the community farewell, explained the reason for his suicide, launched an accusation against the discarded lover who had driven K'ma'i to his death, and then amidst a loud wailing jumped from the tree to his death. A fight followed in the village, during which K'ma'i's rival was wounded.

* Another example of predominantly altruistic suicide is that among the Yuit of St. Lawrence Island (Leighton & Hughes, 1955). Among the Yuit, one does not kill oneself alone. The custom is to ask a family member at least three times to help with the suicide. At first the family member is expected to refuse this request. However, if this request is repeated at least three times (similar to getting a divorce among Orthodox Jews), the relative is expected to honor the wish of the would-be suicide. The Yuit are a hunting and gathering society, and hunting and killing are highly valued. If a family member is infirmed or injured and not able to hunt, then that person becomes a burden for the family. Among Yuit hunters, the ultimate killing is of oneself. Thus, suicide is an indication of courage, wisdom, and respect for those whom the person's infirmity puts at risk.

Before the suicide, the victim dresses as if he or she were already dead: The clothes are turned inside out, with the fur side of the clothing against the skin. If possible, the victim walks unassisted to "the destroying place." There the victim addresses the surviving relatives, saying that they will be able to care for themselves after the death, and then gives a brief statement of his or her philosophy of life. Then either the wife shoots her husband (or vice versa), or a number of relatives hang the victim. The latter method of death is particularly unpleasant, since it may take up to 30 minutes for the victim to die, and the victim may defecate and urinate on the hanging site. Usually there is a period of isolation and purification for those who have participated.

 • There are other examples of culture and suicide that are more ego-anomic (see Firth, 1961). For example, among the Tikopia (a Polynesian community in the western Pacific), the suicide rate has always been relatively high (50 per 100,000). The Tikopia believe that to take one's life is merely to anticipate what will inevitably happen anyway. Whether or not risking one's life actually results in suicide depends on many contingencies, such as the status of the suicide attempter or the degree of enthusiasm in rescue attempts. Suicide does not violate any religious prescriptions or norms. The methods of suicide reflect the geography and lifestyle of the Tikopia. Young women swim out to sea, and young men put out to sea in a canoe.

 • Once it is known that someone is attempting suicide, the search and rescue effort is usually immediate and enthusiastic, particularly if the attempter is of high social status. However, rescuers will not go out beyond the sight of land. Thus, most serious suicide attempters are not found, if they leave secretly and paddle steadfastly out to sea. If (another contingency) a suicide attempter loses sight of land but returns, or if the attempter is rescued before losing sight of land, then he or she is completely reinstated within the community; all is forgiven by everyone. Other contingencies in suicide include the changeable natural forces of wind, sea, and storms, which also affect the level of enthusiasm of the rescue effort. If weather conditions are unfavorable, and if the community feels the attempter should suicide, then their efforts to rescue him or her may be less.

Anomie has been found to be a distinguishing trait of many Japanese suicides (Iga, 1993). Iga contends that few Japanese suicides since World War II have been obligatory or altruistic suicides. There is not much egoistic suicide either, since conformity and dependency are widespread traits among young Japanese. New economic opportunities since World War II have reduced fatalistic suicides. This leaves primarily anomic suicide, which is characterized by unrealistically high aspirations resulting from weakening social restraint, and even a sense of greed and jealousy.

This brief sojourn into cultural variations in suicide has been far from exhaustive (see also Chapter 8 and White, 2014). The intention has been to call attention to the values and meanings that selected cultures have given to death and suicide. Depending on cultural differences, social and psychological forces may have very different influences on suicide among different peoples of the world.

In Chapter 18, I turn to how the concept of suicide has evolved over time by examining suicide in history and art.

CHAPTER 18

Suicide in History and Art
How Did Suicide Evolve?

> Why did human civilization begin somewhere between
> 40,000 and 45,000 B.C., but our first graphic depiction
> of suicide was not until about 540 B.C.?
>   —ANTON J. L. VAN HOOFF

History and art are rare topics in suicide books. However, I am including works of art depicting suicide in this chapter, to remind readers of the historically ubiquitous nature of suicide and self-destruction. Giving self-destruction a historical context helps us avoid suicidological myopia. As Santayana says, those who forget the past are often doomed to repeat it. Much of very early civilization is simply unknown or uncodified, but most societies we know about allowed some form of self-inflicted deaths. Under rare circumstances, suicide could be preferred to life; it might even be required in some conditions, such as soldiers giving up their lives in battle or after defeat in battle, infirm hunters and gatherers suiciding so as not to jeopardize the welfare of other family members, or persons ending their lives as a last resort to avoid intolerable pain and suffering.

The word *suicide* was first used in English by Sir Thomas Browne (1642) and Walter Charleston (1651) (Maris, 1993). It is derived from the Latin *suicidium,* to kill one's self or "*felo de se.*" See also *mors voluntaria* in Latin and *heukousios thanatos* in Greek. Shneidman (1993, p. 137) has defined suicide as "the human act of self-inflicted, self-intended cessation." Worldwide, suicide is rare, but fairly ubiquitous. Box 18.1 lists a sample of famous suicides.[1] The list reveals that suicide is democratic and widespread. It encompasses many different cultures and nationalities from 399 B.C. to 2012. These suicides include men (mainly), and women, young and old (mainly). The study of suicide often focuses on the celebrated because more is known about celebrities. One has to be careful in doing so, however, since celebrity suicides may be different from noncelebrity suicides.

---

[1]See also *https://en.wikipedia.org/wiki/List_of_suicides,* which contains at least 750 suicides.

BOX 18.1. Selected Famous Suicides

- Ryunosuke Akutagawa (1927, Japanese writer, *Rashomon* author)
- Ricky Berry (1989, NBA Sacramento Kings basketball player)
- Bruno Bettelheim (1990, American psychoanalyst and World War II concentration camp survivor)
- Eva Braun (1945, wife of Adolf Hitler for 24 hours, cyanide poisoning, she had prior suicide attempts)
- Brutus (42 B.C., assassin of Julius Caesar)
- David Carradine (2009, U.S. actor, *Kung Fu* and *Kill Bill,* autoerotic asphyxiation in a hotel room)
- Seung-Hui Cho (2007, Virginia Tech mass murderer, then suicided)
- Cleopatra (30 B.C., Queen of Egypt, self-induced snake bite)
- Ray Combs (1996, host of *Family Feud* TV show)
- Dorothy Dandridge (1965, U.S. actress and singer, first black female nominated for an Academy Award for Best Actress)
- George Eastman (1932, founder of Eastman Kodak, his suicide note said: "my work is over, why wait?")
- Kurt Gödel (1978, German mathematician)
- Joseph Goebbels (1945, Nazi propaganda minister)
- Hannibal (182 B.C., Carthaginian military commander)
- Adolf Hitler (1945, Nazi leader)
- William Inge (1973, U.S. playwright)
- Yasunari Kawabata (1972, Japanese Nobel Prize writer)
- Jerzy Kosiński (1991, Polish American writer)
- Primo Levi (1987, Auschwitz camp survivor and author)
- Meriwether Lewis (1809, U.S. explorer with William Rogers Clark, shot self, but lived for hours)
- Jack London (1916, U.S. novelist, *The Call of the Wild* author)
- Joseph Merrick (1890, Britain's "Elephant Man")
- Donnie Moore (1989, relief pitcher for California Angels)
- Cesare Pavese (1950, Italian poet and writer)
- Freddie Prinze (1977, Puerto Rican comic in TV's *Chico and the Man*)
- George Reeves (1959, U.S. actor, played Superman on TV)
- George Sanders (1972, English actor)
- Junior Seau (2012, San Diego Charger all-pro NFL football linebacker with a history of traumatic brain injury)
- Anne Sexton (1974, U.S. poet)
- Anna Nicole Smith (2007, model)
- Jim Tyrer (1980, all-pro NFL tackle)
- Sid Vicious (1979, British musician with the Sex Pistols)
- Virginia Woolf (1941, British novelist)

Source: Original list by Maris. For a history of suicide in the cinema, see Stack and Bowman's *Suicide Movies* (2011).

In other countries and times, suicide has had low rates or been virtually unknown. Perhaps in extremely rare cases, a culture with low suicide rates might have few, if any, words for suicide. Here are some of these very-low-rate countries, cultures, or groups:

- Andaman Islanders (residents of an island in the Indian Ocean, near Burma and India).
- The Yaghans of Tierra del Fuego (an island at the southern tip of South America,, near Cape Horn).
- The Tiv of Nigeria.
- African American females.

The earliest human civilizations are usually said to be those that developed in Mesopotamia and Egypt around 3200 B.C. But far before that, humans used tools, made beads, created pigments, and engaged in organized warfare and hunting. Human civilization probably started in Africa around 44,000 B.C.[2] Cave paintings depict hand stencils, abstract colored signs, use of bows and arrows, drawings of animals, and stick figure humans, but none clearly illustrate any suicides. As we shall see later in this chapter, one of the earliest depictions of suicide in art—on a Greek vase dated 540 B.C.—was that of the legendary warrior Ajax falling on his sword after a public humiliation (and later for defeat in battle) . But this raises an interesting question. Were there no suicides in the 40,000 years before the Ajax vase, and, if so, why? Was suicide a luxury at a time when most people lived about 35–40 years and were preoccupied with avoiding death from predators, hunger, disease, or injury?

The Suicidal Animal[3]

Our primate ancestors started to evolve differently from gorillas and chimpanzees about 6 million years ago. Modern humans (*Homo sapiens*) first appeared in Africa between 200,000 and 100,000 years ago. Was there suicide in animal or precivilized hominid beings? For the most part, we simply do not know. Suicide requires willful, intentional self-destruction, not just instinctive self-destructive preservation of genes (such as sacrificing one's self for the sake of children or to preserve a species) or self-sacrifice (usually of male animals and insects) during copulation. A minimum level of self-consciousness and the ability to conceive of death as biological cessation are necessary preconditions to suicide. How can one know what an animal intended?

Nonhuman animal self-destructive behaviors can be seen in whales beaching and lemmings drowning themselves; Malaysian fire ants blowing themselves up for the good of the colony, and worker bees dying after stinging; male honeybees,

[2]There have been "uncivilized" humans on earth far before 45,000 B.C. For specific citations of books about more ancient suicide, see van Hooff (1998, 2000).

[3]I am indebted to van Hooff (2000), on whom I relied in rewriting this section.

male Australian redback (and other) spiders, and male praying mantises all dying after copulation; betta Siamese fighting fish and male lions destroying themselves in battle; rhesus monkeys biting themselves; dogs refusing to eat after their owners die; and many more (cf. Joiner, 2010, p. 204ff). But are these behaviors really suicide? Such self-sacrificial behaviors, even though adaptive (e.g., to perpetuate genes or ward off predators) are animal instinct, not willful, intentional suicide. Aside from refusing food, throwing oneself off heights, or drowning, most suicide requires tools as means of self-destruction. In Africa, where humans evolved, the overwhelming means of suicide was the noose or halter used to hang oneself (Bohannan, 1960). Thus suicide probably evolved in part as tools were created, such as ropes, poisons, firearms, high buildings, and knives that could be sharpened. Probably early hominids lacked both the necessary abstract self-awareness and the lethal means to commit suicide.

Suicide in Greek and Roman Antiquity

Suicide appears relatively late in the development of human civilization, although this may be due to prehistory's lack of a record. With the creation of tools like swords and knives for warfare, hunting, and agriculture, new means were available to commit suicide. Before then, self-hanging probably prevailed. In the relevant literature, about 40% of all suicides used swords, daggers, and knives (van Hooff, 2000, p. 98). Around 3500 B.C., swords were made of copper and bronze in Egypt. But it was not until around 800 A.D., that the traditional double-edged sword appeared.

Ajax

Self-killing in ancient Greece was called *hekousios thanatos* (voluntary death). Ancient Egyptians, Romans, and Greeks all allowed suicide in place of execution. The ancient prototypical suicide was probably that of Ajax. Ajax, who like his fellow warriors was probably a mythological figure, was heralded as the second greatest fighter in Greece at the time of the Trojan War (circa 1194–1188 B.C.). His strength and courage were second only to those of his more famous cousin, Achilles. During the Trojan War, Ajax recovered the body of Achilles and returned it to a Greek camp. Greek leaders then had to decide who would receive Achilles's armor. The final two candidates for the armor were Ajax and Odysseus.

Ajax then spoke, simply reporting his deeds, which included upholding the Greek cause on several occasions by fighting Troy's greatest champion(s). But when Odysseus spoke, he did so with great eloquence and won Achilles's armor. Ajax was infuriated and planned to murder his rival and the kings who wronged him, but in his distraught madness he instead hacked and slashed a herd of sheep. When he awoke, his head cleared, and he saw what he had done, Ajax was overcome with shame and fell on his sword rather than live in dishonor. Out of more than 100 Greek, Etruscan, and Roman representations of suicide, Ajax alone accounts for more than half that number (see van Hooff, 2000, pp. 100 ff.). Among the first

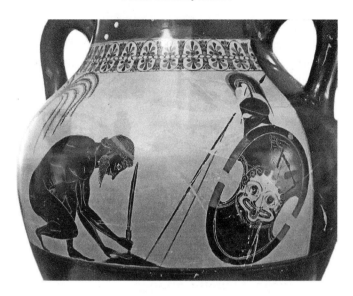

FIGURE 18.1. Suicide of Ajax. *Source:* Musée Boulogne-sur-Mer, Boulogne, France. Photo by Ptyx.

visual references to suicide is Ajax preparing to fall on his sword, as depicted on the vase shown in Figure 18.1.

Socrates

Socrates's death circa 399 B.C. was immortalized in one of Plato's *Dialogues* ("Phaedo"). Socrates's death was an execution, not actually a suicide. He was sentenced to die for corrupting the youth of Athens and introducing new, strange gods. Plato can be seen in Jacques Louis David's famous oil painting *The Death of Socrates* (1787, now displayed in the Metropolitan Museum of Art in New York City), sitting at the foot of Socrates's deathbed (although in actuality Plato was young at the time, not old).

Although his death was an execution, Socrates calmly (stoically) accepted his sentence by voluntarily drinking the hemlock, a poison that he knew would kill him. Note that the organization promoting assisted suicide in California and Oregon, founded by Derek Humphry (1991/1996), was originally called the Hemlock Society. In theory, Socrates was opposed to suicide. Socrates saw death as a separate actual realm, different from life, but not the end of being.

Lucrece (Lucretia)

The Roman female counterpart to Ajax was Lucrece (Lucretia in Latin). From 1430 until 1922, over 150 artists painted her stabbing herself to avenge her rape by Sextus Tarquinius, son of the Roman despot Lucius Tarquinias Superbus, in 509 B.C. The artists included Botticelli, van Cleve, Hans Holbein the Elder, Rembrandt, and

Raphael. There is also a poem by Shakespeare titled "The Rape of Lucrece," published in 1594. Lucretia became a model of the heroic female suicide: using suicide as a means to preserve honor, morality, and social justice, and to avoid shame. Her death caused a revolt and led to the establishment of the Republic.

Dido

Another heroic female suicide who inspired over 50 paintings was Dido. When her brother Pygmalion killed her husband, Acerba, Dido took her husband's treasures, sailed to Africa, and built the city of Carthage. She was the first queen of Carthage. Dido became renowned throughout Africa for her courage and feminine leadership. When she was asked to remarry, she resolved her loyalty and conflicts related to her deceased husband by suiciding (see Figure 18.2).

Ixtab, Mayan Goddess of Suicide

Mayan civilization began circa 2600 B.C. in Central America. From about 200 to 800 A.D., the Mayans had a goddess, Ixtab, who presided in the afterlife over those

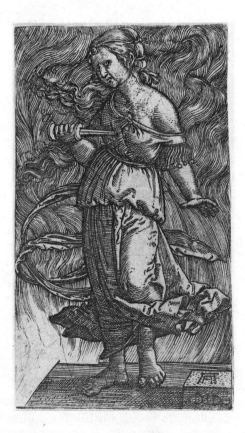

FIGURE 18.2. *The Suicide of Dido. Source:* Courtesy National Gallery of Art, Washington, D.C. Image is in the public domain.

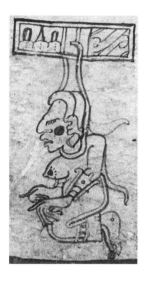

FIGURE 18.3. *Ixtab, Goddess of Suicide. Source:* Saxon State and University Library, Dresden.

who died by suicide (usually by hanging). This Yucatec goddess would accompany suicides, those who died in battle, sacrificial victims, women who died in childbirth, and members of the priesthood to a paradise under the shade of a pleasant tree (Yaxche), where they would have ample food and drink and be free from want. Ixtab was portrayed as a woman with a noose or rope ("Rope Woman") around her neck (see Figure 18.3). She typically had a black ring on her cheek to symbolize decomposition.

Heart sacrifice (death by removal of the heart) was a common Mayan custom in which the best, strongest, and most beautiful young women were sacrificed to appease a god. Although others carried out the sacrifice, these deaths were technically suicides, since the women consented to the ritual. To be chosen was an honor, which resulted in special favors for the eventual suicides, sometimes for up to a year before the sacrifice.

From Christ to the Middle Ages

The Judeo-Christian scriptures depict about seven to nine men and one woman dying by suicide, with various motives. These include Samson (revenge); Saul and his sword bearer, as well as Abimalech and his sword bearer (military defeat or battle; see van Hooff, 2000, p. 105); Achitophel; Zimri; one of the Macabee brothers (and his mother); Judas Iscariot (shame for betraying Jesus); and perhaps even Christ himself (self-sacrifice for a higher good). The Talmud (a commentary on the Torah) also notes a mass suicide similar to Masada, as mentioned in Chapter 17.

The commandment "Thou shalt not kill" or "Thou shalt do no murder," early on, was not interpreted to include suicide. The Bible is matter-of-fact about the suicide of Judas Iscariot (he "went and hanged himself"; Matthew 27:5) and all the others. In the British Museum, there is an ivory casket panel of Judas's hanging himself. The casket dates to about 450 A.D., By the time of St. Augustine (354–430 A.D.),

"Thou shalt not kill" was interpreted to include both homicide and suicide. The first known Christian prohibition of suicide by a Roman Catholic Council does not occur until 454 A.D., (Council of Arles) and again in 563 A.D., (Council of Braga).

Christians seemed to believe that some suffering was instructive and even necessary. It built religious character and could be God's will. Suicides were thought to commit the sin of *hubris* or pride, in putting their individual human desire to die over God's life plan for us, including trials and tribulations. The Catholic Church could deny Christian burial to suicides (van Hooff, 2000), and it still regards suicide as a grave sin. As we have seen in Chapter 17, Muslims also severely condemn suicide except in rare, strict *jihad* conditions.

Early Modern Times (16th and 17th Centuries)[4]

The 16th and 17th centuries included the periods of the Renaissance, the Protestant Reformation, the Roman Catholic response to the Reformation, and the Baroque. Thomas More (1477–1535) was a representative of the Renaissance in northwestern Europe. In his *Utopia* (the word literally means "Nowhere"), members of the ideal state are expected to care for the weak. More wrote:

> However, those who suffer from incurable diseases that are accompanied by continuous pain are urged by the priests and magistrates not to endure their sufferings any longer. . . . But they dishonor a man who takes his own life without the approval of the priests and senate. They consider him unworthy of decent burial and throw his body unburied and disgraced into a ditch.

Thus, in More's ideal society, proper suicide required approval or sanction of the church and state. When More was jailed in the Tower of London, as a devout Catholic he rejected suicide as an option. While in jail More wrote "A Dialogue of Comfort against Tribulation," in which he adhered to the traditional view that thoughts of suicide were inspired by the devil.

By contrast, Michel de Montaigne (a French essayist who lived from 1533 to 1592) came down on the side of human autonomy and not the Church's control. He wrote, "The most voluntary death is the finest. The wise man is not one who lives as long as he can, but as long as he should."

The plays of William Shakespeare (1564–1616) mention suicide 14 times. Lady Macbeth's suicide occurs offstage, but Shakespeare stages the suicides of Othello, Brutus, Antony, Cleopatra, Romeo, and Juliet. Romeo and Juliet's suicides represent death (suicide) for or because of love. Juliet, upon learning of Romeo's exile, says: "Come, cords, come, nurse, I'll to my wedding-bed,/And death, not Romeo, take my maidenhead!" (III.ii.136–137). Hamlet's famous soliloquy is a contemplation of suicide: "To be or not to be, that is the question: / Whether 'tis nobler in the mind to suffer / The slings and arrow of outrageous fortune, / Or to take arms against a sea of troubles, / And by opposing, end them. To die, to sleep—" (III.i.55–59).

---

[4]Again, I am indebted to van Hooff (2000), on whom I relied in rewriting this section and the two following sections.

In the early modern period, for the first time, people tried to find rational explanations for the act of suicide. For example. Robert Burton (1577–1640), in *The Anatomy of Melancholy* (1621), attributed suicide to an excess of black bile and the imbalance of the four bodily humors or fluids. These fledgling rational causes of suicide, however, did not influence how most suicides were treated. The corpses of suicides were still dragged through the streets on a sledge, displayed and hanged on gallows, and denied burial in a churchyard; a pole could even be driven through a suicide's body to prevent the self-murderer from arising from the grave.

The major figures of the Protestant Reformation were Martin Luther (1483–1546), from whose work the Lutheran religion developed, and John Calvin (1509–1564), whose teachings gave rise to the Presbyterian Church. Luther had been an Augustine monk and adopted the Catholic view that Satan was behind the act of suicide. Luther wrote to his wife (July 10, 1540) that the devil was active in Eisenach in inciting people to suicide. However, Luther refused to regard a suicide's soul as condemned forever. If men were driven by melancholy or madness, then they were not responsible for their actions. John Calvin did not discuss suicide directly, but he did say in 1536 that Judas's loss of hope was not real remorse and was "no better than [a] kind of threshold to hell." In Calvin's doctrine of predestination, an individual's future was foretold regardless of his actions. Those who opposed Calvinism argued that this doctrine led to melancholy and a tendency to suicide.

The Roman Catholic theologian Juan Caramuel (1606–1682) wrote *Theologia Moralis Fundamentalis* (1656). Caramuel argued that the commandment "Thou shalt not kill" included both homicide and suicide. He then went on to discuss four cases of suicide. In the first case, Caramuel repeated that "nobody is allowed to kill himself." But if the person suicides in delirium, he or she does not sin. In the second case, Caramuel was asked to pass a verdict on the corpse of a priest who thought he had three heads and strangled his real head while trying to remove the two imaginary heads. Caramuel opined that the priest acted from illness and deserved Christian burial. The third case also involved mania and delirium, and it too was not thought to be sinful. The fourth case concerned a priest who suffered from chronic masturbation and hated himself because of it. The priest hanged himself and left his Bible open to Job 7:15, "So that my soul chooseth strangling, and death rather than my life." When his body was found, it was disfigured and dumped into a river.

The Czech Jan Amos Comenius wrote *Orbus Pictus* (1658). Under the title of "Patientia," he said that "the impatient person . . . rageth against himself . . . at last despaireth, and becomes his own murderer." Samuel von Pufendorf (1623–1694) expounded on the Christian view that "No one gave himself life; it is a gift of God." Thus human beings cannot terminate their lives at their own pleasure or will.

John Donne (1572–1631) anticipated the Age of Reason. The first English defense of suicide was probably his *Biathanatos* (the title is a Greek word combining the concepts of "violence" and "death"), published between 1644 and 1647. Donne saw suicide as acceptable in some circumstances and made the heretical argument that Jesus Christ himself was a suicide. He wrote, "To me there is no external act that is naturally evil"; that is, the merits or demerits of the act depend upon the person's intention. Donne argued that the Christian martyrs, even Christ, were appropriate suicides. Martyrs sacrificed their lives for an excellent cause. However, most of his contemporaries saw Donne as heretical.

The Age of Reason (18th Century)

During the Enlightenment or the Age of Reason, there was a marked shift away from condemning suicide and its victims. If a person were *non compos mentis* (not in his or her right mind), then suicide could be excused and was not sinful. The old practices of desecrating the corpses of suicides were no longer carried out.

British philosopher David Hume (1711–1776), in his work *On Suicide* (1770), pointed out that suicide is not explicitly condemned in the Bible. However, the founder of Methodism, John Wesley (1703–1791), urged the British Prime Minister to discourage suicide by hanging the corpse in chains for all to see. Hume argued that if it is moral to disturb or avoid some operations of nature (such as the weather), then it is permissible (for example) to divert blood (exsanguination) from its natural course in human vessels. The French philosopher the Baron de Montesquieu (1689–1755) agreed with Hume. He claimed that life is given to us as a favor, and that we may return it the moment it is no longer a favor.

In 1723, a Dutchman, Jacob Weyerman (1679–1747), argued for the right of free disposition of one's life. Weyerman's view was this: "Let a bold man not stay so long the sparrow of death comes and munches on the overripe cherries." Like Thomas Joiner (2005) much later, Weyerman claimed that to end one's life is an act of courage and not easy to accomplish. These views paved the way for a reassessment of suicide in the French Revolution of 1789.

George Cheyne (1733) wrote in *The English Malady* that England was the country of suicide. Also, in the last decades of the 18th century, Prussia (now part of Germany) witnessed many cases of suicide: 136 drownings, 53 hangings, 42 suicides by firearms, and 8 throat cuttings. About half of these suicides were by soldiers. In 1774 Johann Wolfgang von Goethe (1749–1832) wrote a romantic novel about suicide, *The Sorrows of Young Werther,* which apparently caused several copycat or contagion suicides. The 18th century also saw the opening of many institutions for the mentally ill, as opposed to simply punishing suicides.

A late-18th-century (circa 1780) type of suicide in India was the institution of *suttee* or "widow burning," mentioned in earlier chapters. The faithful wife of a deceased husband was immolated (burned) on his funeral pyre or bier (she could also be buried alive or drown herself in the River Ganges), along with his other possessions (see Figure 18.4). This custom reflects the Indian/British law that a wife was part of her husband's property. The sacrificial wife could also atone for her husband's sins through *suttee*. The first mention of suttee is that of Sati, the consort of Shiva (so *suttee* is sometimes called *sati*).

The American television news show *60 Minutes* reported (in 1993) that a version of *suttee* still happens in modern India to avoid payment of dowries for female children (see *The New York Times,* December 27, 2000). Marriageable females can be burned. Female infanticide as well has been practiced in India, preceded by ultrasound imaging in clinics to determine the sex of the fetus.

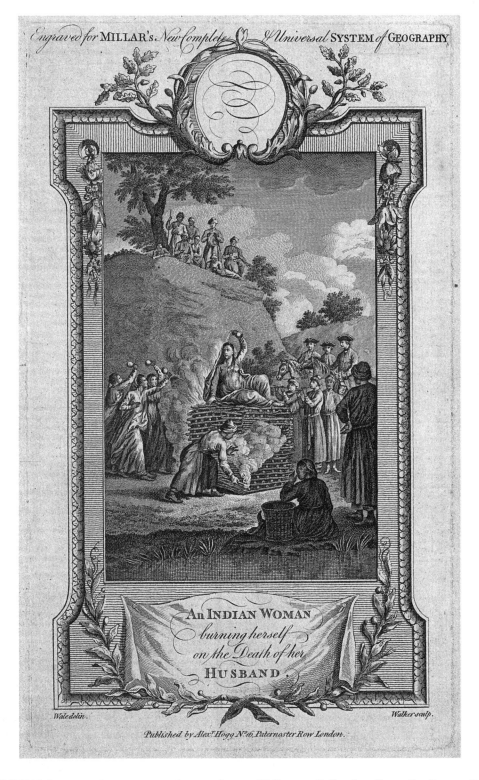

FIGURE 18.4. The Indian custom of *suttee. Source:* Wellcome Collection (*https://wellcomecollection.org/works/bxk6jd3e*).

Suicide in the Metropolis (19th and 20th Centuries)

The French Revolution for the most part abolished punishment for suicide. In England, burial of suicides at crossroads was ended in 1824, but from 1854 to 1961 suicide was still considered a crime in English law. Alvarez (1971) related a bizarre case in which a prisoner condemned to death slit his own throat the night before his execution. His wound was closed, and he was still hanged the next morning. But the wound opened upon hanging, giving him a makeshift tracheotomy. Punishment for suicide could still include estate fines, defiling the suicide's body, burying the body at a crossroad (ensuring perpetual unrest), and denying Christian burial. English law assumed that a death was not a suicide unless proven, a variant of "innocent until proven guilty." Thus, the law stated that a questionable or equivocal death was not by that fact alone a suicide. The plaintiff had to prove in court that a suicide did in fact occur.

In the 19th century, suicides came increasingly to be seen as ill sufferers, not as sinners. For the first time a medical doctor was called when there was a suicide, not a pastor. One big shift that began in the 19th century was industrialization, accompanied by a move from a relatively simple life in rural villages to major cities. People now lived in more stressful, competitive, faster-paced, and densely populated urban areas. Metropolises like London, Paris, Vienna, and St. Petersburg were considered to be unnatural and alienating. All of these major cities were notorious for their high suicide rates.

Innocent, naïve young women from the countryside moved to industrialized cities to find work. Many of them became anxious and emotionally disturbed (often depressed) by this strained new life in big cities. Some of these troubled young women drowned themselves in the Seine (in Paris) or the Thames (in London). Edith Wharton (1862–1937), in her 1905 novel *The House of Mirth,* describes a woman, Lily Bart, in search of an affluent husband in New York City. As Lily moves down, not up, the social ladder, she becomes unable to sleep or be calm; she takes a chance to sleep by using drugs, but instead dies from an overdose. This was a new historical pattern—gambling with drugs, resulting in accidental or suicidal deaths. In England in 1861, 7% of suicides were by drugs, but by 1911 drug suicides had doubled to 14%.

Another shift accompanying the Industrial Revolution (about 1760–1830) was that technological development changed the means for attempting suicide. Although early forms of guns had been around since 1364, the first Colt revolver was invented in 1835, and the first cartridge revolver in 1871. Pistols or revolvers became the suicide means of choice (see Chapter 9) for most modern suicides in the United States. In Europe, however, hanging rates remained higher than rates of gun use. Gunshot wounds to the head were also very lethal. Figure 18.5 shows Edvard Munch's (1864–1944) drawing of a man dead by gunshot on a sidewalk. Munch was an alcoholic Norwegian artist who painted several classic depressed, suicidal scenes; these negative images of the human condition included *The Suicide* (1896), *The Scream* (1893), *Despair* (1892), *Anxiety* (1894), and so on. Munch's drawings and paintings were depressive, cynical, and negative. Many of them have been used by suicidologists to illustrate the common mentality of suicides.

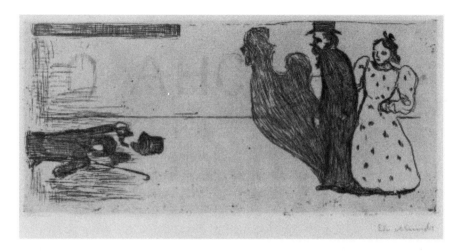

FIGURE 18.5. Edvard Munch, *The Suicide. Source:* National Gallery of Art, Washington, DC.

With the arrival of modern metropolises came the construction of multistory high-rise buildings, high towers, and bridges like the Eiffel Tower (completed in 1889, 324 meters high, 108 stories) in Paris, the Empire State Building (1931, 1,250 feet high, 102 stories) in New York City, and the Golden Gate Bridge (1937, 186–270 feet high) in San Francisco. I have noted in Chapter 9 (Table 9.2) that in the United States as a whole, about 5% of suicides jump to their death from high places, but in New York City about 40% of suicides jump (that's where the tall buildings are). See Andy Warhol's 1962 silkscreen print *Suicide (Fallen Body),* available from the Castelli Gallery in New York.

In the 19th and 20th centuries, we see for the first time in history the argument that urban mass society tends to make people sick and suicidal, such as that made by the Czech sociologist and statesman Tomas Masaryk (1850–1937). One of the founders of contemporary empirical suicidology, Emile Durkheim (1858–1917; see Chapter 7), argued that suicide has social causes. In Durkheim's view, what causes suicide is not so much the mental disorder, substance abuse, or other conditions of individuals, but rather failures of social integration or regulation. For example, *anomic* suicide is the result of the sudden disruption of social regulation (e.g., the 1929 U.S. stock market collapse). *Egoistic* suicide results from extreme individuation (e.g., being homeless in the inner city). Modern urban life tends to increase failures of both social integration and social regulation, which in turn increase the social suicide rate. *Altruistic* suicide, discussed in earlier chapters, results from self-sacrifice for a higher social good or cause rather than just personal troubles of the individual.

A good example of Durkheim's altruistic suicide in the Japanese ritual of *hara-kiri* or *seppuku* ("belly cutting"), originating in the 12th-century Samurai warrior culture. *Hara-kiri* signifies that the individual is dying for a higher or greater (usually social) cause (cf. the related acts of *kamikaze* pilots in World War II sacrificing their lives for the Emperor and Japan), such as loyalty to the Emperor or a leader, to atone for the shame of defeat in battle (there are airplane photographs by

American pilots of Japanese officers assembling their troops after defeat in World War II and committing *seppuku),* as self-punishment or execution, for their failure to accomplish an assignment, to express grief, and so on.

Rather than be captured, a defeated Japanese soldier would often stab himself in the left belly, draw the blade to the right, and then pull it upwards. Then he could pierce his own throat or have a colleague behead him after the stabbing. Obviously, *hara-kiri* is a very slow, painful death requiring great courage and resolve. Figure 18.6 shows a warrior about to commit the act.

A more recent example of *hara-kiri* is that of the Japanese writer and filmmaker Yukio Mishima, who killed himself in 1970 at age 45 (many Japanese suicides occur early in the life cycle, as opposed to late in life in the West). As described in Chapter 8, Mishima had his own private army take over a Japanese military base and assemble all the troops; he berated and lectured them for not following Samurai values, and then committed *seppuku* in front of them (one of his officers subsequently beheaded him). Mishima was runner-up (to Yasunari Kawabata) for the Nobel Prize in Literature and was a well-known millionaire, body builder, and actor in Japan. There were on average about 1,500 instances of *seppuku* per year in Japan until 1873, when the Emperor abolished obligatory *seppuku.* However, voluntary *seppuku* continues in Japan even today, as evidenced by the death of Mishima.

In Chapter 15, I have noted the prominence of drug overdose suicides among modern Western women. One example is the overdose suicide (or perhaps accidental death) of film actress Marilyn Monroe. Monroe was a tortured, troubled beauty queen and actress who overdosed on August 5, 1962, in Los Angeles. Some have claimed that Bobby Kennedy had her killed to silence her about their affair, but this seems far-fetched. Again, too, her overdose might have been accidental.

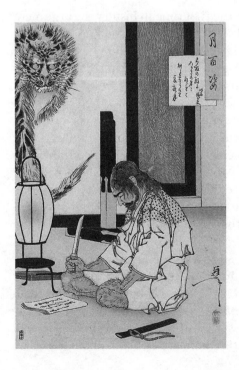

FIGURE 18.6. *Hara-kiri. Source:* Wiki Commons.

Monroe had overdosed or attempted suicide at least four times with drugs, but each time she had called for help and was rescued. Her toxicology report said she had the barbiturates Nembutal, Seconal, and chloral hydrate in her body at death. One account of her death states that she was found with her hand on, or reaching for, her bedside phone. Robert Litman, a famous suicidologist based in Los Angeles, did Monroe's psychological autopsy for Medical Examiner Theodore Curphey. I discuss Monroe further in Chapter 26 (Case 26.2).

Finally, H. C. Westermann's (1922–1981) sculpture *Suicide Tower* (1962), shown in Figure 18.7, summarizes many of the themes of suicides in the metropolis. This sculpture is thought-provoking about the nature of modern suicide. For example, it suggests ultimately that life leads to oblivion, that we are boxed in, and that life requires effort and achievement in a process of climbing up various ladders or steps. We cannot see what is coming; there is no escape from death on our life course; and life has many blind corners.

The Dark Side of Creativity

Throughout history several artists, comedians, writers, and performers have been especially self-destructive (Jamison, 1993, says that this is particularly true for poets). This raises the interesting question as to whether or not artistic creativity, fame, wealth, or success are related to suicide. In August 2007, comedian and actor Owen Wilson (known for his roles in *Wedding Crashers* [2005] and two *Night at the Museum* movies [2009, 2014]) made a serious self-cutting suicide attempt, which I discussed on *Good Morning America* (ABC Television, August 13, 2007). It seemed

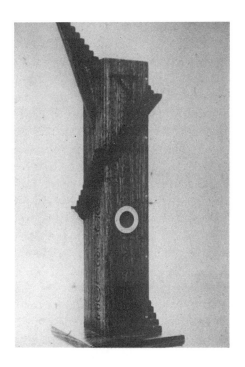

FIGURE 18.7. H. C. Westermann, *Suicide Tower.* *Source:* The Museum of Contemporary Art, Los Angeles. Art © Dumbarton Arts, LLC/ Licensed by VAGA, New York, NY.

on the surface that Wilson had a lot going for him. The next year (2008), actor Heath Ledger (*Brokeback Mountain* [2005] and *The Dark Knight* [2008]) overdosed and died (see Case 18.1), followed by Philip Seymour Hoffman (2014; see Chapter 15, Case 15.1) and Robin Williams (2014; see Chapter 12, Case 12.2). They were not alone. Other famous suicides are listed in Box 18.1 near the start of the chapter.

CASE 18.1. Heath Ledger

Heath Ledger was born April 4, 1979, in Perth, Australia, and died on January 22, 2008 in Manhattan of an accidental overdose of pain medications and benzodiazepines, which he took for sleep problems and an anxiety disorder. Ledger was best known for his role as The Joker in the 2008 film *The Dark Knight,* for which he received a posthumous Academy Award for Best Supporting Actor. Before that, Ledger was nominated for an Oscar for his role in the film *Brokeback Mountain* (2005). He got his big film break in the 2000 film *The Patriot,* in which he played Mel Gibson's son. Ledger said he slept on average about 2 hours a night and had a restless mind that he just could not shut down, even though he was physically exhausted. Ledger also tended to be a perfectionist and was always unhappy or dissatisfied with his performances. He said that he "never figured out who he was."

Source: Compiled by Maris from various public news accounts.

What, if anything, do the artists in Box 18.1 and in many of this book's cases have in common? Two traits jump out at us: mood disorder and substance abuse. Owen Wilson had been in drug rehab twice. Kurt Cobain (Chapter 26, Case 26.3) and John Belushi (Chapter 15, Case 15.2) had opiate abuse problems. Ernest Hemingway (Chapter 1, Case 1.1) and Styron were both alcoholics. Sylvia Plath (Chapter 6, Case 6.1) and Hemingway were both treated for major depression with ECT. Hoffman abused heroin.

A third trait of artists' suicidality is loss of boundaries (compare Durkheim's anomic suicide). With wealth and fame can come a loss of structure and restraint that helps keep us centered (perhaps such a loss is exemplified by golfer Tiger Woods's excessive money and his many extramarital affairs). Elvis Presley once told his personal pilot to rev up the jet at 2 A.M. so he could fly from Memphis to Nashville to get a peanut butter sandwich he especially liked. We cannot do whatever we like all the time without consequences, as Belushi's polydrug abuse on the *Saturday Night Live* set indicates. Novelist Kurt Vonnegut was fond of reminding us that we all live in our own "body bags"; that is, we have limits and boundaries that we cannot exceed whimsically without increasing our mental strain and even our risk of dying (see Klausner, 1968). Al Alvarez (1971), who had an affair with Sylvia Plath, was struck by how unbalanced Plath was at the end of her life and how obsessed she was with images of death and feelings of exaggerated anger just before she gassed herself in London.

Many rich and famous people (such as musical producer Bob Fosse; see the discussion of *All That Jazz* in Chapter 6) continually push their boundaries (e.g., through sexual acting out, substance abuse, and creative overwork, as Fosse did). But a metaphysical problem cannot be resolved physically. They may eventually start to come unglued and perhaps fall apart. Cutting oneself (as Owen Wilson did) tends to result in temporary tension reduction (see Kettlewell, 1999).

Notice that creative people often see the world differently than the rest of us do. One result of their uniqueness is a sense of profound isolation. How many people can get a Pulitzer or Nobel Prize, win an Oscar, or be billionaires? This isolation (being an "outlier") can lead to unstable interpersonal and sexual relationships and far-out ideologies. In May 2007, before that year's August suicide attempt, Wilson had broken up with actress Kate Hudson. Tom Cruise and John Travolta—who have had erratic personal lives, although neither has made a suicide attempt—are both believers in Scientology. If you don't have at least one other person who loves and sticks by you no matter what (like your mother, best friend, or partner), then it is difficult to live well—or to live at all, for that matter. As noted in earlier chapters, I call them "significant udders," to remind us of the image of total dependence on our surrogate mothers.

The life of an artist is often unstable, and like unstable vital signs, it can lead to death. Performing artists are often traveling often, living in strange places where they don't have what comedian George Carlin called "their stuff" with them. They can have bizarre ideas, and feel as if they are just one step away from disaster (in the form of a bad review, a failed movie, a divorce, a book that fell stillborn from the press, etc.). I am reminded of the behavior of the comedian Louis C. K. in his HBO comedy specials and his sexual inappropriateness which came to light in 2017.

Artists are often impulsive—a trait that may be tied to mood disorder and to neurobiological dysfunctions of brain serotonin, dopamine, and/or norepinephrine. When I first heard that Owen Wilson tried to kill himself, it was not surprising to me; in fact, for many artists, survival past 35–40 years of age is itself surprising. Wilson's scripted affect was very labile (think of his comedy movies with Jackie Chan or his film *Wedding Crashers*). It does not take very much for such exaggerated, slapstick comedic affect to swing to the opposite end of the mood continuum off camera. Wilson himself said that his humor was born of sadness.

To take another example, Vincent van Gogh (see Chapter 12) probably had bipolar disorder (Jamison, 1991). He painted starry nights and brilliant sunflowers only when he was having a manic episode. When he was depressed, he did nothing; except cut off his own ear, shoot himself in the stomach (of all places), or chase fellow artist Paul Gauguin around with a knife.

Suicide can represent both an effort at problem solving and a transformation drive: The suicidal person wants his or life to change, not necessarily to die. Many suicides just want to alter the conditions of their lives, even if they have to die to do so. Artists seem to "live on the edge" and sometimes just fall off. In a short film, a New Orleans cornet player was straining to hit high C. When he did, he just disappeared in a puff of smoke. Certain things you just cannot do repeatedly and expect to stay alive. In fact, that may even be the objective.

In Chapter 19, I consider ethical issues, euthanasia, and rational suicide. Is suicide ever the right thing to do?

CHAPTER 19

Ethical Issues, Euthanasia, and Rational Suicide
Is Suicide Ever the Right Thing to Do?

My mother said, "If I had life, I'd want it. I don't want this." My mother was naïve enough to think that once she made that decision—a decision that in her view was rational and reasonable, she would somehow be able to die. . . . For my mother life had become a trap, an imprisonment, and she managed to escape, but almost didn't make it. Physician after physician turned down our pleas for help

—DEREK HUMPHRY

Up to now we have assumed that suicide is always wrong or irrational, and thus something to be prevented. But can suicide be appropriate in some circumstances (Battin & Joiner, 2018)? Is there such a thing as *rational suicide* (Joiner, 2005, pp. 186ff; and 2010, pp. 70ff. and 192ff.)? Should we ever assist someone to suicide? Do our lives belong just to us, or also to those who love us or even to God? In his book *Final Exit* (1991/1996), Derek Humphry sidesteps crucial moral, ethical, religious, and philosophical issues that logically precede the mechanics of suiciding. For a fuller discussion, see my book review of *Final Exit* (Maris, 1992a).

A major ethical debate exists as to whether or not suicide is *ever* the right thing to do. I debated Humphry once in Washington, D.C., where he was accused by an angry young woman in the audience of causing the suicidal death of her college roommate. The roommate was found dead with an open copy of Humphry's recipe in her lap. Humphry's own state, Oregon, was the first state to legally allow assisted suicide in 1997. Even there, one has to be certified by a medical doctor as being "terminally ill" and within 6 months of natural death (plus meeting other conditions) to be permitted to obtain suicide assistance from a physician. However, I do not wish to do a disservice to Humphry. He is a sensitive, gentle, compassionate, bright man, attempting to confront an extremely complex, deeply ingrained controversy with a resolution that challenges many of our fundamental human values.

Another issue to be explored in this chapter is this: Can suicide ever be rational? Some people contend that *rational suicide* is an oxymoron (like *thunderous silence* or *jumbo shrimp*), in part because the mood disorders, social pathology (like Joiner's thwarted belongingness or perceived burdensomeness), impulsivity, agitation, intoxication, or even psychoses present in the vast majority of suicides preclude rationality. But I have argued (Maris, 1982) that suicide can be rational in some circumstances. This is an important topic that I examine closely later in this chapter.

A third major issue considered in this chapter is this question: Should physicians help their patients to suicide? Doctors helped their patients die long before Jack Kevorkian appeared on the scene. Many people do not realize that Viennese psychoanalyst Sigmund Freud's death (see Case 19.1, below) was a physician-assisted suicide. What is new is legalized, active euthanasia in several of the United States, the Netherlands, Switzerland, and Germany; for example, see the assisted suicide clinic in Switzerland, Dignitas (*http://dignitas.ch/*). We need to remember, though, that many physicians take the Hippocratic Oath, which obligates them to abstain from doing harm—a promise often rendered as "First, do no harm." Kevorkian (1991) went so far as to propose a new medical specialty that he called "obitiatry," devoted to physician-assisted suicide, which Kevorkian called "medicide."

Derek Humphry and Jack Kevorkian tended to focus on the mechanics and legal ramifications of assisted suicide, glossing over crucial ethical issues in their rush to provide lethal recipes and explain the technical practicalities of suicidal deaths. Before one decides to commit suicide, assisted or not, the important controversies raised above need to be considered carefully:

- Is suicidal death ever appropriate?
- Can suicide be rational?
- Can euthanasia and physician-assisted suicide ever be right?
- To whom do our lives belong?

Is Suicide Ever Appropriate?

Many people believe that suicide is never justified. For example, religious groups typically conclude that even though we all have to die eventually, none of us has to suicide (cf. the epigraph in Chapter 1). However, one has to question whether such dogmatic, rigid thinking is not overly simplistic and perhaps, because of that, irrational. At the other extreme, psychiatrist Thomas Szasz argued that suicide is an unalienable right of individuals, and in that sense suicide is always right (see Box 19.1).

To suggest that suicide may be right, ethical, or legal in certain circumstances raises the question of whether suicide is ever appropriate—and, indeed, of what might constitute an appropriate death. *Euthanasia* literally means "good death," which implies that there may also be bad or inappropriate death, or that some deaths (perhaps natural deaths) are more appropriate than others (such as suicides). Avery Weisman (see Kastenbaum, 1993) has defined an *appropriate death* as "a death that someone might choose, if he or she had a choice."

BOX 19.1. Psychiatrist Thomas Szasz on Suicide Prevention

- If suicide is not an illness . . . but an act of a moral agent, the only person ultimately responsible for it is the actor himself.

- . . . insofar as suicide is perceived as an undesirable act or event, people will insist on holding someone or something responsible for it.

- Psychiatrists now stigmatize suicide as much as priests did before them [see Chapter 17] . . . psychiatrists patronize their patients and promise more than they can deliver . . . psychiatrists ally themselves with the police powers of the state.

- A person cannot be held responsible for something he does not control. . . . This is why persons who want to assume control over others typically claim to be responsible for them [this is called *paternalism*].

- The physician is committed to saving lives. . . . He thus reacts . . . as if the suicidal patient had affronted, insulted, or attacked him.

- There is neither philosophical nor empirical support for viewing suicide as different, in principle, from other acts; such as getting married or divorced, working on the Sabbath, eating shrimp, or smoking tobacco.

- Insofar as suicide is a physical possibility, there can be no suicide prevention; insofar as suicide is a fundamental human right, there ought to be no such thing.

- . . . policies aimed at preventing suicide . . . imply paternalistic attitude toward the "patient" and require giving certain privileges to a special class of "protectors," vis-à-vis a special class of "victims."

- If the "patient" does not want such help and actively rejects it, the psychiatrist's duty ought to be to leave him alone.

Source: Notes taken by Maris from his 1985 debate with Szasz (see also Szasz, 1985).

An appropriate death might include several conditions' being met. For example:

1. The dying person should be free from pain as much as possible (if desired).
2. No unnecessary medical procedures should be performed, especially if they entail high risk for the patient and low gain.
3. The person should be allowed to die where and with whom he or she chooses.
4. If possible, interpersonal conflicts should be resolved.
5. Preparations for death should have been made, including good-byes (notes or person-to-person); funeral plans (obituary, music, in-ground burial or cremation, etc.); wills and other legal arrangements (e.g., power of attorney); financial arrangements (insurance policies, contact numbers and names, account numbers and lock box keys, accounts in beneficiaries' names, funeral home preferences and expenses, bills and debts paid, etc.).
6. The dying person should share control of the dying process with, or yield it to, trusted others—as Freud did to his doctor and his daughter Anna Freud (see Case 19.1).
7. The dying person should have the degree of consciousness desired.

8. The dying process should be the desired length of time, if possible (neither too short nor too prolonged).

9. The method of suicide should not be violent or disfiguring. (Humphry has advised using barbiturates and a plastic bag over one's head, and Kevorkian used pure carbon monoxide, not vehicle exhaust.)

10. If possible, death issues and choices should have the input of the dying person, not just a third party (such as a doctor or a relative).

CASE 19.1. Sigmund Freud

Freud [at age 82] had come to England [from Vienna to escape the Nazis] . . . "to die in freedom." But . . . [oral] cancer . . . had been his intimate enemy for fifteen years. . . . Not surprisingly, he was experiencing intervals of depression. . . . There were alarming signs that his malignancy was active once again. . . . Dr. Pichler from Vienna performed major surgery on September 8, 1939, followed by radiation treatments. . . . The man who distained medications . . . now lived on pain killers, like Pyramidon. . . . He wrote: *"Since September I have been suffering from pains in the jaw."*

Max Schur, his personal physician, established himself as a figure almost as central to his life as his daughter, Anna. . . . He disregarded Schur's advice to give up his blessed necessary cigars. . . . Freud's prosthesis was hard to put in and take out and the smell from his cancerous tissue . . . was most disagreeable. . . . On August 1 . . . Freud had closed his medical practice. . . . On September 21, as Schur was sitting by Freud's bedside, Freud took his hand and said to him, "Schur, you remember our 'contract' not to leave me in the lurch when the time had come. . . . Talk it over with Anna, and if she thinks it's right, then make an end of it." . . .

On September 21, Schur injected Freud with three centigrams of morphine. . . . Schur repeated the injection, when Freud became restless, and administered one final dose the next day, September 22. . . . He died at three in the morning, September 23, 1939. . . . [In a letter to a friend years earlier, he had written:] "I have one wholly secret entreaty: only no invalidism, no paralysis of one's power through bodily misery. Let us die in harness, as King Macbeth says."

Source: Excerpted by Maris from Gay (1988).

Death is seldom appropriate when something short of death would have resolved the individual's life problems or had the same effect. Each suicide has unique legal, medical, social, ethical, religious, and even political implications. Let us now examine some of these considerations.

Pain Control

Everyone has to die eventually, and many of us will suffer technologically prolonged disability and pain (even if treated) that may diminish the quality of our last days. Death is an effective but drastic means of pain control, if we assume that it entails a permanent annihilation of consciousness and that there is no afterlife. I speak here not just of physical pain, but also of psychological or emotional pain—Shneidman's "psychache"—which can be excruciating, too. Can pain always be controlled short of death? No, clearly not. Most opiate narcotics (like morphine, hydrocodone, and hydromorphone [Dilaudid]) risk respiratory death. Furthermore, pain medications often cause altered consciousness, panic, nightmares, transient psychosis, long periods of unconsciousness, nausea, constipation, and addiction, withdrawal, and dependency issues.

To be sure, pain control technology is progressing rapidly. Many hospices now use classical pain-killing drinks, similar to the well-known "Brompton Cocktail" (gin, chlorpromazine [Thorazine], cocaine, heroin, and sugar). It is also possible to block nerves or to use sophisticated polypharmacy (some localized, such as with implanted spinal pumps) to deaden pain. But some pain is relatively intractable, such as that involved in bone cancers, lung disease with pneumonia, emphysema, congestive heart failure, gastrointestinal cancers, amputation stump pain, and so on. Not everything can be fixed short of death. We do not always get well or feel better. Sometimes (as Freud said) we may need to die, not to be kept alive to suffer pointlessly just to please others. We deserve to be helped with our pain, even if it means dying.

Depression and Other Mood Disorders

Obviously, many people who suicide are clinically depressed and deserve effective antidepressant treatment or ECT before deciding to suicide. We have seen that as many as 90% of all suicides are mentally disordered, most with affective (mood) disorders. Over one-third of people with early Alzheimer's disease have major depression. A study in North Carolina of asphyxia by medications and a plastic bag over the head (one of Humphry's methods) revealed that 50–60% of them were clinically depressed (D. Radisch, personal communication, 2016). People probably should not suicide if their depression is temporary, treatable, or reversible. They owe it to themselves to reconsider such a monumental decision when they can see all the reasonable alternatives to suicide more clearly (Brandt, 1975; Battin & Mayo, 1980; Battin & Joiner, 2018).

But not all depressive illness is temporary. Most suicides have recurring depressive illnesses and eventually can become hopeless (both chronic depression and hopelessness are parts of a suicidal career). A person may be sad, even clinically depressed, if and when he or she decides to suicide. This does not necessarily mean that the depression caused the suicide, that the person could not think clearly, or that nonsuicidal alternatives had not been considered. Many people suicide after their depression or psychosis is ameliorated. Nevertheless, the concept of *terminal illness* probably should include emotional illness, not just physical illness.

Terminal Illness

Initiative 119 in the state of Washington in the fall of 1991 (Proposition 161 in California in 1992 was quite similar) permitted "aid in dying" to be provided for persons if (1) two medical doctors certified them to be within 6 months of a natural death (i.e., to be "terminally ill" or injured); (2) they were conscious and competent; (3) they signed a voluntary written request to die witnessed by two impartial, unrelated adults; and (4) their wish to die was enduring, persistent, and noncoerced. The first

Initiative 119 vote failed on November 7, 1991, with 54% against and 46% in favor (the first Proposition 161 vote also failed). However, as of 2018, assisted suicide is now legal in both Washington and California. In June 1990, when PBS discussed Jo Roman's suicide (see Roman, 1980/1992) after she contracted breast cancer, a live poll of viewers showed that 71% agreed that "suicide is sometimes justified when a person has a painful terminal illness." Roman's cancer was not terminal, but she suicided anyway.

When one is near death, life often lingers at great financial expense and psychosocial discomfort to the dying individual, the family, the hospital, and even larger society. With modern medical technology, many terminally ill patients are kept alive indefinitely (my own sister has been in a nursing home with Alzheimer's for about 10 years now), even though they are brain-dead, are in great pain, and/or have no realistic hope of recovery.

At first blush, it would seem easy to get help in dying. But clearly it is not. Doctors, nurses, hospitals, and family members are all often reluctant to help patients or loved ones die, given the complicated ethical issues and the many legal suits that can follow (e.g., consider the famous cases of Karen Ann Quinlan, Nancy Cruzan, and Elizabeth Bouvia). But why should we be forced to live, or to die slowly, expensively, and painfully, when we are ready to go as Freud was? Except in those states where it is legal, doctors, nurses, and family members currently have to sneak around at great personal and professional risk to help another human being die appropriately.

Religion

As we have seen in Chapter 17, most religions oppose assisted death or suicide (Battin, 1992). The argument is that God has an inscrutable plan or purpose for our lives, and that we should not interfere with it. A large part of the religious taboo against suicide has nothing much to do with the fact that someone dies. What is forbidden is to stand apart, to be separate—in short, to be a self-determining individual. What most religions object to is the *hubris* (self-centered pride) of a suicide. A few religions argue that suicide is a mortal sin that damns the soul, and perhaps even the body, to eternal suffering in the afterlife (like Dante's *Inferno* or a Hieronymus Bosch painting). Any suicidal end to suffering on earth is thought to be short–sighted and ill advised, since the person may suffer eternally in Hell or its equivalent.

Individual versus Social Responsibilities

For psychiatric radicals like Thomas Szasz (see Box 19.1), the individual's life belongs to him- or herself alone, not to God, the state, family, or friends. He has argued that suicide is a highly personal matter concerning just the suicide. Szasz (1961) wrote, "The only person ultimately responsible for suicide is the actor himself." And, again, "Society does not have the right to interfere by force with a person's decision to commit suicide."

We do not or should not have (e.g., be forced by others) to suffer great pain just to please others, if the prospect of relief is miniscule and others' preferences are whimsical. On the other hand, no one ever only kills just him- or herself. Every suicide can be seen as an indirect claim that life itself is not worth living under some circumstances. Suicide diminishes the life force, demoralizes those who love and depend on the person who suicides, stigmatizes family members, and can even threaten the social order.

All responsible persons who commit suicide should consider the meaning and implications of their suicide for those who love and depend on them. They must also be reasonably assured that their survivors can indeed *survive* without them. Ideally, they ought to discuss their suicide plan with their loved ones. To paraphrase John Donne, the suicide bell tolls for every other still living human being.

One way to explore the appropriateness of suicide is to take a few minutes to read and consider the case of the eminent Dutch suicidologist Nico Speijer (Case 19.2). Was Speijer right to suicide? Like Freud, he had terminal cancer, was in great pain, and could not find adequate relief from the pain. Speijer had been ill for a long time. He had thought a lot about his decision to suicide, discussed it with his wife, and did not act impulsively. He had an "enduring wish" to suicide. He was not mentally disordered, although he was understandably sad. Just because one wishes to die does not mean *ipso facto* that one is clinically depressed or mentally disordered.

CASE 19.2. Nico Speijer

On September 28, 1981, Nico Speijer—the grand old man of suicidology and long-time champion of suicide prevention in the Netherlands—himself committed suicide. He wrote this note to Rene Diekstra, who had been his pupil and friend:

Dear Rene:
     When you receive this letter, I will no longer be alive. As you know, I suffer from a carcinoma and a lot of metastases. Up to now I have been relatively capable of controlling the pain, but I cannot cope with it any longer—as you yourself will very well understand—I have decided to put an end to my life. . . . My wife has decided to go with me. After a marriage of forty years she prefers to die with me over having to stay behind all on her own.

As Diekstra (1986) wrote, "How could it have happened that a man who had virtually all of his 76 years been a protagonist of suicide prevention committed suicide himself?"

Actually, in 1980 Speijer and Diekstra had published a book, *Aiding Suicide*, which gave some of the answers. In this book, they described the conditions when suicide might be permissible as follows:

- The choice of ending life by suicide is based on a free-will decision and is not made under pressure.
- The person is in unbearable physical or emotional pain with no improvement expected.
- The wish to die can be identified as an enduring one.
- At the time of the decision, the person is not mentally disturbed (*compos mentis*).
- No unnecessary and preventable harm is caused to others by the suicide.

- The helper should be a qualified health professional—an MD, if lethal drugs are pre-scribed.
- The helper should seek professional consultation from colleagues.
- Every step should be fully documented and the documents given to the proper authorities.

Source: Rene Diekstra (personal communication, 1986). See also Diekstra (1986) and Speijer and Diekstra (1980). Diekstra contributed this case to Maris.

Speijer had sought counsel from his professional colleagues (and, indeed, had even written a book on assisted suicide with Professor Diekstra). In short, Speijer met all eight of his own conditions for an appropriate suicide. But was Speijer's suicide rational? In the next section, I consider rational suicide, define it, and argue that although the vast majority of suicides are not rational, suicide in some circumstances or conditions can be rational.

Rational Suicide

> Whenever Richard Cory went down town,
> We people on the pavement looked at him:
> He was a gentleman from sole to crown,
> Clean favored, and imperially slim. . . .
> And he was rich—yes, richer than a king—
> And admirably schooled in every grace:
> In fine, we thought that he was everything
> To make us wish that we were in his place.
> So on we worked, and waited for the light,
> And went without the meat, and cursed the bread;
> And Richard Cory, one calm summer night,
> Went home and put a bullet through his head.
> —E. A. ROBINSON (1897)

Rationality can be defined as follows: "Exercising one's reason in a proper manner; having sound judgment; sensible; sane; reasonable; not foolish, absurd, or extravagant . . . the tendency to regard everything from a purely rational point of view" (Maris, 1982). Rationality implies the ability to reason or think logically, as in drawing valid conclusions from inferences, and often connotes the absence of emotion. As I have noted earlier, for many *rational suicide* is an oxymoron (like *jumbo shrimp*). Probably the main reason for this view is that so many suicides have a mental disorder, which is often thought to preclude rationality (cf. Werth, 1996). There also appear to be many alternatives to suicide. Irrational suicide might include suiciding while being impulsive or agitated, intoxicated, psychotic, or severely depressed; making a decision not based in fact (such as one based in faith rather than reason); or being unable to see realistic alternatives to problem solving short of suicide.

We have a regrettable tendency to see suicides only as emotionally and physically ill, confused, unloved, unable to work, substance-abusing, products of broken homes—in short, as deprived of essential life amenities and supports. We assume that if would-be suicides only lived better, then they would not be suicides. But this assumption is obvious and wrong.

The human condition is such that even for people with the best that life can offer, like Richard Cory,[1] suicide can still be understandable. Life is short, often painful, and unpredictable, and it can be lonely. In addition the lives of some individuals are in effect suicidal careers, in that the harshness of normal life is combined with extra suicide catalysts (e.g., an unfortunate family history, mental disorder, or alcoholism). Even for the best among us, suicide can make sense. Suicide can be a solution to the problem of life itself, not just some perverse response to a life gone awry. To understand suicide, we must imagine abandoning life at its *best*.

Life itself—the human condition, not merely life gone awry or astray—is the basis for suicide. Human beings are not primarily creatures striving toward acquisition of property, money, pleasure, and other material sources. Rather, we are anxious mortals always looking back to see if entropy and death are gaining on us. Sexuality, aggression, money, power, religion, work, health, art/music, and drugs/alcohol are relatively ineffective defenses against death.

Under the best of conditions, life is relatively short, periodically painful, fickle, often lonely, and anxiety-generating. All of us share the basic givens of life. These include a finite life span with an upper limit of about 85–100 years and other, smaller deaths, such as loss of meaningful work, eroticism, love relationships, health, and strength; periodic unavoidable sickness, pain, and fatigue; a fickle and unpredictable life course; and the psychological burdens that are associated with human traits, such as anxiety, stress, and depression. The harshness of the human condition varies from individual to individual and across societies. Harshness has a complex relationship with suicide. People do not suicide simply because their lives are hard.

The vast majority of individuals and groups deal with the problem of life through nonsuicidal alternatives and have good enough lives. Common resolutions include love, work, religion, art/music, acquiring wealth, alcohol/drugs, sex, denial, friends and family, humor, play, travel, and diversion/distraction. Nevertheless, nothing short of death can truly end the problems associated with being human. Under such conditions, surely suicide can sometimes be rational. Suicide is at least an effective means for resolving common life problems, although usually not the best means.

Elsewhere I have argued (Maris, 1982) that rational suicide includes four ambiguities:

1. Having a reason versus a right to suicide.
2. Whether or not rational suicide excludes affect.
3. Whether suicides are "crazy" if they are irrational.
4. Whether suicides are always or sometimes irrational.

I discuss these ambiguities in turn below.

---

[1]There is some evidence that Cory's creator, poet E. A. Robinson and Cory himself, did not in fact have the best of lives.

1. Cesare Pavese (1908–1950) has said that "no one ever lacks a good reason to suicide." Even if this is true, suicide may still not be right, proper, or ethical. Suicide never just concerns the would-be suicide. Suicide may resolve a person's own problems but cause lifelong problems for their loved ones. What about the rights of others affected by the suicide? If something short of suicide would have the same problem-solving effect, then suicide is perhaps irrational overkill: "You didn't have to do *that!*" What about God's rights? If life belongs to God, then the person may have a reason to suicide, but not a right. If suicide is illegal or immoral, it may not be an individual's right.

2. It is hard to imagine that rational suicide excludes all affect. One can be emotional and rational at the same time. Sometimes we need to heed affect, to avoid becoming slaves to unfeeling reasoning or a dry, sterile, purely logical calculus. A person might say to him- or herself, "I have every *reason* to suicide, but it just does not feel right in my gut." Disemboweled, decathected reason or mind may not be sufficient by itself.

3. Often suicide is taken as *prima facie* evidence for insanity or mental disorder. But one can be not crazy and yet be irrational, and one can be mentally disordered and yet still capable of reasoning correctly. Most people who suicide are sad, but they may not be clinically depressed. However, mentally disordered people often cannot consider their best alternative to suicide; that is, they cannot be rational. One reason to wait a while, when a person decides to suicide, is that he or she might not want to suicide a few weeks or months later: "I can't believe I almost did that!"

4. Most people who argue against suicide believe that suicide is *always* irrational and never justified. Such people tend to be dogmatic and rigid. Most of us would not like to see people cavalierly or whimsically killing anything—themselves, others, or animals. Yet we all have to die eventually. Sometimes death, even suicidal death, is natural. Although suicide may often be irrational, it is not *always* irrational.

If there is no God or afterlife, then to commit suicide is to end the world for the individual committing it. However, life does not *seek* death. Death is not the purpose of life. The goal of life is simply to live as well and be as free from unwanted pain and misfortune as possible. We often forget that a good enough life is okay; we do not need a perfect life. The truth that we age and atrophy is not in itself cause for despair. As we get older, in fact, it can be kind of nice that people stop expecting much from us. The process of loving, living, producing, and reproducing is not invalidated by the final product of our personal death.

Euthanasia and Assisted Suicide

Should we help some people die, and if so, who and under what circumstances? We all have to die. So why not make dying as free from pain as possible, as quick as desired, without unnecessary mutilation (such as by gunshot), and not alone?

Euthanasia is not one simple thing (DeSpelder & Strickland, 2015). Euthanasia can be at least (1) active or passive; (2) voluntary or involuntary; and (3) direct or indirect.

Active euthanasia is an act that kills, whereas *passive euthanasia* is the omission of an act that results in death. Giving someone a lethal dose of barbiturates would be active euthanasia; not resuscitating a patient with terminal cancer or a serious heart condition, or not doing cardiopulmonary resuscitation (CPR), would be passive euthanasia.

Voluntary euthanasia is a death in which the patient makes the decision to die, perhaps by drafting a will or making an explicit, witnessed, written statement of intent. *Involuntary euthanasia* is a death in which someone other than the patient makes the decision—perhaps a family member, doctor, or nurse, when a patient is in a coma. *Direct euthanasia* is death when it is the primary intended outcome. *Indirect euthanasia* is death as a by-product of, for example, administering narcotics to control pain. It secondarily and unintentionally causes respiratory and/or cardiac failure.

Consider this vignette: Sam Kowalski is in a motorcycle accident, which results in a serious head injury and coma. A motorcycle club friend visits Kowalski at the hospital and shoots him in the head, knowing that Kowalski had told him previously that he would not like to continue living in such circumstances. This death would be *active, voluntary, direct* euthanasia (and, of course, murder).

Elizabeth Bouvia, a California woman with quadriplegia resulting from cerebral palsy, sued to avoid being force-fed as a noncomatose patient. The California Supreme Court upheld Bouvia's right to refuse treatment, but others called this decision "legal suicide." See the description of Bouvia in Case 19.3 for another perspective on assisted suicide.

CASE 19.3. Elizabeth Bouvia

During the closing months of 1983, Elizabeth Bouvia, a quadriplegic woman severely disabled by cerebral palsy, brought legal action in a Riverside County, California court, asking for custodial hospital care and simple treatment for pain while she starved herself to death.

Elizabeth Bouvia's disabilities date from her birth. She has no motor function in her limbs or skeletal muscles, except for very limited use of her right arm. She cannot change her own bodily position. This, together with pronounced spasticity and muscle contractions, aggravates the associated arthritis that she suffers from, and produces almost constant pain for which she requires medication.

Bouvia requires complete assistance in all matters of bodily hygiene, dressing, feeding, and other care functions. She is subject to multiple infections. However, she is able to speak quite well, to hold a cigarette in two fingers, to chew, and to operate her motorized wheelchair by means of a joystick.

She was able to complete a BA degree at San Diego State and started work on an MSW. In August 1982, she married Richard Bouvia, a machinist. After a year, he left her and filed for divorce. When Elizabeth was visiting her father in September 1983, she asked him to drive her to Riverside (California) General Hospital, where she requested that she be allowed to starve herself to death and filed suit. Her case involved ethical issues of force-feeding a noncomatose patient and her right to refuse this treatment (DeSpelder & Strickland, 2015; cf. *Cruzan v. Director, Missouri Department of Health,* 1990).

Bouvia said, "I know what's available to me out there and don't need or want it. My only outlet is talking or screaming. I am trapped in a useless body. Unfortunately, I have a brain. It makes it all the worse." (Note that many hospital patients who might be considered by some as potential candidates for euthanasia are just the opposite—i.e., brain-dead or brain-damaged.).

I was an expert witness for the defense (the hospital) in Bouvia's case, opining as to whether or not her request amounted to "legal suicide." The California Supreme Court eventually upheld Bouvia's right to refuse treatment. She voluntarily decided to eat on Easter morning, in April 1984, after checking out of the hospital and into a local motel. At last report, she is still alive.

Source: California court case from Maris. All information cited here was public.

Jack Kevorkian

In the United States, Jack Kevorkian was one of the most controversial, even radical advocates of physician-assisted suicide, which he called "medicide" (see his book *Prescription—Medicide;* Kevorkian, 1991; cf. Al Pacino in the HBO movie about Kevorkian). In the late 20th century, public awareness of physician-assisted suicide was focused largely on him. By early 1999, Kevorkian had assisted more than 100 suicides.

Initially, with the death of Janet Adkins, Kevorkian used a suicide machine that he dubbed a "Mercitron." This machine (described briefly in the discussion of barbiturates in Chapter 15) provided a motor-driven, timed release of the contents of three IV bottles. In succession, the bottles contained (1) thiopental or sodium pentothal (an anesthetic producing rapid unconsciousness); (2) succinylcholine (a muscle paralyzer like the curare used by African pygmies to poison darts in blowguns to hunt monkeys); and (3) potassium chloride, which stops the heart. The Mercitron was turned on by the would-be suicide. There were some malfunctions of this suicide machine, and so almost all of Kevorkian's later suicides were accomplished with a simple facial mask hooked up to a hose or tube and a canister of pure carbon monoxide. The carbon monoxide flow was initiated by the patient, not Kevorkian, to try to avoid legal ramifications.

Kevorkian's first eight clients were women, mostly single, divorced, or widowed. This is worth noting, since male suicide rates are about four times those of females. Almost all of Kevorkian's clients were not terminally ill, or at least would likely have not died within 6 months. Their toxicology blood reports showed that only two of the first eight assisted suicides had detectable levels of antidepressants in their blood at the time of death. It might be concluded that most of Kevorkian's clients were not first being treated for depression before suiciding.

Given Kevorkian's zealous pursuit of active assisted euthanasia, one suspects that at least his early assisted suicides were not adequately screened or processed. For example, Hugh Gale is reputed to have asked Kevorkian to take his mask off and abort the procedure, but he was ignored by Kevorkian. It also seems likely that

Kevorkian did not insist on a trial of psychiatric treatment (such as for depression) before agreeing to assist in some of his suicides.

Kevorkian lost his medical license in 1998 (he was a pathologist trained at the University of Michigan Medical School). He was charged with manslaughter and convicted in 1999 after videotaping an assisted suicide for the CBS television program *60 Minutes*. Kevorkian died on June 3, 2011, at the age of 83. Paradoxically, he may have set euthanasia and doctor-assisted suicide back several years. Michigan, South Carolina, and several others states introduced bills to make assisted suicide into a felony with concurrent fines and imprisonment, when it had previously been legal or a minor offense. In Kevorkian's home state of Michigan, it is now a felony to assist a suicide. These laws may have a chilling effect on both active and passive euthanasia, even for legitimate pain control (palliative care) previously offered to dying patients.

Euthanasia in the Netherlands

Legal physician-assisted suicide began outside the United States in the Netherlands (cf., Dignitas, founded 1998 in Switzerland and Germany). On February 10, 1993, the Dutch Parliament voted 91–45 to allow euthanasia. To be eligible for euthanasia or assisted suicide in the Netherlands, one must:

1. Act voluntarily.
2. Be mentally competent.
3. Have a hopeless disease without prospect of improvement.
4. Have a lasting (or persistent) wish for death.
5. Have the assisting MD consult with at least one colleague.
6. Require the assisting MD to write a report afterward.

The Dutch law opened the door for similar legislation in the United States.

Herbert Hendin, former executive director of the American Foundation for Suicide Prevention (AFSP), painted a bleak picture of assisted suicide in the Netherlands in his book *Seduced by Death: Doctors, Patients, and the Dutch Cure* (1997). Hendin claimed excessive reliance on the judgment of physicians; a consensual legal system that placed support of the physician above the rights of patients in order to protect euthanasia policy; the gradual extension of the practice to include administration of euthanasia without consent in a substantial number of cases; and abuses of power in the doctor–patient relationship.

Hendin claimed that 60% of physician-assisted Dutch suicides cases were not reported, and that in America a significant percentage of doctors were practicing assisted suicide without their patients' consent. A doctor named Samuel Klagsbrun, who was a plaintiff in a New York case that challenged laws prohibiting assisted suicide (see *www.patientsrightscouncil.org/site/rpt2005-part1*), said of Hendin's argument: "He is wrong . . . suffering needs to be addressed as aggressively as possible to stop unnecessary suffering." One also wonders about all those patients being forced to live and suffer without their consent.

Derek Humphry

Derek Humphry's best-selling book *Final Exit* (1991/2002) is basically a how-to book on the practicalities of suicide for the terminally ill. One of the big concerns about it has been its potential abuse, especially by those who are young and those with treatable depressions. Having the lethal methods of suicide described in such vivid, explicit detail worries many people, who fear that suicide will become too easy, and thus often will be clearly inappropriate (Stone, 1999). Yet Humphry is right that it is hard to get help with suicide without fear of penalties for those providing the help (e.g., physicians' losing their medical licenses or incurring federal narcotics charges). He has long argued that the laws in the United States need to be changed to permit assisted suicide and specify its procedures for the terminally ill under highly controlled circumstances.

Derek Humphry waged the first assisted-suicide battle in Oregon, initially as president of the Hemlock Society and later as president of the Euthanasia Research and Guidance Organization) and the Oregon Right to Die organization. On November 4, 1994, Oregon became the first U.S. state to permit a doctor to prescribe lethal drugs expressly and explicitly to assist a suicide. However, the National Right to Life Committee effectively blocked the enactment of the Oregon assisted-suicide law until 1997, when the measure again passed overwhelmingly. On March 25, 1998, an Oregon woman in her late 80s stricken with cancer became the first known person to die in the United States under a doctor-assisted suicide law.

A few other states have undertaken reforms to permit legal assisted suicide. Both Washington and California held referenda in the early 1990s that narrowly failed by votes of about 45% in favor to 55% against. But the proposals in both states were later approved, in Washington in 2009 and in California in 2016. These laws provide "aid in dying" for a person if the following conditions are met:

1. Two physicians certify the person to be within 6 months of a natural death (i.e., to be terminally ill).
2. The person is conscious and competent.
3. The person signs a voluntarily written request to die, witnessed by two impartial, unrelated adults.
4. The person is 18 years old or older (stipulations 4–6 were originally Oregon stipulations).
5. The patient must wait 15 days ("an enduring wish") before getting the prescription.
6. The patient can rescind a request at any time.

As this book goes to press (2018), the following states (plus Washington, D.C.) had passed assisted-suicide legislation:

- Oregon, 1997.
- Washington, 2009.
- Montana, 2009.
- Vermont, 2013.

- California, 2016.
- Colorado, 2016.
- Washington, D.C., 2016.
- Hawaii, 2018.

Other states that have had assisted-suicide legislation under review are Tennessee, New York, Massachusetts, and New Jersey.

From 2011 to 2014, 70% of a sample of 66 assisted suicides in the Netherlands were women (Young, 2016),[2] About half of these suicides had depressive disorders, and almost 70% had psychiatric histories of at least 11 years. In another study (*Time Magazine*) from 1998 to 2014 of 1,173 assisted suicides in the United States, their median age was 71 years; 70% were female; 79% had a malignant tumor; and 46% of them had at least a BA degree. The reasons they gave for suiciding were (1) fear of loss of autonomy, 91%; (2) feeling like a burden (cf. Joiner, 2005), 40%; and (3) not wanting to be in pain or inadequate pain control, 24%. During this time period, 62 MDs wrote prescriptions for assisted suicides, mainly for barbiturates. The median time from barbiturate ingestion to death was 25 minutes.

Although assisted-suicide laws are enacted by individual states, the authority of MDs to prescribe narcotics is federally licensed, and those who prescribe such drugs for assisted suicides risk losing their licenses in many states. People in states where assisted suicide is not legal will may be more likely to mutilate themselves, to die alone, and to feel generally abandoned in their time of greatest need.

Whose Life Is It Anyway?

Let's consider the movie *Whose Life Is It Anyway?* (Badham & Clark, 1981) as a specific case in which the issues of ethics, euthanasia, and rational suicide are illustrated. The film, based on a 1972 television play by Brian Clark, tells the story of Ken Harrison, a 35-ish sculptor in Boston who is gravely injured in a car wreck, becomes a quadriplegic, and wants to die, but is unable to commit suicide by himself. Since Ken's brain is fully alive, but his body is dead from the neck down, he needs assistance to die. The key theme of this play is the question of who decides life and death; that is, power is the main issue. Readers are invited to consider the following synopsis (or view the film) and then think about some of the issues raised in this chapter.

The film begins with Ken (played by Richard Dreyfuss) riding in his convertible in Boston, just after completing a city sculpture. When he is distracted by adjusting his radio for a Red Sox baseball game, he drives under an 18-wheeler stalled at an intersection, breaking his neck and becoming a helpless quadriplegic. In the hospital Ken slowly is stabilized medically, but eventually has to accept the fact that his life is now abruptly changed forever. At first Ken tries to distance himself by joking about his situation. Other attempts at coping with his dire condition (through sexuality, using marijuana and drugs, music, dictating books about his art, etc.) also

---

[2]See also *www.deathwithdignity.org/learn/researchers*.

fail. But in the end in an effort to gain some control over his life and not be totally dependent upon others for his care, he hires an attorney and sues the hospital for the right to die. He intends to starve himself (like Elizabeth Bouvia in Case 19.3). There is actually a trial for a writ of *habeas corpus*. Ken wins the trial, but the movie ends before we can learn whether Ken is going to commit suicide or adjust to his condition and keep trying to start a new life.

The movie's characters in addition to Ken include Pat (Ken's girlfriend), Dr. Clare Scott (an internist who treats Ken at the hospital), Dr. Emerson (the chief of Ken's treatment team), Mary Jo Sadler (a student nurse), Nurse Rodriguez (the head nurse on Ken's ward), John (an orderly who has a punk rock band and takes Ken to hear it), Mrs. Boyle (a social worker and occupational therapist), Dr. Jacobs (psychiatrist for the hospital as the defendant; he claims that Ken's depression clouds his judgment), Dr. Barrow (psychiatrist for Ken as the plaintiff; he argues that Ken can be depressed and still be rational), Judge Wyler (the judge who hears Ken's plea for writ of *habeas corpus*), Carter Hall (Ken's attorney), and Mr. Easton (the hospital's attorney).

One of the issues the film raises is humor as a psychological defense against death, dying, and difficult life situations (see Chapter 11, Figure 11.2). Can humor distance us from a dire situation like Ken's? Still, Ken's humor is childish and maddening at times. You almost want to shake him and say, "Grow up!" Note, too, that Ken is a rigid thinker. He tells Mrs. Boyle (the hospital social worker) that he *cannot* change, and he actually has a panic attack while telling her this. But Ken's mind need not be his enemy (as he claims). Long life is a succession of compromises, although usually not as severe as those Ken must make. What about the argument that if a person is depressed, then he or she cannot decide (rationally) to commit suicide or euthanasia? Can the person even consider the best alternatives when depressed? There are tests that can measure the level of depression (e.g., the BDI-II and the HAM-D). Is mild depression very different from severe depression? Depression need not be determined only by psychiatric clinical judgment. Also, many depressed people can still make rational decisions.

Note the *Catch-22* in this film: If you want to suicide, then you must be crazy; but if you are crazy, then you cannot make rational decisions. But not all suicides are crazy, even if they are mentally ill. When Ken breaks up with his girlfriend, Pat, Dr. Emerson forces Ken to have a 10-mg IV injection of Valium, since he is so agitated. In one sense, this is an abusive, coercive, bad act by Dr. Emerson. But it also has good consequences. Ken has gotten agitated because he has decided that he should break up with his girlfriend and set her free. When the girlfriend leaves Ken's room, a vase falls and breaks, which is symbolic of Ken and Pat's ending relationship. There are a lot of innuendos about death and sex in the movie. Why is Ken always making sexual jokes? Does sex in a sense equal life (Freud thought so at one time)? Is all energy sexual energy? If you are not sexually active or sexually capable, are you as good as dead? Why does Ken tell his internist, Dr. Clare Scott, that her breasts are "wonderful" after he objects to feeling sexual about his own girlfriend?

It is important to notice that only Ken's brain is alive, versus the more typical euthanasia situation in which the patient is brain-dead (has a flat EEG), but the body is alive. In a sense this makes Ken's situation more difficult to tolerate, since he is acutely aware of his helplessness. At one point in the film Ken says, "If I were a cat or a dog, you'd put me to sleep." What are the differences between mercy killing of animals versus killing human beings? Why can we easily euthanize pets, but not family members when they have intractable pain? The attending physician at the hospital, Dr. Emerson, tells Ken after the trial before a judge, "We will not even feed you, if you want to stay at the hospital." Note, however, that the 1981 movie predates a 1990 U.S. Supreme Court decision (*Cruzan v. Director, Missouri Department of Health*), according to which a hospital does not have to allow a patient to starve to death, even if the patient or his or her guardians want it.

It is not clear what Ken will do at the end of the film. He has ambivalence once he gets the power he needs to suicide. Although he wins the trial, will he now actually suicide? Would it be rational for Ken to commit suicide, given his circumstances? The film closes with a shot of Michelangelo's sculpted hand pointing upward. Ken has told Clare that he is sure he wants to die. But will he actually do it, now that he has control of his life and death? Maybe the issue here is not so much living or dying, but rather being able to make that decision.

This chapter completes Part V of the book. The chapters in Part VI consider the special topics of war, murder–suicide, and jail and prison suicides.

SPECIAL TOPICS

CHAPTER 20

Suicide in the Military
War, Aggression, and PTSD

Older men declare war. But it is youth that must fight and die.
—HERBERT HOOVER

From the legendary Greek warrior Ajax to the Islamic State of Iraq and Syria (ISIS), suicide has always been part and parcel of the military (Defense Suicide Prevention Office, 2017). Being a soldier means being willing to die for your country (Durkheim's [1897/1951] altruistic suicide). In ancient history and myth, military suicide was related not just to sacrifice in battle, but also to shame or defeat (as in the case of Ajax; see Chapter 18). In World War II, 2,500–3,860 *kamikaze* pilots had their fighter planes loaded with explosives, then flew them into Allied ships for the sake of the Emperor and Japan. Many of the pilots expressed ambivalence about *kamikaze* suicides, but once they got into their planes, there was no way to return alive (Ohnuki-Tierney, 2006). Typically officers refused to become *kamikaze* pilots, and young men had to be trained specially for the job. Japanese officers not only committed *hara-kiri,* but also jumped off cliffs to their deaths in front of their assembled troops to atone for losing the war. Hitler and several of his leading officers and other associates committed suicide rather than be captured and tried in court. These included Hitler's mistress, Eva Braun, as well as Joseph Goebbels, Hermann Goering, and Erwin Rommel. Interestingly, suicide rates of natives in Nazi-occupied countries like France, Belgium, and the Netherlands actually decreased during the war, especially from 1941 to 1943 (Rojcewisz, 1971).

The suicide rate among Jews in Nazi-occupied countries, however, was high. As discussed in Chapter 17 (see Table 17.1), I examined Jewish suicides (Maris, 1981; 246) during World War II who were buried in the only Jewish cemetery in Berlin; I found a dramatic increase in the number of Jews suiciding as the war progressed, and a decrease as it declined (Maris, 1981). The Jewish suicide rates in the concentration camps were very low. Most camp prisoners were concerned just with surviving and getting enough to eat. "Suicide by Nazi" was easy; all it took was running into the lethal electrified barbed-wire fences or getting shot (Bettelheim, 1943). Bettelheim, who was in a camp, later suicided in 1990, long after World War II.

Why do suicide rates of countries often drop in times of "Great Wars" such as World Wars I and II? This happened in the United States in roughly 1917 and 1918, and from 1941 to 1945 (Rojcewisz, 1971). One theory is that nations at war become more socially integrated and united when they confront a common external enemy or threat (and that social integration and suicide rates are negatively related). Another hypothesis is that external aggression (e.g., fighting in a war) and internal aggression (e.g., suicide rates) vary inversely. That is, usually the more people aggress externally, the less they aggress against themselves (and suiciding is the most drastic form of self-aggression). It is worth noting that among physicians, surgeons usually have low suicide rates, while psychiatrists tend to have higher suicide rates. However, the causes of suicide are obviously more complicated than generic social or economic forces. Suicide rates tend to peak in times of economic depression, such as those in the United States in 1929–1933.

Karl Menninger (1938) argued that individually external aggression (which many soldiers are trained to commit or actually commit when deployed) *increases* self-destruction in the long run (he cites a case of an executioner who later suicided). Menninger examined the psychodynamics of self-destructive behaviors short of suicide (indirect self-destructive behavior), such as alcoholism, antisocial personality, self-mutilation, multiple surgeries, accident-proneness, and asceticism. Menninger claimed that that all suicides are made up of three components; (1) hate (which he called the "wish-to-kill"), (2) hopelessness (the "wish-to-die"), and (3) guilt (the "wish-to-be-killed"). Notice that the wish-to-kill is highly related to self-destruction, and that killing and training to kill are major activities in the military. At one point in his life, Freud (by whom Menninger was heavily influenced) claimed that all suicide starts out as murder, which then (for various reasons) is retroflexed back against the self.

Suicide also plays a major role today in terrorist Islamic military groups like ISIS or Al-Qaeda. For example, suicide bombers sacrifice their own lives for the sake of the Muslim religion or its cause, and are told that they will go straight to heaven (Paradise) to be with Allah. The Muslim heaven is for most very sensual and sexual (a common myth is that 72 virgins are promised for male suicide bombers), with ample, abundant food and water, and beautiful, serene surroundings.

Merari (2010) studied the lives of 15 would-be Palestinian suicide bombers; his control group was made up of nonsuicide bombers (who were otherwise matched with the bombers). He reviewed 2,622 suicide attacks from 1981 to 2008. Most of the suicide bombers were male, under age 25, single, and (of course) Muslim. Compared to the nonbomber terrorist controls, the suicide bombers had more dependent–avoidant and impulsive–unstable personalities. The suicide bombers tended to be shy, had often been school failures, and felt as if they were a disappointment to their parents. The majority of the bombers did not have suicidal wishes, nor were they mentally ill. Only about 12% of ISIS recruits became suicide bombers, compared with about 50% of Al-Qaeda militants. Recently more females have been recruited and trained to be bombers, since they are less suspicious, attract less attention, and perhaps are more effective. Some young females are forced to be suicide bombers (see, e.g., *www.nytimes.com/2018/01/17/world/africa/nigeria-boko-haram-suicide-bombers-attack.html*). Although some bombers were like Durkheim's altruistic suicides, most of the bombers' motivations derived from their own personal lives.

When I discuss the *military* in this chapter, I mean mainly U.S. soldiers in either the Army (the largest single military group), Marine Corps, Navy, Air Force, or Coast Guard. Suicide data and prevention programs vary among these five military groups. I traveled to six American military bases in Germany from July 26 to August 21, 1986, to speak to Army troops about suicide and its prevention. Since then, I have also testified in 14 U.S. Department of Veterans Affairs (VA) Hospital medical malpractice cases. I was an expert witness in a San Francisco-based trial, *Veterans for Common Sense v. Peake,* in 2008. Peake was a lieutenant general and cardiovascular surgeon who at the time directed the VA. I have also testified before the U.S. Congressional Committee on Veterans Affairs in Washington, D.C. (Maris, 2008).

One last introductory comment: Police suicide is closely related to military suicide (Maris et al., 2000, pp. 200–211, 364; see Aamodt & Stalmaker, 2006). The police also tend to have high suicide rates and share many suicidogenic risk factors with the military—such as the use of guns in their work, alcohol abuse problems, high levels of stress and danger, a heightened probability of being killed while working ("A good day is when I come home at night"), and the likelihood of being white males.

Aggression and Suicide

Suicide is not easy. All suicides involve at least some minimal aggressive action (Giner et al., 2014). A person who is just depressed and hopeless may lack a sufficient aggressive catalyst to be able to suicide. Remember, too, that soldiers are trained to kill or be aggressive. A motto of a Marine Special Forces unit is "Swift, Silent, Deadly." In fact, aggression may be a more basic suicide risk factor than depressive disorder, since aggression (but probably not depression) occurs in all species, animal and human, and at all ages.

Neurobiologically speaking, suicide is just one of several aggressive malfunctions of the serotonergic system (but remember that other neurotransmitters are involved in suicide and that the brain is complex). These other malfunctions include sleep difficulties, impulsivity, disinhibition, headaches, mood volatility or lability, poor peer relationships, and glucocorticoid abnormalities (Brown et al., 1992). In spite of attempts to romanticize death or suicide, there is also an element of aggressive obscenity in suicide (e.g., a prematurely wasted life, a mind shut down forever).

Freud at one time saw all suicides as displaced or disguised murders (Brown & Goodwin, 1986). Hate or the wish-to-kill is strongest in younger suicides and involves interpersonal dynamics. The average soldier is 28 years old. See also Sylvia Plath's poem "Daddy" (written in 1962 and published in 1966). One theory suggests that since Plath's father died when she was a young girl, her anger and aggressive energy toward him got turned back on herself (technically, he was already gone, so she symbolically killed an introjected object). Sometimes suicidal anger is directed at the terms of the human condition; it becomes a kind of protest of the pain, decline, atrophy, and failure built into being human and finite with even the best life can offer.

The suicidal triad consists of mood disorder, loss of hope, and aggression. Suicide is an act that requires energy, as noted above. People have to acquire the ability to suicide over time (Joiner, 2005). Sometimes this necessary aggressive catalyst is anger, irritability, frustration, hatred, anxiety, desperation, or dissatisfaction (Maris, 1981). Think back to Henry and Short's (1954) frustration and aggression theory of suicide, discussed in Chapter 7. To oversimplify, the more frustration there is, the more aggression accumulates, and so on. The target of aggression may be determined by other factors. Frustration can be economic, as in business cycle variation or poverty and financial problems (which many vets have). Chapter 21 focuses on a specific kind of aggression, murder followed by suicide (see West, 1966, and Joiner, 2014). Some murder–suicides may result from unexpended or leftover aggressive energy after murder.

Note that three of the five leading causes of death of young to middle-aged people (say, ages 15–45) are violent and aggressive, not natural. These three are homicide, suicide, and accidents (most often motor vehicle accidents). Among black males up to age 45, homicide is the leading cause of death.

What about aggression in animals? Animals tend to behave aggressively under the following conditions: (1) predation for sex or food, (2) male–male interaction, (3) fear, (4) irritability, (5) territoriality, (6) maternal protection of the young, or (7) instrumentality (e.g., to obtain another end, such as escape from perceived threats or dangers). We study animals in part because usually we cannot do suicide experiments on humans. Some laboratory experiments show that individuals with lower brain/CSF serotonin are more likely to commit violent suicides, such as using guns to shoot themselves in the head.

There are some unanswered questions about aggression: (1) Why is it not possible to provoke suicide by lowering CSF serotonin? (2) Why does raising serotonin levels not automatically prevent or lower suicide rates? (3) Why does lithium lower suicide rates? Does it stabilize mood and minimize impulsivity? (4) Is self-destruction in individuals with lower brain serotonin levels just waiting to be provoked by the right kind of environmental stress? (5) What other biological factors are involved with aggression (e.g., XYY chromosomes and maleness, sexuality in general, testosterone, plasma cortisol, steroids, dopamine, GABA, or glutamate)?

War and Suicide

It is hard to get a clear, unbiased, and accurate understanding of military suicide rates and how they might be affected by war. This problem is shrouded in varying political agendas, inconsistent or missing data, and even a little hysteria. To start with, the five different U.S. military groups each have somewhat different data. With some wildly different estimates of the incidence and prevalence of military suicide, whose data are correct? Is there really an epidemic of military suicide or not? Bates et al. (2012) conclude that "the true incidence of suicide among veterans is unknown."

Table 20.1 reflects the ambiguity of the U.S. military suicide problem (cf. Box 20.3, below). Note the question marks in the table for wars in the remote past. Moreover, no data were available from 1958 to 1975, so the effect of Vietnam on the military suicide rate is in fact unknown. We do know that Vietnam vets had a slightly higher relative suicide risk than other vets of the same era who were not in Vietnam. Suicide rates for Army vets peaked in 1910 (68 per 100,000) and 1932 (50), then declined dramatically until about 1945 (8 per 100,000) and stayed relatively low from 1945 to 1985.

Concern with a possible veteran suicide problem probably started about 1980, when the U.S. Army began collecting data on the issue, and also when the diagnosis of posttraumatic stress disorder (PTSD) was created in DSM-III (American Psychiatric Association, 1980). As far back as the U.S. Civil War (1861–1865), Da Costa (see Black & Andreasen, 2014) spoke of a military anxiety disorder that he called "soldier's heart" (see also Maris, 2015, p. 98). However, it was not until the 1950s that the first true anxiolytics (antianxiety drugs) became available for generalized anxiety, panic disorder, agoraphobia, social phobia, OCD, and PTSD.

In Table 20.1, we have to compare *male* general population suicide rates with those in the military, since men have suicide rates about four times higher than

TABLE 20.1. U.S. War Death Statistics

Major U.S. wars	U.S. deaths	Wounded	Years	Male suicide rate (per 100,000)	Military suicide rate (per 100,000)
Iraq War	4,800	31,965	2003–2016	19.2 (2009)	18.5 (2009)
Afghanistan	2,344	19,675	2001–2016	18.3 (2007)	18.5 (2007)
Gulf War	258	849	1990–1991	20.4 (1990)	15.3 (1990)
Vietnam War	58,209	153,303	1955–1975	19.8 (1970)	16.0 (1970)
Korean War	36,516	92,134	1950–1953	20.0 (1950)	11.0 (1950)
World War II	405,399	670,846	1941–1945	20.0 (1942)	10.0 (1942)
World War I	116,516	204,002	1917–1918	19.2 (1918)	13.0 (1918)
Civil War	625,000	281,881	1861–1865	? (1865)	? (1865)
Revolutionary War	25,000	25,000	1775–1783	? (1780)	? (1780)
All U.S. casualties	1,343,812	1,529,230 (Missing in action = 38,159)			

Sources: Original table by Maris. Data in "U.S. deaths," "Wounded," and "Years" column from *www.statisticbrain.com/u-s-war-death-statistics.* Male suicide rates from U.S. Vital Statistics. Military suicide rates from U.S. Army and National Institute of Mental Health data. Most of the military suicide data are Army rates from Rothberg et al. (1987). Several of the listed military suicide rates in the table are approximations. Data for nonveteran male suicide rates in 1918 and 1942 are from the National Center for Health Statistics (Massey, n.d.). All U.S. government statistics in public domain.

those of females, and most of the military is male. If we do not make this correction, then the mean U.S. suicide rate (not controlled for gender) has been about 11–12 per 100,000 since about 1900, with some troughs during major wars and some peaks in economic downturns. This would lead us to believe (falsely) that the military suicide rate exceeded that of the general U.S. population by a ratio of about 1.5 times (i.e., 18.5 divided by 12).

But once we have made the male gender adjustment, it seems that military suicide rates and those of a comparable general population group are about the same—namely, 18.5 per 100,000 per year (Donnelly, 2013). Military suicide rates are not statistically significantly higher than the mean for U.S. male suicide rates in general. Thus, in one sense, we do not have a special suicide problem in the military to explain, control for, or treat. Rothberg et al. (1987) stated, "Military service in itself does not carry an extra risk for suicide." Of course, any suicide can be a problem that deserves attention and possible intervention. Given the data in Table 20.1, there seems to be a certain hysteria in the United States today about a veteran suicide problem.

Even if we concede that military suicide rates may be somewhat higher than those of the general population, this does not mean that combat stress or PTSD is causing the increased suicide rates. Daniel Lippman (personal communication, May 14, 2012) has data indicating that the suicide rates of deployed combat veterans are not higher than those of veterans who were never deployed. If soldiers were never in combat or a war zone, how could PTSD make their suicides, or suicide rates, in general, higher?

Similar data have been reported by Reger et al. (2015). In Reger et al.'s data on all U.S. troops who served from October 7, 2001 until December 31, 2007 ($N =$ 3,945,099), 31,962 soldiers died, and 5,041of these suicided. However, of the suicides, 3,879 service members were not deployed (77%) versus 1,162 who were (23%). The rate was 17.8 per 100,000 for the not-deployed, versus a rate of 18.9 for soldiers who were deployed. Soldiers with multiple deployments had a suicide rate of 19.9. The deployment suicide rate is slightly higher than the suicide rate of the not-deployed, but this difference is not statistically significant. Thus something other than combat stress or PTSD caused the suicides of the not-deployed soldiers who made up most of the suicides (cf. Kime, 2015). Lippman has suggested that the military suicide rate may have more to do with soldiers' selection and recruitment than it does with military stress, combat, or PTSD. That is, *soldiers are recruited from a population that has more suicide risk to start with,* independent of their military or combat experience.

The typical military recruit is young (22–30 years old, with a mean age of 28), white (75%, vs. 18% black), male (about 14% of soldiers are female), and single. Only 53% of enlisted soldiers are married, versus 70% of all officers. Most only went to high school (93% stopped school by 12th grade), and are of lower-middle to lower SES. Only 1% of Ivy League graduates or sons and daughters of members of the U.S. Congress go into the military. Recruits tend to have alcohol or other substance abuse problems (Maris et al., 2000), as well as more mood disorders. Once these recruits enlist, they are given guns (Bates et al., 2012), trained to kill, and often separated from their friends and families. They do not get paid much for being soldiers; later, they often have trouble getting nonmilitary jobs, and have financial problems after being discharged.

PTSD and Military Suicide

In 1980 in DSM-III, PTSD was classified as one of the many anxiety disorders. Anxiety includes both fear (an emotional response to threat(s) and anxiety (anticipation of future threat(s). In DSM-5 (American Psychiatric Association, 2013), PTSD has been removed as a type of anxiety disorder and is now in the new psychiatric diagnostic category of trauma- and stressor-related disorders. PTSD includes the diagnostic criteria summarized briefly in Box 20.1. A question remains about the relationship of PTSD to suicidality (Spitzer et al., 2018).

Kang (2007) stated that as of September 2007 among vets in health care at VA facilities, 40% had diagnoses of major depression, and 20% had a diagnosis of PTSD. PTSD is important among combat veterans because it is apparently common. From 15 to 50% of vets have PTSD (about 33% of female veterans experience sexual trauma, which can also cause PTSD), and it is interactively related to other suicide risk factors (*Veterans for Common Sense v. Peake,* 2008). It has been estimated that 15% of Vietnam vets had PTSD (Maris, 2015). Rathbun (2008) reported that 28.3% of Iraq vets had mental health problems. Kang (2007) claimed that of the approximately 1.6 million troops deployed to Afghanistan and Iraq, 3,444 to over 4,000 have been killed, and 90% have been "traumatized" but do not necessarily have PTSD.

It must be pointed out that vets have more suicide risk factors than just PTSD. For example, among all patients who used the Veterans Health Administration (VHA) services in 1999, a total of 7,684 died by suicide in the following 7 years (Ilgen, 2010). Of the suicides, 47% had a psychiatric diagnosis, the most common ones being depressive disorder (31.2%) and substance abuse (21.3%). Other veteran conditions related to suicide include combat-related guilt and physical injuries,

---

BOX 20.1. Summary of Posttraumatic Stress Disorder (PTSD) Criteria

- Being exposed in one of several ways to one or more traumatic events in which a serious injury, sexual violence, or death occurs (there also can be feelings of intense fear or hopelessness).
- The event is reexperienced repeatedly, often in nightmares or intrusive memories.
- The person avoids stimuli associated with the original trauma.
- Symptoms of increased arousal (such as irritability, hypervigilance, etc.) are experienced.
- Negative changes in mood and cognition are experienced.
- The symptoms last 1 month or more (i.e., are chronic vs. acute) and are characterized by social, and occupational, or other dysfunction.
- The disorder is not due to substance use/abuse or a medical condition.

Source: Original table by Maris, considerably abbreviating the American Psychiatric Association (2013) criteria. Note that the criteria are different for children age 6 or younger.

especially if a vet was wounded multiple times or sustained major injuries, like loss of a limb or traumatic brain injury (Bates et al., 2012).

PTSD is one of the unique suicidogenic factors among veterans (especially those who have been in combat) and is interactively related to other suicide risk factors. Note that the percentage of all U.S. yearly suicidal deaths is 2.1% (American Association of Suicidology [AAS], 2008). But among 15- to 24-year-olds, 12.3% of all deaths are by suicide. Kang (2007) reminds us that the median vet suicide age is 20–29, and that 18- to 24-year-old soldiers' suicides make up 26.3% of all suicides— about twice the percentage of the nonsoldier population. Obviously, the prompt and accurate diagnosis and treatment of vet PTSD (and related depressive and substance use disorders) are important conditions for vet suicide prevention.

Having said all this, Donnelly (2013) concluded:

> The science of military post-traumatic stress is also less settled than conventional wisdom has it, there is no doubt about the mental suffering that too many combat veterans endure, but there is confusion about the extent of the anguish and how to treat it. Yet, with hundreds of millions, if not billions of health-care dollars at stake, the rush toward more treatment, therapies, and medications is accelerating. Something like a "PTSD" industry—and an accompanying and powerful political lobby—has spring up over the last decade. Our feelings of appreciation for military service, perhaps mixed with more than a little guilt, may be overruling better judgment. Compared with other countries, the United States diagnoses PTSD cases at improbably high rates. Recent military PTSD rates in the U.S. have reached as high as 30% according to the Congressional Budget Office. By contrast, only 2% of Danish soldiers are diagnosed with PTSD.

Not only are the estimates of PTSD in the U.S. military improbably high, but if 77% of military suicides never even saw combat, then obviously other suicidogenic risk factors than PTSD have been contributing to military suicides.

Is the U.S. Veteran Suicide Rate an Epidemic?

One problem in getting a consistent answer to this question is that there are shifting veteran populations—all vets, vets in different military branches, vets in different wars (World War II, Korea, Vietnam, Gulf War, Afghanistan, Iraq), and so on— as well as shifting time frames (2001–2005, 2006–2008, 2003–2014, etc.). Various samples are also based on different data sets (e.g., incident briefs; root cause analyses, which are legally protected data; death certificates; Department of Defense data; and VA/VHA data). Consequently, the range of estimates of veteran suicides is very wide.

For example, in Table 20.1 there were no significant differences in Iraq or Afghanistan in military suicide rates versus those of the general U.S. nonveteran general population of males (viz., about 18.5–19.0 per 100,000 for both groups). Certainly, the military suicide rate excess (if any) is not an epidemic (Donnelly, 2013). For example, in 2012 there were 349 military suicides versus 295 nonsuicidal deaths.

All of the VA suicide data are suspicious, since they were created or quoted mainly by VA personnel, who have a vested interest in whether or not the veteran suicide rates are high. Also, the vet suicide rate comparisons tend to be to a general population rate of 12 per 100,000, not to the U.S. male suicide rate of about 18.5–19.0 per 100,000. Some of the VA estimates of veteran suicide rates and how much higher they are than those of the general population are listed below.

- Katz (2008) said that vets have a suicide rate 3.2 times higher than that of the general population: The suicide rate was 34.6 in a population of 8,218 VA patients from 2001 to 2005. (The rate is 1.8 times higher, if the general population rate is 19.0 per 100,000.)
- The VA Office of the Inspector General (Daigh, 2007) said that the vet rate is 7.5 times higher: a suicide rate of 83 divided by 11–12. (The rate is 4.4 higher, if the control rate is 19.0.)
- Rathbun (2008) said that the vet rate is 1.8 to 2.3 times higher: A survey of 6,256 vets of any war in 45 states indicated about 120 vet suicides per week.
- Zivin et al. (2007) said that 1,683 of 807,694 vets suicided, which equals 208 per 100,000, or about 19 times higher. (The rate is 11 times higher, if the control rate is 19.0.)
- Katz (2008) said, "VA suicide prevention coordinators are identifying about 1,000 suicide attempts per month among vets seen in VA medical facilities." But is that high? Suicide attempts exceed completions by a ratio of about 25:1. So 1,000 divided by 25 equals a rate of 40.0 per 100,000.
- Kang (2007) reported 18 suicides per day out of 25 million total vets. That works out to a suicide rate of about 26.0.
- Kang (2007) simply said, "The risk of death for vets from suicide and motor vehicle accidents is higher that than for the general population."

These VA data seem to suggest that the veteran suicide rate is somewhat higher than that of the general population, but probably not enough to constitute an epidemic.

If we concede that the military suicide rate is significantly higher than that of the general population (and the data suggest that we should not necessarily concede this), how high does a vet suicide rate have to be to merit national concern? Of course, even one suicide can be one too many. A decade ago, Michael Kussman, the Deputy Under Secretary for Health Care Operations in the VA said in a deposition that "suicide occurs like cancer occurs" (U.S. Committee on Veterans' Affairs, 2008). It is not clear what Kussman meant; we all have to die. Does this mean the VA thinks that a certain number of vet suicides are inevitable and there is not much we can do about them?

An *epidemic* can be defined as a disorder or condition that is prevalent and spreading rapidly among many people in a community (like the U.S. military) at the same time. It does seem that veteran suicides are the product of a disease process and may be increasing. For example, Kang (2007) claimed the following percentages for Operation Iraqi Freedom (OIF) or Operation Enduring Freedom (OEF) vet suicides from 2002 to 2005 (each percentage represents the rate of increase of suicides compared to the preceding year):

- 2002 = 7%
- 2003 = 21%
- 2004 = 48%
- 2005 = 68%

One could easily argue that these figures look a little like an "epidemic," but to be certain one would have to control for the number of vets and calculate rates per 100,000. Sometimes percentage increases can be very misleading, if the prior prevalence was low. For example, at Johns Hopkins University many years ago, 50% of coeds (as female students were then called) were married to their professors—but there were only two coeds at that time, one of whom one married her professor.

The VA Mental Health Strategic Plan for Suicide Prevention

The purpose of the VA Inspector General's Mental Health Strategic Plan (MHSP) for Suicide Prevention was to assess implementation of action pertaining to suicide prevention in the VHA (Daigh, 2007). Overall, the 2007 report on the MHSP was a systematic, well-organized survey, but it also pointed out many of the VA's shortcomings in suicide assessment and prevention. Since 2007, changes have been made. In 2008 in the VHA, there were (1) 21 regions (veterans' integrated service networks or VISNs), (2) 154 hospitals or medical centers, (3) 875 community-based outpatient clinics (CBOCs), and (4) 136 nursing homes (Feeley, 2008). The plan overview indicated that "At present, MHSP initiatives for suicide prevention are [only] partially implemented" (Daigh, 2007, p. iv). For example, the overview summarized the findings at the time for six major objectives as follows:

Areas	Findings
A. Crisis availability and outreach	24-hour mental health services in 94.5% of facilities
B. Screening and referral	98% for depression, a major suicide risk factor
C. Tracking and assessment	70% of facilities do not have a tracking system
D. Interventions and research	61.8% of facilities do not target special groups
E. Development of a suicide prevention database	See the Serious Mental Illness Treatment Research and Evaluation Center at Ann Arbor, Michigan (data were not available to Daigh)
F. Education	61.4% of facilities did not make information on suicide risk mandatory

Other documents (e.g., the *Suicide Risk Assessment Guide Reference Manual,* VA 001510, in the trial record of *Veterans for Common Sense v. Peake* on May 21, 2008, p. 1) have stated that suicide attempts are a major risk factor in vets. The problem with this finding is that (in one study) about 90% of suicides age 45 or older make only one fatal suicide attempt, usually because they shoot themselves in the head

(Maris, 1981). Thus, for many vet suicides, a prior suicide attempt cannot be used to prevent their suicides. It is too late.

Importantly, when the VA measured the crucial risk factors of depression and hopelessness (see Box 20.2), as far as could be determined it just mainly used self-report data, not reliable and valid scales such as the Hamilton Rating Scale for Depression (HAM-D; Hamilton, 1960), the Beck Depression Inventory–II (BDI-II; Beck et al., 1996), the Beck Hopelessness Scale (Beck et al., 1974a), and the Beck Suicide Intent Scale (Beck, 1990) (see Chapter 3 for a discussion of these instruments). All of these scales are relatively short (17–21 questions), have the advantage of indirection (the veterans completing the scales cannot be sure what they measure), have known reliability and validity, and can be administered in 15–20 minutes. Since hopelessness and depression are key suicide risk factors, they should be measured objectively and systematically, not just by subjective self-reporting. Finally, some veterans may not even know if (and how much) they are depressed, hopeless, or suicidal.

Daigh (2007), in his review of the MHSP, stated that 90% of the VA facilities do not have suicide case managers (this has changed since then). Why identify vets with suicide risk, if no one monitors them? Recently, in fact, there were *suicide coordinators* in all 21 VISNs in the medical centers, but few at the 875 CBOCs (the outpatient clinics). It is unclear who these people are, what their suicide prevention training is, what their exact job descriptions are, or how effective they are. There is also a question about the level of staffing of CBOCs, where most staff members are LPNs, RNs, MSWs, and MA psychologists, and not usually psychiatrists or other MDs.

Psychiatrists are important, since two psychiatric drugs have proven very effective in reducing suicidality in patient populations. One of these is lithium (Baldessarini et al., 2012) for bipolar patients. It is not clear how many veterans get lithium treatment. Likewise, with suicidal psychotic patients, the drug Clozaril has been shown to be effective in clinical trials in reducing the suicide rate. In the vast majority of VA clinics (about 90%), fewer than 10% of their psychotic patients are on Clozaril. Thus most of the MHSP initiatives (at least in 2007) were only partially implemented after about 4 years, and some of the operational definitions of key risk factors were below the standard of care.

Measuring Suicide Risk Factors and the Suicide Risk Assessment Guide/Template

There is no reason why all veterans could not have all significant suicide risk factors measured at clinical VA visits, deployment, or discharge. For example, see the 15 suicide risk factors I have described in Chapters 3 and 4. The VA's Suicide Risk Assessment Guide (a card template; U.S. Department of Veterans Affairs, 2012), the contents of which are shown in Box 20.2, is woefully inadequate to detect veterans' suicidality. For example, section 3 of the card— asking if vets (1) are feeling hopeless about the present/future; (2) have thought about taking their lives; (3) if so, when, and whether they have a plan; and (4) have ever made a suicide attempt— does not measure suicidality adequately.

BOX 20.2. VA Suicide Risk Assessment/Template Guide

1) LOOK FOR THE WARNING SIGNS

Presence of any of these warning signs requires immediate attention and referral. Consider hospitalization for safety until a complete assessment can be made.

- Threatening to hurt to kill self
- Looking for ways to kill self
- Seeking access to pills, weapons, or other means
- Talking or writing about death, dying, or suicide

Additional warning signs (if any, refer for treatment or appointment): hopelessness; rage, anger, seeking revenge; acting recklessly or engaging in risky activities; feeling trapped; increasing alcohol or drug abuse; withdrawing from friends, family, and society; anxiety, or agitation, inability to sleep, or sleeping all the time; dramatic changes in mood; perceiving no reason for living.

2) ASSESS FOR SPECIFIC FACTORS THAT MAY INCREASE OR DECREASE RISK FOR SUICIDE

Factors that may increase suicide risk: Current ideation, intent, plan, access to means; previous suicide attempt(s); alcohol/substance abuse; previous history of psychiatric diagnosis; impulsiveness; hopelessness; recent losses; recent discharge from an inpatient unit; family history of suicide; history of abuse; comorbid health problems; age, gender, race; same-sex orientation.

Factors that may decrease suicide risk: positive social support; spirituality; sense of responsibility to family; children in the home, pregnancy; life satisfaction; reality-testing ability; positive coping skills; positive problem-solving skills; positive therapeutic relationship.

3) ASK THE QUESTIONS

- Are you feeling hopeless about the present/future? (If yes, ask . . .)
- Have you had thoughts about taking your life? (If yes, ask . . .)
- When did you have these thoughts, and do you have a plan to take your life?
- Have you ever had a suicide attempt?

4) RESPONDING TO SUICIDE RISK

Ensure the patient's immediate safety and determine the most appropriate treatment setting.

- Refer to mental health treatment or ensure that a follow-up appointment is made.
- Inform and involve someone close to the patient.
- Limit access to means of suicide.
- Increase contact and make a commitment to help the patient through the crisis.

Provide the number of an ER/urgent care center to the patient and significant other.

Source: Adapted from U.S. Department of Veterans Affairs (2012). This card template is in the public domain.

Veterans can easily deny depression or suicide ideation (Berman, 2018), especially if they think that admitting either one might affect their promotions or military careers, or are ashamed to admit mental health issues. When I worked for the U.S. Army in Germany doing suicide prevention training, the staff psychiatrist in Berlin told me that he had little to do, because soldiers (particularly males) would not admit to any mental health problems for various career reasons. Vannoy (2017) found that Army soldiers showed rates of mental health concerns two to four times higher on anonymous surveys; 56.4% of soldiers who reported suicide ideation anonymously told nobody of their thoughts. Many males (not just soldiers) do not even seek mental health treatment. Soldiers may not even realize that they are depressed or self-destructive, or how serious the conditions are. In short, all the questions on the Suicide Risk Assessment Guide card need to be asked and answered, and put into objective formats that do not make it obvious what is being measured. An earlier (2008) version of the card had questions about the following:

1. A suicide plan.
2. Whether the plan includes firearms.
3. What psychiatric symptoms the vet is having, if any.
4. Any lack of social support.
5. The age, sex, race, and family history of the vet.
6. Whether there have been any prior suicide attempts.
7. Levels of impulsivity.
8. Past psychiatric diagnoses or treatment.
9. Chronic pain.
10. Protective factors like religion.
11. Additional suicide risk factors.
12. Quantification of suicide risk.
13. Any immediate action and treatment needed.

Every veteran should have every one of these risk and protective factors assessed, not just one or two of them, and in a manner that is effective and standardized. As of 2017, these other questions only get asked if a veteran responds positively to the section 3 questions and gets a "high" suicide risk rating. Note, too, that moderate and low suicide risks are not operationally defined in the Suicide Risk Assessment Guide.

Systematic Health Care Deficiencies in the VA Incident Briefs

In the *Veterans for Common Sense v. Peake* (2008) trial, there were only 170 incident briefs provided to me out of the estimated 15,000 briefs in which VA patient suicides and/or suicide attempts were described. Nevertheless, they offer a sample of systematic health care and treatment deficiencies identified by the VA itself. Below are some of the VA's treatment failures in assessing and managing veterans, as reported in these 170 briefs:

- Treatment was delayed.
- Patients with suicide ideation were not evaluated for suicide risk (section 2 of the Suicide Risk Assessment Guide card).
- There was no coordination of patient care (even though there were suicide coordinators).
- A vet should have been admitted to a hospital but was not.
- The response to a vet's expressed wish-to-die was inadequate.
- The VA needed a suicide hotline. (The VA now does have a hotline, but some research shows that only a small percentage of actual suicides even call clinics or hotlines.)
- There was no referral of veterans for severe antisocial behavior.
- No psychiatric evaluation of a vet was done in the emergency room.
- Suicide assessment policies and procedures on the Suicide Risk Assessment Guide card were not followed.
- A hopeless vet was not identified as such.
- A vet was not rescheduled for a follow-up appointment within 1 week, as per official policy.
- A vet's suicide risk assessment was negative, but the vet suicided anyway.
- A patient was denied access to a VA hospital and then suicided.
- A doctor at a VA hospital who was fired for inadequate treatment of a soldier was later found dead.
- Inadequate health care was provided for a homeless vet with suicidal ideation and threats.
- The VA was not meeting the needs of a suicidal vet.
- A vet actually shot himself on the grounds of a VA outpatient clinic.

These bulleted items reflect the VA's own admissions of health care problems or failures in treating suicidal vets. One can only imagine how much more investigators could have learned about VA assessment and treatment failures, had they been given all of the redacted incident briefs and root cause analyses (*root cause analyses* are protected VA postmortem documents analyzing possible causes of the suicide). Since the U.S. Congressional hearing in 2008 at which I testified was entitled "The Truth about Veteran Suicides," it only makes sense that all incident briefs be made public. For current research and prevention programs for the military, see Box 20.3.

In addition, the following facts were reported in a public deposition for *Veterans for Common Sense v. Peake.* The VA Deputy Under Secretary for Healthcare Operations and Management is third in the chain of command when it comes to VA vet health care.

- The Deputy Under Secretary said that all 21 VISN directors reported to him at least once a week, but when asked about vet suicide rates, he said he "did not talk to directors about their suicide rates."
- When asked about implementing the MHSP, his reply was "I did not read the plan from cover to cover."
- When asked if there was a systematic national plan for suicide prevention from 2004 to 2008, he answered, "No."

BOX 20.3. Recent U.S. Military Suicide Research and Prevention Programs

The suicide rate among members of the U.S. Armed Forces has traditionally been lower than the age- and gender-adjusted suicide rate of the U.S. general population (Kuehn, 2009). Beginning in 2004, however, suicides among military personnel started to increase, most notably in the Army and Marine Corps, and have since surpassed the adjusted general population rate for the first time in recorded history (Kuehn, 2009; Smolenski et al., 2014). In response to this troubling trend, research and prevention efforts focused on understanding and reducing military suicide have rapidly expanded.

Military-specific risk factors were initially assumed to be primary drivers of this change, based in large part on two related lines of thought: (1) The rise in military suicides followed the onset of military operations in Afghanistan and Iraq, and (2) there was no comparable rise in the U.S. general population suicide rate. One of the earliest hypotheses developed was that increased deployments were leading to elevated suicide risk. Epidemiological data from military medical surveillance and personnel record systems did not support this link, however. Contrary to expectations, the majority of military personnel who died by suicide had never deployed, and suicides were not overrepresented among military personnel who had died by suicide (Kinn et al., 2011; LeardMann et al., 2013; Luxton et al., 2012; Reger et al., 2015; Smolenski et al., 2014). Other lines of research have suggested that some forms of combat exposure *were* correlated with increased risk (Bryan et al., 2015; Maguen et al., 2011). These seemingly contradictory findings were fueled in large part by confusion about *deployment* and *combat,* which are distinct constructs that are often mistakenly assumed to be equivalent. A service member might deploy to a location with no active combat, however. Deployment in and of itself therefore may not be a risk factor for suicide, but certain traumatic experiences that occur while deployed (e.g., exposure to death and killing) may be (Bryan et al., 2015).

The combat–suicide link can only account for fewer than half of all military suicides, however; as noted previously, the majority of military personnel who die by suicide have no history of deployment. If the problem of military suicide is not attributable to deployments or combat exposure, why do military personnel die by suicide? To answer this question, we can turn to what we know about suicide in general across various populations. Research during the past decade has largely confirmed that the risk factors for suicide among military personnel are by and large the same as those among nonmilitary populations, such as psychological distress, life stressors, social isolation, demographic factors, and inpatient hospitalization (Kessler et al., 2015; Nock et al., 2014). Research has additionally confirmed that the primary motive for suicidal behavior among military personnel is the same as that among nonmilitary samples: to escape from or alleviate emotional distress (Bryan et al., 2013).

Given these similarities, suicide prevention among military personnel can reasonably be understood from the perspective of contemporary theories and models of suicidal behavior, albeit with culturally relevant adaptations that reflect the unique values and characteristics of the military. For example, the military is a collectivist institution that values mental toughness, self-sufficiency, fearlessness, pain tolerance, and sacrifice for the greater good (Bryan et al., 2012; Bryan & Morrow, 2011). These cultural values can potentially moderate or influence an individual service member's risk and protective factors. The collectivist orientation of the military, for instance, can serve to enhance belonging and social support in most cases. If a service member violates cultural norms (e.g., disciplinary action, failure to meet expectations), however, this collectivist orientation could instead lead to ostracism and rejection by the group. Risk and protective factors must therefore be understood within the larger context of the military culture.

(continued)

BOX 20.3. *(continued)*

In addition to identifying and describing risk and protective factors associated with military suicide, numerous efforts have aimed to reduce suicidal behaviors and associated risk factors among military personnel. Positive results to date have come in large part from mental health treatment studies. Of note, brief cognitive-behavioral therapy (BCBT) has been found to contribute reduce suicide attempts among active duty soldiers by 60%, as compared to treatment as usual (Rudd et al., 2015). Soldiers treated with the 12-session BCBT were also significantly less likely to be hospitalized during the 2-year follow-up period. BCBT shares many treatment components with the 10-session cognitive therapy for suicide prevention previously shown to be effective in a nonmilitary sample: emotion regulation, problem solving, and cognitive reappraisal skills training. Cognitive processing therapy, a trauma-focused psychological treatment, has also recently been shown to be associated with decreased suicide ideation among active duty soldiers diagnosed with PTSD (Bryan et al., 2016), similar to earlier findings from a study of the treatment in a nonmilitary sample of trauma survivors (Gradus et al., 2013).

Taken together, these studies demonstrate that principles of suicide prevention shown to be effective in nonmilitary samples can be successfully and effectively adapted to meet the cultural values and institutional demands of the military. Though research continues to develop and refine effective suicide prevention strategies within as well as external to the health care system, these early findings clearly demonstrate that suicide risk can be mitigated among military personnel. Several notable research studies and programs include the following:

- *Army Study to Assess Risk and Resilience in Servicemembers (STARRS).* Army STARRS is an interdisciplinary, epidemiological research study aimed at identifying risk and protective factors for mental health and suicide risk among Army personnel (*www.starrs-ls.org*).
- *Military Suicide Research Consortium (MSRC).* The MSRC runs cutting-edge empirical studies focused on the assessment, treatment, and prevention of suicidal behavior among military personnel and veterans across all branches and eras of service (*www.msrc.fsu.edu*).
- *Millennium Cohort Study (MCS).* The MCS is a large-cohort study aimed at describing long-term health outcomes of military personnel from all branches of service over the course of and following military service (*www.millenniumcohort.org*).

Source: Craig Bryan, University of Utah. Used with permission.

- One of the policies that has been fully implemented in the MHSP was 24-hour VA health care. When asked to name that policy, his answer was "I don't know that policy."
- He was asked, "Well, where are these policies?" Answer: "I don't know."
- Question: "Has the idea of screening every service person coming back from Iraq or Afghanistan for PTSD been a subject of discussion?" Answer: "I really could not give you an answer on that."
- Question: "Is there a national screening program for every returning

serviceman or woman to meet with a mental health professional?" Answer: "I don't know the answer to that."

- "The MHSP at page A-14 says that 'Every military person . . . will meet individually with a mental health professional as part of post-deployment and separation.' Has that happened?" Answer: "I don't believe it has."
- Question: "Have you read the National Strategy for Suicide Prevention and Institute of Medicine report *Reducing Suicide* [2002]?" Answer: "No."
- Question: "What methods are there for tracking at-risk [for suicide] veterans?" Answer: "I'm not sure, sorry."
- Question: "Is there any relationship between the number of times a vet is deployed and suicide?" Answer: "I don't know."

From such answers, one could easily conclude (at least from the trial data just cited) that if the suicidal "buck" stops with the Deputy Under Secretary for Healthcare Operations and Management, then the VA could be in serious trouble when it comes to assessing and preventing veteran suicides.

Remaining Related Issues

There are a few other important issues in military suicide that deserve mention.

Recruitment and Screening in the Military

It is entirely possible, if not likely, that soldiers become suicidal largely or in part due to conditions predating their military recruitment. If so, their baseline vulnerabilities (see the discussion of stress–diathesis theory in Chapter 4) may interact with the stressors of military service and especially with combat deployment to exacerbate their suicide risk. One example might be the DSM diagnosis of antisocial personality disorder (ASPD, code F60.2) among young males ages 18 and older. There is evidence (*Veterans for Common Sense v. Peake*, 2008) that some soldiers may have been induced to accept a discharge diagnosis of ASPD, rather than (say) PTSD. A diagnosis of any personality disorder precludes a vet from receiving disability benefits, since the psychopathology was presumed to have been present prior to military recruitment and enrollment. Even if this presumption is true, the Department of Defense needs to improve its recruitment screening procedures to keep vulnerable recruits out of the military in the first place.

Psychopharmacology

There is surprisingly little mention in the VA's mental health policies and procedures of treating mood disorders psychopharmacologically (see Maris, 2015). It is axiomatic in suicide prevention that much of the treatment of suicidality (but not all) requires prompt and precise diagnosis of mood disorders, followed by appropriate pharmacological treatment with one or more of the SSRI antidepressants (e.g.,

Lexapro, Zoloft, Celexa, Prozac, Luvox, Paxil), the SNRIs (e.g., Cymbalta, Effexor), anxiolytics (e.g., Xanax, Klonopin, Tranxene, Ativan, Buspar), and perhaps even a major second-generation antipsychotic (like Risperdal or Zyprexa) or an augmenting atypical antipsychotic (like Latuda or Abilify). ECT may be required in some cases.

Note that many of the VA's 875 CBOCs in 2008 often did not even have a physician on staff, who could write prescriptions that suicidal vets may have needed. There may be advanced practice nurses at these outpatient clinics, but they do not have the same training that physicians do. Since in 2008 there were about 875 CBOCs but only 154 VA hospitals or medical centers, a depressed or agitated vet was likely to get only psychotherapy, rather than both psychotherapy and pharmacological treatment.

Suicide Coordinators

The VA rightly takes pride in the fact that there are suicide coordinators in its medical centers (Feeley, 2008). However, serious questions remain about these suicide coordinators. In 2008 (this is no longer true at this writing), none of the 875 CBOCs had suicide coordinators; the 154 VA hospitals and medical centers did. Thus the vast majority of VA treatment facilities (82%) did not have suicide coordinators. If a vet goes randomly to one of the VA's 1,029 treatment centers, the probability of the vet's seeing a medical doctor is just under 18% (154/875).

There are several other questions about VA suicide coordinators: (1) What do these coordinators actually do? What is their job description (e.g., do they do clinical care, or are they only administrators)? In some of my legal VA suicide cases, coordinators tried to avoid liability by claiming that they were just administrators (not clinicians). (2) How are they trained to do suicide assessment and prevention? (3) What are their professional credentials and licensing, especially if many of them are nurses (LPNs and RNs), social workers (MSWs), MA psychologists, mental health technicians, and so on? (4) Who supervises the suicide coordinators? To whom do they report, and how often? (5) Do suicide coordinators themselves interact directly with suicidal vets in VA clinical care, and if so, how often? (6) What exactly are they coordinating (clinical care, suicide data, suicide policies and procedures, etc.)?

Treatment Delays

There are a whole set of questions concerning diagnosis, treatment, and benefit delays. To even get mental health treatment for up to 2 years a suicidal veteran in 2008 had to fill out a 23-page application form, which could be daunting if the vet was depressed or had PTSD. Then he or she received a disability rating from 0 to 100% from a "Compensation and Pension" examination.

If a vet's disability was denied, the rating was too low, or the disability was found not to be related to the vet's military service, then the appeal process could be long and drawn-out, which in turn could encourage a suicidal resolution of the vet's problems. Some vets have died during their appeal process. As of 2017, a vet can have direct, immediate care without extensive screening, if in a suicidal crisis. Finally, note that many of the VA suicide prevention initiatives described by Daigh (2007) have only been partially implemented. One wonders how many vets have died due to assessment and treatment delays.

Chapter 21 considers a second special topic, murder–suicide. How are suicides preceded by murder different from suicides alone, what varieties of murder–suicide are there, and what causes them?

CHAPTER 21

Murder–Suicide
Why Take Someone with You?

I think in a way I wanted it to end,
even if it meant my own destruction.
—JEFFREY DAHMER[1]

Up to this point, the focus has been on self-destruction, its types, and its causes. But what about *other-destruction* before suicide? It is one thing to kill yourself, but quite another to take someone with you. This does not necessarily mean that suicide and murder–suicide are fundamentally different. In fact, Joiner (2014) has argued that suicide and murder–suicide have a lot in common, and less in common with murder. Suicide and murder–suicide even tend to occur on the same days of the week—Monday and Tuesday—while homicides tend to occur on Saturday and Sunday (Joiner, 2014). Joiner argued that suicide (not murder) is the primary motive in murder–suicides. So, except for the time lag problem, maybe *murder–suicide* could be called *suicide–murder.*

Superficially, the concept of murder–suicide seems pretty straightforward and simple: One or more perpetrators kill one or more others, after which they kill themselves. But, as with most concepts, a moment's reflection reveals important subtleties. For example, what types of suicides and murders are we talking about? Suicides are intentional self-destruction, which can be motivated by altruism, escape, or revenge. The concept of murder is complex, especially in the law. Usually in murder–suicide there is first-degree murder, which involves premeditation and malice of forethought. However, murder can also be committed without premeditation (second-degree murder) or without any intent at all (manslaughter). For the most part, *murder–suicide* means premeditated killing(s) followed by intentional self-destruction.

---

[1]Technically, Dahmer was a murder–suicide ideator, since he never actually killed himself.

There is also a question about the suicide time lag after murder. Most suicides after murders occur in minutes or hours after the murders, not years (Joiner, 2014; Malmquist, 2012). Suicides can also occur when murderers are about to be apprehended. However, there is a serious question about apprehension suicides, since the murderers may have intended to escape and not even to commit suicide at all; their plans may simply have been foiled.

Murder–suicide tends to be the rarest of the rare. As we know, suicide itself in the United States occurs only at a rate of about 1 in 10,000 per year. But just 1–2% of those already rare suicides are murder–suicides. Joiner has argued that suicide is rare in part because it is hard to do; suicides have to develop what Joiner (2005) has called "the acquired ability to inflict lethal self-injury." If suicide is hard, then murder–suicide is harder still. Most killing in animals is cross-species. In the military only about 20% of combatants shoot to kill the enemy, and among the police that percentage shrinks to 10% of criminals (Joiner, 2014).

No national murder–suicide data are kept systematically, as there are for deaths or suicides (Malmquist, 2012). In 2015 in the United States, there were about 44,193 suicides, which translates into about 884 murder–suicides in that year (2% of all suicides). But since usually 2 people at least die in each murder–suicide, there were roughly 1,768 murder–suicides in the year in question. About 80% of murder–suicides involve one victim; 20% involve two or more. Ninety percent of the perpetrators are males, and 75% of the victims are females. This is particularly true for domestic murder–suicides. Malmquist (2012, p. 502) estimated that if a spouse is murdered, this alone increases the murder–suicides by a factor of 12.68. In a sense, domestic violence ending in murder–suicide tends to overvalue a relationship (Malmquist, 2012); it implies, for example, "I cannot live without you, nor will you be able to live without me."

Most murder–suicide victims are older. Only 14% are age 18 or younger. Worldwide in a recent year, there were 10,578 murder–suicides. As for suicides alone, the preferred method for murder–suicides is firearms, at least in the United States. One study claims that 55–70% of U.S. murder–suicides involve firearms; Malmquist (2012) says that the U.S. percentage is even higher, 88%. But there are cultural and ethnic variations in other countries. As in suicide alone, depressive disorders are common (Malmquist, 2012), with any mental disorder being present in over 90% of the cases; Joiner (2014) says that the figure is closer to 100%. Alcohol is common in murder–suicide as well. About 30% of the murderers at least test positive for alcohol (Malmquist, 2012); Joiner (2014) says 25–30%.

Murder–suicides can be classified by type of victim or by motive. In Table 21.1 there are three main types of victims, a type of perpetrator, and about three to four subtypes per category. The four primary types of murder–suicide are (1) domestic violence, usually a male killing his female spouse or lover, who has rejected him, filed for divorce, or gotten a restraining order; (2) murder–suicide perpetrated by the elderly, in which normally an aged male kills his terminally ill or infirm wife, then himself; (3) murder–suicide with victims who are minors—the subcategories include feticide (killing one's unborn fetus), neonaticide (killing one's baby within 24 hours of birth), infanticide (killing an infant up to 1 year old), and pedicide

TABLE 21.1. Murder–Suicide Classifications

  I. Domestic violence
     A. Spouse
        1. Male
        2. Female
     B. Partner
        1. Male
        2. Female
 II. Elderly perpetrators
     A. Spouse
     B. Offspring
     C. Companion
III. Minors
     A. Feticide (murder of fetus)
     B. Neonaticide (murder of infant in first 24 hours)
     C. Infanticide (murder of child up to 1 year)
     D. Pedicide (murder of child older than 1 year)
 IV. Mass murder–suicides
     A. Familicide (murder–suicide of an entire family)
     B. Workplace murder–suicides (murder of fellow workers)
     C. School shootings
     D. Religious, cult, political murder–suicides

Source: Adapted from Malmquist (2012, p. 502). Adapted with permission from *The American Psychiatric Publishing Textbook of Suicide Assessment and Management,* Second Edition. Copyright © 2012 American Psychiatric Association. All Rights Reserved.

(killing offspring older than 1 year), and (4) mass murder–suicides, such as those in Jonestown, Guyana.

The most common type of murder–suicide is that engendered by dissolution of a relationship, usually a female breaking up with a male (Malmquist, 2012). Examples of mass murder–suicides include the Columbine school shootings, killing one's entire family before suiciding, workplace murder–suicides, and Jim Jones's murder–suicides at Jonestown, Guyana. As I have discussed in Chapter 17, it was as if Jones had an extended sense of self, in which his suicide required killing his followers—Jonestown as well as Jones.

Joiner on the Perversion of Virtue

Why do murder–suicides occur?[2] In an impressive, ambitious book, Joiner (2014) has argued that to truly understand murder–suicide, we need to classify not only the types of victims, but also the types of motives of the perpetrators, most of whom

---

[2]Henry and Short (1954) argued, in their classic book *Suicide and Homicide,* that the broad social and personal conditions or traits favoring higher suicide rates are weak external restraint and strong internal restraint, while strong external restraint and weak internal restraint increase homicide risk or rates.

are male. What are the murderers' motives in murder–suicides? Joiner claims that murder–suicides involve a perversion of four basic human virtues. *Virtues* refer to aspects of moral excellence or character; they are traits or qualities deemed to be morally good and thus valued. Examples of virtues include prudence, justice, temperance, courage, faith, hope, and charity. The opposite of virtue is vice. The four virtues perverted in Joiner's theory of murder–suicide are (1) justice, (2) duty, (3) mercy, and (4) glory (Joiner, 2014). Of these four, justice and mercy are thought to be the most common types.

1. *Justice.* The implication is that in the suicide's mind, murdering others first is good and proper in certain conditions. For example, Seung-Hui Cho murdered 17 Virginia Tech students and wounded 17 others on April 16, 2007. He believed that his behavior was just. He had contempt for the rich students there, whom he viewed as unfairly privileged and engaged in debauchery (Joiner, 2014). He felt that he was the savior of the oppressed, poor, and downtrodden.

Joiner (2014) has claimed that the logic of justice was intact in the Virginia Tech murders. In Cho's mind, it was unjust for one spoiled group to have privileges just because their parents were wealthy and powerful. However, Joiner also claimed that Cho's logic was perverted. His murders were in fact not justified. Cho's behavior was not only a narcissistic vice, but was also illegal and immoral.

2–3. *Mercy and duty.* Some older married persons (again, usually men) claim that it is sometimes merciful and dutiful to help their long-time spouses die, when the spouses are in pain with no hope of survival or improvement. Although he did not suicide, 78-year-old Bertram Harper helped his 69-year-old wife, Virginia, die by an overdose of sleeping pills combined with a bag over her head on August 18, 1990. Harper was charged with second-degree murder (i.e., murder with intent, but no premeditation). The jury acquitted Harper on May 11, 1991. Derek Humphry (who testified in Harper's trial) said that the jury ignored the law and brought a moral victory. Harper could have had to spend the remainder of his life in prison, which is similar to suiciding.

Almost all people, especially mental health workers and clinicians, are committed to suicide prevention and contend that neither suicide nor murder–suicide is ever rational, just, merciful, dutiful, or glorious; they protest that in fact, both types of acts are perversions of virtue. However, one could easily argue the opposite. For example, are not some suicides rational? Is it not merciful to help a terminally ill wife or husband in great, unrelenting pain die, or to bring evildoers and criminals to justice? In short, some murder–suicides may be virtuous and not perversions of virtue. But part of the problem with murder–suicide is that a few individuals (many of whom are mentally disordered) just assume the unilateral right to determine morality without the checks and balances of the law, collective judgment, or custom.

In most murder–suicides involving minors, parents also believe that it is merciful and dutiful to kill their dependent children in certain circumstances, rather than leave them behind without a mother and father. Joiner (2014) cites the 2009 case of Ervin Lupoe in southern California, who murdered his five children, ages 2–8 years, and then suicided with his wife (see Case 21.7, below). Lupoe had lost his job and did not want anyone else to raise his children. Mercy and duty with minors are more complicated issues than with a spouse, in part because the children's own wishes are ignored.

4. *Glory*. Other murder–suicides believe that their murder–suicides are courageous and will bring them glory and fame. On April 20, 1999, Eric Harris and Dylan Klebold murdered 12 students and a teacher, injured 21 others, and then shot themselves at Columbine High School in Colorado. They believed that their murder–suicides would make both of them famous forever, and it probably did, even though most of us would agree that they had a perverted sense of glory. The Columbine shootings are discussed further in Case 21.13, below.

Joiner's (2014) *Perversion of Virtue* is well written, readable, and interesting—almost like an essay or novel. Notice how Joiner argues: He begins with hypotheses, then presents selected quotes from well-known people, in an attempt to support the theory of murder–suicide he is constructing. One could just as easily argue in the opposite direction from Joiner, however. For example, why are murder–suicides always "perversions" of virtue? Derek Humphry could cite many murder–suicides he believes are virtuous. A lot of people contend that the killing of Osama bin Laden was just and heroic, even if the Navy SEALs who did this could have been on a suicide mission.

Most people assume "wrongly" (says Joiner, 2014) that suicide occurs impulsively. In another example, he says that Freud and Menninger are "wrong" about humans' having a death wish. Joiner has written an entire book (*Myths about Suicide*, 2010) in which he, in effect, argues that much most of what many people believe about suicide is "wrong." Edwin Shneidman (1985) also wrote about suicide myths. A lot of murderers who later kill themselves do not start out with a suicide plan, but Joiner would probably say that this is "wrong."

Joiner's data do not necessarily support his theory of murder–suicide. Everyone is entitled to have opinions, but often they are just that—opinions. Having said this, I must add that Joiner often has tremendous insight. For example, in what Joiner (2014) labels an "opponent process," he claims that serial murderer Jeffrey Dahmer learned to kill. Most of us are repulsed by killing (murder or suicide), and only a few of us will do it or even be able to do it.

In the remainder of this chapter, I present several cases to illustrate the types of victims listed in Table 21.1 and some of Joiner's types of perverted virtues. Almost all of these are cases that have been made public in some manner (court cases, the news media, etc.), and no confidential or protected information is given for any case.

Domestic Violence

The first case (Case 21.1) is one of domestic violence, and it is a little unusual in two ways. First, it is a case of a woman murdering her husband, then killing herself. Usually in murder–suicides men murder their wives or unmarried female partners.

Second, this was a case that occurred at my own university; this was also true of Case 21.2, in which a professor intended to murder the university president and did kill himself. Case 21.3 was an instance of more typical domestic violence (a husband's murdering his wife and then suiciding), in which the husband was taking an SSRI antidepressant.

CASE 21.1. Raga Fayad and Sunghee Kwon

At about 1 P.M. on February 5, 2015, at the University of South Carolina (USC) School of Public Health, Raga Fayad, a 45-year-old professor of anatomy and physiology, was murdered by his ex-wife, Sunghee Kwon, age 46. She shot him several times in the upper body, then shot herself once in the stomach with a 9-mm handgun. That he was shot several times suggests rage and/or desperation by Kwon. That she shot herself in the stomach and not in the head could indicate her own ambivalence about dying. Chest and stomach shots are more characteristic of females. The FBI records the number of times a victim is shot or stabbed as one indicator of anger or rage.

Kwon and Fayad had been divorced for a few years, but they had continued to live together until he recently rented a motel room. Kwon felt that Fayad's leaving her was terribly unjust and inconvenient, and it made her incredibly angry. His leaving their home caused her to lose not only her husband, but also his income, their home, and her reputation. Divorce is not well regarded by Korean women. The fact that they had been divorced for years but continued to live together is strange in and of itself. Unfortunately, there is a lot about Fayad and Kwon that we just do not know. Was he having an affair? Did she have dependent personality disorder?

Fayad was a physician and medical researcher from Syria, and Kwon was from South Korea. One wonders whether Kwon had adequate social and familial support in the United States during her crisis. They had met and married in Chicago at the University of Illinois. Apparently they had no children. They moved to Columbia, South Carolina, in 2008, where he directed a colon cancer research lab at the USC School of Public Health and was head of an Applied Psychology Division. They bought a house together on a nearby lake before they divorced. After Fayad moved out, Kwon stayed in the couple's home, but could not pay the utility bill and had lost her heating and lights. It had recently been cold, and this may have been another factor in her desperation.

Kwon had previously stalked Fayad at his lab, and he had called the police in the last month to have her forcibly removed. He did not tell the police that she was his ex-wife. It sounds as if the couple had been in a love–hate relationship for some time, which may have contributed to Kwon's suicidal career, along with her evident psychological disturbance.

Most of the university did not know Fayad, and so the depth of the university's public response to his murder was striking: Numerous bouquets of flowers were sent to the School of Public Health; there was a campuswide religious service at the university's chapel; and counseling sessions were held for students. Maybe it was as John Donne said: "Never send to know for whom the bell tolls; it tolls for thee." Death, murder, suicide, and violence remind us all how fragile and precarious life can be. For all of us in the long run, life eventually ends in death. However, fickle, violent death is terrifying for everyone.

Source: All information about this case came from public information presented in the news media; none of it was confidential.

CASE 21.2. Philip Zeltner and James Holderman

There was an attempted murder–suicide case at USC in the mid-1980s: Philosophy profes-sor Philip Zeltner tried to murder the university's president at the time, James Holderman. This domestic violence within the USC "family" was unusual in that it involved two men. It is probably more accurately categorized as workplace violence. Zeltner was a friend of mine. He won the top university teaching award and had published a book, but was still denied tenure by President Holderman. Zeltner felt something way beyond a lack of justice—perhaps even betrayal. Zeltner was bright, but he also struck me as aggressive, self-centered, sometimes inappropriate in pursuing his own interests, and probably unaware of his own disqualifying faults. It was not clear why he was denied tenure, but when that happened, he felt hopeless and believed that his career was ruined.

He decided to take his anger out on Holderman, who had been a friend of his. He went to the president's office with a gun, but Holderman was out at the time, which saved his life. Zelt-ner left 30 silver dollars on Holderman's desk, suggesting betrayal like Judas Iscariot's betrayal of Jesus Christ. Zeltner barricaded himself in the president's office, but ended up shooting himself even after his wife and others came to plead with him not to suicide.

Source: I was acquainted with both parties in this case.

CASE 21.3. Bill and June Forsyth

Bill Forsyth was a robust, 61-year-old, white male millionaire living in his dream house on the beach in Maui with his wife of 37 years, June. After retiring from his Los Angeles airport car rental business and moving to Maui, however, he became clinically depressed and was started on 20 mg of an SSRI antidepressant (Prozac). After only 1 day of treatment, he reported feeling 100% better—but by day 2 he felt 200% better, became agitated (did he experience akathi-sia?), and requested to be hospitalized. After being in a psychiatric hospital for 7 days, Bill was released and came home. At some time during the night, he stabbed June 17 times, and then stabbed himself to death.

Source: All case information was publicized in *Forsyth v. Eli Lilly,* a trial in U.S. District Court in Honolulu, Hawaii, in 1999. See Box 21.1 for details.

In a subsequent trial, one legal issue in the Forsyth case was whether Bill Forsyth's antidepressant caused or contributed to the murder–suicide (see Box 21.1 for a discussion of two similar cases involving Prozac). The Forsyth jury said no, but that was not the end of the matter. Discussion and research studies have continued to investigate whether psychiatric medications may have contributed to suicides such as these. As noted throughout this book, most depressed individuals have lower CSF and brain serotonin (5-HT) levels than normal controls do (Maris, 2015). SSRIs (like Prozac, Paxil, Zoloft, Luvox, and Lexapro) block serotonin reabsorption postsynaptically. This, theoretically, makes more serotonin available in the brain and should reduce depressive disorders. Not only SSRI antidepressants, but also the herb St. John's wort and certain diets high in tryptophan (tryptophan is the dietary precursor to serotonin), are thought to raise brain 5-HT levels and functioning—and thus to prevent or alleviate suicide ideation and depression.

BOX 21.1. Can Domestic Violence Be Caused by Antidepressants?

The antidepressant fluoxetine (Prozac) was first marketed in the United States in 1988 by the drug company Eli Lilly. Early in the marketing, Lilly was the defendant in two cases in which the plaintiffs contended that Prozac triggered violence, including suicide. Lilly claimed victory in both cases. The first win was in the December 1994 case *Fentress (Wesbecker) v. Eli Lilly*. After the verdict, the trial judge learned that Lilly had secretly settled the case during the trial, to keep damaging evidence that Lilly had withheld from being heard by the jury. The *American Lawyer* branded it as "Lilly's Phantom Verdict." The Kentucky Supreme Court observed with regard to this case: "There was a serious lack of candor with the trial court and there may have been deception, bad faith conduct, and abuse of the judicial process."

Lilly's second win came in April 1999, with a seemingly unanimous verdict on *Forsyth v. Eli Lilly*. However, on June 7, 2000, the Forsyths filed a new suit to set aside the prior verdict, on the grounds that it had been obtained via fraud on the court. That suit alleged, as in the *Fentress* case, that critical information was withheld from the judge and jury. Specifically, it claimed that despite Eli Lilly's having paid $20 million for a patented new Prozac molecule (an isomer) that it claimed would reduce certain side effects of the original Prozac, a Lilly patent lawyer sat mutely in the courtroom while Lilly's trial counsel told the judge and jury that that suicide was not a side effect of Prozac.

Source: Notes from Maris's personal experiences in the two public trials described above.

Paradoxically, though, SSRIs have also been accused of increasing both suicide ideation and actual suicide (Teicher et al., 1990a, 1990b; Maris, 2015). The purported causal mechanisms of increased suicidal behaviors in serotonin-enhancing drugs include (but are not limited to) (1) akathisia, a diffuse inner and outer psychomotor restlessness; (2) increased anxiety, agitation, and decreased impulse control; (3) switching depression to mania or hypomania; and (4) reducing vegetative (biological) symptoms of depression before they reduce the patient's depressed mood, thus energizing patients who still have suicide ideation. That is, improvements in depression and amelioration of suicide ideas have different cycles, such that if depression is lessened, it may produce a window of opportunity for suicide.

Admittedly, it is hard to sort out drug-related and non-drug-related effects, especially since the drug companies who manufacture and profit from antidepressants and their sale tend to minimize adverse effects. One might reasonably suspect that drug companies tend to be biased in favor of their products and tend to fund clinical trial studies that favorably assess possible side effects of drugs. Not only is murder–suicide about justice; it is also perhaps about neurochemistry. The final case I use to illustrate domestic violence, Case 21.4, describes a celebrity murder–suicide in which the murderous spouse appears to have consumed multiple substances.

CASE 21.4. Phil and Brynn Hartman

One last case of domestic violence murder–suicide is interesting because it involved Phil Hartman of *Saturday Night Live* fame, and because his wife killed him and then herself. On May 28, 1998, Phil Hartman was shot to death by his wife, Brynn, while their son, Sean, age 9, and daughter, Birgen, 6, were asleep. Brynn, Hartman's third wife, was a 40-year-old model and aspiring playwright whose birth name was Vicki Jo Omdahl. She had about a 10-year history of on-and-off cocaine and alcohol abuse. Their marriage had been tumultuous. Brynn was jealous of Hartman's second wife and threatened her. She was emotionally volatile, and Hartman's fame made her feel insecure. There were many arguments at home, including the day of the incident. In the spring of 1997, Brynn was treated for cocaine abuse at Arizona's Sierra Tucson facility. One week before Phil's death, Brynn tried to book herself into Promises (a Malibu rehab center where Robert Downey, Jr., and Charlie Sheen were treated), but the facility was full.

The day Phil Hartman died, he had bought a boat (he enjoyed sailing) in Newport Beach, near Los Angeles. That evening Brynn went to dinner at an Italian restaurant one block from her home with a friend, Christine Zanders. Brynn drank two Cosmopolitans (a vodka mixed drink) and left about 10 P.M. to return home. When she got home, Brynn and Phil argued; it is not clear about what. Their two children slept. Then Phil went to sleep. Brynn came into the bedroom and shot Phil three times, twice in the head and once in the torso with a .38 revolver Phil kept at home for protection. Son Sean heard the shots, but went back to sleep.

Brynn left her children sleeping alone and Phil dead, and went to the home of Ron Douglas in Studio City (about 10 miles away) at about 3 A.M. Friends whom she called during the drive reported that she was disoriented. Douglas was a singer, actor, and stuntman (and perhaps a lover of Brynn's). He apparently supplied Brynn with cocaine. Brynn fell asleep at his house, after telling him that she had shot Phil. Douglas and Brynn returned to the Hartman home around dawn.

Douglas confirmed that Phil was dead, called 911, and was starting to take Sean out of the house when the police arrived. Brynn locked herself in the bedroom and called her sister, Kathy Wright, who later reported that Brynn was acting "weird" on the phone. The police, who were walking Birgen out of the house, heard an inhuman wailing, followed by a single shot. Brynn had shot herself in the mouth.

An attorney was retained by the executor of Brynn's estate. Brynn's brother, Greg, was questioned, to see if Brynn's "weird" behavior might be due in part to the SSRI that she had been taking. The SSRI was not prescribed to her, but rather to her son, Sean, who had ADHD. At autopsy, Brynn had a 0.12% blood alcohol level and trace amounts of cocaine and the SSRI in her body.

One issue for the Hartman family was to try to determine whether Brynn's homicide–suicide might have been the result of an SSRI-induced drug reaction, perhaps akathisia (as in the Bill Forsyth case; see Case 21.3). Her housekeeper, Lorraine Blanco, reported that Brynn had felt like she was going to "jump out of her skin," had diarrhea, and had called a physician 2 or 3 days before the murder–suicide.

Source: Compiled by Maris from *TV Guide* (July 18–24, 1998) and other news media accounts.

The Elderly

When the elderly murder, suicide, or commit murder–suicide, it is often in response to their own or their spouses' poor and declining health (Malmquist, 2012). Bourget et al. (2010) found that in murder–suicides over age 65, 80% of the murdered partners had a preexisting medical condition, but only about half the murderers did. Typically, an older white male spouse puts an end to his wife's suffering, presumably out of mercy (Berman, 1996). Case 21.5 illustrates this dynamic.

CASE 21.5. Nelson and Evelyn Harvey

Nelson Harvey, age 91, shot his wife, Evelyn, 93, in the back of the head (an interesting site) on December 20, 2015, in El Paso, Texas. They had been married for 65 years and had fought her terminal illness for the last 9 years. Nelson told the police that he "was tired of her suffering, so I shot her." He was charged with murder. There has been no verdict at this time, but often juries do not send elderly spousal "mercy killers" to jail or prison; in Nelson's case, this would be in effect a death sentence. Normally, the elderly killer's life is so intertwined with that of the spouse that the killer commits suicide as well. Elderly murderers are often unable or unwilling to be separated from their spouses and cannot imagine life without them.

Source: This case account is based on information in the public domain.

Closely related to such murder–suicides are *suicide pacts*, which usually also occur among aged couples; in a pact, the husband and the wife decide to die together. In effect, such cases are often symbolically murder–suicides, since the male spouse routinely decides for his wife to die (Malmquist, 2012). Case 21.6 describes the suicide pact between the writer Arthur Koestler and his third wife.

CASE 21.6. Arthur Koestler and Cynthia Jeffries

A well-known case example of a couple's suicide pact is that of Arthur Koestler, age 78, and his (third) wife, Cynthia Jeffries, only 55 and in good health, in London on March 3, 1983. Arthur Koestler was born on September 5, 1905 in Budapest, the only child of Henrik and Adela Koestler. The first trauma for Arthur was an unexpected tonsillectomy without anesthesia in 1910. Because of the father's poor business sense and his mother's dislike of Hungary, the family moved to Vienna in 1914, amidst much conflict between his parents.

Shy and insecure, Koestler studied science and engineering, but became involved in a Zionist dueling fraternity at a polytechnic college in Vienna. The 3 years he spent in this group were very happy and began his involvement with politics. He became a follower of Vladimir Jabotinsky, burned his matriculation papers, and left for Palestine in 1926. After a hard period of adjustment there, he obtained a job as Middle East correspondent for a German publishing company.

In 1929, disillusioned with Palestine, he returned to Europe, where he continued to work as a newspaper correspondent. He joined the German Communist Party in 1931 and lost his job as a result. He traveled to Russia to report on events there and returned to Paris to write, though the Communist Party disapproved of many of his articles and books and greatly restricted his freedom. He married Dorothy Asher, but they separated a few months later and were divorced in 1950.

Koestler made three trips to Spain during its Civil War and was arrested and imprisoned for 3 months by Franco's Nationalists as a spy. He was sentenced to death but freed after British protests. Disillusioned now with Communism, he resigned from the Communist Party. He was detained and imprisoned in both England and France, but after the publication of *Darkness at Noon* (1940), he was released and worked for the Ministry of Information in England during the war.

After the war, Zionism again captured his attention, and he traveled to Israel and both reported on events and wrote novels that incorporated his experiences. In 1950 he married Mamaine Paget, but she separated from him in 1951 and died in 1954, soon after their divorce. His third and final marriage was to Cynthia Jeffries in 1965, who had been his secretary since 1950.

He settled in England in 1952 and became a British citizen. He continued to work for and write about political issues. His writings, including novels, essays, and biographies, always explored the important social issues of the times, and his work has been compared to that of George Orwell's in its impact on the times.

Cynthia Jeffries was 22 when she started working for Koestler. She was from South Africa and had gone to Paris with the aim of working for a writer. There had been stress in her life; her father committed suicide when she was 13, which is noteworthy, given her own suicide pact later on. She had had a brief, unsuccessful first marriage. From the time she joined Koestler, her life was rarely distinct from his.

One of the causes for which Koestler worked was euthanasia. As he grew older, he developed Parkinson's disease and then leukemia. When the effects of these illnesses worsened, he decided to commit suicide. Cynthia decided (according to Arthur) that she could not live without him, and she suicided as well.

Source. Adapted from Lester (1996). Adapted with permission.

Minors

Children in murder–suicides are innocent victims of their parents' decision to suicide. The parents' decision to suicide is what comes first; then, out of what Joiner (2014) would describe as a perverted sense of mercy and compassion, the children are murdered. Case 21.7, the case of the Lupoe family mentioned earlier, involved both parents' murdering all five of their children; Case 21.8 was an instance in which depression and related problems caused a mother to attempt murder–suicide with her only son (but both parties survived); Case 21.9, which caused a media sensation in the 1990s, involved a mother's murdering her two young sons and apparently intending to commit suicide but changing her mind at the last moment.

CASE 21.7. The Lupoe Family

On January 26, 2009, Ervin A. Lupoe, age 40, killed his wife, Ana, and the couple's five children: Brittney (age 8) and two sets of twins, Jasoman (5) and Jessely (5), and Benjamin (2) and Christian (2). Ana had planned the murder–suicides. Ervin shot himself in the head the next morning.

Ervin and Ana had both just been fired from Kaiser Permanente, for which they worked as radiology technicians in a hospital. The hospital accused them of fraud when they lied about their income in order to get cheaper child care. Because of the firings, the Lupoes pinpointed Kaiser Permanente as the cause of their murder–suicides. The Lupoes were also deeply in debt. They had three mortgages on their $250,000 home in a suburb of Los Angeles and had filed for bankruptcy earlier. Recently a check they wrote to the IRS had bounced. They were also a month delinquent on their mortgage payments.

All of this and more (there is a lot we do not know about the Lupoes) triggered what the Lupoes called a horrible "ordeal." Not wanting their children to be put through this ordeal, out of what they thought was compassion and mercy (Joiner, 2014), Ana planned the murder–suicides and Ervin carried them out. In anticipation of the event, the school-age children were taken out of school a few days earlier.

Joiner (2014) argued that it was a mistake, and thus a perversion of mercy, for the Lupoes to assume irremediable agony and needless suffering for their children. Regardless of how the parents may have felt, they also decided on murder for their young children without giving them an opportunity to live. Although it would be trying, the children themselves were not hopeless about the future, and their lives could have been salvaged with some support, perhaps from Social Services or extended family. Lupoe had called his brother-in-law after the murders and before his suicide.

A strange suicide note, addressed "To Whom It May Concern," suggested that the Lupoes did not feel that they had any support or anyone to turn to for help. The note went on and on about their perceived workplace injustice. An administrator may have suggested that now the Lupoes would not be eligible for employment after admitting to fraud. Ervin claimed that Kaiser Permanente would not release their licenses, so they could not even look for other work. Two days before they were fired, Ervin said that his supervisor perhaps told him, "I don't know why you even showed up for work; you should have blown your brains out." If just the Lupoes had suicided and had not killed their children, this would have been a suicide pact like the one by the Koestlers (see Case 21.6).

Source: This case account is based on information in the public domain.

CASE 21.8. Nancy and Samuel Simpson

Nancy Simpson (not her real name) was a bright, attractive, 45-year-old plastic surgeon. A few hours after midnight on September 9, 1996, she injected her 8-year-old son, Samuel, with Xylocaine, and cut his throat with a scalpel. Then she cut her own carotid artery and fainted on the bathroom floor. Covered with blood and screaming, Sam stumbled upstairs and awoke the housekeeper, who called 911 and saved both Sam and his mother. Thus, technically, the case was an attempted murder–suicide.

Nancy was arrested and jailed after recovering from her wound in a regional medical center. She exsanguinated several pints of blood and required two transfusions. Her charge was assault and battery with intent to kill. Her medical license was suspended, and her divorced husband got custody of Sam. When Sam explained the incident to the police, he said, "Mommy mistook me for someone else and cut me."

This is a very sad story about how depression (and perhaps its treatment), anxiety, and physical illness can transform a caring physician into a hopeless, desperate mother. Nancy had a long history, at least since medical school, of outpatient treatment for depression. At various times she took Paxil, Zoloft, Effexor, and Serzone (all antidepressants), with only modest improvement in her mood. She also had severe anxiety attacks, for which she took Ativan. For 6 weeks before her attempted murder–suicide, Nancy had been suffering from physical illness (diarrhea, dysentery, and dehydration) and taking antibiotics.

Since she had also been on an SSRI for weeks and was severely depressed, she retained an attorney to get experts to testify how depressive disorder and its treatment can turn competent, compassionate, loving individuals into desperate people, who see no way out of their troubles but to die. There was a possible product liability issue as to whether or not Nancy had an adverse drug reaction that transformed her (e.g., lowered her impulse control).

Nancy won her criminal trial, in part by arguing that major depression is a serious medical disease that caused her to act out of character, in a way she would never behave when she was healthy. Nancy is now slowly putting her life back together and trying to live with what she did to her only child (whom she loves dearly) in the grips of depression.

CASE 21.9. Susan Smith and Children

A case of minors' being murdered (pedicide) and the perpetrator's attempting suicide was the infamous case of Susan Smith, publicized by many news media outlets. One commentator branded the Smith case as "Münchausen's-by-proxy"—that is, causing the injury or death of others in order to get attention for oneself. Twenty-three-year-old Susan Smith told the nation that a black man hijacked her car and abducted her two small sons, Michael and Adam, ages 3 and 1, on October 25, 1994. She and her husband, David, made repeated pleas to their abductor to return the boys. A little over a week later, Susan confessed that she herself had drowned her young sons by rolling her car down a boat ramp into a lake with her sons strapped inside. Her attorney's hypothesis was that Susan Smith intended to kill herself and take her children with her—that is, to commit murder–suicide, not murder. Indeed, the record showed that Susan initially released the hand brake with all three of them inside the car, but at the last minute reset the brake, got out, and then rereleased the brake.

There was a lot of suicide, attempted suicide, suicide ideation, and depressive disorder in Susan Smith's family background. Her own father committed suicide on January 15, 1978, when Susan was 6 years old. Her grandmother and her brother both attempted suicide. Susan herself had two prior suicide attempts at ages 13 and 18 by overdosing on aspirin. Susan spent 8 days in a medical center after her second suicide attempt and was diagnosed with depression with adjustment disorder.

Susan also suffered many other stresses and negative life events in her young life. Most notably, her stepfather sexually assaulted Susan from at least March 1989, when she was 17, until shortly before she murdered her sons in 1994. Susan had a series of promiscuous sexual relationships. For example, she had sex with her boss (from 1989 to 1994) and, at the same time, with her boss's son. All this promiscuity by her and her husband, David, apparently wrecked her marriage; on September 21, 1994, she sued David for divorce.

Mothers who attempt suicide sometimes attempt to or succeed in murdering their children, as in the case of Nancy Simpson (see Case 21.8). For some young women, sexual acting out and nonfatal suicide attempts can be a desperate effort not to suicide, but rather to keep living (see Maris, 1971). The fact that Susan had sex mainly with older men suggested a perverse attempt for intimacy and fatherly affection that she never got. As heinous as Susan's crimes were, her father and stepfather perhaps share part of the blame for helping create a young woman capable of such unthinkable behavior.

Sources: N. Gibbs (1994) and other news stories at the time.

Mass Murder–Suicides

Mass murder–suicides include the following four types:

1. *Familicide.* The husband usually kills his entire family or extended family and then himself. The Lupoe case (see Case 21.7) was an example of familicide as well as the murder of minors.
2. *Workplace murder–suicides.* Examples include the Joseph Wesbecker case in 1989 (see Case 21.11) and possibly the crash of EgyptAir Flight 990 in 1999 (see Case 21.12).

3. *School shootings.* Two famous examples, the Columbine High School (1999) and Virginia Tech (2007) shootings, have been mentioned earlier in this chapter. Case 21.13 adds more details about the Columbine murder–suicides.
4. *Cult, religious, or political murder–suicides.* Examples include Jonestown, Heaven's Gate, and *jihad,* all discussed earlier in Chapter 17.

Most of these types of murder–suicides have been considered elsewhere in this text and are not elaborated upon much more here. Although the fit is not perfect, the primary perverted virtue in both the Jonestown and *jihad* murder–suicides is probably duty. Jim Jones's congregation felt a duty to obey his wishes, and he and his followers felt a duty to their religious principles. Terrorists in *jihad* have a duty to protect Islam from evil and heretics, and are glorified in heaven for doing their duty. An interesting question arises in religious or cult murder–suicides, due to the fact that the suicides often do not believe that they will actually die. If the persons intend to go to heaven and be transformed, but do not believe that they will cease to be, are their deaths really suicides?

The most recent case discussed in this chapter, and by far the deadliest, is the Las Vegas mass shooting of October 2017 (see Case 21.10). The motives of the shooter, Stephen Paddock, are as yet unknown and may never be known. Some instances of murder–suicide will always elude easy classification.

CASE 21.10. The Las Vegas Mass Murder–Suicide

One of the most recent and deadliest mass murder–suicides was 64-year-old Stephen Paddock's killing of 58 and wounding of 546 concertgoers at a music festival on the Las Vegas strip on October 1, 2017. For about 10 minutes, Paddock fired into the crowd below with modified automatic rifles from a rented suite on the 32nd floor of the adjacent Mandalay Bay Hotel, then killed himself. No motives were found, but the American Association of Suicidology (Joiner, 2010) has contended that in murder–suicide, suicide itself is the primary driving motive among complex factors.

Paddock made extensive preparation for the mass shootings, checked out alternative sites and events, and had about 20 rifles and handguns with large amounts of ammunition in his room. This was not an impulsive incident. Paddock himself was a retired millionaire from the Las Vegas area, former IRS agent, pilot, and real estate salesman. Although he had no criminal history, his father was a notorious bank robber who had been on the FBI's Ten Most Wanted Fugitives list. Stephen was a heavy drinker and a high-stakes poker (mainly video poker) player; he was twice divorced.

Source: This case account is based on public news stories of the event and its circumstances.

CASE 21.11. Joseph Wesbecker

On September 14, 1989, Joseph Wesbecker, age 47 (who had been put on disability), went to the Standard Gravure printing plant in Louisville, Kentucky, where he had previously worked. He took with him an AK-47 and other guns. He then shot and killed 8 of his coworkers and wounded 12 others before he shot himself. The estates of the injured and deceased workers sued Eli Lilly, the manufacturer of Prozac, which Wesbecker had been taking. They claimed that the drug had caused or substantially contributed to Wesbecker's violence and homicides. Even though 9 of the 12 jurors exonerated Prozac and Lilly from blame, the judge ruled that Lilly had "bought" the verdict and had secretly settled the case.

Source: All case information was publicized in *Fentress (Wesbecker) v. Eli Lilly,* a trial in Kentucky in 1994. See Box 21.1 for details.

CASE 21.12. EgyptAir Flight 990

EgyptAir Flight 990 crashed on October 31, 1999, at 01:50:38 hours, approximately 30 minutes after takeoff from a stopover at New York's John F. Kennedy International Airport. It crashed about 60 miles south of Nantucket Island, Massachusetts. The plane was a Boeing 767 with 217 people aboard. Of the passengers, 100 were Americans, 89 Egyptians, and 22 Canadians; the remaining 6 were of mixed nationalities and crew members. Among the Egyptian passengers were 7 oil professionals, 3 nuclear experts, and 33 Egyptian military officers (ironically, all pilots).

The senior pilot on the flight was Ahmad El-Habashi, age 57. There were two copilots, Adel Adwar and Gameel El-Batouty. Captain El-Habashi went to the toilet, so copilot El-Batouty took control of flying the plane. Twenty-one seconds after Habashi left the cockpit, El-Batouty said, "*Tawakkelt Ala Allah*" ("I rely on God") 11 times.

At 01:49:45, the autopilot was disconnected; at 01:49:53, the throttle level was set to idle; at 01:49:54, there was an abrupt downward elevator movement leading to a steep dive. The captain returned to the cockpit and said, "What's happening?" and "Pull with me." At 01:50:21, the right and left elevators were in split directions. Another crew member returned to the cockpit. It appeared that the pilot and copilot were not working together. There was no evidence of mechanical failure.

A key issue in the case was whether or not El-Batouty deliberately crashed the plane (i.e., suicided and killed all of his passengers). Reports were filed by the FBI, the National Transportation Safety Board, and Egyptian officials. One of the people interviewed about suicide in Egypt was the president of the Egyptian Association for Mental Health. You may recall from Chapter 8 that typically Egyptians are not likely to suicide, and that the entire country has a very low suicide rate.

The profile of El-Batouty indicated that he was upper-middle-class. He was lively and without suicide ideation; nor was there any family history of suicide or mental illness. Like most Egyptians, he did not drink alcohol. El-Batouty graduated from the Egypt Air Academy and was a pilot instructor in the Army for 14 years. Nothing unusual happened the day he died. He spoke with his wife on the phone, who wanted some clothes. El-Batouty replied, "I got them."

While in the United States, he had also gotten some medicine for one of his five children, who had lupus; he was bringing the medicine back home with him. El-Batouty and his wife had no marital problems. One of his sons had graduated from a police academy just before El-Batouty left on his flight. His mother and father were both dead, but he had five sisters. In short, there was no clear evidence that Gameel El-Batouty had committed suicide by airplane.

There was no trial (all issues were settled or dropped). The only real anomaly was El-Batouty's saying, "I rely on God" 11 times just before the crash. However, if something major had gone wrong with the airplane, it would have been reasonable for El-Batouty in his agitated state to say, "I rely on God," or "*Ya Sater Ya Rub*" ("Oh my God!"). It is more likely that a suiciding Muslim would probably say, "*Allahu Akbar*" ("God is great").

The evidence for murder–suicide is stronger for the Germanwings Flight 9529 plane crash on March 24, 2015, in which copilot Andreas Lubitz killed himself and 150 passengers. Phillips (1980) has argued that there is a significant rise in airline suicides 7–10 days after a publicized mass murder followed by a suicide, suggesting a contagion or copying effect.

Source: This case account is based on public news stories of the event and its circumstances.

CASE 21.13. Eric Harris and Dylan Klebold

Of the many cases of school mass murders followed by suicides, perhaps the best known is the one that took place at Columbine High School in Colorado on April 20, 1999. Eric Harris (an 18-year-old with a psychopathic personality) and Dylan Klebold (a depressed 17-year-old) killed 13 students and a teacher, and injured many others, using various firearms. They also had bombs that failed to detonate.

The public perception of the Columbine murder–suicides was, and still is, mainly that the shooters were social outcasts who had been bullied by others at school (especially by athletes). But Joiner (2014), as discussed in the chapter text, has said that the Columbine shootings followed by suicide were about perverted glory, not justice. Eric Harris said in an audiotape, "People will die because of me. It will be a day that is remembered forever."

Harris and Klebold did not kill athletes and were not especially bullied. Joiner claims that in murder–suicide, suicide is the primary intention, not murder. Klebold stated in his journals that he expected to be dead before the school shootings, and Harris had faked his suicide 3 years before the school shootings.

Source: This account is based on public news stories of the event and its circumstances.

In Chapter 22, I conclude the consideration of special suicide topics by examining jail and prison suicides. Do the dynamics or rate of suicide change for those behind bars?

CHAPTER 22

Jail and Prison Suicides
Confinement, Rage, and Target Reduction

> Since jails are *de facto* housing for largely undiagnosed and untreated
> mentally disordered white male inmates, it should come as no surprise
> that suicide is the leading cause of death there.
>
> —PRISON POLICY INITIATIVE

Confinement increases irritability, rage, and aggression (Heyerdahl, 1950)—but for the inmates of jails and prisons, they themselves are the only viable targets to aggress against, especially in segregation. Consider the case of Bob Morris (Case 22.1), who suicided after being put into segregation and a restraint chair. Overall, the jail suicide rate in particular is three (to nine) times higher than that of the general, nonincarcerated population; it is even higher than that of the prison population. Clearly, something specific is going on with jail populations and suicide that needs to be explained. Most discussions of jail and prison suicide just attend to the *what* (the facts), not the *why*—the causes of suicide in incarceration (Metzner & Hayes, 2012). And sometimes even the *what* cannot be completely explained, as in the death of Kenneth Trentadue (see Case 22.2).

CASE 22.1. Bob Morris

Bob Morris (5'10" and 170 pounds) was a 25-year-old white male, who hanged himself with a torn sheet in a Southeastern U.S. jail in October 2012. The time of hanging was early Sunday morning (1 A.M.). He was found sitting behind his cell door with a knotted sheet around his neck affixed to grated cell bars. Morris was probably hanging for about 4–5 minutes. He was still alive when initially found, but had anoxic brain damage. He had come to the jail in early May 2012 for armed robbery. At that time, Morris had been diagnosed with bipolar disorder and treated with the antipsychotic Seroquel. He also had several substance abuse diagnoses (methamphetamine, heroin, Xanax, and cocaine). The jail had a contract with a medical agency to provide medical treatment for jail inmates.

Morris tried to kill his guard and escape during treatment at a medical center for an alleged seizure. He had tried to take the guard's weapon after hitting her on the head with a pipe from a bathroom, but she pepper-sprayed him. He fled, only to be captured later. He said repeatedly that he had intended to shoot his guard, if he had been able to get her gun. He was then charged with attempted murder on May 10, 2012.

At the jail he was prescribed Risperdal, but refused to take it. Morris had made a prior suicide attempt, when he cut his wrist. Given his history of a prior suicide attempt, he was put on suicide watch at the jail from May 10 to 24, 2012. On May 11, Morris cut himself and tried to drown himself in a toilet. After this attempt, he was temporarily put in a restraint chair for a short time.

He seemed to calm down for about 5 months, but then his wife filed for divorce, and he punched his hand through a piece of sheetrock in a wall. In October 2012, Morris was put back on suicide watch. On October 16, he cut himself and was seen by the jail doctor, who gave Morris a 5-mg injection of Haldol and prescribed Geodon. But, again, Morris refused to take his psychiatric medication.

In a progress note on October 19, 2012, he told the mental health liaison, "No, sir, I don't feel suicidal," even though he was caught hiding a razor blade in his mouth. On October 21, 2010 he said, "I still don't want medications." The next day (October 22, 2012), the doctor discharged Morris from suicide watch, and he was assigned to administrative segregation. His discharge note said, "Has not reacted aggressively for 5 days." Morris hanged himself with a torn sheet on Sunday, October 24, 2012 while segregated, a little over a day after being taken off suicide watch. Morris's widow filed a complaint alleging violations of the Eighth and Fourteenth Amendments to the U.S. Constitution, gross negligence of serious medical needs, deliberate indifference by a nurse, violations of the jail's own written policies and procedures, wrongful death against the sheriff, and vicarious liability by a medical subcontractor. The case was eventually settled.

Source: Public information. All names, dates, and identifying information have been changed to protect the privacy of the people, agencies, and places.

CASE 22.2. Kenneth Trentadue

Kenneth Trentadue (the decedent's real name) was a middle-aged white male who was found hanged about 3 A.M. on August 2, 1995, in the special housing unit of a federal transfer center (FTC). The federal government argued that Trentadue suicided. However, his body had numerous injuries that made his alleged suicide unusual, if not suspicious. For example, he had three acute lacerations on his head; his throat was cut on the right side; his knuckles on both hands were bruised; and he had other bruises all over his body (on his right eye, nose, lower left leg, his biceps, the bottom of his left foot, and his left wrist). This did not look like a typical hanging suicide. After Trentadue's body was photographed, the family filed suit against the FTC, the Bureau of Prisons (BOP), and the U.S. Department of Justice (DOJ), among others, claiming that the BOP guards murdered Kenneth.

The case turned into a very high-profile media event. Then Attorney General Janet Reno and Senator Orrin Hatch (Head of the Senate Judiciary Committee) argued about the case; there were two articles in *Gentlemen's Quarterly* (in September 1996 and December 1997); Leeza Gibbons did a TV feature on Trentadue (February 3, 1998); and NBC's *Dateline* covered it as well (April 11, 1997). At least eight different agencies—the FTC, BOP, DOJ, and FBI; the Office of the Inspector General; the Oklahoma City district attorney's office; and the Oklahoma

City Police Department—did independent investigations, generating mountains of evidence. For example, the FBI alone took 302 depositions. After several continuances, the trial finally took place at the end of 2000.

It was hypothesized that Trentadue wrote a suicide note on his cell wall and attempted to hang himself (but the sheet broke). He then hit his head on the cell wall and a metal desk, when he fell and tried to get up. After that, he took the crimped end of a toothpaste tube and tried to cut his throat. When that failed, he reattached the bedsheet and rehanged himself. The other bruises on his body were days old. As for the homicide hypothesis, there was no evidence of a struggle in his cell, and the blood patterns were not cast-off blood (as would be expected in a fight). There was no clear motive for a homicide, as Trentadue had just arrived at the FTC.

The judge agreed that Trentadue suicided, but still awarded the estate over $1 million because of the trauma suffered by the Trentadue family (e.g., the guards did not cut Trentadue down for 8 minutes, and the FTC sent a grossly disfigured body to the family).

Source: All the information is public. There was a public trial. The information came from the news media stories mentioned in the case.

First, let me differentiate among jails, prisons, and other types of confinement. *Jails* are short-term facilities (usually confining their inmates for no more than 1 year), run by counties, cities, or the police. Hayes (2010) reported the jail population in the United States as 767,620. There are 3,096 U.S. counties, but 3,163 jails, with a total inmate capacity of 810,966 (American Jail Association, 2010). *Prisons* are long-term facilities (normally confining inmates for 1 year or more) run by states or the federal government.[1] Of federal prisons, there are 20 high-security, close-control penitentiaries; 65 lower-security correctional facilities; 6 prison camps; and 20 administrative facilities (West et al., 2011). There are approximately 1,190 state prisons and 102 federal prisons (these numbers may change, depending on the year). In addition, there are about 80,000 inmates a year in juvenile detention, plus another 400,000 in immigration detention, Department of Defense detention, and Bureau of Indian Affairs facilities.

It is estimated that there are about 2.3 million inmates incarcerated in any given recent year. Of these, 203,233 are federal inmates, 1,326,549 are state inmates, and 767,620 are jail detainees. If you add these up, you get 2,297,400 inmates. There are some detention facilities for which the numbers of inmates are not included here, but if these were included, there are close to 2.3 million inmates. Although the Bureau of Justice Statistics (West et al., 2011) estimates the total state and federal incarcerations at 2,297,000, another data source (Metzner & Hayes, 2012) estimates yearly total incarcerations at 2,374,000, which seems more likely because these data are more recent.

The highest numbers of state and federal prison suicide deaths from 2001 to 2013 (Noonan et al., 2015) were, in order, in these four states: (1) California (425), (2) Texas (326), (3) New York (165), and (4) Florida (91).

Incarceration encompasses many different situations, all likely having different suicidal impacts (if any) on the prisoners. Types of incarceration include (1) being

---

[1]Six states (Alaska, Connecticut, Delaware, Hawaii, Rhode Island, and Vermont), all with fairly small populations, have combined jail and prison systems.

in 23-hour-a-day solitary confinement or segregation, often in a cave-like cell with no windows or clocks; (2) being isolated behind bars; (3) being behind bars, but in the general jail or prison population; (4) being in jails versus penitentiaries versus correctional facilities; (5) being in short- versus long-term incarceration; (6) having to wear an ankle bracelet while on bond at home; and (7) having to report to a probation officer—and the list could go on. In most types of incarceration, the inmates' lives and behavior are controlled; there are rules; and the prisoners are given jobs to do on specified schedules. For the most part, the nonincarcerated are free to choose their own lifestyles and schedules.

Perhaps jail and prison suicide is related more to the type of people who tend to be incarcerated than to their lives behind bars. Recall my argument in Chapter 20 that military suicides are more a function of the recruitment process than of combat or PTSD. It is very likely that many jail inmates' suicidal careers started far before the inmates were jailed. Who tends to be in jail? Table 22.1 indicates that the jail population includes many young white males with a history of mental disorder, especially of substance use and depressive disorders. They are often trying to adjust to segregation and control of their lives in jail.

As Table 22.1 shows, the only excessive suicide rate is found in jails (for a European comparison, see Editorial, 2018). The suicide rate in jails (36 per 100,000) is over twice as high as those in any other group studied, including prisons. According to Hayes (2010), jail suicide rates 20 years before his report were nine times higher than those of the nonjailed population. Since suicide rates in prisons are not significantly different from the rate in the general population, it is not just being incarcerated that elevates suicide rates. The only study group in which suicide is the number one cause of death is the jail population. Suicides make up 34% of all deaths there. In the general and prison populations, the leading causes of death are essentially the same—heart disease, cancer, stroke, and (in prisons) liver disease.

Males (especially white males) make up the bulk of the jail population who suicide: 93% in jails and 94% in prisons. In jails, the men who suicide tend to be young (a mean age of 35 years). Prison inmates who suicide tend to be much older; 54% of them are age 55 or older. In the general population, being a white male is a significant suicide risk factor. Although suicide is the 10th leading cause of death overall, for people ages 15–24, particularly men, it is the 2nd leading cause of death.

Like suicides in the general population, suicides in incarcerated populations tend to have depressive and substance use disorders. In jails, 38% of inmates who suicide have a history of mental disorder, as do 26% of the prison inmates. Elsewhere (Maris, 2015), I have estimated the prevalence of any mental disorder to be 18.5% in the general U.S. population. Thus, in the jail suicides, the prevalence of mental disorder is roughly twice that of the nonincarcerated general population. This is noteworthy, since mood disorder is probably the single most important suicide risk factor.

Outside of jails and prisons, a little over 50% use firearms to suicide. But inmates obviously do not have access to firearms. Instead, hanging is the method used by 93% of jail inmates who commit suicide, and 85% of suicides in prisons. In the United States, only 27% of the noninstitutionalized who suicide do so by

TABLE 22.1. Suicide in U.S. Jails, Prisons, and the General Population

	U.S. pop. (2000)	U.S. suicides (2014)	Jail suicides (2010)[a]	Prison suicides (2015)[b]
Suicide rate (per 100,000)	13.4	13.4	36	16
Causes of death	Heart 192 smr[c] Cancer 185 Stroke 42 Suicide 13.4	NA[d]	34% suicide (#1 cause)	Cancer 27% Heart 25% Liver 10% Suicide 6%
White race	75%	90%	67%	40%
Male gender	49%	77%	93%	94%
Age (mean yrs.)	35.3	12% < 25	35	6% = 25–34 54% = 55+
Marital status	62% marr.	16.5–20.9 per 100,000 single	42% single	78% never marr., sep., div.
Hx SA[e]	1 in 309 mil.	70% = 1 SA	DK[f]	62% past suicidal behav.
Hx mental disorder	3%; 15% diagnosable	Bipolar 25 smr Sev. depr. 21 smr Sub. abuse 20 smr	38%	26%
Time of SA	NA	5–6 P.M. = #1 time	32%, 3–4 P.M.	
Method of SA	NA	27% hanging	93% hanging	85% hanging
Isolation	NA	98–99% alone	38% isolated	46% segregated
Near court hear.	NA	DK	80% 2 days	DK
15-minute watch	NA	DK	87%	DK
Suicide early in confinement	NA	NA	50% first week	DK

[a]Data in this column from Hayes (2010).
[b]Data in this column from Noonan et al. (2015).
[c]Standard mortality rate.
[d]Not appropriate or not available.
[e]Suicide attempt(s).
[f]Don't know.
Source: Original table by Maris, with data from other sources as indicated separately.

hanging. I come back to the topic of suicide method later in this chapter, since it relates to suicide watch and precaution standards in incarceration.

Other relevant facts from Table 22.1 are: (1) Inmates tend to be alone when they suicide (e.g., 38–46% of them are in single-cell isolation);[2] (2) 80% of jail suicides occur within 2 days of a court hearing; (3) 87% of jail suicides are on 15-minute suicide watch, if they are on a watch at all; and (4) 50% of jail suicides occur in the first week of incarceration.

If one wants further detailed data on jail and prison suicide, three of the best sources for a general overview are Hayes (2010), Noonan et al. (2015), and Metzner and Hayes (2012).

The Jail Standard of Care

In the Bob Morris jail suicide (Case 22.1), his widow, the plaintiff, alleged that the defendants (the jail and its staff) were *negligent*, were *deliberately indifferent*, and violated their own policies and procedures. These allegations raise important questions. What is the jail standard of care, especially for suicidal inmates? What do the basic legal concepts of *negligence* and *deliberate indifference* mean? Where are the relevant jail policies and procedures stated?

The *standard of care* in general is "what a reasonable and prudent professional or practitioner would have done in same or similar circumstances" (*Black's Law Dictionary*, 2009). Operationally, the standard of care is defined in part by the opposing testimony of qualified experts for the plaintiff and defendant in court, based on their education, training, experience, and certification, and on their review of the specific facts of the individual case in question. This can be confusing, since both the plaintiff and defendant usually are able to find qualified experts that disagree on the standard of care and whether or not it was met. Judges and juries often have to resolve disagreements.

Local jails also have stated specific standards (usually coded or numbered in a manual) that the jails are operating under and must be responsive to. For example, in the sheriff's office where Morris was jailed, the jail published a long list of standards called *Detention Directives*. Most of the relevant suicide standards were in a section on "Medical Care." This section included standards for suicidal inmates, how to identify suicidal inmates, suicide watch, suicide prevention, and so on.

Policies and procedures exist generically, statewide, and locally (e.g., in the manuals of specific county jails). Sometimes jail and prison standards are combined, but there are also separate prison standards (such as those created by the Bureau of Prisons or the American Bar Association). In the state of South Carolina, there is a document titled *Minimum Standards for Local Detention Facilities in South Carolina* (abbreviated here as MSLDF; South Carolina Association of Counties, 2013). As the title suggests, these standards are generic for all county jails in the state. The MSLDF has sections on administration, admission and release, security,

---

[2]However, about 60% were in nonisolation single cells.

classification, separation, discipline, physical plant, inmate programs, medical services, clothing and hygiene, bedding, food, work programs, and many other topics.
Each topic is listed in a specific coded, numbered category.

As for the legal concepts mentioned above, *deliberate indifference* is the failure
to provide proper treatment or the intentional denial of medical treatment. It is
shown by measuring the adequacy of jail officers' and staff members' responses to
the inmates' known serious medical needs. It exists if an individual inmate like Bob
Morris in Case 22.1 is prevented from receiving prescribed treatment or is denied
access to medical personnel and/or treatment.

Negligence can be defined by four D's: Dereliction of Duty leading Directly
to Damages. *Gross negligence* is a relative term in the law, generally meaning "the
absence of care that is necessary under the circumstances." Gross negligence
involves an intentional conscious failure to do something that is incumbent upon
one to do, or doing something intentionally that one ought not to do.

Finally, the U.S. Constitution states (under the Eighth and the Fourteenth
Amendments) that an inmate is entitled to *due process* and to be free from *cruel and
unusual punishment* during the period of his or her incarceration and detention.

Suicide Risk Assessment and Screening in Jails

Since jail inmates are different from the general population, their risk factors for
suicide are somewhat different, too. Given that suicide is the leading cause of death
in jails, it is imperative that jails systematically and thoroughly assess all inmates
for suicide risk. For example, the MSLDF document (South Carolina Association of
Counties, 2013) states: "Each facility shall have a written manual of all policies and
procedures for the operation of the facility" (item 1021, p. 13). More specifically, it
states: "Each facility shall have current written procedures to be followed in emergency situations," including "suicides and attempted suicides" (item 1022, p. 14).

The correct procedure for assessing the suicide risk of jail inmates includes
knowing the salient, specific jail suicide risk factors and then applying them to the
particular inmate being assessed. Normally the assessor arrives at a quantified,
standardized suicide score, typically ranging from 1 (low) to 10 (high). According
to Hayes (2010), the primary suicide risk factors for inmates in U.S. jails are those
listed in the left column of Table 22.2.

Before the act of suicide, Bob Morris had 58% (7 out of 12) of the known risk
factors for jail suicides, for a moderate suicide risk. On a 10-point risk scale, he was
at 6. Plaintiffs have to be careful not to engage in "Monday morning quarterbacking"—that is, knowing the outcome with 100% certainty; it is easy for a plaintiff to
say (without scientific justification) that a defendant jail should have seen the suicide coming (i.e., foreseen it). That is unfair to the defense, since before the fact,
suicide is rare and often unpredictable.

Individual suicides cannot be predicted with any degree of accuracy. Even
when risk factors are known to be present, suicide prediction tends to result in
false positives; that is, we predict suicide, but get a nonsuicide. What the plaintiff is
doing in a case of "Monday morning quarterbacking" such as the Bob Morris case

TABLE 22.2. Jail Suicide Risk Factors

Risk factors	Present in Bob Morris?
1. White race	1. Yes
2. Male gender	2. Yes
3. Young age (average is 35 years)	3. Yes (25 years)
4. Marital status single (42%)	4. No (but divorce coming)
5. Past suicide attempt	5. Yes (four of them)
6. History of mental disorder	6. Yes (bipolar disorder)
7. Common time of suicide attempt (3–9 P.M.)	7. No (1 A.M.)
8. Hanging (92%)	8. Yes
9. Isolation (60% single occupancy)	9. Yes
10. Close to court hearing (80% less than 2 days)	10. No
11. On 15-minute watch level (87%)	11. Yes
12. In early stages of confinement	12. No (in jail for 5 months)

Sources: Hayes (2010) and Maris (trial for Bob Morris jail suicide case, 2014; identifying information changed).

is formally known as *postdiction* (see Simon, 2006). We can assess the probability of a jail suicide, but we cannot predict it.

The jail and medical agency did correctly assess Morris's suicide risk. They knew that he had a moderate risk of suicide, and they did take proper precautions against his suiciding. However, even with prevention precautions at or above the standard of care, suicide cannot always be prevented. The jail personnel knew that Morris had made four prior suicide attempts. They appropriately put Morris on suicide watch twice. Note that inmates cannot be kept on suicide watch indefinitely without violating their constitutional rights. Plaintiffs often seem to want it both ways. That is, they want more, longer, and closer suicide watches, but also complain about cruel and unusual punishment and loss of due process.

Another part of assessing jail suicides are the written standards in the manual that the state and local jails operate under. As mentioned earlier, the Florida jail in which Morris was housed published a long, detailed specification of jail standards called *Detention Directives*. Most of the relevant standards concerned "Medical Care." Standard 7.1 said that suicidal inmates must be assessed by the judgment of a qualified mental health professional, here primarily the jail psychiatrist. There was a jail mental health screen of Morris, and suicide observation checklists were completed in regard to Morris's mood, behavior, suicide ideations, hallucinations, appetite, and medical needs. Since medical and mental health care is usually sub-contracted to medical agencies, these agencies' own policies and procedures are relevant to the care of Bob Morris at the jail. Hayes (2010) has written:

> Intake screening and ongoing assessment of all jail inmates are essential to a correctional facility's suicide prevention efforts. Screening should not be just a single event but a continuous process. . . . [For example,] inmates can become suicidal

[or more suicidal] after receiving bad news [such as Morris's wife's intention to divorce him]. Screening should include: was the inmate a mental health risk, had the inmate ever attempted suicide [or] ever had suicide ideation, [was there] a recent loss, [or did the inmate have] nothing to look forward to [i.e., hopelessness]? Do not just rely on the inmate's own statement that he is not suicidal.

Mental health screening specifies that the following should be noted in the inmate's history of psychiatric treatment: suicide ideas; violent behavior (e.g., Morris once beat his guard with a pipe while in jail); the use of psychotropic medications (at various times Morris was on Depakote, Paxil, Geodon, Celexa, Risperdal, and Seroquel); past psychiatric diagnoses (if any); substance abuse; and current suicide ideation (e.g., as recorded in progress notes). There should be a quantified mental health screening intake form completed by a mental health professional. If the inmate is acutely suicidal or psychotic, then this constitutes an emergency.

Suicide Watch and Observation Levels in Jail

Once an inmate has been assessed or screened as suicidal, the question naturally arises as to how closely to observe or monitor him or her. It is worth noting that almost half (44.8%) of all jail inmates who commit suicide are dead within the first 6 hours of their confinement (Hayes, 2010). So close initial watch of suicidal inmates is crucial for suicide prevention (Metzner & Hayes, 2012). An inmate needs to be observed at the assigned time intervals, such as every 15 minutes (and observation times logged), although reasonable staggered observations (Metzner & Hayes, 2012) may be used to avoid predictability of the watch (Hayes, 2010).

Not all observations are suicide watches, and watch levels may vary in particular jails. Standard levels of watch or observation may include the following (Maris et al., 2000), although typically bona fide suicide watches constitute just the first three observation levels below and usually occur in special housing units, as in the Kenneth Trentadue prison case (Case 22.2).

- *One-to-one constant observation.* A staff member usually stays within arm's length of the inmate 24/7, so that physical contact can be immediate if necessary. There are no exceptions to this rule. The bathroom door remains open, if there is a bathroom. The inmate is usually restricted to special housing while on constant watch.
- *Continuous or line-of-sight observation.* A staff member must have the inmate in view continuously 24/7. There are no exceptions, although video cameras are sometimes used.
- *Suicide precautions or close watch.* Staff monitors inmate at least every 15 minutes during both waking and sleeping hours. Watch times and conditions are logged.
- *Open observation.* Staff monitors inmate every 15 minutes during both waking and sleeping hours. Bathroom observation is optional. Inmate reports to staff when changing geographical locations.

- *Close supervision.* Staff monitors inmate every 30 minutes when awake and every 15 minutes when asleep. Inmate reports changes in location to staff.
- *Open supervision.* Staff monitors inmate every 60 minutes during waking hours and every 30 minutes during sleeping hours. Inmate reports changes in location to staff.

Note that both open and close supervision usually occur when the inmate is in the general population. Standards may vary to some extent among psychiatric inmates, inmates with mental problems, or those having special needs. Hayes (2010) reminds us that 92.5% of jail suicides were not on suicide watch status when they suicided. Most jails in which there were suicides used 15-minute observation times; only 2% used constant observation.

Jails tend to use 15-minute watch time intervals. Yet the vast majority of inmates hang themselves, and 15 minutes is too long a time to prevent most hanging suicides. Death by hanging is generally due to the compression or constriction of the neck, which either obstructs the blood flow in the carotid arteries, blocks the windpipe, or causes cardiac arrest. The resulting interference in the uptake or utilization of oxygen, together with the failure to eliminate carbon dioxide, produces a subnormal level of oxygen in the blood supply. Loss of consciousness occurs virtually instantaneously. Complete arterial occlusion may occur when the hanging victim is in a sitting, kneeling, or lying position (Maris et al., 2000).

The tension on the rope or stricture needs only to be 7–8 pounds to block the carotid arteries. In 4–5 minutes anoxic brain damage or death results, which makes the typical jail's 15-minute suicide watches not very effective. An inmate in a cell often ties or tears one end of a piece of undershirt or t-shirt, pulls it over the head, and affixes an armhole on a doorknob; or the inmate may tie one end of a shoelace, a pants belt, a robe or sweatpants belt, a laundry bag string, or the like around a cell bar and the other end around the neck, and then just lean forward while sitting or kneeling. A sheet or cloth may be attached to a door jamb (after the inmate ties a knot in the cloth), a vent, an overhead sprinkler pipe, a shower rod, or any other protruding object that cannot be broken off easily.

The standard times for suicide watches or observation also do not answer these questions: For whom and when should watches be utilized, and what stipulations should apply? In the Morris suicide, the jail's *Detention Directives* said the following regarding "suicide watches": Such watches are for close, direct supervision of suicidal inmates; suicidal inmates must first be identified; suicide watches will be every 15 minutes; there will be constant personal or electronic observation by deputies; all inmates will have their personal property removed; an inmate will be stripped (and given a comforter or smock that cannot be torn; this jail called the smock a "turtle suit") only if the inmate is overtly suicidal at the time; there will be no shaving with a razor blade while an inmate is on suicide watch; and, finally, the inmate must be cleared medically before being moved out of special housing and suicide watch. Again, however, even though suicide watches usually help prevent jail suicides, inmates cannot be kept on suicide watch indefinitely, as that itself might constitute cruel and unusual punishment.

Housing, Isolation, and Suicide-Proofing in Jails

Once the jail and mental health staff have screened and assessed an inmate, and established suicide watch and observation protocols, it is necessary to stipulate where all this takes place. Typically, when an inmate is assessed as imminently dangerous to self or others, he or she is placed for a time in isolation, administrative segregation, or solitary confinement, until (for example) the inmate is no longer acutely suicidal, violent, or aggressive, as determined by a qualified mental health professional.

Although sometimes isolation is necessary, it is seldom good for the inmate, even if it may make the jail staff feel better. Isolation increases inmate alienation (Metzner & Hayes, 2012) and may paradoxically increase suicide risk. For example, 60% of jail suicides were in single-occupancy cells, and over one-third of inmates were in isolation or segregation, when they suicided (Hayes, 2010).

Most knowledgeable commentators (Metzner & Hayes, 2012) argue that whenever possible, suicidal inmates should be housed in the jail general population or in a mental health unit. If a suicidal inmate is not violent, psychiatrically agitated, or reacting to a substance (such as alcohol, opiates, other street drugs, or psychiatric medications), it is preferred that the inmate have a cellmate. Morris was in administrative segregation just 1 day before he suicided.

As a rule, a segregated inmate is alone 23 of 24 hours each day, but is allowed 1 hour outside the cell for a 15-minute shower (at least three times a week) or for exercise. Most segregated cells have a bunk, toilet, and sink, and perhaps a fixed desk, a stool, and one exterior window. Meals are served at the cell door. When being escorted to a recreational or exercise room, inmates are often in restraints. I actually observed another segregated inmate when I visited the Morris jail, and I found the situation very sad.

As for restraints, one should only use the force necessary to protect an inmate from bodily self-harm. For example, Morris had been trying to cut himself for a little over 2 hours. He was put in three-point restraints (i.e., head and arms) rather than five-point restraints (which add the legs). Restraints can also include *chemical confinement,* which means sedation. When Morris continued to struggle, he was given 5 mg of haloperidol (Haldol) to calm him down. Usually Morris refused medication when he had that option and put his refusals in writing. Restraint chairs, boards, and leather straps can also be used, but should be avoided whenever possible (Metzner & Hayes, 2012).

Safe housing can also include *suicide-proofing* a cell (Hayes, 2010). Short of totally immobilizing an inmate physically or chemically, complete jail suicide-proofing is impossible and is not required by the standard of care. Of course, suicide-proofing can also violate the inmate's Fourteenth Amendment rights.

Table 22.3 lists several procedures and policies to limit *architectural* (i.e., housing-related) suicide risk. Since hanging is the preferred jail suicide method, protruding objects or bars to which something can be tied should be avoided. Any bedding or clothing that can be torn and stuffed down an inmate's throat should be eliminated. There was a jail suicide in South Carolina where an inmate swallowed the pants leg of his jogging suit. Toilets should not permit drowning, and all

TABLE 22.3. Suicide-Proofing Jails

• Supervise inmates when and if it is necessary to use "sharps." Use only electric razors.

• Remove from the inmate any items that could be used in a suicide attempt (belts, neckties, shoelaces, matches, lighter, scissors, glass, jewelry, etc.). Sometimes inmates are stripped and given suicide smocks (called "turtle suits" in the jail where Bob Morris was held; see Case 22.1). Bedding may be removed, and/or a thick quilt that cannot be torn may be given.

• Unless inmates are violent or mentally disturbed, seldom place them on suicide precautions in seclusion. If they are placed in seclusion, there should be constant observation by cameras or staff.

• Allow inmates to take showers only, not baths.

• Install breakaway (and nonprotruding) shower heads, rods, and toilet paper holders; remove exposed pipes and cover vents (and keep them at floor level); remove uncovered bars from seclusion cells.

• Keep electrical cords short, such as personal computer cords. Remove phone cords.

• Install windows of unbreakable glass, like Lexan or Plexiglas. Remove exposed light bulbs. Keep all windows locked. Locate psychiatric or mental health units on bottom floors to prevent inmates from jumping.

• Lock all storage closets, supply closets, cleaning fluids, utility rooms, stairwells, and offices.

• Train all staff in security precautions, and have emergency tools (like cutting tools) available.

• Clear all gifts brought in by visitors, and search inmates after visitations.

• Train all new staff in the necessary procedures (such as radio or intercom alert codes) or alert policies, and conduct annual staff update training.

• Make sure all electronic devices have fresh batteries and are functioning properly.

Source: Adapted from Maris et al. (2000). Copyright © 2000 by The Guilford Press. Adapted by permission.

"sharps" must be controlled. Kenneth Trentadue (Case 22.2) reportedly even tried to cut his throat with the crimped end of his toothpaste tube.

Training in Jail Suicide Prevention

The jail personnel who most need suicide prevention training are the front-line correctional officers who are present in the jail 24/7, weekends and nights. Mental health professionals, physicians, and nurses also need training, but usually not administrators (Hayes, 2010). Hayes (2010) has pointed out that most jail suicides tend to occur in July and August, when many mental health professionals are on vacation. Suicide timing tends to be from 1 to 3 A.M. and from 6 to 9 P.M., when most medical and mental health staffers have gone home.

Jail personnel minimally need at least one 8-hour initial suicide prevention training session (Metzner & Hayes, 2012), followed up each year with 2-hour refresher seminars. However, only 6% of jails offer even one 8-hour-day initial training (Hayes, 2010). Most jail employees (70%) get a total of under 2 hours of initial suicide prevention training. So even though 61.8% of jails provided some suicide prevention training, it was too short to be very effective (Hayes, 2010).

What should be included in an 8-hour training session? An agenda for such a session can be found in Hayes and Rowan (1995), and the Suicide Prevention

Resource Center (2017) offers a number of suggested materials and trainings. Most of these 8-hour, 1-day training sessions review the following:

- Specific suicide risk factors for jail populations, such as the list in the left column of Table 22.2.
- The highest jail suicide risk times—for example, in the first week of incarceration, early evenings (6–9 P.M.) and early mornings (1–3 A.M.).
- Warning signs for imminent jail suicide, such as the mnemonic "IS PATH WARM?"
  - I = suicidal ideas
  - S = substance abuse
  - P = purposelessness
  - A = anxiety
  - T = trapped feelings
  - H = hopelessness
  - W = withdrawal
  - A = anger
  - R = restlessness, impulsivity
  - M = mood changes
- Situational risk factors, such as being near the date of a court hearing, being in the first week of being jailed, being a young single white male, having a history of mental illness, being intoxicated, having undergone a recent negative event or loss, and so forth.
- Recent high-stress periods, like family problems, sentencing problems, or an impending divorce.
- The history of suicides and attempted suicides in the specific jail (case reviews).
- Suicide prevention strategies and precautions.

Training sessions should also include (1) CPR certification (80% of jails have it); (2) emergency responses if an inmate is found hanging (including mock practice drills); (3) having emergency equipment readily accessible (e.g., a rescue bag with a cutting tool, a video camera with live batteries); (4) testing the employees' knowledge of their own jail's suicide prevention policies and procedures (e.g., giving a short exam); (5) strategies for supervising and managing suicidal inmates; (6) aspects of jail design conducive to increased versus decreased suicide risk; and (7) follow-up and postmortem review and report after a jail suicide.

Follow-Up and Postmortem Reviews

Staff members need to learn from their mistakes and unfortunate outcomes, to help prevent them from happening again. When an inmate suicides, an interdisciplinary review team needs to be assembled to try to figure out what went wrong, if anything. Could the staff have done something differently and prevented this suicide? Does the institution need to make any changes in its policies and procedures? Were any of the employees liable for this outcome?

All of the relevant correctional officers, mental health professionals, and jail staff need to give at least one-page signed affidavits describing the details of the incident from their own perspectives. Did anyone fail to do a cell check or not do it on time? How did the inmate get access to the means for suicide? Was prescribed psychiatric medication not given as ordered? Was the response to the suicide or hanging prompt and effective, and did it follow protocol?[3] The first responders (emergency medical services [EMS], etc.) also need to be involved. Was the staff suicide prevention training adequate and up to date? Should any architectural modifications be made in the jail or prison?

The decedent's family needs to be notified sensitively and humanely as soon as possible, perhaps by a chaplain, social worker, or medical or mental health staff member. Crisis therapy and social support needs to be offered to all employees involved.

Metzner and Hayes (2012) suggest that the mortality review and death investigation at least include the following:

- A critical review of the incident.
- An evaluation of all relevant policies and procedures.
- Determination of whether the staff members were adequately trained and up to date.
- Debriefing of the medical and mental health staff, and review of their reports and progress notes for the decedent in the file.
- A list of the possible precipitating factors.
- Any recommendations for changes.
- Development of a discharge form that summarizes all of the above, similar to discharge summaries in hospitals.

Doing a retrospective psychological autopsy is strongly recommended. One form people are free to use can be found on my website (*www.suicideexpert.com/forms*); it is entitled "Psychological Autopsy and Death Investigation." (See Chapter 26, Box 26.1, for an outline of this form.) Its reliability or validity is not guaranteed.

It is useful for the jail or prison to catalog all past jail suicide attempts and completions, and to keep these records on file. Sometimes collecting newspaper reports can be helpful. Most of the time, a postmortem review will be considered by the court as confidential and privileged information that cannot be used against the jail or prison if there is a lawsuit. Experts, if they are involved in litigation, seldom if ever get to see a postmortem review.

Preventing Jail Suicides and Treating Suicidal Inmates

Suicide prevention and treatment involve most, if not all, of the topics already considered. To summarize, prevention and treatment of jail suicide should include the

---

[3] It took 8 minutes for the guards to cut Trentadue down (see Case 22.2).

following (Metzner & Hayes, 2012; National Commission on Correctional Health Care, 2015):

- Training.
- Intake and ongoing risk assessment.
- Communication among custodial, transport, mental health, and correctional staff, and between all staff and the inmate.
- Housing.
- Observation or watch.
- Intervention and treatment, especially for mental health.
- Reporting, mortality review, psychological autopsy.

Intake and ongoing risk assessment and suicide screening should include questions about an inmate's past and current suicide ideation. Clinicians should not just let inmates deny suicide ideation, but rather should probe for details. They should ask about prior suicide attempts or threats and whether or not they have a plan to commit suicide again. How would they do it, and under what circumstances? How lethal is the plan? Do they have the means to do it? In addition, clinicians should evaluate current mental status and mood, recent loss or stress, family history of mental disorder and/or suicide, and feeling hopeless. They should discuss possible suicide watches and segregation, and ask how the inmates would tolerate it. Clinicians should also ask about protective factors such as religion; adherence in taking psychiatric medications; having a supportive family, spouse, or partner; availability of social support; and having a place or job to go to after release. There should be a treatment plan that is specific and detailed about doctor visits, medication, follow-up times (and with whom follow-ups are conducted), and psychotherapy appointments. This plan should be made up by a treatment team of different professionals (doctors, nurses, social workers, psychologists, occupational therapists, drug counselors, etc.).

I have not yet said much about mental health treatment in jail and prison. Suicide is usually seen by most people as a mental health problem—for example, "You'd have to be crazy to do that!" or "You'd have to be depressed, psychotic, or abusing alcohol and drugs to do that!" A. E. Daniel (2007, p. 406) quoted this question and answer: "So where did all the [state hospital] patients go?" "Jails and prisons."

Medical and mental health care of incarcerated inmates is usually farmed out to medical organization subcontractors. Mental health workers in jails and prisons consist of psychiatrists, medical doctors, psychiatric nurses (especially), psychologists, counselors, and mental health techs. Unfortunately, most of these (particularly the doctors) work in the correctional setting only part-time. For example, at the jail Morris was in, there was a part-time psychiatrist on Mondays and Fridays only (0.3 of full-time equivalent or FTE); a part-time medical director (0.6 of FTE); a few RNs (14), some of whom were psychiatric nurses; and a lot of less qualified LPNs (39). There was also one nurse practitioner.

So what happens if an inmate needs to be put on psychiatric medications or have a medication adjustment? Likely the inmate waits or is driven to a local emergency room. Given the scarcity of medical doctors in jail and prison, we may well suspect that most inmates are undiagnosed, undertreated, or inadequately treated psychiatrically. This could result in a big problem, since mental health is highly related to a suicide outcome.

To what extent are mental health problems present in jails and prison? A good source for answering this question is James and Glaze (2006). Here are some of the most important data they produced:

- Sixty-four percent of jail inmates have mental health problems.
- Forty-nine percent of jail inmates have depressive or manic episodes (and presumably would often need antidepressant, anxiolytic, and/or antipsychotic medication).
- Of the DSM criteria for major depression, the two most common in jails were (1) disordered sleep (49.2%) and (2) persistent anger (49.4%), both of which are highly correlated with suicide outcomes.
- 24% of jail inmates have symptoms of psychotic disorders (and would presumably need antipsychotic medications).
- 76% of jail inmates with mental health problems have comorbid alcohol and other substance use disorders (and would presumably need drugs like Antabuse or methadone).

Morris was on the antidepressants Paxil and Celexa, and the antipsychotics or mood stabilizers Risperdal, Seroquel, and Geodon. One could argue that allowing his refusal of psychiatric medications and inadequate medical management of his mental health problems contributed to his eventual suicide (Maris, 2015).

A few concluding thoughts about suicide prevention in jails are in order. Metzner and Hayes (2012, pp. 392–393) quote correctional officers whose attitudes toward jail suicide discourage prevention efforts:

"If someone really wants to kill themselves, there's generally nothing you can do about it."

"Statistically speaking, suicide in custody is a rare phenomenon, and rare phenomena are notoriously difficult to forecast due to their low base rate."

In one sense, these comments are correct: Particular jail suicides, especially in the short run, are *not* predictable. As with any rare phenomenon (such as an earthquake or an individual suicide), when it's predicted, it usually doesn't happen; it's a false positive. On the other hand, jail staff should not assume that an inmate might not suicide (a false negative), only then to have him or her suicide.

If suicide occurs at the rate of 1 in 10,000 per year, and the prediction is *no suicide,* then, on average, the prediction would be right 9,999 times. Or if 10% of depressed inmates kill themselves (usually over more than 1 year), and the prediction is *no suicide,* then it would be right 90% of the time. So why should we even try to assess or predict jail suicide?

The goal of suicide risk assessment, however, is not suicide prediction. It is reducing the number of jail suicides that are most likely to happen. It is about identifying those who are really in *high-risk groups.* Effective suicide prevention is costly. For example, jail or prison staff may need to be assigned to watch an inmate 24/7 within arm's reach. If too many false-positive potential suicides are identified, there will not be enough resources to manage all of them, and most of them will not suicide anyway. So the goal of suicide assessment and screening is not to predict suicide, but rather to reduce to a manageable size the jail population at high suicide risk. Intervention and treatment then become more feasible.

For purposes of simplicity, let us assume that there are 100 inmates in a local jail. Pokorny (1983, 1992) has argued that if the usual jail suicide risk factors (like those in the left column of Table 22.2) are used, then on average about 30% will be false positives. That is, suicide is predicted for 30 inmates, but it doesn't happen. Jails and prisons cannot afford the financial or personnel costs of having 30 of their 100 inmates put on suicide watch, chemically confined, or put in restraints.

But if accurate screening and suicide risk assessment are in place, then the number of inmates who are truly at risk for suicide is likely to be much fewer than 30. For example, if 10–15% of depressed inmates eventually suicide, or if 15% of prior suicide attempters go on to suicide later, then the size of the inmate group at risk for suicide is reduced to 10–15 out of 100, not 1 out of 10,000. All of a sudden, intervention and suicide prevention now become more practical.

Suicide prevention is costly both to jails and to their inmates. Think of inmates like Bob Morris, in solitary confinement because they are thought to be acutely at risk for suicide. Such confinement can be cruel, unusual, punitive, inhumane, and unnecessary—particularly if an inmate is not likely to suicide anyway. However, if nothing is done and an inmate suicides, the facility is going to be sued, and the inmate will lose his or her one and only life. Given the seriousness of the outcome (unnecessary death), often it is better to be safe than sorry, even if the outcome is rare.

In the next section of this book, Part VII, treatment and prevention issues are examined. What can we do to prevent suicide? Is there an optimum suicide rate? How does suicide affect the survivors? What about liability and litigation after a suicide?

TREATMENT
AND PREVENTION

CHAPTER 23

Treatment and Intervention I. Pharmacology

What Are We Going to Do about Suicide?

I'm going to walk to the bridge. If one person smiles at me on the way, I will not jump.

— SUICIDAL PERSON QUOTED BY JEROME MOTTO

Smiling does not prevent suicide any more than titrating cerebrospinal fluid (CSF) with Lexapro does. The highest suicide rates (see Table 5.1) are in midlife (19.3 per 100,000 for ages 45–54) and old age (18.6 for ages 85+). Thus, most suicidal careers take 50–80 years to develop and are not going to be undone simply by a smile or a pill in a few weeks. As Joiner (2005) has written, "The acquired ability to enact lethal self-injury, once in place, does not fade quickly. It is a relatively static quality" (p. 210). In other words, it is not very malleable. You will also recall Shneidman's argument that suicide is an "interactive multidimensional malaise." No one factor causes it, and nothing simple is going to change it, especially in the short run. If it took you 50 years to become suicidal, you are not going to be cured in 6–8 weeks.

Since suicide is a multidimensional outcome, treatment is necessarily complex, takes time, and is specific to each individual case and the person's unique biopsychosocial surround (Stanley et al., 2008). Nevertheless, strangely, the prototypical suicide intervention is mainly pharmacological (Cipriani et al., 2018); that is, it involves simply and generically adjusting the person's neurotransmitters and neurosystems. Medication management tends to be neurobiological reductionism. How can that possibly work by itself? This is not to argue that pharmacology is not important for suicide prevention—only that medication alone is not sufficient.

Remember as well (Chapter 19) that suicide is related to the problems of life itself and the human condition (which are also relatively unmalleable), and not just to life gone awry biochemically or situationally. Although it may be gloomy to contemplate, we are all going to die and have episodic illness, injury, and pain along the way. Even the good life is hard, and suicide can beckon like the "Black Wolf of Psychiatry" described in Chapter 1, Box 1.1.

Distinguishing Treatment, Intervention, and Prevention

Suicide treatment, intervention, and prevention are inextricably intertwined, even though this book places the topics in separate chapters. Gerald Caplan (1964) coined the terms *primary, secondary, and tertiary prevention*. Most suicide prevention is tertiary—that is, detecting and limiting the suicidal damage after it has already occurred. Primary suicidal prevention stops the initial creation of the hazard, similar to a polio or measles vaccination. Thus, ideally, treatment is not necessary, because the disease (suicide) never happens. Put differently, you can have prevention without treatment.

Note that it is possible to *intervene* in suicide, but not to try to prevent it. One could intervene by just keeping the person who wishes to commit suicide as comfortable and free from pain as possible, but not trying to prevent the suicide. This is the idea behind physician-assisted suicide (which at this writing is legal in the states of Oregon, Washington, Vermont, Montana, Colorado, Hawaii, and California, and in the District of Columbia). Most of us assume that all intervention is or should be prevention.

Much of suicide treatment involves taking the edge off the individual's pain or "psychache" (Ducasse et al., 2018; Brown et al., 2018; Joiner, 2005; Shneidman, 1993). Joiner contends that this mainly involves reducing what he calls "perceived burdensomeness" and increasing "feelings of belongingness" (Joiner, 2005, 2010). Suicide intervention can also distract a person or make life more tolerable (without curing the suicidality) by reducing suicide risk factors like depression, substance abuse, isolation, negative family history, nonfatal suicide attempts, pain, and availability of lethal means (O'Neill et al., 2018).

This chapter begins with a brief overview of generic suicide treatment (which has been described previously, specifically in Chapters 11–14; *some redundancy is inevitable*) before moving on to more detailed considerations of treatment options. Most treatment of suicidal patients starts with a longish (1–2 hours) clinical assessment (see Chapter 4 and Rudd, 2012), history taking, diagnosis, and the formulation of a detailed interdisciplinary treatment plan (Maris et al., 2000). In the hospital, this assessment is done by the patient's treatment team—usually a psychiatrist, nurse, social worker, and/or psychologist (Goodwin, 2003).

An internist or family practice physician should do a thorough physical examination as part of the assessment, including perhaps ordering lab tests, x-rays, or other imaging, as well as obtaining past medical records and so on. One always needs to rule out conditions like thyroid malfunction, tumors, drug abuse, adverse medication reaction, alcoholism, and other diseases or injuries that may cause psychiatric symptoms or disorders.

Suicide is not a mental disorder (at least not yet) or a DSM diagnostic category. I have argued that a person can be suicidal without being crazy. In treating the suicidal patient, the sequence below is often followed (where Hx = history, Sx = symptoms, Ax = assessment, Dx = diagnosis, Tx = treatment, and Rx = pharmacology):

$$Hx \rightarrow Sx \rightarrow Ax \rightarrow Dx \rightarrow Tx\ (Rx)$$

Most psychiatric suicide treatment today is psychopharmacological management of mood disorders (especially), anxiety disorders, and substance use disorders (particularly alcoholism). Antisocial and borderline personality disorders (ASPD and BPD) are also often treated, but usually with psychotherapy and perhaps some anxiolytic or selective serotonin reuptake inhibitor (SSRI) medications (Maris, 2015).

Unfortunately, today psychiatrists are mainly medication managers, and suicide treatment is primarily psychopharmacology (Carlat, 2010). At Johns Hopkins Medical School in the early 1970s, most of the well-known psychiatrists (like Jerome Frank, Joel Elkes, and Seymour Perlin) all did psychotherapy. However, also at Hopkins, Solomon Snyder prepared the neurobiological groundwork (on *synaptosomes*) that allowed researchers to identify neurotransmitters (Kramer, 1993; Maris, 2015).

Most suicidal patients are treated with one or a number of psychotropic medications (a "cocktail"), mainly antidepressants (see Part IV; what follows is somewhat redundant and can be skimmed). The antidepressants are usually SSRIs (like Lexapro or Zoloft); serotonin–norepinephrine reuptake inhibitors (SNRIs, like Cymbalta or Pristiq); or an atypical antidepressant (like Wellbutrin, which is mainly a dopamine and norepinephrine agonist). There are always newer antidepressant medications, like Viibryd (2011), Fetzima (2013), or Brintellix (2013), or adjunctive treatments for depression, like Rexulti (2015), Abilify (2007), or ketamine (2017; cf. Grunebaum et al., 2017). Lately, atypical antipsychotics are often used adjunctively with antidepressants[8]

If the patient has a bipolar disorder, then lithium, Lamictal, Depakote, Tegretol, Latuda, or Neurontin may be used. Neurontin is used mainly off-label for pain control and is problematic for treating mood disorders, since it reduces serotonin, epinephrine, and dopamine (monoamines) and can enhance depression, aggression, and impulsivity in vulnerable patients. Lithium is the only mood stabilizer that has been demonstrated in clinical trials to reduce suicide rates (Baldessarini, 2002; Baldessarini et al., 2012).

If psychotropic medications fail to produce an antidepressant response (and 30–40% of them fail to do so) and/or the suicidal crisis is acute, then the patient may receive electroconvulsive therapy (ECT; cf. Gambino, 2018) every other day for up to 2 weeks, even as an outpatient (Maris, 2015). ECT is quicker than taking antidepressants and is very effective (about 80%), although side effects often include posttreatment short-term memory loss, temporary headaches, and muscle soreness (cf. Anderson, 2018). ECT probably operates on the serotonin system. The anesthetic ketamine can also be used for short-term relief.

Psychotherapy is usually used conjointly with pharmacotherapy to treat suicidal patients, although it is normally provided nowadays by psychologists, social workers, or counselors and not by psychiatrists. Psychotherapy is normally a variety of either cognitive therapy (Beck et al., 1979b; Brown et al., 2012) or dialectical behavior therapy (DBT; Linehan et al., 2015), in which the therapist attempts to persuade or teach the suicidal patient to avoid catastrophizing, dichotomizing, or other forms of fallacious reasoning; to see more nonsuicidal alternatives; to become more hopeful; and to design a plan with the therapist to engender hope (Marchalik & Jurecic, 2018).

To sum up, the treatment of suicidal patients can include psychopharmacology; other biological approaches (treatment of physical illness, sleep disorders, and disturbances of appetite or sexuality, as well as physical exercise, technical procedures such as ECT, TMS, etc.); psychotherapies (especially cognitive therapies and DBT); crisis intervention or brief therapies (such as emergency room or suicide prevention center [SPC] services, as well as suicide hotlines and online services); family therapy, group therapies, or sociotherapy; behavioral modification schedules; or psychodynamic therapies (not used much today). Even diet, exercise, sleep therapy, and other physical therapies can be important. Treatment modalities (see Table 23.1) can involve the suicidal individual, a group, or an institution (such as a school, a business, or even a country), and can occur in outpatient (Maltsberger & Stoklosa. 2012) or inpatient (Xiong et al., 2012) settings.

TABLE 23.1. Treatment Modalities for Suicide

- Outpatient treatment with a private psychiatrist, psychologist, social worker, or counselor.
- Inpatient treatment for about a week with a psychiatrist and a treatment team.in a psychiatric ward of a local hospital, psychiatric hospital, or medical school psychiatry department.
- Emergency room of a local hospital. (The personnel there can find the patient a specialist, or the patient's own psychiatrist or family doctor can meet him or her there.)
- The patient's family doctor or internist. (These physicians prescribe most antidepressants.)
- Student health service or school counselor, if the patient is a student.
- Community mental health center (CMHC), even in rural areas.
- Suicide prevention center (SPC), usually crisis intervention and referral.
- National Suicide Prevention Lifeline (1-800-273-8255, English; 1-888-628-9454, Spanish; 1-800-799-4889, TTY/hard of hearing; or *https://suicidepreventionlifeline.org*).
- Group therapies and various support groups, such as those for survivors after a suicide (e.g., Survivors of Suicide [SOS]; *www.survivorsofsuicide.com*).
- Counseling from the patient's pastor, rabbi, priest, or imam/mullah, or other religious counseling (including prayer).
- Family (mother, father, siblings, friends, peers).
- Employee assistance program (EPA) at work or by medical insurance referral.
- Calls to 911 or 211.
- Internet searches (via Google, etc.) for *suicide treatment* or *suicide prevention*.
- Local United Way and other agencies.
- American Association of Suicidology (AAS; *www.suicidology.org*).
- American Foundation for Suicide Prevention (AFSP; *www.afsp.org*).
- Self-help books (a book is not the same as a person, nor is reading the same as therapy).

Source: Adapted from Maris (2015). Copyright © 2015 the University of South Carolina. Adapted with permission.

Almost all suicide treatment today involves prescribing pills (often with conjoint psychotherapy and/or other technical procedures), especially the antidepressants and anxiolytics. But psychopharmacology does not target suicidal behavior per se. There is no antisuicide pill. Rather, pharmacological strategies are diagnosis-specific and aim to regulate the biochemistry associated with predisposing, suicidogenic risk factors. As mentioned earlier, there is evidence linking diminished serotonin (5-HT) metabolism and low CSF 5-HT levels with depressive disorders. This suggests that the administration of SSRIs should effect reduction of suicidality.

Antidepressant and mood-stabilizing medications (Cipriani et al., 2009, 2018; Maris, 2015), particularly the less toxic SSRIs (like Lexapro) or SNRIs (like Cymbalta) for depressive disorders and lithium for bipolar disorder, are basic pharmacological interventions in suicidal patients. These medications (especially lithium) may reduce episodic impulsive and aggressive behavior. Antipsychotics are used to manage chronic schizophrenia and other psychotic disorders (and as adjunctive therapy for depressive disorders), as is the short-term use of benzodiazepines (like Klonopin) for acute anxiety, or even of major tranquilizers (like Risperdal or Zyprexa).

The effectiveness of psychopharmacological suicide interventions has been widely debated in the literature (Kirsch, 2010; cf. Cipriani et al., 2018). For example, clinical trials studying depression typically exclude individuals who have made a suicide attempt or currently have significant depression. So clinical trials may be studying the wrong people—that is, those who are *not* highly suicidal. There also can be high dropout rates in clinical trials, further compromising the validity of such trials' data. There has been little conclusive scientific evidence demonstrating that antidepressant treatment of suicidal patients is much more effective than placebo treatment (says Kirsch, 2010) or psychotherapy.

Even the newer antidepressants like the SSRIs and SNRIs can show little gain in effectiveness relative to the older tricyclic antidepressants (TCAs) like Tofranil. However, the clear benefit from SSRIs is the reduction of suicidogenic adverse side effects. There are adverse effects like insomnia and irritability, and paradoxical reactions like rage or akathisia, associated with using antidepressants (particularly older antidepressants, which can also be fatal in overdose). Sometimes there is even *de novo* suicide ideation in patients taking antidepressants (Maris, 2015; Teicher et al., 1990b).

As noted above, perhaps the most effective medication in reducing suicide rates is lithium (Baldessarini et al., 2012; Baldessarini, 2002). Most studies that examined suicide rates with lithium maintenance consistently found suicide rates to be lowered during lithium maintenance therapy.

Antidepressant Treatment

Prozac was the first SSRI to be introduced in the United States (in 1988), and at one time it was the most widely prescribed antidepressant in the world. For example, in 1990 Prozac had an 18.9% market share, followed by 7.9% for Pamelor and 3.3% for Desyrel. Prozac was an effective, safe antidepressant (it is still the only SSRI recommended for children), with few of the side effects of TCAs or monoamine oxidase inhibitors (MAOIs). However, Prozac was not without controversy. Teicher et al. (1990a, 1990b) at Harvard had six of their depressed patients develop intense violent, paradoxical suicide preoccupations after 2–7 weeks of Prozac treatment. It should be noted that five of Teicher et al.'s patients had considered suicide *before* taking Prozac, that a very small portion of Prozac patients ever actually suicide, and that Teicher et al.'s research was anecdotal (not a randomized clinical trial). It should also be noted that when Teicher's group discontinued Prozac treatment, the patients' suicide ideation stopped, and that when it was restarted, they once again felt suicidal. This procedure is called a *challenge–dechallenge–rechallenge* research design.

The antidepressants of choice include the SSRIs, such as fluoxetine (Prozac), paroxetine (Paxil), sertraline (Zoloft), escitalopram (Lexapro), and fluvoxamine (Luvox); the SNRIs, such as duloxetine (Cymbalta), venlafaxine (Effexor), desvenlafaxine (Pristiq), and mirtazapine (Remeron); and atypical antidepressants, like bupropion (Wellbutrin), trazodone (Desyrel), and the augmenter aripiprazole (Abilify). The three newest (as of 2018) antidepressants are vilazodone (Viibryd), levomilnacipram (Fetzima), and vortioxetine (Brintellix).

Patients with bipolar disorder are likely to be on lithium carbonate (Esklith, Lithobid, Lithane), lamotrigine (Lamictal), valproate acid (Depakote), carbamazepine (Tegretol), lurisadone (Latuda), or gabapentin (Neurontin). If none of these antidepressants are effective or a suicide attempt is perceived to be imminent, then ECT may be used (see Maris, 2015). Other antidepressants include the older heterocyclics like amitriptyline (Elavil), imipramine (Tofranil), amoxapine (Ascendin), doxepin (Sinequan), and nortriptyline (Pamelor). Less commonly used nowadays (given their side effects) are the MAOIs, like phenelzine (Nardil), isocarboxazid (Marplan), and tranylcypromine (Parnate).

Modern psychiatry tends to assume that depressive disorders result from or are characterized by various dysfunctions or chemical imbalances (Carlat, 2010; Whitaker, 2010) in our brains (as opposed to our minds) and neurochemical systems. The latter include neurotransmitters (and neurosystems) like dopamine, serotonin, epinephrine, and norepinephrine; other neurotransmitters include histamine, neuropeptides, endorphins, tyramine, and so on. About 30–100 neurotransmitter molecule types (it depends on how you count them) have been identified so far, although (as noted above) about 10 of them do most of the neurological work (King, 2017). A *neurotransmitter* is a chemical that transmits signals from a neuron to a cell across a neuronal gap called a *synapse* or *synaptic cleft* (see Chapter 16). The human brain has about 100 billion neurons (Black & Andreasen, 2011, p. 55), far more than the total number of people on earth. Most of the modern psychiatric treatment of depression consists of, or at least starts out with, titrating or adjusting these alleged dysfunctions with one or more of the antidepressants listed in Table 23.2 (Trimble & George, 2010; Black & Andreasen, 2014). Of course, concomitant psychotherapies, ECT, and polypharmacies are used in addition to single medications to treat depressive disorders.

Often patients get "cocktails" of various antidepressants, benzodiazepines, mood stabilizers, and/or augmenting drugs. The augmenters can include lithium, aripiprazole (Abilify), lurasidone (Latuda), brexpiprazole (Rexulti), or even

TABLE 23.2. Antidepressant Medications

Generic name/ brand name	Dosage in mg/day (half-life in hours)	Company (year first manufactured)	Adverse events/other characteristics	
			Generic	Specific
Tricyclics (TCAs)				
Imipramine/ Tofranil	150–250 (5–25)	Ciba (1958)	Dry mouth, blurred vision, constipation, urinary retention, fatigue, tremors, sexual dysfunction; respiratory failure in OD; weight gain	"Gold standard" for AD effect; used frequently in 1960s
Amitriptyline/ Elavil	150–250 (20–50)	Merck (1961)		
Doxepin/ Sinequan	150–250 (8–24)	Boehringer Mannheim (1968)		
Nortriptyline/ Pamelor	25–150 (18–44)	Eli Lilly (1960s)		
Clomipramine/ Anafranil	150–250 (20–50)	Novartis (1960s)		
Monoamine oxidase inhibitors (MAOIs)				
Tranylcypromine/ Parnate	10–60 (2.5)	SmithKline (1959)	Must limit meat, cheese, fava beans, ripe fruit, Chianti, pain meds, chocolate; sexual dysfunction, orthostatic hypotension, headache, nausea, racing heart, chest pain	
Phenelzine/Nardil	30–60 (11.6)	Pfizer (1959)		
Isocarboxazid/ Marplan	20–40 (unk)	Hoffman-LaRoche (1959)	Not used much today, except for atypical depression	
Selective serotonin reuptake inhibitors (SSRIs)				
Fluoxetine/Prozac	20–80 (24–72)	Eli Lilly (1988)	Nausea, increased suicidality up to age 24, sexual dysfunction, jitteriness, somnolence, dizziness, headache, akathisia?	First SSRI, first kids' AD
Paroxetine/Paxil	20–50 (20)	SmithKline (1992)		Withdrawal, short half-life; voted "most acceptable";[a] anxiety Tx
Sertraline/Zoloft	50–200 (25)	Pfizer (1991)		

(continued)

TABLE 23.2. *(continued)*

Generic name/ brand name	Dosage in mg/day (half-life in hours)	Company (year first manufactured)	Adverse events/other characteristics	
			Generic	Specific
Selective serotonin reuptake inhibitors (SSRIs) *(continued)*				
Citalopram/ Celexa	20–40 (35)	Lundbeck (1989)	SSRIs = most widely prescribed for AD Tx	
Escitalopram/ Lexapro	10–20	Lundbeck (2002)		Isomer of Celexa; fewer AEs
Fluvoxamine/ Luvox	100–300 (15)	Solvay (1993)		OCD Tx
Serotonin–norepinephrine reuptake inhibitors (SNRIs)				
Venlafaxine/ Effexor	75–350 (3.5)	Wyeth (1993)	Anticholinergic, sedation, nausea, sexual dysfunction, dizziness	Panic/phobia Tx
Desvenlafaxine/ Pristiq	50–100 (11)	Wyeth (2008)		Serotonin syndrome
Duloxetine/ Cymbalta	40–60 (12)	Eli Lilly (1990)	SNRIs = prescribed more recently	Also used for pain Tx
Mirtazapine/ Remeron	15–45 (20–40)	Oragnon (1996)		Voted "most effective"[a]
Atypical and newer antidepressants				
Bupropion/ Wellbutrin	100–150 (20)	Burroughs Wellcome (1989)	Nausea, headache	Dopamine + NE, ↓ cigs.
Trazadone/ Desyrel	150–200 (3–6)	Auglini (1981)	Sedating, antihistamine	Used HS
Nefazodone/ Sersone	300–500 (2–18)	Bristol-Myers (1994)	Similar to Desyrel	Does not suppress REM sleep
Vilazodone/ Viibryd	10–40 (25)	Trovis-Forest (2011)	Lower effects on sexual dysfunction	Affects 5-HT$_{1A}$
Aripiprazole/ Abilify	1–5 (75)	Bristol-Myers (2007)	5-HT$_{1A}$ agonist; akathisia?	Augmenter & adjunct Tx

Note. No foreign-brand drug names are given. Since new antidepressants are constantly being marketed (such as Fetzima/ levomilnacipran, Brintellix/vortioxetine, and Viibryd/vilazodone), this table is almost by definition an incomplete list. Abbreviations in table: OD, overdose; AD, antidepressant; Tx, treatment; AEs, adverse effects; dopamine + NE, increases dopamine and norepinephrine; cigs, Wellbutrin marketed as Zyban for controlling cigarette smoking; HS, hours of sleep or at bedtime; REM, rapid eye movement; 5-HT$_{1A}$, a specific serotonin neuroreceptor.

[a]Votes for "most effective" and "most acceptable" in *The Lancet,* June 29, 2009 (Cipriani et al., 2009).

Source: Adapted from Maris (2015). Copyright © 2015 the University of South Carolina. Adapted with permission.

ketamine. Some patients take five or six psychoactive drugs (not just antidepressants) a day (Angell, 2011a, 2011b). Since the SSRIs often have related sexual dysfunction side effects, they can be given concomitantly with a small (20- to 30-mg) dose of Wellbutrin on a day when sexual activity is expected, or there can even be an SSRI "drug holiday" to promote sexual function.

Psychiatrists normally "start low and go slow" with medications. Typically, a depressed patient is started (often on a low dose for a week or so—say, 10 mg of Prozac or Lexapro, or 150 mg of Wellbutrin) of an SSRI, an SNRI, or Wellbutrin (see Table 23.2) for 4–8 weeks. If the desired antidepressant effect is not achieved, or if the unintended adverse effects are too bothersome, then the antidepressant type may be switched, or the dose may be increased or decreased. One needs to be careful not to increase the dosage mindlessly if there are serious adverse effects, which could then be made worse or even possibly cause or contribute to suicidality. Serious adverse effects can include mania, agitation, *de novo* suicide ideation, sleep disorder, and serotonin syndrome. If any of these occurs, the patient is instructed to call the doctor immediately or go to a local emergency room.

Once a desired antidepressant effect is achieved (as determined by clinical judgment or a score below 7 on the Hamilton Rating Scale for Depression [HAM-D]; Zimmerman et al., 2017), the patient may remain on the antidepressant for 3–8 months after remission of symptoms. If there have been multiple prior depressive episodes (so-called "kindled" depression), the patient may stay on the antidepressant indefinitely. The time varies, and appropriate follow-up is important. Except for Prozac (or other antidepressants with a long half-life), stopping an antidepressant "cold turkey" can be problematic, especially with antidepressants like Paxil that have a very short half-life. There can be withdrawal or discontinuation syndromes, including symptoms or adverse effects specific to the particular antidepressant (nightmares, nausea or other gastrointestinal problems, "electric shock" sensations, muscle stiffness or spasms, nervousness, etc.). A lot of antidepressants can contribute to nausea. Sometimes the antidepressant effect itself just stops or wanes (*tachyphylaxis*). Sometimes drug treatment of suicide can have paradoxical effects and even make depression or suicide ideation worse (Maris, 2015). The antidepressant package inserts have up-front black-box suicidality warnings.

The TCAs tend not to be used much any more, since they can be fatal in overdose and cause annoying anticholinergic side effects. The same goes for the MAOIs (see Table 23.2), which have dietary restrictions that normally make them not worth the trouble. Violating these restrictions can result in severe hypotension, stroke, or even death. The SSRIs tend to have fewer adverse effects than the TCAs. Lately, SNRIs (Table 23.2) such as Pristiq, Cymbalta, and Remeron have become more popular, as have dopaminergic agents like Wellbutrin, which have fewer sexual side effects. Other antidepressants getting more recent attention are Viibryd (a 5-HT$_{1A}$ agonist, also with fewer sexual side effects) and Brintellix.

Antidepressants are often used conjointly with long-acting benzodiazepines (like Klonopin) or other minor tranquilizers (or even with major tranquilizers, like Risperdal or Zyprexa). Anxiety needs to be controlled until, or even after, the desired antidepressant effect is achieved (Fawcett et al., 1997, 2012). There are even some drugs that combine an antidepressant with an antipsychotic, such as

Symbyax, which combines Prozac with Zyprexa. Sometimes at bedtime, an antihis-
tamine like Desyrel or Serzone is also given to aid sleep.

Augmenter medications like Abilify, lithium, Latuda, Rexulti, or ketamine may
be administered as well. Abilify is a third-generation antipsychotic that often is used
to boost or augment the effects of antidepressants. However, it can result in serious
problems, such as weight gain and diabetes, extreme restlessness, insomnia, and constipation. If time is short (e.g., the patient is in an acute suicidal crisis), or the antidepressants are not having the desired antidepressant effects, then ECT is still the "gold
standard" treatment for depression (Black & Andreasen, 2014; Behrman, 2002).

The choice of an antidepressant is often based on clinical judgment and individual patient idiosyncrasies, not just on science. An antidepressant that worked for
one of a patient's parents, for instance, might give the clinician a clue to what might
work for the patient. After all, mother and father each contribute 50% of their
child's genes. It is interesting how much of the recent research on suicide concerns
genetics. For example, see the work of Virginia Willour and Mary Anne Enoch
(discussed in Maris, 2015). An article in the prestigious British medical journal *The
Lancet* (Cipriani et al., 2009; see also Cipriani et al., 2018) rated the most effective
(i.e., they delivered the desired antidepressant effect) and most acceptable (patients
kept taking them) antidepressants worldwide. The results have been shown in
Chapter 11, Table 11.2. (Remember that *The Lancet* is published in Great Britain,
and drug usage in Western Europe may be different from that in the United States.)

For theories of neuropharmacology, see Chapter 16 of this book, as well as Cooper et al. (2003) and Trimble and George (2010). As we have seen, the run-of-the-mill
antidepressant theories like the serotonin hypothesis are overly simplistic (Carlat,
2010) and hotly contested. The neurobiology of depression is extremely complex.

In early research, a Swedish researcher and her colleagues (Äsberg et al., 1976)
developed a theory on serotonin and suicide. To oversimplify, Äsberg et al. found
that suicidal individuals (not suicide completers) tended to have statistically significantly lower levels of serotonin and its metabolite, 5-hydroxyindoleacetic acid
(5-HIAA), in their CSF, as measured by spinal taps (the two hemispheres of the
brain float in CSF). Later research by John Mann and his colleagues found that
actual postmortem studies of completed suicides' brains showed too little serotonin
in the prefrontal cortex (Mann & Currier, 2012). Important recent neurobiological suicide research is also being done by Maria Oquendo and her colleagues (see
Gananca et al., 2017).

Of course, suicide is not just a function of serotonin and serotonergic system
dysfunction, but rather of a number of neurotransmitters and neurosystems operating together in a complex synthesis and occurring in various concentrations in various anatomical sites in the brain (e.g., the Brodmann areas). Nevertheless, starting
with the marketing of Prozac in 1988 and continuing today, the drug companies
have marketed antidepressants as designed to boost the serotonergic system, by
blocking presynaptic reabsorption of serotonin in the gap between neurons (the
synaptic cleft), leaving more serotonin in the CSF and promoting or enhancing
neural transmission of serotonin.

An antidepressant like Prozac or Lexapro blocks the presynaptic reabsorption
(into the axonal reuptake pump) of serotonin—thereby increasing the amount of
active serotonin that can be delivered to the receiving (postsynaptic) nerve cell,

and boosting serotonergic transmission, the serotonin system, and serotonin levels. Since lowered serotonin levels and transmission are thought to be related to depressive disorders, enhancing the serotonergic system should elevate mood. However, if one has too much serotonin, this can cause a serious adverse event called the *serotonin syndrome,* which can involve confusion, agitation, mania, anxiety, muscle incoordination, spasms, twitching, cramps, headache, sweating, and even coma (Angell, 2011a, 2011b).

Mood Stabilizer and Antiepileptic Treatment

Since mania is the polar opposite of depression, one would think that the treatment of mania should be different from that of depression, and it is (see Chapter 12). Medications to treat mania are called *mood stabilizers, anticonvulsants,* or *antiepileptics.* Although the mechanisms of mood stabilizers (especially lithium) are not completely understood, some of them seem to affect the neurotransmitter gamma-aminobutyric acid (GABA) and sometimes influence glutamate, acetylcholine, and serotonin or have a structure like TCAs (e.g., Tegretol). In this section, I argue that these GABA effects are precisely what can cause or contribute to suicidogenic adverse effects (however, see Rothschild, 2017).

Treatment of manic or hypomanic episodes in bipolar disorders can consist of a combination of lithium, anticonvulsants or antiepileptics, antidepressants, and sometimes minor tranquilizers (like benzodiazepines) and/or major antipsychotics(like Risperdal, Zyprexa, or Latuda). Table 23.3 is a partial list of mood stabilizers and antiepileptics. Of course, concomitant psychotherapies may be advised as well (see Chapter 24). Any individual patient should discuss his or her specific case and its treatment with a qualified mental health professional.

Gabapentin (Neurontin)

Some mood stabilizers are *GABAergic;* that is, they increase the neurotransmitter GABA and stimulate the GABA neurosystem. Because they do, there are possible suicidogenic implications of treating mania and bipolar disorders with them. Therefore, I focus first here on the GABAergic mood stabilizer/antiepileptic gabapentin (Neurontin), although Neurontin is usually not the first-line treatment for mania. Some of the claims about Neurontin are theories, based especially on the research of Trimble (2007; Trimble & George, 2010). Other, more first-line anticonvulsants are discussed later.

As its generic name suggests, gabapentin (Neurontin) is a GABA agonist; that is, it raises human brain GABA (Trimble, 2007). Increase in brain GABA leads to negative effects on mood and behavior (Trimble, 2007). Glutamate is the brain's main excitatory transmitter. Neurontin reduces glutamate release at cortical synapses (Trimble, 2007). Depletion of monoamines (particularly serotonin and norepinephrine) can lead to significantly increased risk of depression (or can make a preexisting depression worse), dysphoria, depersonalization, agitation, and aggression. It can also increase suicidal behaviors (e.g., including suicide attempts), and even possibly completed suicides (Trimble, 2007; Brown et al., 1992).

TABLE 23.3. Mood Stabilizers and Antiepileptics

Generic name/ brand name	Dosage in mg/day (half-life in hours)	Company (year first manufactured)	Adverse and beneficial effects/other characteristics
Lithium carbonate/ Eskalith	900–2,400 (20)[a]	Generics (1970)[b]	Intoxication effects (inc. death); need to monitor blood levels,[c] salt; thirst, tremors, weight gain, renal complications, hyperthyroidism; blocks acetylcholine; augmenter with ADs; RCTs indicate suicide prevention
Lamotrigine/ Lamictal	200 (25)	GSK (1994)	Stevens–Johnson syndrome, rash; blocks sodium channels; delays occurrence of depressive episodes.
Valproic acid/ Depakote	1,250–2,500 (8–17)	Sandoz et al. (1993)[d]	GI problems, tremor, sedation, weight gain; take with food; enhances GABA; rare hepatoxic reaction; first used as epilepsy treatment; birth defects
Carbamazepine/ Tegretol	600–1,200 (20–65)	Taro/Validus (1974)[e]	Structure like TCAs; rash/skin disorders, drowsiness, ataxia, dizziness; dampens kindling; rare hematological effects, fetal malformations?, dizziness
Gabapentin/ Neurontin	900–2,400 (5–7)	Pfizer (1994)	Enhances GABA, lowers monoamines; may contribute to depression; somnolence, nausea; used off-label for pain control
Topiramate/ Topamax	400 (21)	Ortho-McNeil (2011)	Nausea, fatigue, weight loss, dizziness, ataxia

Note. This table is not a complete list. Other mood stabilizers, anticonvulsants, or antiepileptics include pregabalin/Lyrica, oxcarbazepine/Trileptal, tiagabine/Gabitril. vigabatrin/Sabril, levetiracetam/Keppra, zonisamide/Zonegram, clobazam/Onfi, lurasidone/Latuda, and others. Abbreviations in table: ADs, antidepressants; RCT, randomized clinical trials; GI, gastrointestinal; GABA, gamma-aminobutyric acid; TCAs, tricyclic antidepressants.

[a]The half-life in manic patients is about 8–12 hours, since they tend to be overactive.

[b]First antimanic effects discovered by Cade in 1949; used as early as 1843 for bladder stones and 1859 for mood disorders.

[c]0.9–1.4 mEq/L.

[d]Depakote has been around since 1882.

[e]Synthesized in 1960.

Source: Adapted from Maris (2015). Copyright © 2015 the University of South Carolina. Adapted with permission.

Lithium Carbonate

As discussed in Chapter 12, lithium is a naturally occurring salt that is often used for suicidal bipolar patients and for the initial stabilization of mania (Maris et al., 2000), although many patients will not take it. We still do not know exactly how lithium works to treat mania (Black & Andreasen, 2014). It may be related to decreased cellular responses to neurotransmitters. Some have argued that in mania there is an increase in protein kinase C (PKC), and that lithium inhibits PKC.

Lithium is tricky to administer, and some patients cannot tolerate it, in which case they may be put on other anticonvulsants (Goldsmith et al., 2002). There can be lithium intoxication, in rare cases even resulting in death. One has to monitor blood plasma levels carefully to achieve a therapeutic lithium level (initially 0.9–1.4 mEq/L) and maintenance levels (0.5–0.7 mEq/L). The typical patient is started on 300 mg of lithium twice a day, and then the dose is titrated upward until a therapeutic plasma level is achieved (see "Lithium: Patient Drug Information," 2013). There is a slow-release preparation of lithium to reduce gastric irritation.

Given that lithium is a salt, there can be side effects of polyuria or thirst, weight gain, edema, diarrhea, and tremors. As many as 15% of patients taking lithium develop get hypothyroidism, which can be treated, for example, with Synthroid. Lithium is sometimes used as an augmenter with antidepressants for the treatment of major depression. Lithium (like Prozac) can be stopped without tapering dosages. One strikingly consistent result from clinical trials is that lithium appears to lower suicide risk significantly in bipolar patients (Baldessarini & Tondo, 1999; Baldessarini et al., 2012; Goldsmith et al., 2002; Tondo et al., 2001). The reduction in suicide risk is most pronounced after a minimum of 2 years of lithium treatment. Sometimes bipolar patients can develop schizoaffective disorder, in which case treatment with Tegretol may be preferred to lithium treatment.

Valproic Acid (Depakote), Carbamazepine (Tegretol), and Lamotrigine (Lamictal)

Even though lithium treatment is one of the most effective and common medications for bipolar disorder, it is not for everybody. Some bipolar patients cannot tolerate lithium or do not want the associated weight gain (Goldsmith et al., 2002). Most such patients take one of three anticonvulsants: Depakote, Tegretol, or (most likely) Lamictal. There are also several other drugs to treat bipolar disorder (see Table 23.3), such as Latuda.

Valproic Acid (Depakote)

Valproic acid was first synthesized in 1882. It was found naturally in the herb valerian. Like Neurontin, Depakote enhances the neurotransmitter GABA. It was first used to treat epilepsy and later was approved as a mood stabilizer. Most patients receive from 1,250 to 2,500 mg each day. Depakote can cause a rare, severe hepatotoxic (toxic to the liver) reaction, possibly leading to death. It needs to be taken with food and may cause gastrointestinal problems. Many patients will not take it, since it causes weight gain (i.e., it offers no advantage here over lithium). Patients can feel sedated or develop tremors, and pregnant women should not take it, since it can cause birth defects.

Carbamazepine (Tegretol)

Carbamazepine was first synthesized in 1960 and was later marketed as an anticonvulsant. Its molecular structure is similar to that of the TCAs. Most patients take

200 mg of Tegretol three times a day, up to 1,600 mg/day. It has a dampening effect on kindled depression. Tegretol can have rare hematological effects, such as infection, anemia, and *petechiae*. Like Lamictal, Tegretol can cause rashes or skin disorders. It may result in drowsiness, dizziness, ataxia, or possibly fetal malformations.

Lamotrigine (Lamictal)

Lamotrigine was first marketed as an anticonvulsant by GlaxoSmithKline in 1994. Its target therapeutic dosage is 200 mg/day, through a slow titration in 25-mg increments. Lamictal blocks sodium channels and delays the occurrence of depressive episodes in bipolar patients. Many patients not on lithium take Lamictal.

Although Lamictal has relatively few adverse effects compared to Depakote and Tegretol, it does have a black-box FDA warning (the strongest warning available) for rashes and skin disorders, including the rare but dreaded Stevens–Johnsons syndrome. With Stevens–Johnson syndrome, the skin becomes necrotic (like shedding a snake's skin), and the throat can swell and impair breathing. Other serious adverse effects can include damage to vital internal organs, such as the liver.

Anxiolytic Treatment

Like most psychiatric disorders, anxiety disorders are treated with a variety of medications and psychotherapies, including cognitive therapies, DBT, behavior modification, eye movement desensitization and reprocessing (EMDR), hypnosis, distraction, breathing procedures, and occasionally psychoanalysis or ECT. Patients with anxiety disorders are advised to limit or avoid caffeine intake, sodium lactate, carbon dioxide, or any drugs that increase catecholamine levels (norepinephrine and dopamine), as well as antipsychotics or antidepressants that may stimulate mania or akathisia.

The first-line treatment for anxiety disorders is often one of the SSRI antidepressants (Table 23.2), like Zoloft, Luvox, Lexapro, Paxil, or Prozac, or an SNRI like Effexor. It may seem strange to treat anxiety with an antidepressant. However, anxiety and depression overlap considerably (Black & Andreasen, 2014), and the names of many major types of psychiatric medications are misnomers. For example, Prozac is used to treat anxiety much more than depression.

Most SSRIs take several weeks to have antidepressant efficacy, and only then in about 60–70% of patients. Kirsch (2010) suggests using an antidepressant only when a patient has a moderate to severe depression (e.g., as measured by the BDI-II or HAM-D). There may be a relatively long period of antidepressant trial and error to find the optimal antidepressant(s) for an individual and/or the most appropriate dosage. Consideration of interaction effects with other medications and diet is also needed. On the positive side, most SSRIs are relatively well tolerated, even if used for longer periods, unlike benzodiazepines.

For short-term use and/or acute or time-limited situational anxiety, generally either a benzodiazepine or a nonbenzodiazepine anxiolytic like Buspar or Desyrel (see Table 23.4) is normally prescribed, either alone or (more often) along with an antidepressant. Some benzodiazepine and nonbenzodiazepine minor tranquilizers for short-term use include alprazolam (Xanax), diazepam (Valium), chlordiazepoxide (Librium, also used for alcohol detoxification), flurazepam (Dalmane), triazolam (Halcion), temazepam (Restoril), clonazepam (Klonopin), oxazepam (Serax), lorazepam (Ativan), and some sleep aids (like Ambien, Lunesta, and Sonata, all of which have FDA warnings as of August 31, 2006). Unlike antidepressants, benzodiazepines act relatively quickly and have rapid rates of onset of tranquilizing or sedating effects (see Table 23.4). Acute, highly agitated patients in emergency rooms or psychiatric inpatient wards may be given a drug cocktail sometimes referred to as "5–2–25" (i.e., 5 mg of Haldol + 2 mg of Ativan + 25 mg of Benadryl). Klonopin has a long half-life and is often recommended for suicide prevention while a patient is waiting for an antidepressant effect to kick in (Fawcett, 2006, 2012).

Unfortunately, benzodiazepines, unlike SSRIs or SNRIs, should only be prescribed for a few weeks or months. Many benzodiazepines can induce or worsen depressive disorders, cause oversedation, create addiction, and cause physical and psychological dependence. Stopping them abruptly (especially if they have a short half-life) can lead to insomnia and other adverse effects. In one report, it was claimed that as little as 10 mg of Valium taken every day for as little as 2 weeks could itself induce a clinical depression.

We now know (Trimble & George, 2010) that GABA-enhancing drugs (like the benzodiazepines or Neurontin; see above) tend to deplete central nervous system serotonin and norepinephrine, and that lowered levels of monoamines are positively associated with depression, perhaps even with increased suicide risk (Maris, 2007, 2015). There are other adverse effects of antianxiety medications. Clinicians need to consider the possibility that benzodiazepines might produce paradoxical effects, especially during withdrawal (e.g., aggression, violence, or even suicide attempts instead of sedating or calming effects).

Nonbenzodiazepine anxiolytics (see Table 23.4) include Buspirone (Buspar); antihistamines (like trazadone [Desyrel] or diphenhydramine [Benadryl]); beta-blockers (like propranolol [Inderal]); barbiturates; the nonbenzodiazepine hypnotics (like Ambien, Sonata, and Lunesta); or even major tranquilizers (like Zyprexa or Risperdal). Buspar is used to treat generalized anxiety disorder, but it apparently is not effective for panic disorders, phobias, or obsessive–compulsive disorder (OCD). Buspar is relatively nonsedating, is not a muscle relaxant (as, e.g., Valium is), and does not interact with alcohol. In the famous case of Karen Ann Quinlan (see Maris et al., 2000), she ingested Valium along with alcohol and went into a coma for about 10 years.

Antipsychotic Treatment

In patients with schizophrenia or other forms of psychosis, suicide is not so much the result of antipsychotic medications (antipsychotics are sometimes also called *neuroleptics*) as it is of the disease itself. In very few cases is antipsychotic medication alleged to be a cause of suicide. In fact, most studies show that antipsychotics

TABLE 23.4. Antianxiety Medications

Benzodiazepines,[a] generic name/trade name	Dosage in mg/day	Company (year first manufactured)[b]	Adverse effects/other characteristics
Diazepam/Valium	5–40	La Roche (1963)	Paradoxical rage, aggression, and depression;[c] very fast onset
Chlordiazepoxide/Librium	15–60	Hoffman (1955)	Used in tapered doses for ethanol withdrawal
Alprazolam/Xanax	1–4	Pharmacia (2006)	Dependency issues; fast onset; not first Tx
Oxazepam/Serax	30–120	Wyeth (1965)	Slow onset; metabolite of Valium
Temazepam/Restoril	15–30	Novartis (1964)	Short duration of action
Lorazepam/Ativan	0.5–10	Wyeth (1971)	Fast onset; parenteral adm. available[d]
Clonazepam/Klonopin	1–6	Roche (1997)	Long-acting (with ADs); moderate onset
Triazolam/Halcion	0.125–0.25	Upjohn (1982)	Old sleep aid; some paradoxical aggression

Nonbenzodiazepine anxiolytics,[e] generic name/trade name	Dosage in mg/day	Drug type/other comments	
Sertraline/Zoloft	50–100	SSRI (SSRIs are the preferred Tx)[f]	
Buspirone/Buspar	20–30	5-HT$_{1A}$ agonist (Bristol, 1986)	
Trazadone/Desyrel	300–800	Antihistamine, HS (often with SSRI)	
Imipramine/Tofranil	50–300	TCA	
Fluvoxamine/Luvox	100–300	SSRI	
Propranolol/Inderal	20–80	Beta-blocker (Wyeth, 1960s)	
Venlafaxine/Effexor	75–350	SNRI	
Zolpidem/Ambien[g]	0.25–12.5 (extended release)	Hypnotic (Sanofi-Aventis, 1992)	

Note. This table is not a complete list. Given the volatility and rapid change in drug research and marketing, some newer antianxiety medications may not be listed here. See Tables 23.2 and 23.3 for abbreviations.

[a]For short-term and acute, situational treatments, benzodiazepines enhance GABA, which results in anxiolytic, hypnotic, and sedative effects.

[b]After patents expire, of course many antianxiety drugs have many different manufacturers.

[c]Depression can result in as little as 2 weeks after treatment at 10 mg/day; be careful about concurrent ethanol consumption and interactive effects.

[d]That is, it can be given intravenously.

[e]Nonbenzodiazepines also include sleep or hypnotic agents like zolpidem (Ambien), zalepon (Sonata), and eszopiclone (Lunesta). All of these may have suicidogenic effects (see the FDA's, safety review of August 31, 2006).

[f]Including, for example, Lexapro, Prozac, and Luvox.

[g]See also Sonata and Lunesta.

Source: Adapted from Maris (2015). Copyright © 2015 the University of South Carolina. Adapted with permission.

reduce suicide risk, especially Clozaril. It is true that some of the older phenothi-azine drugs like Thorazine can cause akathisia (a drug-induced profound inner and outer restlessness), which is related to suicide; they can also cause other suicido-genic effects, including psychosis itself (particularly so-called "command hallucina-tions" to kill oneself). People with schizophrenia have a 5–10% lifetime suicide out-come, versus 10–15% for patients with depressive disorders (Hor & Taylor, 2010). The suicide rate in the general population is only about 1 in 10,000 a year. Thus schizophrenia itself is a major risk factor for suicide outcome.

With psychotic disorders (like schizophrenia and psychotic depression), anti-psychotic medication treatments are usually necessary (i.e., psychotherapy by itself generally does not work). Most suicidal psychotic patients start out with one of the second-generation atypical antipsychotics, like Clozaril, Zyprexa, or Risperdal (Angell, 2011a, 2011b), or adjunctive antipsychotics, like Rexulti or Abilify; the ear-lier first-generation typical antipsychotics have some fairly serious adverse effects, especially long-term effects (Whitaker, 2010).

Low-potency antipsychotics such as chlorpromazine (Thorazine), thioridazine (Mellaril), and chlorprothixene (Taractan) may be used for their sedative effects, but they can also lower blood pressure dangerously and result in tardive dyskine-sia. One might also consider intermediate-potency antipsychotics, such as perphen-azine (Trilafon) or loxapine (Loxitane), or newer second-generation antipsychotics, like clozapine (Clozaril), risperidone (Risperdal), olanzapine (Zyprexa), ascenapine (Saphris), or ziprasidone (Geodon). Clinical trials show that Clozaril is effective in reducing suicidality and treatment-resistant psychosis and does not cause tardive dyskinesia. However, it tends to be expensive and can cause seizures, as well as agranulocytosis (failure of the body to produce white blood cells that fight infec-tion, in about 1% of patients). See Chapter 13, Table 13.4, for a list of antipsychotic medications along with their adverse effects.

Psychotic patients may be on antipsychotics, antidepressants, and anxiolytics at the same time. They may even take more than one of each medication type, such as two antidepressants or even two different antipsychotics. Compliance with medi-cation regimens is important; presumably patients get better if they keep taking their medications. When the *British Medical Journal* (Tiihonen et al., 2006) rated the various antipsychotics by rates of discontinuation (which are usually indicators of higher levels of side effects), the lowest rates of discontinuation in order were for (1) Clozapine, (2) Trilafon, and (3) Zyprexa. (See also Chapter 13.)

Neurochemically, psychosis is thought to be related primarily to dopamine excesses and dysfunctions of the dopaminergic system in the brain (Black & Andreasen, 2014). Most antipsychotic drugs are dopamine blockers or antago-nists; that is, they block excess dopamine. (An *agonist* is a substance that promotes a receptor-mediated biological response.) Although the dopamine hypothesis of schizophrenia (described in more detail in Chapter 13) is overly simplistic, all anti-psychotic drugs tend to block dopamine (D_2)receptors in the brain, thereby reduc-ing dopamine excesses in the brain.

One of the more serious adverse effects of (mainly first-generation) antipsy-chotics is a movement disorder called *tardive dyskinesia,* an irreversible writhing of the mouth, tongue, and face, often seen in patients with chronic schizophrenia who have been taking Thorazine a long time. Other movement disorders related to antipsychotics include parkinsonism (flattening of facial expression, stiffness of gait, rolling tremors of the finger, excessive salivation); acute dystonic reactions (tightening of facial and neck muscles, jaw tightness, difficulty opening mouth); catatonia (bizarre posturing, rigidity/immobility, withdrawal); akathisia (restless legs, fidgety, pacing, rocking, inner restlessness); akinesia (decreased motor movements); so-called "rabbit syndrome" (fine, rapid tremors of the lips); tremor (rhythmic alternating movements, mostly of the fingers); and athetotis (slow, writhing purposeless movements).

Antipsychotic patients can also have anticholinergic adverse effects, which reduce the effects mediated by acetylcholine in the central and peripheral nervous systems. Some of these symptoms include dry mouth, urinary retention, constipation, ataxia, increased body temperature, double vision, tachycardia, shaking, lack of perspiration, and respiratory depression. Finally, as noted earlier, about 1–2% of patients taking Clozaril get agranulocytosis (an inhibition of white blood cell production that can lead to infection and even to death).

Because of the adverse effects of many antipsychotics, patients may need to take antiparkinsonian agents along with their antipsychotic medications. Some of these agents are Cogentin (1–2 mg), Artane (1–15 mg), over-the-counter Benadryl (25–200 mg), various beta-blockers (like Inderal, Corgard, or Tenormin), or vitamin E.

Finally, note that sometimes treatment for psychosis is ordered not because a person is ill, but rather because the person is eccentric, different from most others, or annoying. See the Academy Award-nominated movie *A Serious Man* (Coen & Coen, 2009), in which the main character likens his neighbors' killing deer to killing motivated by xenophobia.

ECT and Other Technical Treatment Procedures

In 2000, I wrote:

> Electroconvulsive therapy (ECT), in its modern form, is generally considered safe [even preferred for acute suicidal crises] and effective [it is about 80% effective in 1–2 weeks, versus an effective rate for antidepressants of 60–70% in 6–8 weeks] in the treatment of major depression and mania and should be considered for suicidal patients whose disorders are refractory to psychopharmacological interventions. However, perhaps because there is a paucity of randomized controlled studies to document its effectiveness—or because of negative public perceptions, fueled by such popular books/films as *One Flew Over the Cuckoo's Nest*—it has not gained widespread use or acceptance. . . . [It] is often [an intervention] "of last resort," only for those difficult-to-treat patients. . . . The mechanism of its action remains shrouded in mystery [less so today], although it is believed that ECT affects serotonin function. (Maris et al., 2000, pp. 525–526).

When Sylvia Plath's alter ego character, Esther Greenwood, is "shocked" in *The Bell Jar* (1963/2005) to treat her refractory depression, she sees it as an awful punishment (for what, she does not know), similar to the electrocution of Soviet spies Julius and Ethel Rosenberg on June 19, 1953.

If psychiatric medications fail to produce an antidepressant response and/or the suicidal crisis is acute, then the patient may receive ECT every other day for up to 2 weeks. ECT has been described in detail in Chapter 11, and this description is not repeated here (however, see Gambino, 2018). Also, see Chapter 16 for a review of other technical treatment procedures, such as vagus nerve stimulation, transcranial magnetic stimulation (Weisman et al., 2018), bilateral cingulotomy, and imaging.

The Limitations of Psychopharmacology

Pills are inert, impersonal chemical compounds that cannot listen to you, care about your well-being, give you a hug, or in any significant way undo the pathological conditioning of your long suicidal career. If a part of being suicidal is a tortured, obsessive, narcissistic pathology, pills can do little to help you get outside of yourself. At most they can deaden your pain, without curing it. Pills cannot be a caring significant other (although they could help facilitate or make you more receptive to such care), help your social and mental isolation, or repair a history of negative interaction and interpersonal trauma.

What if one did not treat mild (or even some moderate) psychiatric disorders with medications at all, other things being equal? John Maltsberger (personal communication; see also Maltsberger & Stoklosa, 2012) has said to me, "Ron, do not forget that before there were antidepressants, we used to manage depression fairly well."

There are before-and-after magnetic resonance imaging (MRI) and single-photon emission computed tomography (SPECT) studies of psychiatric drug treatment versus psychotherapy (usually some form of cognitive or cognitive-behavioral therapy), which suggest that psychotherapy actually can make changes in our brains similar to those of psychiatric medications (Roffman et al., 2005). Often psychiatric medications are used simply because they are in vogue; they are cheaper and quicker than talk therapy; and insurance plans will pay for them, or at least for some of them.

A cartoon by Gahan Wilson depicts two figures resembling Catholic cardinals, with huge capital "N's" on their towering caps, looking quizzically at several other individuals with "N's" on their robes who are bowing down in front of a pillar labeled "Nothing." One of the two figures says to the other, "Is nothing sacred?" An alternative to psychiatric medications, especially early in the development of mental disorders for younger patients, is to do nothing pharmacologically. Sometimes less can actually be more. Do not forget that the Hippocratic Oath includes a promise to abstain from doing harm, often rendered as "First, do no harm."

Children and adolescents have immature, developing brains. It may well be that suicidality has a lot to do with serotonergic function or dysfunction in the prefrontal cortex of the brain—or, as Mann (2008; see also Mann & Currier, 2012) has said, "Low serotonin in the wrong place." But when is the proper time to intervene

chemically in young brains, if at all? Most young people have very low, not high, suicide rates. Even when the adolescent suicide rate in the United States tripled (from
1950 to 1977), it never rose above the average suicide rate (about 11–12 per 100,000,
not controlled for age). Some psychiatric disorders (such as bipolar disorder or
ASPD) cannot even be diagnosed reliably until later adolescence.

Some suicide experts have worried that if we do nothing and discourage the use
of psychiatric medications in young children and adolescents out of concern about
being sued for malpractice, the teen suicide rate may go up. There have been studies
(see Vedantam, 2007) which claim that after the FDA black-box alert warnings on
antidepressants came out in 2004, the number of SSRI prescriptions for adolescents
declined, and the suicide rate of people below age 19 rose 14% from 2003 to 2004.

However, the actual U.S. Vital Statistics data for 15- to 24-year-olds from 2004
to 2010 show a very different pattern. The data indicate the following suicide rates
(per 100,000 per year): 2004 (10.3), 2005 (10.0), 2006 (9.9), 2007 (9.7), 2008 (10.0),
2009 (10.1), and 2010 (10.5). Thus, the U.S. data show that the suicide rates of 15- to
24-year-olds are essentially unchanged, at least from 2004 to 2010. Adolescent suicide rates actually went down for 2–3 years after the FDA 2004 black-box warning,
and were basically the same in 2004 as they were in 2010.

It is difficult to know whether pharmacological treatment of mental disorders
always makes patients better (Whitaker, 2010, p. 335). David Healy (2012) claims
that there are more dead bodies in treatment groups than in the placebo groups
in clinical trials (cf. Whitaker, 2010). In suicidology, there is a saying that "suicide
often results from undiagnosed and untreated or undertreated depression" (Whitaker, 2010). The catch is that such a dictum may unreasonably justify an increase in
the diagnosis of depression and its treatment with powerful psychiatric medications, even in children.

Some have argued that we need to be very careful in continuously medicating
patients who have chronic schizophrenia with antipsychotics (Whitaker, 2010). For
example, does chronic blockage of the D_2 receptors lead to chemical anhedonia?
Can antipsychotics "perturb" neurosystems (e.g., the dopaminergic system), so that
the brain tries to compensate for receptor blockage (Whitaker, 2010)?

It has been argued (Whitaker, 2010) that overall about 50% of those with schizophrenia will eventually "recover" or improve anyway, even if they are not placed
on antipsychotic medications. Furthermore, one of the problems with the efficacy
studies of (say) antidepressants is that unmedicated depression may take longer
than most clinical trials last to lift, and so we may be missing non-medication-
related improvements in mood (Whitaker, 2010).

We cannot always fix things. It is not even clear that fixing mental disorders
is always a good thing. For example, as I have noted in Chapter 12, Jamison (1993)
speculated that when artist Vincent van Gogh painted, he was in a manic phase of
bipolar I disorder. In fact, we can say that van Gogh was only creative when he was
manic. Novelist Kurt Vonnegut may have had schizophrenia, and his son Mark was
hospitalized for schizophrenia. Would we have *Breakfast of Champions* (1973), among
Kurt Vonnegut's many other novels, if he had been taking Clozaril?

In Aldous Huxley's fictional Utopia called the World State, described in his 1932
novel *Brave New World,* suicides are virtually eliminated by properly conditioning

citizens and by encouraging them to ingesting the drug *soma*—but who would want to live there? In *Brave New World,* Shakespeare's plays and the Christian Bible are locked away in safes, because they are thought to be too socially disruptive.

Although at first blush it sounds naive, before (or at least in addition to) beginning a course of medication, people should be sure to eat right, get enough sleep (especially REM sleep), get aerobic exercise (Whitaker, 2010; minimally 20–30 minutes at least three times a week), avoid sexual excesses and indiscretions, and try to minimize unnecessary stress (easier said than done!). There were sociological studies of early New England settlers who had diets low in tryptophan (a dietary precursor of serotonin) in which virtually the whole community ended up becoming depressed (Ullman, 2007). Similarly, exercise has all sorts of physical and psychic consequences that we do not fully appreciate (unfortunately including total knee and hip replacements).

Patients in 19th- and early 20th-century lunatic asylums were frequently out in the country, in protected environments with fresh air. It is often assumed that they were worse off than modern psychiatric inpatients with their average 1-week stays and heavy medication regimens (Healy, 2012). But were they?

Whitaker (2010) notes that in 2004, the British government decided against paying for psychiatric medications for mild depression, and that in 2006, the Alaska Supreme Court sharply limited forced psychiatric medication. According to Whitaker, the psychiatric establishment has failed to tell the public that psychiatric medications often worsen long-term mental health outcomes.

Of course, better mental health through doing nothing but diet or exercise has its obvious limits. A severely depressed patient who cannot sleep or eat, or a mute patient with paranoid schizophrenia in a catatonic state, or an anxious patient with multiple (even serial) panic attacks each day, needs treatment.

Suicide treatment has at least two major components, psychopharmacology and psychotherapy. In Chapter 24 I consider psychotherapy, including psychodynamic treatment (Gabbard et al., 2012), cognitive-behavioral treatment (Brown et al., 2012), DBT (Linehan et al., 2015), brief therapies (e.g., those offered by suicide prevention centers, crisis intervention hotlines, and the emergency room), and family and group therapies. I also consider the two major modalities: outpatient and inpatient treatment, as listed in Table 23.1.

CHAPTER 24

Treatment and Intervention II. Psychotherapy
What Are We Going to Do about Suicide?

> As to how to help the suicidal individual, it is best to look upon a suicidal act as an effort to stop unbearable anguish or intolerable pain by "doing something." Knowing this usually guides us as to what treatment should be.
> —EDWIN S. SHNEIDMAN

John Mann and his colleagues focus suicide treatment on the psychopharmacology of the brain: titrating neurotransmitters and other neurochemicals, and adjusting dysfunctional neurosystems (Mann & Currier, 2012; Mann & Rudd, 2018; Gananca et al., 2017); mapping the levels of neurotransmitters in CSF and their concentrations in different parts of the brain; taking functional MRI scans of the brain; measuring levels of stress hormones; examining disruptive sleep patterns at 4–5 A.M. the day before a suicidal act (see Petersen, 2016a); and reviewing genetic associations. Edwin Shneidman (1993), Aaron Beck (Brown et al., 2012), and Marsha Linehan (1997, 2015) have focused treatment on the intolerable psychic pain ("psychache"; Ducasse et al., 2018) of suicidal individual's mind, and trying to reduce it through human therapeutic interactions aimed at (1) cognitively and behaviorally correcting faulty reasoning, inappropriate problem-solving efforts, catabolic catastrophizing and other rigid, dichotomous thinking, and unduly negative affect; and (2) helping the individual learn to react to suicidal risk through therapeutic social support and behavioral modification schedules, with the help of a competent, empathetic person—not just handing out pills.

Notice the disconnection between the neurobiological and psychological treatment approaches to suicide as described above. Such "split treatment" (Meyer, 2012) is done by two very different types of mental health professionals, usually with little coordination or interaction: psychiatrists and family practice physicians versus psychologists, social workers, and counselors. Often suicidal patients do not even have a psychotherapist—just pills in the medicine cabinet and a medication manager they see occasionally, if there are adverse effects of their medications (Carlat, 2010).

What does psychotherapeutic treatment involve? An individual with a symptom or set of symptoms seeks—or is referred, taken (e.g., by a parent or spouse), or commanded (by a court) to seek—help from a qualified mental health professional with specialized skills. The professional is licensed to observe and evaluate, and to offer (or refer to) treatment for the presenting issues. This is the clinical paradigm. It defines the role of the patient and therapist, and it outlines the patient–psychotherapist relationship. However, with suicidal patients, this therapist–patient relationship is not simple.

The quality of the therapeutic alliance is the single most important factor affecting suicide treatment outcome (Maltsberger & Stoklosa, 2012), and recognizing alliance issues is crucial to developing a treatment plan with any chance of success. High-suicide-risk patients have a number of personality traits, life stresses and traumas, skill deficits, and attachment difficulties that help explain their suicidality and negatively affect their treatment alliances with their caregivers (Maltsberger & Stoklosa, 2012). Among these are psychopathology, limited impulse control, often alcohol and/or other substance abuse, poor communication skills, social isolation, poor emotional regulation or control, and poor problem-solving skills. There are also life-stage-specific developmental deficits that make forming a therapeutic alliance difficult; for example, treatment alliance problems differ for adolescents and the elderly. Suicide treatment dropout rates are also high. Obtaining compliance with a treatment plan is another significant problem in the treatment of suicidal patients.

Berman (1986) estimated that one in six suicide completers were engaged in psychotherapy at the time of their death, and that about one-half of suicides have had experience with the mental health system at some time in their lives. It is important to consider whether or not these suicides were in part the result of some negative iatrogenic effect of a caregiver or treatment (i.e., illness produced by health care). For example, hopelessness could be engendered by lack of response to prescribed antidepressant medications or involuntary hospitalization. Perhaps the most significant contributor to iatrogenesis is *negative countertransference*, which is defined by a range of aversive reactions (thoughts, feelings, behaviors) manifested in a clinician's reactions to working with a psychotherapy patient, and often inappropriately based on perceived similar relationships to prior problematic patients.

Transference is the patient's unconscious assignment to others of feelings and attitudes that were originally associated with important early life figures, like parents or siblings. Both transference and countertransference are crucial factors in the success or failure of psychotherapy. The first task of the therapist must be to establish rapport or a therapeutic alliance with the patient (Maltsberger, 2006). The psychotherapist needs to be able to recognize transference and then point it out to the patient in a nonthreatening, productive way (Carlat, 2010). The following sections of this chapter consider various settings and types of psychotherapy with suicidal patients.

Suicidal First Aid

Much of the initial treatment of suicidal patients is crisis intervention, involving a visit to the local hospital emergency room, brief therapy with a volunteer on the phone, an internet chat line, or other resources like those listed in Chapter 23, Table 23.1 (e.g., the National Suicide Prevention Lifeline, 911, *www.suicidology.org, www.afsp.org,* or the local suicide prevention center hotline). Volunteer treatment is empathetic; it concentrates on listening and referral, sometimes even to the police or emergency medical services. Often the volunteers have "been there" themselves, much as counseling volunteers for Alcoholics Anonymous (AA) or Narcotics Anonymous (NA) are often recovering from addiction themselves. Suicide prevention volunteers are examples of "significant udders"; ideally, a distressed individual can trust and depend on them, as a nursing infant does with a loving mother.

Most would-be suicides have varying degrees of social isolation (Marchalik & Jurecic, 2018). They need somebody, almost anybody, although not suicidal peers who can increase the risk of suicide. Suicide ideators need competent, concerned others to help resolve an immediate problem, and not just a pill. In the hospital, probably a lot of requests for shots of pain medications are as much about the need for human contact as they are about the need for pain relief. Someone else has to touch a patient to give an injection.

Brief therapy or crisis intervention is supportive and hope-engendering, but is mainly psychiatric first aid. Crisis intervention focuses on resolving or defusing acute suicidal situations, not on treating more chronic suicidal careers (e.g., the aim is to get the gun, calm the agitation, or start the detoxification). The main issue often is impulse regulation, as in "You don't have to do *that!*"

Outpatient Therapy

Risk Assessment

Outpatient therapy begins with the assessment of suicide risk and the decision not to hospitalize the patient (Maltsberger, 2006). If the suicide risk is high, the need for monitoring may still be present throughout the period of perturbation or crisis. A person close to the patient and capable of providing vigilance and relief from aloneness may be necessary. The home should be suicide-proofed as much as possible, especially for firearms and medications (Lester, 2012). Frequent contact of the patient with the primary caregiver is important—for example, through increased sessions and/or telephone communications. Pharmacological interventions should be considered for the assessed diagnoses (Meyer, 2012).

The vast majority of psychotherapy for the suicidal takes place in an outpatient setting with a single qualified mental health professional, usually a psychologist, social worker, or counselor. If there are antidepressants involved in outpatient therapy, then many (over 40%) of the prescriptions are written by family practice physicians (Stagnitti, 2008). One of the best short statements about outpatient therapy with suicidal patients is Maltsberger and Stoklosa's (2012) argument that the heart of outpatient treatment with a suicidal client is to establish a treatment alliance or rapport. This process includes building up reasons for living.

Although the patient should have to agree that suicide is off the table, so-called "no-suicide contracts" are of little use (Maltsberger, 2006). Initially in the therapy, the patient's commitment to treatment is fragile—but there is really no treatment until a commitment has been made. The people the patient relies on for support need to be identified, and their names, cell phone numbers, and email addresses should be recorded. Even though the patient is not hospitalized, a treatment team needs to be established, and there should be open, frequent, and regular communication among treatment team members. Since medical doctors cannot delegate responsibility for any patients they are prescribing for, the treatment team "captain" is often the physician. There always needs to be a captain to coordinate care and take primary responsibility. Treatment needs to be tracked and monitored for missed appointments, late arrivals, failure to pay, noncompliance with prescriptions, and the patient's mental status and key treatment variables. Figure 24.1 is an example of a treatment-monitoring form.

Treatment Planning

Treatment planning involves designing interventions aimed at reducing the risk of suicidal behavior and at reducing or controlling the underlying mental disorder, if there is one. It is a truism that the better the assessment is—especially in clarifying the patient's vulnerabilities and pathologies, goals of suicidal behavior, and protective resources—then the easier and more effective the treatment planning is. In addition to deciding structural issues (such as whether treatment should be outpatient, inpatient, or partial hospitalization), treatment planning determines the sequencing of treatment. For example, with *dual-diagnosis* patients (i.e., patients with mental disorders and substance misuse or abuse), planning includes the types of psychosocial interventions, the possible needs for concomitant biological treatment (such as medications and/or ECT detoxification), the frequency and duration of interventions, how to measure interventions, how to determine when to terminate therapy, environmental enhancements to support treatment, and follow-up planning.

Treatment planning further specifies symptom remission goals, such as reductions in the frequency, intensity, duration, and specificity of suicidal ideations; decreased depression or hopelessness (as indicated by a reduced score on an appropriate rating scale); and improved access to supports and monitoring. Throughout treatment planning, there should be ongoing risk assessment and consideration of possible consultation with other professionals. In this regard, Jobes (2016) has introduced a collaborative model for outpatient treatment planning dictated by risk assessment. His Collaborative Assessment and Management of Suicidality (CAMS) model is intended to facilitate building a therapeutic alliance between the patient and therapist to understand the patient's suicidality. When the key constructs that underlie the patient's suicidal state are identified, treatment goals and interventions can be targeted and shaped.

Rate level of disturbance as none (0), mild (1), moderate (2), or severe (3).

Enter date	Date 1	Date 2	Date 3	Date N
Therapeutic alliance	6/14/18 (1)			
Exterior resources				
Interpersonal stability				
Suicide communications				
Sleep quality				
Substance abuse				
Mental state				
Hopelessness				
Anguish				
Rage				
Aloneness				
Anxiety				
Self-hate				
Dissociative experience				
Entrapment				
Anhedonia				
Suicide ideation				
Impulse to self-harm				

FIGURE 24.1. Systematic Monitoring Rating. *Source:* Reprinted with permission from *The American Psychiatric Publishing Textbook of Suicide Assessment and Management,* Second Edition. Copyright © 2012 American Psychiatric Association. All Rights Reserved.

In the multidisciplinary CAMS model, both the patient and the therapist are asked to complete a Suicide Status Form, and then to build specific treatment goals to alleviate intrusive symptoms or strengthen attachments noted in reasons for living (Jobes, 2016). For example, for a patient who has indicated a high level of hopelessness about his marriage, a treatment goal might be to improve marital relations. Interventions to achieve this goal could include some form of cognitive-behavioral therapy (CBT) to address distorted thinking, or couple therapy to improve communication.

The herald of an impending suicide attempt crisis is often a precipitating event that triggers a flood of painful, unendurable affect (Maltsberger & Stoklosa, 2012). However, the therapist must also pay attention to the patient's long suicidal career, which helps produce vulnerability to crises. Some of the affects that can precede a suicide attempt are intense anxiety, hopelessness, desperation, rage, self-hate, and a sense of abandonment (Maltsberger & Stoklosa, 2012). Fawcett (2006) reminds us to treat the patient's anxiety as well as his or her depressive disorder. Management of anxiety is of paramount importance in treating suicidal patients (Maltsberger & Stoklosa, 2012).

Clinicians should beware of patients' self-reports of not being suicidal (as in "denies SI"), since even if they say this, they often make a suicide attempt soon thereafter (Maltsberger & Stoklosa, 2012; Silverman & Berman, 2014; Berman, 2018). Therapists should always probe thoroughly for suicide intent: For example, "If you were ever to be suicidal, how and under what circumstances would you do it?" "Do you have ready access to a means of suicide?" or "Have you ever attempted suicide in the past? If you have, what was going on then?" In addition, what do the patient's family and friends say about the patient's current suicide ideation? Were there any searches on the patient's personal computer about methods of suicide, and if so, what were the dates of those inquiries?

There are scales that purport to predict suicide (Rothberg & Geer-Williams, 1992). Among some of these scales are the Suicide Probability Scale (SPS; Cull & Gill, 1982) and scales measuring factors related to suicide outcome, like the Beck Hopelessness Scale (Beck et al., 1974a) or the Beck Depression Inventory–II (BDI-II; Beck et al., 1996). Unfortunately, all suicide prediction scales have very little validity or reliability and tend to identify false positives; that is, they often predict a suicide that most often does not happen. Often the psychotherapist has to rely on his or her own clinical judgment.

Jerome Motto (1992) speaks of the "suicide zone" or "threshold" that a patient is in just before attempting suicide (see Figure 2.1). It is important to get patients out of this zone of desperation, to prevent suicide attempts. Maltsberger (2006) says that it may be necessary to hospitalize suicidal outpatients, and that such patients should not have the last word about whether or not to go to the hospital. Even though suicide is hard to predict (actually, prediction is almost impossible in the short run for individuals), all that is required is the clinician's judgment that a risk of imminent suicide is high. It is probably better to be safe than sorry. However, we must not forget that suicide is the leading cause of death in psychiatric hospitals; they are not safe places. If a patient cannot make a commitment to treatment, then it may be necessary to terminate and refer the person to another therapist.

Psychodynamic, Psychoanalytic, and Developmental Psychotherapies

A lot of suicides have had faulty, punitive, or absent parenting; early life trauma (such as physical or sexual abuse; Mann & Currier, 2012); early object loss (through divorce or the death or a parent or a sibling); inappropriate socialization or asocialization (e.g., when patients have personality disorders, especially ASPD and BPD); various narcissistic pathologies related to social isolation; and developmental problems contributing to maturation or developmental stagnation. If suicide results from any personality disorder, those character flaws tend to be deeply ingrained and less responsive to medication treatment alone (Linehan, 1997).

Psychotherapy takes hard work and psychosocial support. It involves admitting to and confronting crippling psychological defenses. A lot of patients (especially men) are not up to this hard work, are unwilling to undertake it, or cannot afford it. Psychodynamic therapy often involves partially reparenting, resocializing, and redeveloping damaged suicidal individuals. Such therapy takes time (but how long does normal parenting take?) and costs a lot. Most insurance companies are not willing to pay for it. In the 1973 movie *Sleeper*, Woody Allen's character wakes up 200 years in the future and exclaims, "If I had stayed in analysis, I might have been cured by now!"

Maltsberger and Stoklosa (2012) have argued that the therapists of suicidal patients need to build up their reasons for living (see also Linehan, 1997) and must be ever alert for suicidogenic affects of intense anxiety, hopelessness, desperation, rage, abandonment, and self-hate as precursors to or triggers of imminent suicide.

Sigmund Freud believed that adult psychopathology was often the result of unconscious, repressed conflicts or traumas in infancy or early childhood that led to adult disorders. Through hypnosis, free association, dream interpretation, and reconstructing and reinterpreting the past, theoretically an adult patient could (with the support of his or her therapist) confront and purge unconscious conflict and crippling psychological defenses, and thereby become healthier.

Later developmental psychologists, like Erik Erikson (a Freudian; Erikson, 1963) and Daniel Levinson (Levinson et al., 1978; Levinson with Levinson, 1996), focused on what they called "stagnation" at a chronological life stage. Such stagnation may not allow normal maturation and may contribute to self-destructive behaviors. For example, are adolescent suicides related to abortive transitions to young adulthood? Are elderly suicides due to failure to move from being middle-aged to being elderly? Developmental stagnation raises the interesting possibility of suicide as Darwinian—the simple failure to survive, rather than intentional self-destruction. It may be one mechanism whereby the relatively unfit may fail to be able to keep on living.

Cognitive-Behavioral Therapy or Cognitive Therapy for Suicide Prevention

CBT or cognitive therapy for suicide prevention (CT-SP; Brown et al., 2012) (see also Chapter 14 and Maris et al., 2000) involves training in problem-solving skills short of suicide. Many suicides tend to have faulty cognitions or thinking. For example, a suicidal patient might think, "Either I have to be miserable or I have to kill myself," which is dichotomous and catastrophic thinking. Shneidman referred to what he called "tunnel vision" (in which the light at the end of the tunnel is often on a freight train!) and the "conceptual rigidity of suicides, such as seeing suicide as the one and only way to resolve their life problems. As mentioned in earlier chapters, Shneidman also said that the four-letter word in suicidology is *only*, as in "It [attempting suicide] was the only thing I could do.""

Individuals who are suicidal tend to lack specific cognitive skills for coping effectively with crises (Brown et al., 2012). Suicide is irrational, when something short of suicide would have the same effect—such as getting a divorce, moving out of the parents' house, changing jobs, getting out of a self-destructive relationship, or stopping abuse of alcohol or drugs. Suicide is coping overkill. Suicidal patients need to be educated to avoid fallacious reasoning and to see alternatives to suicide that they themselves might embrace when no longer depressed (Brandt, 1975).

A treatment plan can be designed to engender hope (e.g., Linehan et al., 1983). Some cognitive therapists make up a "hope kit" with two-sided cards. On one side of a card, a suicidal person can write, "I can't take this anymore"; on the other side, the person can write, "I know such situations tend to be short-lived, and I always seem to recover." The patient may need to devise a safety plan, which might include a list of his or her own suicide warning signs, coping strategies, reminders of possible distractions from suicidal crises, names of persons to contact in a crisis (with phone numbers and email addresses), and removal of lethal suicide methods (like guns) from home or car.

CT-SP should start with a complete assessment of the patient's perceived problems and a suicide risk assessment associated with them (Brown et al., 2012). According to Beck et al. (1985), hopelessness is more highly correlated with a suicide outcome than depression is. Hopelessness, problem-solving deficits, perfectionism, dysfunctional attitudes, and irrational beliefs ("I'm a loser and would be better off dead"; cf. the movie *Better Off Dead* [Holland, 1985]) are characteristic of suicidal persons (Beck et al., 1985). Remember the honors student described in the epigraph to Chapter 14, who killed himself after getting his first B+ grade.

Although medications may make a patient feel more euphoric, calmer, or less depressed, feelings do not necessarily change behavior. To avoid suicide, one needs to change a self-destructive lifestyle and avoid being boxed into an increasingly self-destructive corner.

Dialectical Behavior Therapy

Dialectical behavior therapy (DBT) was developed by Marsha Linehan (Linehan, 1997, 2006, 2015; see also Maris et al., 2000; Brown et al., 2012). DBT can be especially effective in treating female suicidal patients with BPD, which Linehan has admitted publicly that she herself has (Carey, 2011). DBT differs from CBT in that it is based on making behavioral (not just ideational) techniques more compatible with the psychodynamic models described above.

DBT is intended to treat the chronically suicidal patient who lives a suicidal career (Maris, 1981; Joiner, 2005; Linehan et al., 2015). These patients are high in suicide ideations, frequently talk about or threaten suicide, and make repetitive nonfatal suicide attempts (such as self-cutting, which is common in women with BPD).

DBT assumes that chronically suicidal individuals lack and must acquire self-regulation of behavior, emotion, and distress tolerance skills, and must be motivated to strengthen these skills in out-of-therapy situations. DBT uses a problem-solving strategy, addressing the patient's behaviors. Possible changes or behavioral solutions are then generated to be tested.

The word *dialectic* probably first occurred in Plato's *Dialogues* (Jowett, 1950), in which two or more philosophers would argue about a subject like justice, to try to arrive at the truth or at least a consensus. Later the philosopher Hegel (1874) spoke of *thesis, antithesis,* and *synthesis* as a dialectical process. Dialectical strategies balance and attempt to synthesize coexisting opposites and tensions. For example, Linehan et al. (1983) created a 72-item Reasons for Living Inventory, in which patients rate their reasons for not suiciding. Patients rate each of 72 items on a scale from 1 to 6, where 6 equals the most important.

The DBT therapist tries to validate the patient's view of life while implementing alternatives to death through problem-solving analyses and responses. Detailed behavioral analyses of situations linked to suicidal behavior are conducted to elicit patterns and to identify alternative solutions. A commitment to learning nonsuicidal behavioral responses while tolerating negative affect is a major target of DBT.

Group and Family Therapies

When an individual is suicidal, it is often helpful to be around others who have experienced similar problematic situations and recovered (however, see Ougrin & Asarnow, 2018). How did they cope? Groups like AA or NA can be supportive and nonjudgmental for those recovering from addictions, as mentioned above, and analogous support for those recovering from suicidality is important. Early in the history of suicide prevention efforts, such support was referred to as "befriending" by the Samaritans in London, founded by Chad Varah in 1953. Survivor groups like Survivors of Suicide (SOS) are useful for the 6–45 others (on average) typically left behind by each suicide (Campbell, 2012).

Death may resolve the suicide's problems, but it creates lifetime problems for those who love the person. Suicide is selfish, but often suicides (especially men) have trouble thinking about the welfare of others when they are agitated and suicidal. Suicide tends to engender a kind of narcissistic pathology, in which would-be suicides are consumed by their own pain and suffering, and don't think much about those who love and care for them. When a person is in severe pain, it is hard to be polite, to remain considerate of others, or to behave appropriately. Of course, in some suicides there may be an active intent to hurt others or get revenge.

Note that family dynamics can themselves be suicidogenic, such that the suicidal individual may not be able to get well or stay well in a pathological family. The whole family may need treatment, or may need to be disassembled and reconstituted, or may have to be avoided altogether.

Which Therapist?

Suicide therapists come in all shapes and sizes. Who is best? Candidates can include males or females, young or old, black or white, gay or straight. A suicide therapist may be a psychiatrist, the family doctor, a social worker, a clinical psychologist, a mental health counselor, a member of the clergy (of any faith), a peer, a best friend, a sibling, a parent, another family member, a teacher, or even a member of a police or fire rescue team. Or a treatment team may be made up of some combination of the above. Clearly, who is chosen depends on many considerations, and a suicidal person may need more than one therapist.

Which Place?

It is fairly clear where to go to get a pill (at a pharmacy), but what if you do not want a pill or want more than a pill? You can seek (or be referred to) outpatient treatment; become an inpatient in a general or psychiatric hospital; go to the local emergency room, a local suicide prevention center, a community mental health center, a church or temple, a school or university health service, a family practice doctor's office, or an employee assistance program; or go online and do a search for treatment.

Inpatient Treatment

Often suicidal individuals are hospitalized because they are not safe at home (Goodwin, 2003). This can be done involuntarily, usually for at least 72 hours, when a patient poses an imminent danger to self or others (and sometimes when there is major property damage risk). The only thing that really prevents suicide is a 24/7 watch in a controlled (suicide-proofed) environment; being given sedating medications (like Haldol); or physical restraints, usually in isolation housing. All of these suicide prevention methods are more likely in inpatient treatment settings, and even there procedures are strictly controlled so as to be humane and not to violate the patient's Eighth or Fourteenth Amendment rights in the U.S. Constitution.

Important aspects of inpatient treatment, some of which are considered in more detail below, include the following:

- A suicide risk assessment and admission summary (Xiong et al., 2012, p. 317; Maris et al., 2000, p. 517).
- The need to beware of suicide risk during hospital shift changes (Sokolov et al., 2006, pp. 407 and 414).
- Knowledge of the profiles of inpatients who are especially suicidal.
- Assessment of depressive ideation and behavior (strong correlates of suicide) in the hospital.
- Multidisciplinary treatment planning: Deciding who should be on the treatment team, who is in charge (the "captain"), how often the team should meet, and how the team should keep progress notes (Maris et al., 2000, p. 517).

- Psychological testing as needed or ordered; this permits quantification (e.g., of depression or hopelessness severity), validation of clinical judgment, and control group comparisons.
- Architecture, the environment, and safety issues related to suicide prevention (Sokolov et al., 2006, p. 413).
- Psychiatric diagnoses related to suicide outcome, including mood disorders, anxiety disorders, BPD, and ASPD (Xiong et al., 2012, p. 317).
- Making detailed interdisciplinary progress notes regularly, with verbatim patient quotes.
- Awareness of hanging as a special inpatient suicide method and its control (Xiong et al., 2012, p. 316).
- Pharmacological treatment of inpatient suicide risk, especially lithium and Clozaril (Sokolov et al., 2006, pp. 408 and 412).
- Recording all doctors' orders, including a medication list.
- Filing laboratory reports, neurological records, consultant reports, imaging records, and other testing records.
- No-suicide contracts (Shea, 1999; Xiong et al., 2012): Do they work, and what are their limitations?
- The epidemiology of inpatient treatment (Sokolov et al., 2006, pp. 401–402) and inpatient suicides.
- Suicide watch and observation issues (Sokolov et al., 2006, pp. 407–408).
- Hospital suicide policy and procedures manuals, and training in their contents.
- Standardizing death reporting and investigation of hospital suicides.
- Discharge planning and follow-up (Maris et al., 2000, p. 519).

The immediate goal of inpatient hospitalization is the reduction or elimination of intense current suicidal ideation and intent. Within the parameters of insurer-managed care, this goal must be met relatively rapidly; the average psychiatric inpatient stay is only about 1 week. Thus, there are economic pressures on top of discharge decisions and conditions. When a patient is still felt to be unsafe outside the hospital, an appeal for extended inpatient treatment should be made to the insurer, so that the patient can be stabilized before discharge.

Intake and Suicide Assessment

Inpatient care involves a suicide risk assessment and screening evaluation, including a mental status exam such as the Mini-Mental Status Exam (Folstein et al., 1975) or MOCA (Nasreddine, 2005). The mental status exam is roughly the psychiatric equivalent of the internist's physical examination, and it should be administered regularly throughout treatment. Intake assessment includes taking social, psychiatric treatment, and family histories. The team should try to get all relevant past assessment and treatment records.

A thorough physical examination should be done to rule out physical problems masked as psychiatric disorders (e.g., thyroid malfunction, brain tumors), as well as substance abuse and drug reactions. Nursing assessment includes regular vital sign testing and recording, including sleep and eating records related to vegetative symptoms of mood disorder.

Psychological testing may be done as needed or ordered. As noted above, such testing permits quantification of depression, hopelessness, or other factors; can validate clinical judgment; and can allow control group comparisons. Clinicians should do assessments and histories promptly, within the timeframe specified in the hospital's policy and procedures manual. Sometimes nurses' suicide assessments are more thorough than the physician's are.

As indicated by the evaluations as well as the treatment team's detailed progress notes, precautions are instituted for the patient, with awareness that suicides can occur in the best of inpatient units. Unit policies and procedures (usually written by psychiatric nurses) should define specific steps to safeguard the environment and the patient, in addition to specifying staff responsibilities in various possibly self-destructive situations.

If the presenting problem or chief complaint involves self-destructive ideations or behaviors (including explicit suicide attempts) or if the admitting diagnosis includes a mood disorder, schizophrenia, panic attacks, BPD, or ASPD, then a much more specific, probing suicide assessment is warranted. Many psychiatric hospitals routinely ask detailed questions about suicide ideation or behavior in the intake assessment. Common questions concern prior suicide attempts, current suicide ideas, and current plans (with specific details, including the anticipated method and when and under what circumstances the suicide attempt might take place). Of course, patients are not always truthful or clear-headed about their suicide intentions and circumstances, and suicide plans do change. Thus a clinician cannot rely too heavily on answers to even direct questions about a patient's suicidality (Silverman & Berman, 2014; Berman, 2018), including any no-suicide contract a patient may make.

However, if one of a clinician's patients should suicide, and the clinician has *not* asked about suicide and written the response down in the medical records, the clinician will regret it. The intake evaluation and assessment are crucial, since clinician–patient rapport or a therapeutic alliance is first established then. Many indirect indications of suicidality and assurances of the clinician's ability and willingness to cope with the patient's suicidality turn on the professional's being seen as genuinely concerned and competent.

The assessment of suicide should not be a sterile, self-contained end game, unrelated to treatment. Most of the time, suicide assessment is carried out in the service of suicide treatment and prevention. In addition to what has been described above, the general assessment and treatment records of a potentially suicidal inpatient usually include the following components (Maris et al., 2000): a clear record of who is on the multidisciplinary treatment team, who is in charge, and how often the team meets; a detailed interdisciplinary treatment plan; the treatment team's progress notes, policies, and procedures; all doctors' orders, including a medication list; and laboratory reports, neurological records, any consultant reports, and imaging records.

Intake and Admissions Summary

The intake assessment and admission summary by the attending psychiatrist (and nurses) generally states the patient's chief complaint(s) or presenting psychiatric problem; a provisional DSM/ICD diagnosis and appropriate codes; current and prior psychotropic medications; prior hospitalizations (records may need to be obtained); results of a mental status exam; and the initial treatment plan and doctors' first orders, including medications. Obviously, this initial encounter of physician, staff, and the hospital environment is critical. Even though it is provisional, the admitting diagnosis needs to be both accurate and thorough, since effective treatment plans depend in large part on a correct, detailed diagnosis (i.e., Dx $\rightarrow$ Tx and Rx).

If possible, a complete diagnosis should be given (including possible personality disorders), with any suspected comorbidity or alternative diagnoses to be ruled out listed as well. It must be remembered that suicide is not (yet) a mental disorder per se, although suicidal behaviors are part of the criteria for diagnoses of major depression and BPD. The listing of previous and current medications often suggests what has worked or not worked before. Also, many newer psychiatric medications are not always clearly superior or preferred to older psychiatric drugs (e.g., the MAOIs, TCAs, or first-generations SSRIs; see the interview with Bodkin in *The Carlat Psychiatry Report*, 2016).

Architecture, Environment, and Suicide Prevention

A patient who is in an acute phase of suicide risk should have a treatment environment that promotes protection, safety, and coordinated treatment. This means that the inpatient should be denied access to the means for suicide (which is usually hanging), and that all dangerous, sharp objects should be confiscated at admission. Inpatient housing should include no rigid, protruding fixtures, no breakaway shower heads or toilet paper holders, and windows that are barred and/or made of unbreakable Plexiglas or Lexan. Vents should be covered; bedding and clothing need to be controlled, especially anything that can be tied or draped around the patient's neck. Watch protocols need to be determined for the individual patient, ranging from 1:1 constant observation to logged 15-minute checks (often with varied start times). Normally, constant (and even some 15-minute) watches will take place on a locked ward or in a seclusion room, similar to a hospital intensive care unit. That is, the suicide watch includes elopement precautions. Remember, however, that no humane psychiatric housing conditions can be totally suicide-proofed. (Cf. the discussion of suicide-proofing in jails and prisons in Chapter 22.)

Almost every psychiatric hospital or clinic has a policy and procedures manual in which various types of probable self-destructive behaviors are linked to levels of detailed precautions. These might include also 30- or 60-minute logged observations for patients who have suicide ideas, but are not judged to be imminently suicidal. Unless a patient is violent, agitated, intoxicated, or aggressive, the cause

of suicide prevention is routinely better served if the would-be suicide has a roommate. There have been numerous cases in which patients have committed suicide
while their roommates were away (attending group therapy, having tests done, on
a home pass, etc.).

In some limited and controlled circumstances, physical restraints may be
needed. Usually these conditions are specified in the hospital's policy and procedures manual. Restraints can include one- to five-point restrictions (the four limbs
and the head) or chemical restraints (like Haldol) for highly agitated, psychotic, or
very aggressive patients. Restraints should be used only for short, specified time
periods with 24-hour logged observations. I have had some patients request to be
put in restraints to be kept from hurting themselves or others—for example, when
they have akathisia. However, Maltsberger and Stoklosa (2012) are of the opinion that physical restraints should almost never be used with suicidal patients. Of
course, sharp, dangerous, and fixed protruding objects will also have to be removed
from the place and from the patient's person for safety reasons.

Unfortunately, as noted in Chapter 22, it only takes 4–5 minutes of 6–7 pounds
of pressure on the carotid arteries in the neck to produce death or anoxic brain
damage by oxygen deprivation to the brain (and/or cardiac failure). Thus 15-min-
ute suicide watches tend to allow a patient sufficient time to commit suicide, especially if the patient has a private bathroom with a closable and/or lockable door.
Almost any article of clothing, together with a fixed protruding object. can be used
for self-asphyxiation.

For example, a t-shirt sleeve can be put over a doorknob, with the neck of the
shirt left on while the patient just leans forward without being suspended. Other
actual forensic cases have included lowering an electric bed down on one's throat;
forcing three cellophane-wrapped dinner rolls down one's throat; and first swal-
lowing the leg of one's jogging pants, and then immersing one's head in a toilet.
Such hanging or asphyxiation deaths often occur during shift changes or other
kind of routine changes, such as moving to another room in another unit, going or
returning from a leave or pass, or coming off suicide precautions or seclusion. They
can also occur when a patient experiences a decrease in vegetative symptoms (e.g.,
improvement in sleep, appetite, or libido) before the suicidal mood lifts.

Pharmacological Treatment

Psychiatric medications for potentially suicidal clients need to be considered carefully (see Part IV and Chapter 23). It is well known that many psychiatric patients
attempt suicide by overdosing on the very drugs prescribed to treat their depression, anxiety, psychosis, and sleeplessness. In particular, the older TCAs were often
fatal in overdose. Psychiatrists need to be circumspect about giving patients large
numbers of pills and unthinking automatic refills. These considerations apply
not only to antidepressants, but also to benzodiazepines, opiates, and other drug
classes.

A physician has to decide when to medicate, how long to wait before starting drug treatment; what combination of drugs to use for which patients; when to

increase, discontinue, reduce, or stop medication; what the potential adverse effects and drug interactions might be; and what doses the patient should be on. Many physicians probably undermedicate their depressed patients (Maris, 2015). Psychiatrists are responsible for fine-tuning the psychotropic medications they give their patients and minimizing adverse effects.

Since suicide rates are highest for individuals having one or more of the mood disorders, most suicidal patients will be on one or more antidepressants. See Chapter 23, Table 23.2, for a detailed list of antidepressant medications and their characteristics.

A patient with bipolar disorder may be taking lithium carbonate (Esklith, Lithobid, Lithane). Many inpatient would-be suicides are highly agitated or manic, and sometimes delusional, hallucinatory, or otherwise psychotic. If so, a psychiatrist may need to consider an antipsychotic drug as well as an antidepressant. Sometimes a therapist can place an inpatient in the controlled environment of a psychiatric hospital and wait a few days before initiating any psychiatric medication. However, in most cases, potential suicides who are psychotic or highly agitated and confused will be started at hospital admission on a high-potency antipsychotic (such as Haldol at doses of 0.5, 2, 5, or 10 mg two or even three times a day for a short period). If there is extreme agitation and aggression, doses can be much higher, up to 100 mg a day (this is a description, not a recommendation) in otherwise healthy young adults (be careful with elderly patients). Similar high-potency older antipsychotics include Navane, Stelazine, and fluphenazine. See Chapter 13 (especially Table 13.4) and Chapter 23 for more details about antipsychotic medications.

As noted in the earlier discussions, one must attend to extrapyramidal adverse effects in administering antipsychotic drugs. These can include akathisia, dystonia (involuntary posturing), muscular rigidity, tremors, parkinsonian symptoms (like a shuffling gait), and a host of other movement disorders. High-potency antipsychotics may exacerbate anticholinergic effects like dry mouth, blurred vision, and constipation.

Clinical trials show that Clozaril is effective in reducing suicidality and treatment-resistant psychosis and does not cause tardive dyskinesia. However, it tends to be expensive and can cause seizures and agranulocytosis (failure of the body to produce white blood cells that fight infection in about 1% of patients).

Finally, many suicidal patients will have been prescribed short-term benzodiazepines or nonbenzodiazepine minor tranquilizers; see Chapter 23, Table 23.4, for a list of these medications. Since the benzodiazepines can cause depression, hostility, and paradoxical rage reactions, their use with potentially suicidal individuals needs to be monitored closely. There have been several forensic cases involving Halcion, which has an ultrashort half-life (1.5–5.5 hours) and can produce severe withdrawal effects (like Paxil). Benzodiazepines can cause or contribute to angry outbursts, assaultiveness, anterograde amnesia, clinical depression, suicide ideas, delirium, and rebound insomnia. Benzodiazepines can interact with alcohol or barbiturates to severely depress respiration, as in the case of Karen Ann Quinlan (see *Time*, 1985; Maris et al., 2000).

Interdisciplinary Progress Notes

Interdisciplinary progress notes constitute an extremely valuable record of a patient's course in treatment. Records of treatment team meetings, plans, and other notes can also protect a psychiatrist and hospital in the event of a malpractice lawsuit. There is a clinical/legal dictum that "if you did not write it in the notes, then you did not do it." The treatment team meetings should be documented carefully, including listing who was in attendance. Detailed interdisciplinary progress notes should be made regularly, with verbatim patient quotes relevant to suicide, such as this one: "I have played a lot of checkers in my life, and tomorrow will be my last move."

The notes might follow the so-called "SOAP" format (Subjective, Objective, Assessment, and Plan). Clinicians should also review the vital signs records (such as sleep and eating charts) for signs of vegetative changes in depression. As emphasized earlier, vegetative symptom improvement before depressive affect and suicidal mood lifts should be noted, as it often indicates increased suicide vulnerability. Staff members should be especially attentive to increased suicide risk at times of any treatment changes, such as shift changes, mealtimes, medication changes, changes in seclusion, moves to and from different security levels, and going on and coming off passes. They should also be aware of patients' personal and domestic issues (divorce or child custody proceedings, court hearings, holidays, sleep times, etc.). As part of ongoing suicide risk, activity needs to be monitored for those with depression diagnoses. Figure 24.2 is an example of such a monitoring form.

Date:	Level Depression						Asleep	Activation				
	Lo				Hi			Hi	Mod	Norm	Mod	Hi
TIME	0	1	2	3	4	5		2	1	0	1	2
6:00 A.M.							X					
6:15 A.M.							X					
6:30 A.M.			X							X		
6:45 A.M.			X								X	
7:00 A.M.			X								X	
7:15 A.M.			X								X	
7:30 A.M.			X								X	
7:45 A.M.			X								X	
8:00 A.M.				X								
8:15 A.M.				X								
etc.												

FIGURE 24.2. Depression and Activation Chart. *Source:* Reprinted with permission from *The American Psychiatric Publishing Textbook of Suicide Assessment and Management, Second Edition.* Copyright © 2012 American Psychiatric Association. All Rights Reserved.

Inpatient Suicide

Note that suicides account for 1% of all deaths outside psychiatric hospitals, but 4–5% within such hospitals (Sokolov et al., 2006, pp. 401–402). Most inpatient suicides occur within the first week after admission. In the case of a hospital suicide, the activities and care of the patient in the last hours of his or her life should be described in exquisite detail and cleared with hospital attorneys. This should include resuscitation attempts, as well as other first responses of staff, emergency medical services (EMS), police, and the medical examiner. Who did what, when, and why? Was there a postmortem examination or a psychological autopsy? Were there any policy or procedural changes as a result of the suicide? Obtain a death certificate and any pertinent EMS, medical examiner, autopsy, toxicology, and police reports. Were there pictures memorializing the suicide scene? It is imperative that all staff be familiar with and have adequate training in the hospital's policies, as well as mock practice of suicide prevention procedures.

Discharge Planning and Follow-Up

Discharge planning and follow-up include consideration of the following questions. Is the external (nonhospital) environment toxic? Has suicide risk been sufficiently reduced at the time of discharge? What is an adequate follow-up, and how soon and frequently should it take place? How compliant is the discharged patient likely to be? Will he or she take medication as prescribed? How can substance abuse outside the hospital be controlled? Have the family and friends been warned to suicide-proof the external environment?

The physician should write a careful comprehensive discharge summary and do it promptly. There are many different discharge summary formats (Maris et al., 2000). The items that should be addressed in a discharge summary should include at least the following:

- Client biographical and demographic information.
- DSM/ICD admission and discharge chief complaint, diagnoses, and dates with proper codes, and summaries.
- Doctors' orders.
- Drug administration records.
- History and hospital course of the present illness.
- Treatment plan and a signed list of treatment team members (including providers of other treatments, such as group, occupational, recreational, nutritional, and educational).
- Past psychiatric, medical, family, and social histories.
- Results of mental status exams.
- Summaries of progress notes.
- Review of systems.
- Laboratory data and procedures performed (imaging, blood work, etc.).
- Consultants' reports.
- Discharge medications.

- Discharge instructions, including follow-up data and referrals with dates and addresses or contact numbers for key providers.
- Suicide death report (if any); investigation; root cause analysis; and recommendations for changes in treatments, policies, or procedures (if any).

The frequency of suicides shortly after hospitalization is disturbing. Most occur within the first week after discharge. Did the assessment of suicide risk at the time of discharge adequately consider the toxic effect of the external social milieu (including family discord or conflict) or the loss of constant support provided by the hospital? Was the patient and family sufficiently advised of the need for compliance with the treatment plan, medications, and referral for follow-up outpatient care? Did the patient intentionally deceive the treatment team by falsely appearing well enough to be discharged? Was the family sufficiently advised of the continued need for surveillance and suicide-proofing at home? Were firearms secured?

Finally, an important caveat: Any treatment of a suicidal inpatient is second-rate if it relies on impersonal means alone—the simple prescription of sedating or calming psychiatric medications, seclusion, restraints, checks, and watches. Suicidal patients have been treated without medications, often with fairly good results. The heart of treatment is the relationship of the patient with the therapist. The suicidal inpatient is not receiving adequate care unless he or she is provided with a therapeutic relationship that offers support, hope, accessibility, careful investigation of the patient's current life impasse, and close monitoring of the patient's mood shifts, all done with genuine concern and competence.

Chapter 25 asks these questions: What if suicide could be prevented or the suicide rate reduced, so that treatment was not needed or at least was less critical? Is there an optimum suicide rate, and is it zero?

CHAPTER 25

Prevention
Can Suicides Be Stopped or Reduced?

Unfortunately, most countries free of suicide are fictional Utopias
like Huxley's *Brave New World*, which require coercive medications
(*soma* for Huxley; antidepressants, antipsychotics, and anxiolytics
for the real world) and behavioral conditioning. Who would want
to live there? Furthermore, is the optimum suicide rate zero?

—Anonymous

Whenever possible, it is better to prevent a disease or injury (like suicide) rather than treat it after the fact, such as with medication or psychotherapy (Maris, 2015, pp. 168–169; Goodwin, 2003; Maris et al., 2000, pp. 509ff; O'Connor et al., 2011; cf. Klonsky, 2018). What if there were a vaccine for suicide as there is for polio or tuberculosis, so that no one ever became suicidal? Or what if there were conditions under which suicide was very unlikely, which we could learn from and apply to others? For example, African American women in the United States are almost immune to suicide, and all women have suicide rates about four times lower than men's.

Suicide vaccines may be a far-fetched idea, to say the least—but could we not try to discover why African American women in particular, or women in general, have such low suicide rates? Might the information then be used to prevent suicide without medication or psychotherapy, such as by lowering suicide risk factors? Do black women in the United States have low suicide rates due to their strong extended family ties and their religious involvement (Walker et al., 2018; Nisbet, 1996)? However, as the epigraph to this chapter suggests, countries totally free of suicide are fictional Utopias.

Suicide is preventable in the short run by putting individuals in suicide-proofed safety rooms, perhaps medicating them with antipsychotics and/or anxiolytics, and then observing them 24/7 within arm's reach (see Chapters 22 and 24). These and other prevention measures tend to be inhumane, extreme, punitive, and austere. They may even increase suicide risk in the long run and are generally violations of the constitutional right to be free from cruel and unusual punishment. In short, such drastic suicide prevention measures often just are not practical and cannot be used for long. Eventually such people have to be let out of close watch and confinement.

Gerald Caplan (1964) wrote a classic book on prevention, in which he argued that there are three basic types of prevention:

- *Primary prevention.* It eliminates or reduces the incidence of new cases and tends to occur early—for example, before an individual ever becomes suicidal.
- *Secondary prevention.* It reduces the prevalence of the total number of cases—here, of suicide.
- *Tertiary prevention.* It manages damage of the disease (suicidality) and limits its advance later in the life cycle or suicidal career (Szanto, 2018).

If there were better primary prevention of suicide, then obviously there would be less need for treatment of would-be suicides. Primary suicide prevention involves reducing known suicide risk factors, as well as enhancing suicide protective factors (in the environment, in family relationships and socialization of the young, and in other areas). Trying to prevent people from ever becoming suicidal includes reducing mood disorders, controlling alcohol and other substance abuse, and controlling guns.

For instance, Miller and Hemenway (2008) argued that just having guns in the homes of adolescents, secured or not, increased their suicide rate 5–10 times. Primary suicide prevention also means reducing social isolation or thwarted belongingness, lowering aggression and impulsivity, reducing stress, and trying to prevent multiple problems in families of origin (including reducing poverty, discrimination, and inequality). As noted in earlier chapters, Mann and Currier (2012) claim that suicide is the result of a stress–diathesis model. *Diathesis* refers to a constitutional or hereditary susceptibility to a disease or condition (e.g., suicide in one's family). Both diathesis and stress would need to be controlled or considered.

Unfortunately, most suicide prevention is tertiary, after self-destructive damage is already done and the suicidal career is fairly advanced. At that point one might argue that psychiatric medication is needed to tranquilize, calm, or sedate suicidal patients, but perhaps not cure them. But making suicidal patients easier to live with or able to live better with themselves is not the same as preventing suicide.

We also need to ask: Prevention of what? Are we trying to prevent or control suicidal ideas, nonfatal suicide attempts, completed suicide, or suicidal risk factors (mood disorder, alcoholism, hopelessness, isolation, perceived burdensomeness, etc.)?

Furthermore, when and with whom is suicide prevention indicated? Before suicidality ever develops at all? After the suicidal career is fairly advanced? In adolescents (Plemmons et al., 2018) or the elderly? Or is the objective to reduce the prevalence (secondary prevention)—that is, the total number of suicide cases? For example, one of the goals of the American Foundation for Suicide Prevention (AFSP) is to reduce the annual U.S. suicide rate by 20% by the year 2025. This seems very unlikely, given the overall U.S. suicide rate trend from 2004 to 2014, as depicted in Table 25.1.

Suicide Rate Variations

Table 25.1 shows the overall U.S. suicide rate from 2004 to 2014 and rates for specific age and gender groups. Figure 25.1 graphs the overall rate for the years 1900 to 2014. Note that from 2004 to 2014, suicide rates for all age categories tended to go up steadily but slightly (Tavernese, 2016).

Overall, U.S. suicide rates have been fairly steady, ranging from about 11 to 13 per 100,000 for the last 114 years (Figure 25.1). As noted in a publication of the National Center for Injury Prevention and Control (Kachur et al., 1995), "Nationally the age-adjusted suicide rate has been remarkably constant." Suicide rates of 11–13 per 100,000 are not all that high to start with. For example, a rate of 10 equals 1 suicide in 10,000 population per year. As we have seen in Chapter 8, there were very high suicide rates (per 100,000) in 2012 in Greenland (83.0), Guyana (44.2), South Korea (28.9), and Sri Lanka (28.8), but moderate to low suicide rates in the United States (12.1). However, it should be noted that from 1999 to 2014 the U.S. suicide rate rose 24%, from 10.5 to 13.0 (*www.nimh.nih.gov/health/statistics/suicide.shtml*).

Notice in Figure 25.1 how the curve for suicide rates from 1950 to 2014 flattens out when 10-year intervals are used. In fact, if 10-point intervals had been used for the entire 1900–2014 time period, it would be even more obvious how constant the U.S. suicide rates have been. This suggests that perhaps the U.S. suicide rate is about as low as it is going to get. See below, where the "optimum" suicide rate (the best we can expect or hope for) is discussed.

From 1900 to 1960, when yearly suicide rate intervals, there is more rate fluctuation. Kachur et al. (1995) said, "Despite the stability of suicide rates overall, suicide rates have changed for some groups." The rates have also changed at some specific times. For example, there were rate peaks just after the 1929 stock market crash and, to a lesser degree, after the 1987 Black Monday stock market crash. The years 1900–1914 were the peak of immigration through Ellis Island, and in 1910, 3 million acres of woodlands burned in the Northwest in wildfires (which may have

TABLE 25.1. Suicide Rates per 100,000 Overall, by Age, and by Gender: United States, 2004–2014

	2004	2005	2006	2007	2008	2009	2010	2011	2012	2013	2014
Overall	11.0	11.0	11.1	11.5	11.8	12.0	12.4	12.7	12.9	13.0	13.4
15–24 years	10.3	10.0	9.9	9.7	10.0	10.1	10.5	11.0	11.1	11.1	11.6
45–54 years	16.6	16.5	17.2	17.7	18.7	19.3	19.6	19.8	20.0	19.7	20.2
85+ years	16.4	16.9	15.9	15.6	15.6	15.6	17.6	16.9	17.8	18.6	19.3
Men	17.7	17.7	17.8	18.3	19.0	19.2	20.2	20.2	20.6	20.6	21.1
Women	4.6	4.5	4.6	4.8	4.9	5.0	5.2	5.4	5.5	5.7	6.0

Source: American Association of Suicidology (2015), *suicidology.org/statistics*.

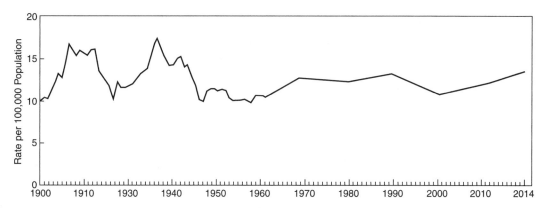

FIGURE 25.1. The overall U.S. suicide rate for the years 1900 to 2014. Note that suicide rates after 1950 are less detailed and varied, due to use of only 10-point interval data. *Sources:* "Deaths by Suicide . . . " (n.d.); American Association of Suicidology (2015).

been irrelevant to suicide rates). Notice, too, that there were troughs in the suicide rate during World War I (1914–1919) and World War II (1939–1945).

Table 25.1 shows that from 2004 to 2014, there was a significant increase in the suicide rates of the middle-aged (from 16.6 to 20.3 for 45- to 54-year-olds or 22% and the very old (from 16.4 to 19.3 in those over age 85 or 18%). As of 2014, the middle-aged had the highest suicide rates of any other age group. Over the same 10-year period, male suicide rates went up from 17.7 to 21.1. Female suicide rates were low, but also had a slight upward trend from 2004 to 2014.

The Prevention Paradigm

Similar to the clinical treatment paradigm, the prevention paradigm or model encompasses the concepts of risk reduction (here, the risk of suicide) and resiliency (health promotion). Thus suicide prevention can proceed by reducing the prevalence of known suicide risks and vulnerabilities, and/or by increasing protective, immunizing factors. But whereas the clinical paradigm rests primarily on a mental health model and too often concerns tertiary prevention, the prevention paradigm rests on a public health model and involves primary prevention (viz., conducting surveillance, understanding etiology and pathways, and then intervening before the disease process develops).

The field of prevention has evolved from simple tripartite models, such as Caplan's (1964) primary, secondary, and tertiary prevention, to complex, multifactorial systems that recognize the complexity and varieties of self-destructive behaviors and individuals. In recent years suicide prevention has come to embrace a melding of mental health and public health thinking, as traditional paradigms have proved insufficient in addressing these real-world complexities. Clinical models, such as the medical model, assume that suicide is a behavioral manifestation of underlying pathology; this assumption calls for treating the underlying disorder, such as depression. A more complex model understands that suicidal behaviors are consequent to both distal (e.g., a long suicidal career and diathesis) and proximal (e.g., acute triggering stressors) antecedent conditions. Both are predisposing conditions, such as depression in males, which then increases acute alcohol intoxication and, in turn, leads to relationship conflicts and loss. The more complex public health variation of this approach is to understand more universal mechanisms and processes that lead to negative outcomes, and then design preventive interventions to reduce long-term vulnerabilities.

The public health approach moves our thinking toward interventions earlier along the suicidal pathway, ideally before the disorder (suicidality) ever develops (Anestis et al., 2017). The public health model encourages our interventions to be "outside the box." For example, instead of simply focusing on the individual or host at risk, interventions also focus on the environment and related agents of self-destruction. Thus early intervention might be designed to increase coping skills in children, restrict access to means of suicide (such as firearms), and/or increase community or parental education about the importance, for example, of safe gun storage (an environmental factor).

Gordon's (1983) model further shifts our thinking. His model (see Figure 25.2) identifies target groups for interventions, ranging from the broad-based *universal,* to the more *selective,* to the yet more specific *indicated* interventions. Universal interventions are focused on the entire population, incorporating specific subgroups at risk. Improving easy access to health care for all, and promoting suicide risk awareness training in schools, are examples of the universal approach. Selective interventions specifically target those at greater risk for becoming suicidal, such as older white males. Indicated interventions target a more focused at-risk group or a condition putting group members at increasingly high risk for suicide, such as those who have made a prior suicide attempt.

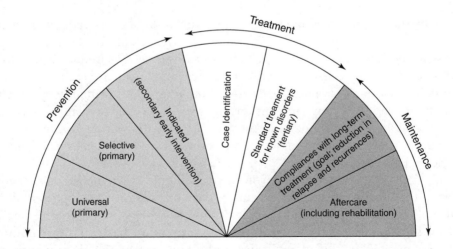

FIGURE 25.2. The mental health intervention spectrum. *Source:* Reprinted with permission from *The Mental Health Intervention Spectrum* (1994) by the Institute of Medicine, National Academy of Sciences. Courtesy of the National Academies Press, Washington, DC.

Beginning with inclusion of agents and the environment in its preventive focus, public health models have incorporated injury control strategies into suicide prevention approaches. The Centers for Disease Control and Prevention (CDC) has subsumed suicide into its public health agenda by distinguishing between injuries that are unintentional (like accidents) and those that are intentional (like suicides). With evidence that reducing the availability of popular means of committing suicide (such as guns) can lower suicide rates, the application of accident prevention to suicide prevention has become more promising. Expanding on Haddon and Baker's (1981) model, a colleague and I (Silverman & Maris, 1995) presented an outline, shown in Table 25.2, of preventive interventions linked to measurable outcomes of phases of prevention.

TABLE 25.2. Adaptation of Injury Control Strategies to Suicide Prevention

Primary prevention (reduces incidence).

  1. Prevent initial creation of hazard.
     * Do not manufacture handguns for nonsecurity civilian use.
     * Improve social support systems.

  2. Reduce amount of hazard created.
     * Control sale of handguns.

  3. Prevent release of already existing hazard.
     * Set standards for purchasing handguns.
     * Limit access to alcohol (amount, frequency, and timing).

Secondary prevention (reduces prevalence).

  4. Modify rate of release or spatial distribution of hazard from its source.
     * Package medications as individual tablets to minimize rapid consumption of large quantities.

  5. Separate hazard from person in time and space.
     * Legislation to prevent access to firearms of severely mentally ill persons.
     * Separate ammunition from firearms.

  6. Interpose a barrier between hazard and person.
     * Place barriers on high bridges and buildings.
     * Promote "safe guns," such as requiring palm print identification for use.

  7. Modify contact surfaces to reduce injury.
     * Prevent access to bridges and building rooftops.

  8. Strengthen resistance of persons who might be injured.
     * Offer school-based health promotion programs.
     * Train parent firearm owners in safe firearm storage methods and necessity.

Tertiary prevention (manages advanced illness and the suicidal career).

  9. Rapidly detect and limit damage that has occurred.
     * Improve professional education to assess and treat suicidal individuals.

 10. Initiate immediate and long-term reparative actions.
     * Improve follow-up treatment for and compliance behaviors among suicide attempters.

Source: Maris et al. (2000), based on Haddon and Baker (1981). Copyright © 2000 The Guilford Press. Reprinted with permission.

This approach to prevention involves altering the external environment to protect individuals at risk. This contrasts with more traditional public health approaches, which rely on education and legislation to persuade behavioral change. A difficulty with the educational strategy is that it requires a long-term commitment, frequent messages, and attention to powerful countervailing messages, such as the media's glamorization of unhealthy lifestyles. Consider the time, effort, and cost of trying to initiate successful smoking reduction or AIDS prevention campaigns. One difficulty with the legislative process is that few public health officials are able to lobby effectively enough or to persist in their efforts to gain support for programs to benefit the public.

Suicide prevention efforts must also compete with an ever-shifting landscape of other public health problems that need preventive relief (such as AIDS or homelessness), as well as with ambivalent attitudes about suicide as preventable, and disagreement among suicide preventers as to what is the most effective approach. In truth, to date little is known about what works. This, then, makes for a "hard sell" for large-scale government suicide prevention programs.

Prevention Questions and Decision Points

Prevention programming requires clearly delineated, empirically sound answers to several basic questions that underlie the development of preventive interventions (Silverman & Maris, 1995; cf. Anestis et al., 2017). Consider the following partial list of questions and decision points in focusing on suicidal behavior as a target for effective prevention efforts. These bullet points are offered to help guide prevention decisions, rather than to provide definitive answers.

● *What is the target of the prevention effort?* Is the hope to reduce the rate of suicide, reduce suicide attempts, reduce suicide ideas, or predisposing vulnerabilities to suicide? Alternatively, is the target to build competencies, enhance wellness, strengthen coping skills, and increase protective (vs. risk) factors?

● *Who is at risk for the target behavior?* Is there a well-defined population at risk for suicide or attempted suicide? Is enough known about pathogenesis and disease etiology to establish, for example, which depressed adolescents are most likely to engage in suicidal behaviors, or when an older white male with alcoholism is at increased suicide risk?

● *How should high-risk groups be identified? Which group, where, is at greatest risk?* In what setting might we best reach the population at greatest suicide risk—schools, primary care physicians' offices, offices of other clinical caregivers, hospital emergency rooms, bars, the military? What methods or procedures should be utilized to identify suicide risk (questionnaires, interviews, etc.)? What questions are most effective at screening those at risk for suicide? How can we be sure that the individual interprets questions correctly? Desjardins et al. (2016) offer an in-hospital self-administered suicide risk assessment questionnaire that is both clinically accurate and convenient.

- *When and where is someone most at risk for suicide?* Are there precipitating events or situations that increase suicide risk among those predisposed to suicide? Are these moments or triggers accessible to intervention? Where should clinicians intervene in the suicidal causal chain? Are there particular settings, contexts, environments, and situations that increase suicide risk and that are accessible to intervention?

- *What interventions are most effective at lowering suicide risk?* Should the approach be to intervene with individuals, to manipulate the environment, to educate, to legislate, or to do something else? How can effective interventions be documented? What intervention will result in immediate versus long-term suicide risk reduction? What interventions are most feasible? Which are most cost-effective? Should interventions be universal, selective, or indicated?

- *Which interventions most protect against suicide risk?* Should we teach elementary school children and their counselors depression and substance abuse awareness and management? Should we enhance middle and high school environments to promote social connectedness and relationship skills? Should we reduce the accessibility of firearms? Should we decease the accessibility and toxicity of medications? Should we reach out to elderly people and try to combat their social isolation and loneliness?

The U.S. Surgeon General's Call to Action Recommendations for Suicide Prevention

Jerry and Elsie Weyrauch (parental survivors of a suicide and cofounders of the Suicide Prevention Advocacy Network, or SPAN) spearheaded a conference in Reno, Nevada over 20 years ago to review and evaluative the best practices in suicide prevention. The goal was to establish a national strategy for suicide prevention, based on the growing belief that the time was ripe and that good enough answers existed to the questions posed earlier. The outcome was the listing of 81 recommendations for preventing suicide. These recommendations were passed on to the U.S. Surgeon General; reformulated into a tighter, smaller blueprint for addressing suicide prevention as part of the nation's Year 2010 health objective; and then presented to the public as *The Surgeon General's Call to Action to Prevent Suicide 1999* (U.S. Public Health Service, 1999). These recommendations can be found in Table 25.3. This essential step toward establishing a national strategy embraced suicide prevention fully within public health. The United States thus joined other countries in the world, notably Norway and Finland, that have adopted national plans to prevent suicide.

The recommended strategies includes 14 key recommendations (Table 25.3), grouped under the acronym AIM (viz., Assessment, Intervention, Methodology). Although clear and convincing evidence based on controlled research studies was lacking, these recommendations probably best expressed the state-of-the-art thinking at the time for suicide prevention. To be sure, the need existed to demonstrate their efficacy, but the humanitarian demand was to proceed with or without clear

TABLE 25.3. The U.S. Surgeon General's Call to Action Recommendations

Awareness: Appropriately broaden the public's awareness of suicide and its risk factors.

- Promote public awareness that suicide is a major public health problem and, as such, many suicides are preventable.
- Expand awareness of and enhance resources in communities for suicide prevention programs and mental health and substance abuse disorder assessment and treatment.
- Develop and implement strategies to reduce the stigma associated with mental illness, substance abuse, and suicidal behavior and with seeking help for such problems.

Intervention: Enhance services and programs, both population-based and clinical care.

- Extend collaboration with and among public and private sectors to complete a National Strategy for Suicide Prevention.
- Improve the ability of primary-care providers to recognize and treat depression, substance abuse, and other major mental illnesses associated with suicide risk. Increase the referral to specialty care when appropriate.
- Eliminate barriers in public and private insurance programs for provision of quality mental and substance abuse disorder treatments and create incentives to treat patients with coexisting mental and substance abuse disorders.
- Institute training for all health, mental health, substance abuse, and human service professionals (including clergy, teachers, correctional workers, and social workers) concerning suicide risk assessment and recognition, treatment, management, and aftercare interventions.
- Develop and implement effective training programs for family members of those at risk and for natural community helpers (e.g., coaches, hairdressers, and faith leaders) on how to recognize, respond to, and refer people showing signs of suicide risk and associated mental and substance abuse disorders.
- Enhance community care resources by increasing the use of schools and workplaces as access and referral points for mental and physical health services and substance abuse treatment programs and provide for support for persons who survive the suicide of someone close to them.
- Promote public/private collaborations with the media to ensure that entertainment and news coverage represent balanced and informed portrayals of suicide and its associated risk factors, including mental illness and substance abuse disorders and approaches to prevention and treatment.

Methodology: Advance the science of suicide prevention.

- Enhance research to understand the risk and protective factors related to suicide, their interaction, and their effects on suicide and suicidal behaviors. In addition, increase research on effective suicide prevention programs, clinical treatments for suicidal individuals, and culture-specific interventions.
- Develop additional scientific strategies for evaluating suicide prevention interventions and ensure that evaluation components are include in all suicide prevention programs.
- Establish mechanisms for federal, regional, and state interagency public health collaborations toward improving, monitoring systems for suicide and suicidal behaviors and develop and promote standard terminology in these systems.
- Encourage the development and evaluation of new prevention technologies, including firearms safety measure, to reduce easy access to lethal means of suicide.

Source: Maris et al. (2000), based on U.S. Public Health Service (1999). Copyright © 2000 The Guilford Press. Reprinted with permission.

evidence, until sufficient trials and samples could be measured for the desired changes. With this in mind, the *Call to Action* document became a provisional template for future examination.

Over a decade later, the U.S. Surgeon General and the National Action Alliance for Suicide Prevention (NAASP) published the revised *2012 National Strategy for Suicide Prevention* (U.S. Department of Health and Human Services & NAASP, 2012). It included 13 goals and 60 objectives, and was aligned with a more inclusive *National Prevention Strategy* document (National Prevention Council, 2011). The *2012 National Strategy* reflected major developments in suicide prevention, research, and practice since the original 1999 *Call to Action,* and was to be put into effect from 2012 to 2022.

Although I do not have space here to reprint the entire 2012 document, it contains four strategic directions:

1. To create supportive environments that provide healthy and empowered individuals, families, and communities (4 goals, 16 objectives).
2. To enhance clinical and community preventive services (3 goals, 12 objectives).
3. To promote the availability of timely treatment and support services (3 goals, 20 objectives.
4. To improve suicide prevention surveillance collection, research, and evaluation (3 goals, 12 objectives).

Other federally supported agencies (see also the Substance Abuse and Mental Health Services Administration website, *www.samhsa.gov*) contributed to the 2012 suicide prevention plan. These included the Suicide Prevention Resource Center and the Action Alliance. There have also been Congressional legislation, policies, and mandates such as the National Lifeline, a separate crisis line for veterans; in addition, the Department of Veterans Affairs has conducted suicide prevention demonstration projects, funded by legislation such as the Garrett Lee Smith Memorial Act (2004) and the Joshua Omvig Veterans Suicide Prevention Act (2007).[1] For a summary of the most recent U.S. government responses to suicide prevention, see Ikeda et al. (2018)

Preventing Adolescent Suicides

Two groups at greater suicide risk are often singled out for selective intervention: (1) adolescents 15–24 years old (especially among young women in recent years), and (2) older white males ages 45–85 (especially among the middle-aged and very elderly). In 2013, 15- to 24-year-olds in the United States made up 4,878 of the total 41,149 suicides, or 12%. Although U.S. adolescents traditionally had very low

---

[1]Much of this suicide prevention information came from a personal communication with Morton Silverman (June 2016).

suicide rates (2–5 per 100,000), from 1950 to 1977 the U.S. suicide rate for those ages 15–24 tripled, from about 4 to 12 per 100,000 (Maris, 1985). As discussed in Chapter 5, this increase triggered great alarm, including a Congressional hearing about the adolescent suicide problem. Yet the adolescent rate never exceeded the suicide rate (not controlled for age) for the United States as a whole. In 2014 the 15–24 suicide rate was 11.1, but the overall rate was 13.0. Suicide rates tend generally to be low in young people. Joiner (2005, p. 163) writes, "Suicidal behavior is rare in young children in part because they have not had the experience and time to acquit ether ability to seriously injure themselves" (p. 163). In fact, we may have the youth suicide issue backwards. The real question may be this: Why are young people's suicide rates so low, and what could we learn from that?

Nevertheless, a 300% suicide rate increase in about 25 years merits investigation. The suicides of young people are especially tragic. Their lives are snuffed out before they have hardly lived (Maris, 1985). There is an old adage that you should never have to bury your own children, particularly because of suicide. Parents of young suicides feel great despair, frustration, and guilt. They think, "What could I have done to prevent this awful death?" (cf. Bolton with Mitchell, 1983).

When the suicides of those under age 21 in a large 5-year sample of suicides in Chicago (Maris, 1981, 1985) were separated out, some of the unique characteristics of youth suicide emerged. This, in turn, suggested some potential selective suicide prevention strategies. Older and younger suicides were alike in their depression, hopelessness, use of a firearm for suicide, social isolation, and seeing their death as escape from an intolerable life situation. Young suicides were different from older suicides in their excessive alcohol and other substance abuse; more anger and revenge motivation, risk taking, impulsivity, and negative social relations; more multiple-problem families of origin (including more suicides in their families); more prior suicide attempts (70% had made more than one suicide attempt before completing suicide); a stronger contagion effect (about 7%, vs. 3% in adults); and a tendency to come from larger birth cohorts.

The first generation of youth suicide prevention programs relied primarily on just two strategies: (1) recognition and referral of at-risk youth, and (2) reduction of suicide risk factors. The CDC (1992) criticized these prevention programs as stand-alone models, inadequately linking community resources and risk prevention programs, and rarely focusing on empirically supported means reduction efforts (see Lester, 2012). In general, these early programs rarely measured outcomes and potential iatrogenic effects. Also, they rarely had a primary prevention focus.

Most youth preventive efforts have yet to focus on protective factors among younger children, instead targeting the development of resiliency in the later teen years. Berman and Jobes (1995) outlined a conceptual model of primary prevention that focuses on decreasing children's potential for later suicidality. The strategies included skill-based approaches to manage depression, anger, aggression, and loneliness, and to enhance competencies like decision-making, social, and problem-solving skills (however, see Ougrin & Asarnow, 2018). These approaches are school-based, manualized, teachable, and time-limited (only eight sessions), and they do not require excessive training. They do require "booster shots" over subsequent years.

Some of the youth suicide prevention programs suggested by Berman and Jobes (1995; cf. Berman et al., 2006) include the following:

* *School gatekeeper training.* Education of counselors, teachers, coaches, and other school personnel to identify and refer at-risk students to mental health care providers.
* *Community gatekeeper training.* Education of clergy, pediatricians, police, and other community figures to identify and refer at-risk students to mental health care providers.
* *General suicide education.* Classroom-centered, knowledge-based training of students to increase self-awareness and peer observation of risk and referral skills.
* *Screening programs.* School-based administration of a screening questionnaire to all students, with a follow-up triage of identified at-risk students.
* *Peer support programs.* School- or community-based peer support groups aimed at fostering social and coping competencies, peer relationships, and networking among at-risk youth.
* *Crisis centers and hotlines.* Anonymous 24-hour telephone support systems offering nonjudgmental listening, problem solving, and crisis intervention to callers (however, see Goodwin, 2003).
* *Means restrictions.* Delaying or thwarting access to available and accessible means for self-harm, particularly firearms.
* *Postvention/cluster prevention.* School and community interventions to reduce the potential of imitative (copycat) suicides after a prior school suicide.

Preventing Older White Male Suicides

Without a doubt, prevention efforts in the United States and most of the world need to be focused on suicides of older white males. Joiner (2005) has written, "If I were put in charge of developing a public service announcement, I think I might target older men, since they are the demographic with high suicide rates, and it might be something along the line of: 'keep your friends and make new ones—it's strong medicine'" (p. 220).

Joiner (2005) goes on to add that suicide increases with age, and that older white males are at the most risk for suicide (at least in the United States). The following observations are based on U.S. suicide rates per 100,000 from 2004 to 2014, as shown in Table 25.1:

* The rates for males increased from 17.6 to 20.6.
* The rates for middle-aged men increased from 12.1 to 14.9.
* The rates for those ages 85 or over increased from 16.9 to 19.3.
* The rates for whites increased from 12.1 to 14.9.
* Over the life cycle, the white male suicide rate increases in virtually a straight line. (Today the increase is somewhat bimodal, with peaks in midlife and old age. See Figure 5.1.)

Why focus on white males? The main reason is that they tend to have the highest suicide rates. Suicide rates for black males tend to peak in midlife, although they are not as high as those for white males (see Figure 5.1). However, the black male suicide rate often rises again in late life.

Prevention ought to be focused on middle-aged to elderly white males, because in recent years there has been a dramatic increase in male midlife suicide rates, such that in 2016 the highest suicide rates for any age group were for those ages 45–54. When Murphy and Robins (1967) examined middle-aged male suicides, they found the following distinctive characteristics for that group:

- Increasing divorce rates and object loss.
- Years of heavy drinking (the average alcoholic male drinks for about 25 years before suiciding).
- High risk for depressive disorders.
- Increasing experience with the suicides of others.
- Lack of adjustment to aging (developmental stagnation in an earlier life stage; Levinson et al., 1978).
- Job and work loss.
- Physical illness and failure to control pain adequately (O'Neill et al., 2018; Richman, 1994).
- Cognitive rigidity and inflexibility of thought (Szanto et al., 2018).

Similar, even overlapping, suicide risk factors can be seen in men ages 65–85 and older. Of my 15 suicide risk factors (Maris et al., 2000; see Chapter 4), 10 are more prevalent in aged males. Much of the work on suicide in late life has been done by Yeates Conwell and his associates (Conwell & Heisel, 2012). Some of the characteristics of late-life male suicide include the following:

- Alcoholism and other substance abuse (especially abuse of opiates and pain medications).
- Access to lethal means for suicide (e.g., guns and narcotics) and few other people who could prevent this access.
- Increased rates of depressive disorders that tend to be undiagnosed and untreated or misdiagnosed and mistreated.
- Increased social isolation (Marchalik & Jurecic, 2018; DeLeo et al., 1995), providing both motivation and increased opportunity to suicide.
- Hopelessness increased by being near the end of a natural life expectancy.
- Work and retirement problems and related economic problems.
- Increasing anger at the unfairness and stress of aging.
- Physical illness, more frequent sickness and injury, more trips to the doctor, and an increase in pain problems.
- Having a long suicidal career and acquiring or achieving the ability to suicide.
- Failure of primary care doctors to seize their opportunity to intervene in their elderly patients' suicidal situations (41% of suicides had seen their primary care doctor within 28 days of their suicides; Simon, 2012; Sher, 2015).
- Increasing awareness that near the end of life, death may be the only real

solution to suffering. (That is, the elderly may not feel much better even with excellent care.)

These suicide risk factors for elderly white males suggest the following specific, focused, dedicated preventive interventions for them:

- Better diagnosis and more effective treatment of mood disorders, especially by primary care physicians (Benson et al., 2018). Probably the leading single cause of suicide is undiagnosed, untreated, or ineffectively treated depressive disorders. Many elderly suicides could be prevented simply by maintaining them on appropriate doses of antidepressants (Wellbutrin, Lexapro, Cymbalta, etc.) or initiating ECT, preferably with conjoint CBT.
- Control of alcoholism and detoxification of those with alcohol problems. Remember that the suicide rate in the former Soviet Union went down when vodka sales were controlled by Gorbachev under the *perestroika* reforms (see Chapter 15).
- Improved physical illness and pain control (O'Neill et al., 2018). Many elderly forensic suicide cases involve problems with pain medications (Vicodin, Dilaudid, etc.). There should be a better way to alleviate pain and make late life more tolerable. People should not have to die to stop their physical or psychic pain.
- Primary care doctors need to be trained, and allowed the time, to intervene in suicide prevention for their elderly patients. Family doctors have a unique suicide prevention opportunity.
- Although this suggestion is certainly debatable, patients need to be helped to have a good death and not be abandoned when life is no longer supportable. Physician-assisted suicide is growing in the United States, and that should tell us something. Life is not always fixable. Eventually it is natural and appropriate to die.
- Lethal means restrictions, especially of firearms and drugs, would go a long way in lowering the elderly male suicide rate. This is easier said than done. Lester (2012) talks about making vehicle tailpipes square to discourage carbon monoxide poisoning. Also, we need to pay attention to safety planning, not just means restrictions (see Stanley et al., 2008; Anestis et al., 2017).
- Elders' social relations often need to be improved. As people age, spouses and old friends die. One estimate is that 76% of elder suicides live alone (Maris et al., 2000). Social relations can be improved through retirement communities, churches, nursing homes, and the like. In addition, volunteers can telephone the elderly. That's done every day to try to sell people something, so why not do it to help keep elders alive?
- The process of transition from work to retirement has to be improved. All of us need meaningful daily activities. Social marginalization can be reduced by remaining active and doing something; what that something is does not matter much.
- CBT can help reduce rigid, negative, self-destructive thinking and behavior, and improve problem-solving skills (Szanto et al., 2018). The problems are

the difficulty of getting older men to engage in psychotherapy, and their frequent inability to afford it (Benson et al., 2018).

- Everyone needs hope. One can have hope without cure. Activities can be meaningful and tolerable without being optimal or ideal.
- Improvement in familial cross-generation relationships could help a great deal. Work opportunities and professional ambition tends to separate parents, children, and grandparents. Adult children often take job opportunities that move them far away from their parents.

Reflections on Suicide Prevention Services

What do people experience if they contact a front-line, grassroots suicide prevention center (SPC) or other suicide prevention service? How are suicidal individuals in crisis responded to when they go to a suicide prevention service or agency? When they communicated in person, on the telephone, or online with a suicide prevention "first-aid" worker, did they establish rapport (a "therapeutic alliance")? Were they put on hold, and if so, how long did they have to wait to speak to someone? Was psychotherapy or psychopharmacological therapy discussed? Did the worker make referrals, and if so, when? Did the worker or anyone else call the police or order (through a judge) hospitalization? What kinds of people call what kinds of prevention services? On the whole, are their contacts positive or negative, and why? What could have made the contacts better?

The types of people served by crisis services are not typical suicide completers. They are mainly young people and are more likely to be females, who have low-lethality suicide ideas. In one recent study of the National Suicide Prevention Lifeline, 63.3% of callers were women, and only 11.1% were age 55 or older (Gould et al., 2018). Psychiatrist Robert Litman at the Los Angeles SPC (LASPC) found that in a given year, fewer than 1% of Los Angeles County suicide completers ever called the LASPC. Most suicide completers are older white males, who are not likely to confide in anyone about their suicidality in person, on the phone, or on the internet. Thus, the people most likely to call an SPC are not those who are the most likely to suicide. Nevertheless, 79.6% of the callers in the Gould et al. (2018) study reported that the intervention stopped them from suiciding, and 90.6% said it kept them safe.

Most suicide prevention workers are volunteers, not professionals, physicians, or psychologists, although the volunteers tend to have supervisors who are mental health professionals. SPC counselors' approach to suicide prevention tends to be based largely on their own personal experiences and common sense. It is not especially scientific or academic. If 90% or more of suicides have a diagnosable mental disorder, then they likely need psychotropic medicine, not just good listeners. Empathy does little to change brain chemistry. "I care about keeping you alive" is different from "I am competent to keep you alive." Behind all of this is the question of the level of training of most volunteers. This is not to say that they cannot do important work, if they realize their limits, make timely referrals, and have adequate supervision.

Many suicide prevention workers tend to give simplistic, rigid suggestions like "Stay positive" or "Be hopeful." But life and death are not always simple. For example, is suicide ever justified? Most suicide prevention workers would say "No." Many of these workers are prior suicide attempters themselves; their philosophy and advice not only may be overly simple, but can be biased. What if a caller wanted help to die?

Acute and chronic suicide risk factors are also different. Most SPC workers have a bias in favor of acute suicide risk factors' causing suicide, which both Joiner (2005) and I (Maris, 2015) disagree with. Many people do call an SPC because of acute stress, but acute stress mainly provokes suicide in chronically vulnerable individuals with long suicide careers and the slowly acquired capability to inflict lethal self-injury. Lots of people are in acute stress, but very few of them ever suicide. What factors make the difference? Probably accumulated psychic and physical pain, acquired suicidal capability, social isolation, repeated self-destructive behaviors and lifestyles, and a genuine, persistent loss of hope, among others.

How much can volunteers help? Often they are young, naïve, and not very knowledgeable yet. If callers cannot help themselves, then how can someone essentially just like them help very much? When people are suicidal, they are vulnerable (sexually, financially, etc.).

Let us consider treatment as problem solving. What exactly is the problem? Is it one or many problems? Suicidal people often have different problems, even if they use the same solution (i.e., suicide). Do their CSF and brain serotonin systems need adjustment with medications? If so, talk alone is cheap. Is the problem a time-limited and resolvable crisis, such that endurance and persistence are the main issues? Is suicide a permanent solution to a temporary problem? Most physical illnesses and financial problems are time-limited and tend to get better, often without treatment, even depressive disorder. Precise treatment turns on correct, precise assessment. One size or one pill does not fit all.

People cannot just be asked whether they are suicidal (see Silverman & Berman, 2014). Most will lie or underestimate their risk or intention—for example, in order to stay in or get out of a hospital. Strange as it seems, people themselves often do not know how self-destructive they are or how serious their problem is. Many people do not realize that if they keep living the way they are doing, they will be lucky to make it until age 30. Among celebrities, consider the examples of Kurt Cobain, John Belushi, Philip Seymour Hoffman, Heath Ledger, Bob Fosse, Sylvia Plath, Marilyn Monroe, and others. It is surprising how little insight many people have, or how delusional, paranoid, or even psychotic they are.

Often clinicians need to rely on objective suicide risk factors. Although there are some times when clinical judgment must trump science, gut instincts and subjective feelings are sometimes unreliable. Clinicians need to consider factors like age, gender, psychiatric diagnosis, race, access to lethal methods, repeated suicide attempts and other self-destructive behaviors, repeated substance abuse, social isolation, and so on.

Prevention involves making critical, tailored suicide prevention and treatment action plans. For example, the steps in such a plan might include these: (1) Develop a good treatment alliance; (2) control the gun or prohibit easy access to other lethal means (Lester, 2012); (3) try to take the edge off (not necessarily cure) psychache or physical pain; (4) resolve acute crises (get the stomach pumped or charcoaled, reduce intoxication, calm desperation, lower agitation with Haldol or Klonopin, try to repair or abandon a broken relationship, consider hospitalizing the caller or calling the police, etc.); (5) pay attention to the caller's gender (especially to middle-aged or older men); and so on.

Suicide prevention may take time and persistence; it is not just a matter of short-term crisis intervention. For most would-be suicides, a quick fix will not be enough. If it took a person 20–25 years to become suicidal, then the person is not going to be fixed in a phone call or even in a few weeks. Long-standing suicidal patterns and behaviors (i.e., a suicidal career) need time to be reversed. An important question is this: How can the person stay alive long enough to get better? Long-term suicidal recovery may involve resocialization or reparenting, as well as chemically readjusting and maintaining the brain. There needs to be a plan of action over a fairly long time that has a chance to reverse chronic, self-destructive lifestyles, so that repeated crises will be less likely to reoccur. Even AA has its Twelve Steps, not one.

What Could the Suicide Rate Be?

Suicide prevention entails some idea of what the optimum or lowest suicide rate should or could be. Most of those who would lower the suicide rate act as if the target rate should be zero—no suicides at all. But is zero a reasonable or likely suicide rate? In 2016, the AFSP set a somewhat more realistic target of reducing the overall suicide rate in the United States by 20% by 2025. If we use the 2014 suicide rate of 13.4 per 100,000, this implies that the 2025 U.S. suicide rate would need to be about 10.7. But how likely is even that result? Not very, in my opinion.

Looking at Table 25.1, we see that from 2004 to 2014, the U.S. suicide rate actually *increased* from 11.0 to 13.4—that is by 2.4 points per 100,000, or 22% (Tavernese, 2016). In fact, in the last 100 years in the United States (see Figure 25.1), the suicide rate overall has never been below 10 per 100,000. There are other countries with rates lower than 10. For example, the suicide rates in Italy, Mexico, United Arab Emirates, Philippines, Egypt, Iraq, Jamaica, and Syria have all been below 5 per 100,000 (see Table 8.1). But note that all of these countries are largely either Muslim or Catholic.

The suicide rate is a special case of the general death rate. The world death rate had dropped from about 18 per 1,000 to 8 by 2010. If we use the same base rate as we do for suicides (since they are rarer) of 100,000, then by 2013 the U.S. death rate dropped to 821.5 per 100,000, or about 8 per 1,000 (Xu et al., 2016). Obviously, there are a lot more deaths per year (2,596,993 in 2013) than there are suicides (41,419). In 2013 suicide was the 10th leading cause of death overall. Over the years, death rates from the leading cause of death of heart disease and cancers have come down. The average human life expectancy (not controlled for gender or race) in 2013 was 78.8 years.

Of course, there will always be deaths each year. One question is this: How low can both the death and suicide rates go? In my opinion, a U.S. death rate of 821.5 and a suicide rate of 12–13 per 100,000 probably are about as low as can be reasonably expected. Note that the suicide rate has probably never been zero at any time or in any major place or group. Some important specifications are also being glossed over here. For example, which types of suicide rates (age, gender, race, marital status, religion, etc.) are we considering lowering? Most of the time, the focus is on suicide rates of older white males who are divorced or separated, and who are Protestant or of no religion.

As mentioned earlier, the only countries or major groups with suicide rates of zero are found in fictional Utopias, like the World State in Huxley's *Brave New World* (1932; cf. Marchalik & Jurecic, 2018). A final important thought: Death, even by suicide, is not always bad. When people are very old, infirm, and in unrelenting pain without hope of remission or relief, some of them may feel that they need to die. Modern medicine and technology tends to keep people unnaturally alive and suffering, often against their wishes, mainly to please others often at the expense of the dying patient.

A suicide is far from "complete." There are always ripples and repercussions of almost unbearable pain. In Chapter 26, I consider suicide *postvention*. How can we deal with the grief, guilt, and pain of those a suicide leaves behind?

CHAPTER 26

Postvention and Survivors

Death May Solve the Suicide's Problems, but What about Those Left Behind?

> Many others will be affected by the suicide. In the United
> States suicidologists have estimated that between six
> and forty-five survivors will be affected by each suicide.
> —FRANK CAMPBELL

If there is no afterlife, then suicide is a very effective, albeit extreme, resolution to life problems—no consciousness, no pain. However, suicide creates severe, often lifelong problems for those who are left behind and care about the deceased, and puts a dent in the life force for us all. Most suicides just want to escape from what they perceive as an intolerable, unbearably painful, hopeless, dead-end life. In a depressed mood, suicides may think others would actually be better off without them. But what is the cost to others who love them?

No suicide is simply *complete*. It is a beginning of ever-widening ripples of anguish, scars, and even fatal wounds (Campbell, 2012; Feigelman et al., 2018) to some of those close to the suicide—spouses, partners, lovers, parents, siblings, grandparents, aunts and uncles, cousins, nieces and nephews, classmates, workmates, sport and club mates, other friends (Feigelman said friends outnumbered first degree relatives by 5 to 1), fans, the local community, the religious congregation (church, synagogue, or mosque), therapist, family doctor, those who find the body, neighbors, the EMS crews, police, and many others.

Suicide has a surprising and sad "domino effect." Suicide may be rare, but self- and other-destructive behaviors are not. There were 42,773 suicides in the United States in 2014. If we use Campbell's (2012) survivor range of 6–45 people (see the chapter epigraph), these suicides would have left from 256,638 to 1,924,785 survivors. What exactly does it mean to be "influenced by a suicide" or to be a "survivor of suicide"? Candidates for various types of survivors include the following (Cerel et al., 2014; cf., Cerel et al., 2018):

- Survivors of any type of self-destruction (Cain, 1972). But this definition is unclear. Does it mean survivors of a nonfatal suicide attempt or of a suicide completion?
- Mainly those family and friends who remain after a suicide (Dunne et al., 1987).
- Survivors of both the impact of a nonfatal suicide attempt and a completion (Mishara, 1995).
- Those who experience a high level of self-perceived psychological, physical, and/or social distress for a considerable length of time after exposure to the suicide of another person (Jordan & McIntosh, 2011).
- Those with a traditional familial kinship relationship with a suicide (Campbell, 2012).
- Those who do not have a personal relationship with a suicide, but nonetheless experience the person and the death through the media (such as fans of a celebrity; Cerel et al., 2014).

These various groupings of survivors of suicide can be classified into four broad types (see Table 26.1); (1) *exposed*, (2) *affected*, (3) *short-term bereaved*, and (4) *long-term bereaved* (Cerel et al., 2014). These types can be defined as follows. *Exposed* means anyone who knows or identifies with a suicide; *affected* means those who are experiencing significant distress; *short-term bereavement* requires an attachment (see the discussion of John Bowlby's work, below); and *long-term bereavement* implies the response of a close or intimate family member, close friend, or therapist survivor. Using these definitions, we can calculate the following survivor statistics (American Association of Suicidology [AAS], 2015). In 2014, 147 persons were exposed to each suicide, or 6.3 million for the year 2014. An average of 18 people experienced a major life disruption from each 2014 suicide, and there are 750,000 loss survivors each year. From 1990 to 2014 there were 15.09 million survivors, or 1 for every 21

TABLE 26.1. Types of Individuals Exposed to, Affected by, and Bereaved by Suicides

Exposed	Affected	Short-term bereaved	Long-term bereaved
• First responders • One who discovers body • Family members • Therapists • Close friends • Health care workers • Community members • School communities • Workmates • Fans of celebrities • Community groups • Rural or close-knit communities	• First responders • One who discovers body • Family members • Therapists • Close friends • Classmates • Workmates • Team members • Neighbors	• Family members • Therapists • Friends • Close workmates	• Family members • Therapists • Close friends

Source: "The Continuum of 'Survivorship': Definitional Issues in the Aftermath of Suicide" by Julie Cerel et al., *Suicide and Life-Threatening Behavior, 44*(6), 591–600. Copyright © 2014 by the American Association of Suicidology. Reproduced with permission of John Wiley & Sons, Inc.

Americans. There are about 18 new survivors every 12.3 minutes in the United States. It appears that over 40% of the U.S. population over their lifetime knows at least one suicide (Cerel et al., 2014).

Many topics relevant to survivors have already been examined in other chapters, such as the social relations of suicide, the contagion effects, and treatment of survivors. This chapter looks at classic publications on survivors, research on survivors, ways in which suicide bereavement and grief are unique, ways in which suicide increases the suicide risk of survivors, and survivor group resources (cf. Feigelman et al., 2018). First, however, Case 26.1 illustrates the devastating impact that a suicide (in this case, that of a young adolescent) can have on the family members and others left behind.

CASE 26.1. Fisher Smith

Fisher Smith was an eighth grader. His birthday was just 3 days away when he died. Suicides tend to occur just after or before important social events like birthdays (Phillips, 1970). Fisher had been depressed for about 9 or 10 months prior to his suicide and was being treated with the antidepressant Prozac (one of the few antidepressants recommended for young people). His depression was first noted and treated after he made a nonfatal suicide attempt by asphyxiation. When seen by a psychiatrist for his suicide attempt, Fisher complained of having suicide ideas, being sad, seldom smiling, feeling socially isolated, and having trouble sleeping. Fisher was a straight-A student and was considered a perfectionist. It was very upsetting to Fisher that about 5 years earlier, his mother (Joan) and his father (Bill) had gotten divorced. Fisher suggested in his suicide note that he greatly loved his mom and dad, and that he was troubled by their divorce and continuing conflict (his mother, Joan, had remarried after the divorce). One assumes that Fisher felt caught in the middle of all this marital stress. Fisher's suicide note was written 6 days before his suicide, and so his suicide was not all that impulsive or opportunistic.

There was so much conflict between Fisher's mother and father that the court appointed a coordinator to mediate custody issues. The coordinator stipulated that Joan would have their children (they had three sons, of whom Fisher was the oldest) on Mondays and Tuesdays, and Bill would have them on Wednesdays and Thursdays, with alternating Friday-to-Sunday custody. It might be worth noting that Fisher had been in Joan's custody the Friday, Saturday, Sunday, and Monday before his suicide on Tuesday. Fisher was not supposed to be at his dad's home on the Tuesday that he suicided.

The Tuesday morning of his suicide, Fisher was taken to school by his mother, although he said he felt sick and wanted to stay home. After being dropped off at school, he ditched his backpack, walked about 2½ miles to his father's house, crawled into the locked house (probably through a doggie door; his shoes were found just outside the door), searched the house, found a .22 rifle hidden under his father's bed (it had been there for about 10 days, since the gun safe was crowded or full; the rifle was intended as a birthday present for his younger brother), loaded it, and shot himself between the eyes. Joan sued Bill for negligence (often defined in terms of four D's: "Dereliction of Duty leading Directly to Damages") for leaving a .22 rifle and ammunition within easy access at home, knowing that Fisher was depressed and had made a prior suicide attempt.

Clearly, it would have been better not to have left a rifle and ammunition unsecured in one's house with a depressed 13-year-old son around (Brent et al., 1987; Kellerman & Reay,

1986; and Miller & Hemenway, 2008; Østergaard, 2018; cf. Anestis, 2018). Most studies show that the probability of a teen suicide is 2, 5, or even 10 times higher just when a gun is readily available at home.

But was Fisher's suicide reasonably foreseeable under the circumstances? For Fisher to suicide, he had to decide to leave school, walk unexpectedly the 2½ miles to his dad's home (he was supposed to be staying with his mother that day), get into a locked house, look for and find a gun with no ammunition in it, find the ammunition, load the gun, and use it. The probably of all these contingent events' co-occurring is astronomically low, A "reasonable and prudent person in same or similar circumstances" would most likely never have suspected that Fisher's suicide would happen under these circumstances.

Certainly, neither Joan nor Bill had been negligent in treating the one most likely cause of Fisher's suicide: his depression. If Fisher had been less depressed, then the presence of a gun becomes less relevant. Fisher was taking Prozac and had seen his psychologist counselor just 1 day (Monday) before his death. His psychotherapist testified that he did not evaluate Fisher as being especially suicidal on that Monday. It is even possible, but not likely, that Prozac increased Fisher's suicide risk (Maris, 2015). Fisher would have scored about a 3 on a 10-point suicide risk scale (Maris et al., 2000) on the day of his suicide, which is a low probability of suicide. A score of three means that Fisher shared 30% of the traits of known suicides, not that he was 30% likely to suicide.

Fisher's suicide utterly devastated his parents. This was a life-changing event that they will never fully heal from. No doubt, they both feel guilty. They also have two younger sons; what will happen to them?

On the other hand, one cannot stay in a bad marriage for fear of what might happen to the children. It is often better for someone like Fisher to get out of such prolonged, intense marital conflict. There were likely other suicidogenic factors contributing to Fisher's death that had little to do with his parents' marriage. Given the level of parental conflict, there was a tendency for both the mother and the father to blame each other for causing or substantially contributing to Fisher's suicide. However, it is possible that no one was to blame. Nevertheless, something awful happened to the Smiths, their remaining two sons, and Joan's reconstituted family, not to mention Fisher's psychiatrist, psychologist, family doctor, and other close friends and family.

Source: This was a case in which I testified as an expert witness. The case is disguised, and facts have been altered to protect the family.

A Brief Chronology of Classic Publications on Survivors

The argument that suicide can also be *altercide,* a social-psychological assault on or trauma for others, probably started in the early 1970s. Here is a brief chronology of some of the major publications on survivors to date:

- *Survivors of Suicide* (Cain, 1972) was a groundbreaking collection of writings focusing theoretical and clinical attention on the impact of suicide on family members, including children. In these early professional discussions of the aftermath of suicide and its effects on the living, the terms *suicide survivors* and *survivors of suicide* were established. Before long, this terminology was adopted by the suicide bereaved themselves, finding its closest expression in programs and in mutual support networks providing advocacy and assistance to those coping with the aftermath of this tragedy (Cerel et al., 2014; Cerel, 2018).

● In *My Son . . . My Son . . . : A Guide to Healing after a Suicide in the Family* (Bolton with Mitchell, 1983; cf., Bolton, 2018), Iris Bolton tells the story of her son Curtis, who committed suicide at age 21. Bolton further describes what it was like for her to lose a child to suicide and the steps she needed to take to heal. The book can help those who are grieving a suicide loss, clinicians who were treating a suicide, clergy or funeral directors, school counselors, and police officers or attorneys (see Maris, 2017).

● In *Suicide and Its Aftermath* (Dunne et al., 1987), the term *survivors* was defined as the family and friends who remain after a person dies by suicide. This book brought together the knowledge base on surviving suicide that had accumulated since Cain's book, with a clear realization of how little was known about this form of bereavement at the time (Cerel et al., 2014).

● The contributors to *The Impact of Suicide* (Mishara, 1995) discussed not only survivorship of completed suicides, but also the impact of nonfatal suicidal behaviors (attempts and ideation) on family and others as well as society as a whole. Although a formal definition was not presented, Mishara (1995) argued that "for each person who dies by suicide there are several family members and a number of friends and acquaintances who are profoundly affected by the loss" (p. 2). This expansion of the definition was further adapted by Andriessen (2009, p. 43), who stated that a survivor is simply "a person who has lost a significant other (or loved one) by suicide, and whose life is changed because of the loss" (see also Cerel et al., 2014).

● *Grief after Suicide* (Jordan & McIntosh, 2011) is a compilation of the larger body of research that existed at the time (for an update see McIntosh, 2018a). Jordan and McIntosh provide a summary of definitions used in research over time, and offer a nuanced definition of a *suicide survivor* as "someone who experiences a high level of self-perceived psychological, physical and/or social distress for a considerable length of time after exposure to the suicide or another person" (p. 7). Carrying implications beyond the earlier, widely adopted but broader conceptualization of survivorship, this definition first implies that a suicide survivor can be "someone with any relationship to the deceased, including but not necessarily based on kinship" (Cerel et al., 2014).

● The chapter by Campbell (2012) in the second edition of *The American Psychiatric Publishing Textbook of Suicide Assessment and Management* emphasizes that survivors are at increased suicide risk themselves. They often need an exploration of the *whys* of the suicide, as well as counseling. Guilt is often intertwined with grief. Many big cities have an active volunteer service associated with the coroner's or medical examiner's office. Clinicians who have lost a patient to suicide may also need postvention care. Many communities have survivor support groups like Survivors of Suicide (SOS). Since most suicide completers are whites, survivors will also tend to be white partners/spouses or parents of the suicides, like Iris Bolton (Maris, 2017).

• Cerel et al.'s (2014) article "The Continuum of 'Survivorship': Definitional Issues in the Aftermath of Suicide" reviews prior research on survivors, and then attempts to compile a more nuanced and inclusive definition of *survivors* that encompasses many prior disparate, incomplete, and fragmented conceptualizations (cf. Cerel, 2018).

Research on Survivors

Surviving a suicide is fraught with emotional upheaval. It is not easy to understand what is going on or what to do about it in order to help survivors cope and try to recover. Thus, research and a more objective, scientific approach to survivorship can be useful. Campbell (2012) has written, "For many survivors the psychological autopsy is a method of review that can answer specific questions regarding the deceased behavior, compliance to treatment, and complications in his or her successful treatment" (p. 655).

Box 26.1 provides an outline/table of contents for my own psychological autopsy form (it has not been assessed for its psychometric properties, and readers are not authorized to use it without permission). The entire form is available on pages of my website (*www.suicideexpert.com/forms*). The table of contents gives a rough idea of the information about the decedent (DCD) and the event that will be necessary for a retrospective suicide death investigation. Often initially a survivor will be asked to fill out the form; then there will be one or more follow-up interviews with the survivor on the phone or face to face. There can be multiple informants for the psychological autopsy.

As Box 26.1 indicates, my psychological autopsy form is a forensic instrument, with an emphasis on the psychiatric medications associated with the suicide. There is also a research version of the form, and other versions for other purposes (e.g., clinical). Doing a psychological autopsy well is much more complicated than has been indicated here (Snider et al., 2006). The AAS offers seminars on how to do psychological autopsies and get certification (see, e.g., Berman, 2018).

A lot of the research on survivors (Jobes et al., 2000; cf. Jobes 2018) focuses on so-called "stage models" of bereavement, the different types of bereavement related to different types of loss, and reactions of others to survivors. A seminal theorist of the stages of the bereavement process was psychiatrist Elizabeth Kübler-Ross (1969). Her five-stage model is shown in Figure 26.1. Originally Kübler-Ross argued that the process of grief and bereavement went through a roughly linear progression of stages: (1) *denial,* (2) *anger,* (3) *bargaining,* (4) *depression,* and finally (5) *acceptance.* Most survivors actually fluctuate back and forth among these stages.

At first the survivor is often in denial (e.g., "This can't be happening!"), followed by anger (e.g., "This isn't fair!") and bargaining (such as "Take me instead, God"). In the depression stage, the survivor will often withdraw, will cry frequently,

BOX 26.1. Psychological Autopsy and Death Investigation

(This instrument is intended for the retrospective examination of scientific evidence relevant to manner-of-death determination and to establish the facts related to the death.)

TABLE OF CONTENTS

INSTRUCTIONS: Copy this form to a word-processing program and then enter your answers electronically. It will take you about 1 to 2 hours to complete it. I need complete answers, even if you think the information may be contained in other records or depositions. Assume that this is the only information on your case that I have. Please, take this task seriously and give complete, thorough, detailed, and specific answers. This form is extremely important as it will allow me to form and defend my expert opinions. If you have any questions, you may call me at _____. When you are finished you may, with your attorney's approval (always send a copy to him/her, too), email your completed form to *rwmaris@aol.com*. Be sure to fill in the cover page with your name and the date. I need a color picture of the decedent.

Source: The "Forms" page of my personal website (*www.suicideexpert.com/forms*).

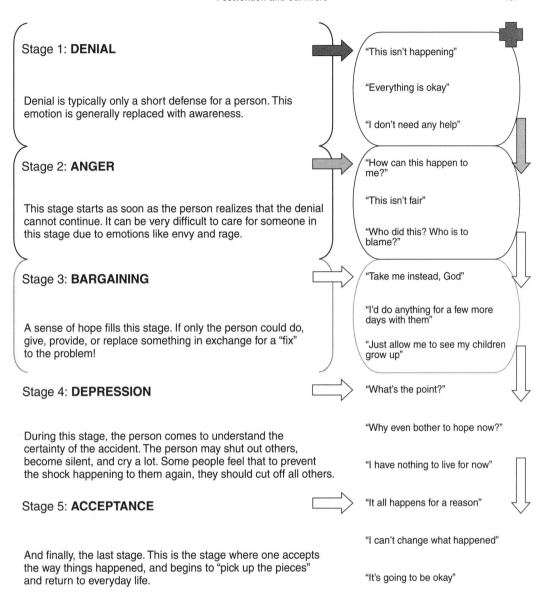

FIGURE 26.1. The Kübler-Ross model (otherwise known as "the five stages of grief"). *Source:* Kübler-Ross (1969).

cannot work or go to school, and may say things like "I have nothing to live for now." Ultimately in the acceptance stage, the survivor reluctantly accepts what has happened and tries to start over without the loved one, saying things like "I'm going to be okay" or "It happened for a reason." Later revisions of Kübler-Ross's five-stage model of grief added an initial stage of *shock* or *emotional paralysis,* and a *testing* stage (seeking realistic resolutions) between the stages of depression and acceptance.

Often survivor research has looked at the following:

1. Cleiren et al. (1994) examined differing recovery processes for suicidal versus accidental or natural deaths.
2. A common reaction of survivors is a desperate attempt to find out why the suicide happened and if it could have been prevented, especially by the survivor.
3. Van Dongen (1993) considered stigmatization by others following a suicide. About 26% of survivors reported negative social reactions to the suicide. Suicide was considered most acceptable by others, if the suicide had a terminal illness, like cancer.
4. Range and Goggin (1990) found that reactions of others to a suicide varied by the ages of the suicide and of those reacting. Most others viewed the suicides of the very young or very old as having less familial impact than (say) the suicides of adolescents or of the middle-aged.

Although survivors often suffer pathological grief, by about 2 years after the death, suicide survivors do about as well in their recovery as do survivors of nonsuicidal deaths.

Survivor Bereavement and Grief

Most suicides are shocking and surprising. Even when the decedents have had longish suicidal careers, survivors often say that they "did not see it coming," at least not then. Suicides almost by definition are premature (not natural) and usually unnecessary. Many suicides deny suicide ideation to their families and clinicians, and even to themselves.

Survivors, justifiably or not, may feel guilt and anxiety for not being able to prevent their loved one's suicide and may even feel somehow complicit or vaguely responsible for the suicide. Survivors can also feel anger for being forced to make major unwanted life adjustments—for example, to their routines, finances, emotions, and the places where they live. They may also feel embarrassment in coping with a still stigmatized event (e.g., "Should I admit to others that suicide was the manner of death?"). There can be reasonable concern for what suicide may mean for the surviving children, since suicide in the family is a suicide risk factor.

Given all this, grief and mourning after a suicide may be prolonged and complicated (Shear, 2015; Zisook et al., 2018). Normally, within 6–15 months after a natural death, the survivors can expect to begin to resume their usual activities, experience joy again, and remember the deceased loved one without intense, crippling, profoundly disruptive pain (Brody, 2015). However, grief after a suicide can continue for years (Jordan & McIntosh, 2011).

Suicide survivors often report feeling stunned, numb, or in shock. They can have an intense yearning for the deceased loved one, feel disbelief ("This cannot be happening!"), and be preoccupied with intrusive thoughts of the person. They may not be able to imagine resuming a meaningful postsuicide life. Such pathological or complicated grief is a psychological or even physical wound that will not heal. There is a Grief Intensity Scale (Prigerson et al., 2009) to help survivors determine whether their grief is severe, and also a Center for Complicated Grief at the Columbia University School of Social Work.

Complicated grief after suicide can be physical as well as psychological. There can be changes in brain activity that impair memory and contribute to depression, sleep disturbances, immunological abnormalities, substance abuse, and even suicidal thoughts and behaviors. Frequently antidepressants and anxiolytics many need to be prescribed. However, with complicated grief, psychotherapy is probably most helpful. Psychotropic medicine alone usually is not sufficient to treat survivors.

Bowlby on Attachment and Loss

Some theoretical roots of the concept of complicated grief can be found in the work of the late John Bowlby on separation, attachment, and loss (Bowlby, 1973, 1980; see also Maris, 1981, 70ff.). Bowlby was one of the most perceptive commentators on the functions of (especially early) object loss, grief, and mourning in the development of psychiatric illnesses such as depressive disorders, and of even suicidal behaviors. Bowlby claimed that attachment to the mother is usually formed in the first half-year of the infant's life. Most traditional psychoanalysts have tended to emphasize identification with the lost object (here, the mother) as the main process in mourning. Often angry efforts are made by the infant (or survivor) to recover the lost object. Bowlby believed that some of the pain following object loss is the result of guilt—for example, feeling vaguely like the cause of the death (the infant or young child may even fear having "eaten" the mother through nursing) or divorce of a parent—and fear of retaliation by the surviving parent.

Bowlby observed that when the mother is temporarily absent, the main symptom is anxiety. However, when the absence is permanent, the usual syndrome is one of grief and mourning. Expressions of grief and mourning by the adult are thought to be related to the more primitive crying or wailing of the infant. Admitting or accepting object loss is sometimes resisted by adults, since they might also have to admit weakness or at least temporary dependence upon others. Bowlby believed that much pathological mourning is fixated in the striving to recover the lost object. On the other hand, healthy adjustment to reality demands abandoning or modifying old libidinal attachments.

Most psychiatrists contend that grief is different from separation anxiety, in that with grief the lost object is or is thought to be irreversible, and thus it is hopeless to recathect the original object. After most separation there is an urge, often accompanied with frantic effort, to recover the lost object. Children separated from their mothers tend to cry, to experience anxiety, or even to become angry. Since most separations are temporary and reparable, such activity and aggression on the children's part is reasonable, even useful. Sometimes in profound, acute, or abrupt irreversible losses of significant others (such as losses through suicide), one sees disorganization or even aimless motion that is not designed to recover lost objects. In fact, depression has sometimes been tabbed the "subjective aspect of disorganization." However, it should be observed that some disorganization is necessary for reorganization, recovery, and growth. The key to whether or not the mourning is pathological or healthy is how the loss is handled.

An important corollary of object loss as it pertains to suicide is the rather common phenomenon of directing anger against a love object that has been introjected into one's own ego—that is, against oneself instead of against the frustrating external object. For example, one possible interpretation of the self-destructive behaviors of children was given by Piaget (1929), who stated that young children tend not to differentiate themselves from their significant others. Furthermore, even if children wish to be aggressive against their parents, the parents are usually too powerful and physically strong (the same might be argued for women responding to men) for the children to aggress against them successfully. When anger cannot be directed against the frustrating or lost object itself—for example, when the object is dead (see, e.g., Plath's [1966] poem "Daddy")—it is often directed at the self or those similar to the lost object (like a therapist), at those thought to be responsible for the loss, or at those thought to be impeding a reunion with the lost object (Berkowitz, 1962).

Treatment of Survivors

Having a general sense of [who survivors are,] the history of
survivorship, and the empirical research related to being a survivor
are critical components to our understanding of the topic. But what
about actually helping survivors of suicide deal with these deaths?
—JOBES ET AL. (2000)

In the treatment of survivors, the following major issues need consideration (cf. Campbell, 2012; McIntosh, 2018b):

1. Should survivors of suicide get treated or not?
2. Is there an increased risk of suicide in survivors?
3. What are some pragmatic issues for survivors?
4. What about clinicians as survivors?

Should Suicide Survivors Get Treated?

Probably not every survivor needs to be treated (Maris et al., 2000; Dunne et al., 1987). Those who do get treatment may wait up to about 4.5 years to seek it, according to one study (Campbell, 2012). Treatment typically includes psychotherapy (e.g., CBT) and/or pharmacological therapy, most often antidepressants and anxiolytics prescribed by a family doctor. Child survivors may have special treatment needs, such as shock, denial, sadness or depression, anxiety, anger, shame/embarrassment, guilt, academic difficulties, and physical symptoms such as sleeping and eating problems (Maris et al., 2000).

Many times survivors will say to me something like this: "My son just killed himself. Could you recommend a good book to help me understand why?" Bibliotherapy by itself is no substitute for psychotherapy or psychopharmacology (Campbell, 2012). With that important caveat, there are many helpful books and other resources. Table 26.2 is a list of recommended books for suicide survivors.

TABLE 26.2. Books for Loss Survivors

1. *Dying to Be Free,* Beverly Cobain (Kurt's cousin) and Jean Larch (2006).
2. *Rocky Roads,* Michelle Linn-Gust (2010).
3. *Suicide of a Child,* Adina Wrobleski (2002).
4. *A Special Scar,* Alison Wertheimer (2001).
5. *In Her Wake,* Nancy Rappaport (2010).
6. *No Time to Say Goodbye,* Carla Fine (1997).
7. *Child Survivors of Suicide,* Rebecca Parkin and Karen Dunne-Maxim (1995).
8. *Real Men Do Cry,* Eric Hipple (a former NFL quarterback) et al. (2008).
9. *Dead Reckoning,* David Treadway (1996).
10. *An Unquiet Mind,* Kay R. Jamison (1995).
11. *Darkness Visible,* William Styron (1990).

Source: American Foundation for Suicide Prevention (AFSP; *www.afsp.org*).

Very often survivors have treatment needs similar to those of the suicide, such as mood or anxiety disorders and a corresponding need for psychiatric medications; the compromised ability to work, take care of their families, or go to school; disruptions in daily living, eating, and sleeping; and so on. Also, there are different types of survivors. For an adult suicide, in addition to adult family members (such as parents, spouses, and siblings) and close friends, there may be child survivors (e.g., offspring, nieces, and nephews) and clinician survivors. One estimate is that roughly half of all psychiatrists and one-fourth of all psychologists will lose at least one patient to suicide over their careers (Maris et al., 2000).

Is There an Increased Risk of Suicide in Survivors?

Does one suicide trigger others in a family or among friends, like dominos knocking each other down (Campbell, 2012; Cain, 1972)? It is well known that a suicide does in fact increase the suicide risk for survivors themselves, either genetically (e.g., there may be a family history of mood disorders like the Hemingways'), contagiously, or through modeling. For example, in Chicago (Maris, 1981), I found that about 11–12% of suicides had another first-degree relative who had also suicided, compared to none of the natural death controls.

Survivors may have *de novo* suicide ideation and self-destructive behaviors. Anniversaries of a suicide can be hard to deal with. Phillips (1970) tells us that survivor suicide rates increase just before or after the death days of loved ones and anniversaries of other important social events. Sometimes a thoughtful clinician will send a survivor a yearly clinical remembrance card (Campbell, 2012).

What Are Some Pragmatic Issues for Survivors?

Suicide survivors confront several pragmatic issues that need to be addressed or resolved. Survivors are often surprised by their challenging financial issues; there can be resultant role adjustments (e.g., a widow may now have to handle the family checkbook). The survivor may become dysfunctional, depressed, and unable to work or go to school. He or she may suffer sleep and eating disruption, as well as either loss of libido or yearning for sexual intimacy (including touching). If the suicide has children, the survivor needs to explain the suicide to them. Survivors may question their religious faith ("How could God let this happen?!"). They may have a pathological preoccupation with the presuicidal past, abuse alcohol and other substances (including pain and sleep medications), lose friends, cope with stigma, and much more. As noted above, they may have *de novo* suicide ideation and self-destructive behaviors and need treatment.

Because the typical suicide is an older white male, this person is often the main family income provider. Therefore, right at the time when a surviving spouse is emotionally unhinged and grieving an unexpected, shocking major loss, there will be financial issues of probating a will and resolving an estate, funeral costs, possibly harassing unpaid therapy and hospital bills, and reduced family income. The loved one's life insurance (if there is any at all) may be denied or deferred, or, if paid, may be insufficient to cover costs. There are likely to be new costs of living, such as bills for the survivor's own treatment. Can college tuitions and school expenses still be afforded? The survivor may need to sell the home or car; many people do not want to stay in the same residence after a suicide at home. All these issues are very daunting to confront.

If they have a choice, should the survivors view the body? A surviving spouse or parent may be the one who finds the body (Campbell, 2012, p. 658). I had a forensic case in which a mother found her son shot under the chin and told the 911 operator, "His tongue is purple and bulging out of his mouth." No one needs to have that lasting final memory of a child.

Survivors may also need to be referred to (1) a local crisis or suicide prevention center (Campbell, 2012), (2) a psychiatrist or psychologist, (3) a counselor, (4) a social worker, (5) a financial advisor, (6) an attorney, or (7) inpatient hospitalization for a while.

What about Clinicians as Survivors?

Clinicians can be devastated by their patients' suicides, especially if they are sued for malpractice (Campbell, 2012; Maris et al., 2000; Tanney, 1995). The AAS (2016) has also published online "Resources for Clinicians Who Have Lost a Patient and/or Family Member to Suicide" (*www.suicidology.org*).

Attendance at a patient's funeral can be an issue for a clinician, especially if the family blames the therapist for the suicide. The therapist would like to be able to support the survivors, show empathy, and deal with his or her own grief—but does attending the funeral have legal implications or increase the probability of being sued for malpractice?

Should a therapist apologize to the family for not being able to prevent the suicide, or should the survivor file a wrongful death lawsuit against the therapist (see Chapter 27)? One survivor said:

> "I brought a wrongful death lawsuit a year after he died because there was a 45-minute gap in the nurses' notes about checking him, and that's exactly when he took the opportunity to kill himself. The psychiatrist had pulled him off all

his medications and was doing tests to determine if there was a chemical imbalance. . . . I was in a courtroom for 12 awful days, on the stand myself for a day and a half, and lost the lawsuit." (quoted in Campbell, 2012, p. 659)

There are also the issues of doctor–patient confidentiality and Health Insurance Portability and Accountability Act (HIPAA) rules. Can the therapist tell the survivors—for example, the parents of an adult child—about the patient's medical condition or records, especially if the patient has previously been assessed to have low suicide risk? There was a forensic case in which the doctor failed to call a father about his son's treatment, even though the father was the listed care partner. Among the problems were that the son was 24 years old, was not clearly a danger to himself or others, and had denied any suicide ideation.

Suicide of a clinician's patient raises the issues of how the clinician's malpractice insurance may be affected and whether or not it is adequate, as well as the emotional stress and time involved in a malpractice lawsuit. A legal case can go on for years, with withering cross-examinations by the patient's attorneys about the clinician's competence and clinical judgment, and time away from the therapy practice and usual routine. At the very least, all this is distracting and viscerally upsetting. Psychiatrist Joan Savitsky (2009) wrote:

> If [a medical mistake] happens, you have to integrate the experience, but for a while you lose your bearings. It is discombobulating. When this is followed by litigation, the effect is paralyzing. And the lawsuit felt like an assault. Being sued, even with the assurance that "it's nothing personal" and that my insurance would likely cover any settlement [and would not result in raised malpractice insurance rates or cancellation of the insurance policy], was in fact deeply personal. The experience was devastating.

We have discussed individual treatment at length, but what about group therapy for survivors? It is often useful to suicide survivors to be with others who have been through many of the same problems and emotions. Social support is important in the suicide bereavement process (Jobes et al., 2000).

Since suicide is relatively rare and often is stigmatized, survivors may feel a special need for group support while attempting to come to grips with the loss of a loved one through suicide. Sometimes it is important just to sit with like-situated others, who can say, "I'm so sorry—but we are going to get through this." Can a pill alone do that? Even when something cannot be changed or fixed, it can nevertheless be adjusted to and at least made more tolerable, allowing life to continue, and the survivor to keep on loving. In the film *Harold and Maude* (Ashby & Higgins, 1971), young Harold says to Maude as she is dying by suicide, "But I love you!" To which Maude replies, "Good, now go and love some more."

Helpful online addresses of suicide support groups include the following:

1. The American Foundation for Suicide Prevention (AFSP) offers a "Find a Support Group" list (*https://afsp.org/find-support/ive-lost-someone/find-a-support-group*). You search by the state and proximity mile radius for a local support group. There are also support group lists for Canada, Australia, China, Brazil, Hong Kong, and Nepal.

2. The AAS has an "SOS [Survivors of Suicide] Directory" (*www.suicidology.org/suicide-survivors/sos-directory*) that currently includes contact information for well over 600 suicide support groups in the United States. You can click on your choice of a specific support group for its address, phone number, email address, contact person, and additional information, such as when the group meets and whether there is a charge for attending.

3. The AFSP also offers "Resources for Loss Survivors" (*https://afsp.org/find-support/ive-lost-someone/resources-loss-survivors*). These include (in addition to the group support resources mentioned above) the date of the National Survivors of Suicide Day, a toolkit for school suicide prevention, suicide in college, postvention in the workplace, and the phone number of the National Suicide Prevention Lifeline (1-800-273-8255).

Postvention versus Prevention

Shneidman (1971) coined the word *postvention* to describe appropriate and helpful acts that come after a dire event, like a suicide. *Postvention* literally means intervention after an event (Brock, 2003). As Shneidman (1971) wrote, "Postvention, then, consists of activities that reduce the aftereffects of a traumatic events in the lives of the survivors. Its purpose is the help the survivors live longer, more productively, and less stressfully than they are likely to do otherwise."

Whereas Shneidman's original use of the term was broad-based and inclusive of any traumatic event, postvention has increasingly been linked to suicide-specific intervention efforts, such as the prevention of suicide imitation effects and provision of overall immediate postsuicide care for survivors.

In effect, postvention adds another column to our general model of suicide (see Chapter 2, Figure 2.1). With this modification, the model's column heads are now as follows, from left to right: Primary Prevention, Secondary Prevention, Feedback Loops (Protective Factors), Tertiary Prevention, Outcome, and Postvention (see Chapter 28, Figure 28.2).

After a suicide, a goal is to ameliorate the negative sequelae of the suicide, especially for the family and close friends of the suicide. For example, in Case 26.3 below, I consider how suicide crisis calls may have lowered the contagion effects of the suicide of Nirvana lead singer and composer Kurt Cobain.

Years ago, I did psychotherapy with a young mother (Ann Lessor)[1] and her two small children, a boy of 8 and a 6-year-old girl. They had all just come home from school at day's end and were sitting together in the front seat of their car. Ann pushed the garage door opener, only to find her husband hanging by his neck from a rope tied to a rafter in the garage. Having to witness this caused enormous shock and trauma to his wife and two small children. I treated them all until the son graduated from high school, a postvention of about 10 years. A few minutes or days of anguish and narcissistic desperation by the husband and father gave rise to years of treatment and emotional scars for his family. Ann decided to sell her house, since

---

[1]Names and other information have been changed to protect the privacy of the family.

she felt strongly that her husband's suicide had tainted the environment and made it impossible for her and her children to stay there.

In brief, then, postvention is aimed at ameliorating all of the suicide sequelae discussed in this chapter. It includes the following:

1. Preventing or reducing imitative suicides of survivors.
2. Coping with the grief and suffering of survivors.
3. Providing resources and support groups for survivors.
4. Doing research to help understand the aftermath of suicide.
5. Focusing special efforts on special groups, such as parents, children, siblings, and clinicians of suicides; fans of celebrities who suicide (like Kurt Cobain); schoolmates and workmates; first responders; and the community as a whole.

Contagion and Media Effects on Survivors

As discussed in Chapter 7, there has been a lengthy examination of how suicides can cause subsequent suicides of survivors (Sinyor, 2018). This is sometimes called *contagion* or the *Werther effect,* after von Goethe's 1774 novel *The Sorrows of Young Werther.* Since the contagion effect has already been discussed, I only comment briefly on imitation or suicide modeling in the aftermath of the suicides of actress Marilyn Monroe (Case 26.2; Summers, 1985) and Nirvana lead singer Kurt Cobain (Case 26.3).

CASE 26.2. Marilyn Monroe

Marilyn Monroe was 36 years old at the time of her death in 1962. She had starred in 22 films and was an internationally renowned actress. A controversial figure throughout her career, Monroe was both beloved by her fans (who sent her up to 5,000 letters a day), and criticized by others as a no-talent blonde bimbo. After her death she became a cultural icon, was the subject of several books, and has been depicted in movies reexamining her life and sudden death.

Monroe was noticeably depressed in the months preceding her death. Toward the end of her life she developed the reputation of being a troubled, petulant, temperamental, pampered star who was almost impossible to work with. Monroe had had psychiatric treatment in an effort to deal with her emotional problems. After two highly publicized divorces (from Yankee baseball great Joe DiMaggio and playwright Arthur Miller), alleged affairs with John and Bobby Kennedy, and the financial failures of her last two movies, Monroe's personal life was in disarray and her movie career in limbo.

In her final weeks Monroe largely lived in isolation in a small Los Angeles bungalow, where she died on the evening of August 5, 1962. Her body was discovered early the next morning (with her hand on her phone, according to some accounts). On the night of her fatal overdose of sleeping pills, Monroe had in fact made calls to her friends and her analyst, all of whom listened, but failed to actively intervene. Psychiatrist Robert Litman did the psychological autopsy for Los Angeles Medical Examiner Theodore Curphey. Litman noted previously failed suicide attempts.

Later, David Phillips (1974) remarked that 7–10 days after Monroe's suicide, the U.S. suicide rate rose 12% over the rate at the same time a year earlier (see Chapter 7, Table 7.2). Phillips went on to claim that "the contagion effect" is about 2–3% on average in adults, but about 6–7% in teens or adolescents. Sanger-Katz (2014) says that it is closer to 5%. The contagion effect following Monroe's suicide was the highest for any celebrity suicide Phillips studied. The systematic empirical study of suicide imitation effects had been launched.

CASE 26.3. Kurt Cobain

The lead singer of the band Nirvana, Kurt Cobain, suicided on April 5, 1994 with a shotgun. He had a heroin abuse problem and other personal and health difficulties. A study of the potential contagion effect failed to support copycat effects of his suicide (Jobes et al., 2000). Jobes et al. (1996) did a time series analysis of Seattle suicide mortality data and utilized a before-and-after study of suicides around Cobain's death in 1994 (Jobes et al., 2000). There was no noticeable increase in suicides following Cobain's death, unlike that of Monroe. The copycat effect thus seems to depend in part on the type of entertainer or celebrity suiciding (Stack, 1987), as well as on the type of responder. For example, the suicide effect for Monroe was greater among white females in their 30s.

However, another study (Jobes et al., 2000) found that suicide crisis calls increased markedly after Cobain's suicide, when compared with the 1993 and 1995 control years for the same time period (see Figure 26.2). This so-called "Cobain effect" speaks to the possibility that Cobain's suicide may have actually inspired young people to reach out for help, rather than to imitate his suicide (see "13 Reasons Why," which seems to have a protective effect).

Source: Compiled by Maris from various sources.

In Chapter 27, I turn to issues involved in suicide litigation, especially those of medical malpractice, jail and prison suicides, contested life insurance claims, psychotropic medications and product liability, manner-of-death determination (e.g., natural, suicide, homicide, or accident), and workers' compensation.

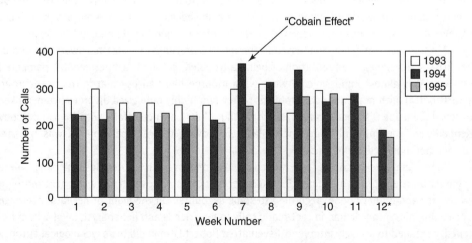

FIGURE 26.2. Suicide crisis calls to the Seattle Crisis Center, 1993, 1994, and 1995. *Source:* Jobes et al. (2000). Copyright © 2000 The Guilford Press. Reprinted with permission.

CHAPTER 27

Forensic Suicidology
A Tort Is the Oldest Antidepressant

> Traditionally, society has felt it was necessary to assign blame
> for every death, either to God (natural or accidental) or to man
> (homicidal or suicidal). If God were the responsible agent, then
> nothing more needed to be done, but if man were to blame,
> there must be punishment for the guilty.
>
> —ROBERT E. LITMAN

For the most part, suicide is not treated as a crime, for the obvious reason that the perpetrator cannot be punished further (Simpson et al., 2015). However, Alvarez (1971) mentions a bizarre case in which a felon sentenced to death slit his own throat the night before his scheduled execution, but was discovered and had his throat sutured, so he could be hanged the next morning. Even though most suicides cannot be punished further, their estates used to be confiscated by the state and their intended inheritances diverted. Today most life insurance policies are rendered null and void, if suicide can be proven within 2 years of the policies' being taken out. Note that the law tends to presume that suicide did not happen (a version of "innocent until proved guilty"). The burden of proof is on a plaintiff who claims that a suicide occurred, and who must demonstrate that the suicide was more likely than not (in civil cases) and/or was the result of malpractice.

In earlier times (see Maris et al., 2000, pp. 480–481, and Chapters 17 and 18 of this book), the suicide's body could be desecrated (e.g., tied to a horse by a rope and dragged around town, or buried at a crossroad to ensure the suicide's soul's perpetual unrest) and denied burial in a Christian cemetery with Christian final rites. Suicides (including priests) were often excommunicated from the Roman Catholic Church. In modern times the church tends to be more compassionate and assert that suicides were temporarily insane (*non compos mentis*), and thus not responsible for their actions.

Although early in Christianity suicide was not condemned or sanctioned (think of Samson, Judas, or even Jesus himself), at least by the time of St. Augustine's *The City of God* (completed by 426 A.D.,), suicide was seen as a violation of the Biblical commandment "Thou shalt do no murder" or "Thou shalt not kill" (see Deuteronomy 5:17 or Exodus 20:13). The assumption was that only God could take a human life, and that his will was often inscrutable (e.g., see the tribulations of Job). Thus, taking your own life was a violation of God's will and plan for you, and constituted the sin of *hubris* (pride). There were also prohibitists of suicide early in church history to discourage overzealous Christian martyrdom.

The epigraph to this chapter by Litman is overly simplistic: People often do blame God for allowing a suicide (especially of an otherwise naïve and innocent young person), and they may even lose their religious faith as a result. Natural deaths are sometimes not all that "natural" and can be hastened due to below-standard medical and/or psychological treatment, for which doctors and counselors can incur liability. Even accidents can be subintentional (as the phrase *accident-prone* suggests) and certainly not the fault of God. Although suicides are intentional, the persons committing suicide may not be in their right minds, and thus may not be accountable for their suicides.

Although suicide is not a crime, assisting suicide is a crime in all but seven states and the District of Columbia. The states are Oregon, Colorado, Washington, Vermont, Montana, Hawaii, and California (this list of states is in flux). There are at least three categories of legal response to assisted suicide (Battin & Mayo, 1980; Humphry & Wickett, 1986; Battin & Joiner, 2018):

1. About 20 states consider assisted suicide murder or a felony (see *People v. Roberts* in Michigan, 1920, and *Gilbert v. State* in Florida, 1986). Occasionally assisting suicide results in sentences of life imprisonment.
2. Twelve states view assisted suicide as manslaughter. Usually the penalty is confinement for 1–10 years.
3. In 11 states, assisted suicide is a separate statutory offense altogether, or it is not illegal under specific circumstances.
   a. Usually assisted suicide is homicide, if the suicide of another is purposely caused by force, duress, or deception.
   b. A person who aids or solicits suicide may be guilty of a second-degree felony (if there is an actual suicide or suicide attempt) or of a misdemeanor (if there is no suicide or attempt).

Usually, but not always, assisting suicide is regarded with empathy by judges and juries. Sentences tend to be minimal. Still, one cannot assist a suicide in most of the United States without fear of legal or professional sanctions.

Scott and Resnik (2012) claim that psychiatrists have about a 50% chance of at least one of their patients' suiciding over their professional careers, and that 22–33% will have at least one medical malpractice lawsuit. Note that about 10–15% of patients with a major psychiatric disorder will eventually die by suicide, especially those hospitalized for major depressive disorder (Bostwick & Pankratz, 2000; Brent et al., 1988).

The Litigation Process

Legal cases involving suicide can be either civil or criminal. Most suicide lawsuits are civil suits or *torts,* which seek financial compensation for individuals who claim to have been injured/damaged or to have suffered losses due to the conduct of others (such as a physician) or a product manufacturer (like a drug company) (Scott & Resnik, 2012). Torts can include (1) strict liability (imposed without proof of due care); (2) intentionality (the individual intended to harm or knows, or should have known harm would result from his or her actions); or (3) negligence (the individual unintentionally caused or substantially contributed to unreasonable risk or harm to another; see the section below on medical malpractice).

In civil cases the standard of proof is more likely than not "a preponderance of the evidence" or "clear and convincing evidence." This is sometimes called in ordinary language the "51% rule." Evidence is presented by the plaintiff/claimant and/or defendant, and may include documents and materials, fact statements, depositions, and expert witnesses' opinions. Then a jury (usually 12 men and/or women selected conjointly by plaintiff and defendant in a *voir dire* process) or a judge (in a bench trial) makes a judgment as to whether the standard has been met and the allegations supported. The judgment can be appealed.

Some suicide cases are criminal, in which the issue is, for example, whether the manner of death was homicide or some variant thereof. Here the standard of proof for the prosecutor and defense is "beyond a reasonable doubt," a much more stringent standard than for torts. It can be called the "98–99% rule."

Suicide cases may be heard in either federal or state courts. Federal cases involve the United States (such as VA medical malpractice claims or suicides in federal prisons) or violations of the U.S. Constitution. Criteria for expert testimony and reporting may vary in federal versus state courts. For example, in federal courts experts must file a Rule 26 expert report and follow specific procedural criteria. In some state courts, no written reports are required.

Most criminal cases are tried in state courts (there are also city, county, and other local courts). Some state courts require that a specific portion of an expert's total time (e.g., at least 51%) be spent in non-litigation-related activities. It is relevant to know how many of an expert's cases are for the plaintiff or defense. Are they biased in favor of one or the other? One could question the credibility of experts' opinions when they testify 100% of the time for either the defense or plaintiff. Possible conflicts of interests are also relevant—for example, if physicians who work for drug companies also testify on behalf of the drug companies' products.

There are variations of the litigation process in different state and federal courts, but in general, the litigation process includes the following:

• *Filing a complaint by the plaintiff(s).* Each complaint lists the plaintiff(s) and defendant(s) (who can be multiple). The facts and chronology of events are also listed (they can be contested by both sides). One or more allegations or *counts* are stated, and the legal basis for them given. Most suicide cases are suits alleging *wrongful death* (which is defined as "the taking of the life of an individual resulting from the willful or negligent act of another person or persons"; in this context, "person" could include a product manufacturer). Later, experts for the plaintiff(s) and defendant(s) testify about whether or not certain actions or omissions caused or substantially contributed to the death or suicide of the decedent. Relevant legal standards may include negligence or gross negligence, deliberate indifference, and violations of the standard of care (all terms are defined below). In some states an attorney has to file an "expert witness certificate of merit report," stating that the lawsuit's claims are worthy of a trial, before a complaint can be filed. Complaints can be amended.

• *Forming and filing answers by both defendant(s) and plaintiff(s).* Various questions are posed by both sides to try to clarify allegations or facts, and the respondents must admit or deny the claims and then give reasons why. Most answers are perfunctory and a waste of time, since respondents tend to say things like "unduly burdensome," "not calculated to lead to useful information," or "see . . ." Early in the litigation process, there can be a *demurrer,* or motion to dismiss.

• *Exchange of interrogatory questions.* Closely related to answers are a series of written questions about specific details of the suicide, the care providers, and/or treatment. Each side is entitled to know in advance the alleged facts of the case and the expected witnesses' testimony.

• *Discovery and assemblage of evidence. Discovery* is a specified period of time during which both sides engage in a systematic exchange of information and anticipated expert and fact witness testimony regarding the standard of care and alleged causation of the suicide, which normally involves the taking of depositions. Depositions can be lengthy and arduous (especially cross-examination). For example, the federal prison case concerning the death in custody of Kenneth Trentadue (see Chapter 22, Case 22.2) involved documents from five different federal agencies, which resulted in enough depositions to fill a garage from ceiling to floor. It was literally impossible to read all the evidence. Expert fees would have been prohibitive; experts can charge from $500 to even $1,000 an hour. In another drug case, there was an expert deposition that lasted for 5 consecutive 8-hour days.

Experts read the evidence, perhaps do interviews (including psychological autopsies) and research, then opine about the lawsuit allegations. Experts may have to be qualified by the court. Interestingly, both plaintiffs and defendants seem to be able to find competent experts for contrary opinions. Experts can have *Daubert* (*Daubert v. Merrill Dow Pharmaceuticals,* 1993) or the older *Frye* (*Frye v. United States,* 1923) hearings to determine the admissibility of their testimony in court. The *Daubert* criteria include about 10 standards for admissible expert testimony (Maris, 2015, pp. 27–33). The court can disallow expert testimony and/or so-called "junk science," but that seldom happens in fact.

Not all documents or testimony may be admitted as evidence in court. Evidence for suicide cases can include medical or hospital records; medical examiners' or coroners' reports (including autopsies, toxicology reports, death certificates, and body and death scene photographs); police incident reports and investigations (with or without scene and body photographs); depositions; psychological autopsies; product descriptions and warnings; computer files; letters and notes (including suicide notes); news accounts; expert reports; policy and procedures manuals of various agencies; pharmacy records; videos; audios of 911 calls; treatment and legal standards; and much more.

Experts often testify whether an action or omission caused or was a substantial proximate factor in an alleged outcome. Causation is hard to prove and is not the same as statistical association (Maris, 2015, pp. 36–37). A psychological autopsy may be used to establish case facts retrospectively (Scott & Resnik, 2012). See Chapter 26, Box 26.1, for items covered in my psychological autopsy form.

- *Motion for summary judgment.* The defense can file a motion claiming that after discovery the plaintiff has not proven or substantiated its claims, and can ask the judge to dismiss the lawsuit. This motion for summary judgment is usually denied and the trial proceeds, although most cases are eventually settled or arbitrated without a trial.

- *Settlement conferences.* Throughout the litigation process, both sides may try to settle the complaint, thus avoiding public guilt, blame, liability and trial expense. Defense attorneys acting as proxies for insurance companies or other clients can have conferences in which monetary awards and damages less than those claimed by the lawsuit can be offered and perhaps agreed to. Experts are not privy to these settlements (especially not the dollar amounts) and in some cases are not even informed that the case has been settled. Frequently settlements will include confidentiality agreements or protective orders prohibiting the parties to the lawsuit from discussing the facts of the case in public. But the intent is often to protect a product or a reputation, not consumers or the public.

- *Case presentation to the court for a trial.* In court, the lawsuit is presented to the *triers of fact,* who are either a jury and judge or just a judge (in a bench trial). Not all lawsuits involve juries; for example, probate cases do not. In the United Kingdom and in Islamic law, all civil trials are heard only by a judge. In the United States, most criminal trials are heard by juries. In a civil trial, a jury of 6–12 members is selected, and then both the plaintiff's and defendant's attorneys present opening arguments and offer fact and expert witnesses who are cross-examined. The judge periodically gives the jury instructions; for example, juries are told not to discuss the case outside of court, not to watch news accounts of the trial, and sometimes to ignore some testimony. The judge may remove the jury from the courtroom at times or occasionally dismiss a juror from a case. After attorneys' closing arguments, the jury deliberates and announces or publishes its verdict. Usually a consensus is required of the jurors. Verdicts must be unanimous in federal court cases and in almost all criminal state trials. However, in civil trials about one-third of states require a simple majority verdict; verdict requirements for civil trials vary in other states. The judge then makes a judgment on the case allegations, essentially finding for the plaintiff or defendant, and determines awards or punishments. Sometimes a jury cannot agree on a verdict (a *hung jury*), and there may be mistrials, retrials, juror removals and substitutions, and appeals.

- *Judgment.* Note that in court, the opinions of attorneys, experts, juries, and judges (in concert with the law) decide an issue or allegations, not science—although the court tries to avoid "junk science" and to be impartial and objective. Thus, a court judgment may be different from what is in fact true.

* *Appeal(s).* The losing party in a decision by a court is usually entitled to appeal to a separate federal or state appellate court. The grounds for an appeal normally involve deviation from due process, distorted or wrong facts, inadequate representation, errors of law, or the like.

Medical Malpractice

Rightly or wrongly, when someone suicides, family members and survivors tend to blame caregivers rather than themselves, fate, or no one. If a caregiver is deemed to have acted below the standard of care, one or more breaches of duty in care have occurred through acts of omission or commission, and the patient's or person's suicide can be argued to have directly and proximately resulted from this breach or breaches, then that action can be considered *malpractice* (literally, "bad practice"; *Black's Law Dictionary*, 2009). Although we commonly say "medical malpractice," malpractice concerns not only physicians, but also psychologists, social workers, advanced practice nurses, counselors, and other care providers.

The legal standard of care is somewhat vague and elusive. It can vary considerably among clinicians. There is no one, unequivocal standard of care agreed on by all practitioners. Usually, the *standard of care* is defined generically as "what a reasonable and prudent professional, practitioner, or person would or should have done in same or similar circumstances" (*Black's Law Dictionary*, 2009). Both plaintiff and defense seem to be able to retain competent experts who say, "I'm a reasonable and prudent professional," and then proffer diametrically opposed opinions about proper clinical care.

Fortunately, in addition to opinions about standards of care by licensed and certified professionals, there are also several formal, fairly consensual lists of standards of care criteria for each professional specialty. Here are some examples:

1. The American Psychiatric Association's *Practice Guideline for the Assessment and Treatment of Patients with Suicidal Behaviors* (Jacobs et al., 2003, 2010).
2. The American Psychological Association's (2014) *Guidelines for Psychological Practice in Healthcare Delivery Systems.*
3. Policy and procedures manuals for various disciplines and institutions, such as the *Minimum Standards for Local Detention Facilities in South Carolina* (South Carolina Association of Counties, 2013).

Most major disciplines (social work, nursing, counseling, public health, etc.) and institutions (hospitals, jails, prisons, outpatient facilities, etc.) all have their own written standards of care, which professionals and staff members are expected to be trained in and to follow in practice.

Often in a medical malpractice lawsuit, a clinician or practitioner can be accused of negligence. *Negligence* occurs when a clinician's behavior unintentionally causes or contributes to an unreasonable risk of harm to a patient or other person

(Scott & Resnik, 2012). The essential elements required to establish medical negligence include four words that all start with the letter *D* (viz., Dereliction of Duty leading Directly to Damages; Scott & Resnik, 2012).

Some possible derelictions of duty include the following (Bongar et al., 1998, p. 156):

1. Failure to predict, foretell, or diagnose the suicide. However, one cannot accurately predict individual suicides in short time frames; there would be too many false positives.
2. Failure to control, supervise, or restrain.
3. Failure to utilize proper evaluations to assess suicide ideation or behavior. For example, usually a clinician cannot just ask a patient whether he or she has suicide or homicide ideation.
4. Failure to medicate properly. This includes being aware of serious adverse effects or events; monitoring the patient or inmate closely at first or whenever changing medications or doses; advising the patient and/or family of FDA warnings; knowing proper dosages and possible drug interactions; knowing the patient's drug history and possible reactions; making sure the patient is complying with the prescribed doses in a timely manner; asking about concurrently ingested street drugs; conducting proper follow-up; and much more.
5. Failure to observe and monitor the patient appropriately. (The best method is 24/7 watch within arm's reach.) This might also include failure to tell the patient when to go to the emergency room, and/or to give the patient the clinician's contact information.)
6. Failure to take an adequate history or get prior medical records.
7. Failure to suicide-proof an inpatient or inmate environment, or to remove dangerous objects and architecture. Failure to put the patient in a secure, safe environment. Does the patient have a roommate or cellmate? As noted in earlier chapters, however, almost no environment is totally suicide-proof.

In Case 27.1, Jacob Fineburg's family practice doctor was accused of causing an unreasonable risk of harm to an elderly depressed patient by allowing him to get about 4½ times the amount of Valium he himself had ordered, and by not even seeing the patient face to face. In Case 27.2, the VA assessed John Roberts to be a "high suicide risk" but then did not treat him accordingly, or so the complaint alleged.

CASE 27.1. Jacob Fineburg

Jacob Fineburg was a 67-year-old white Jewish male who shot himself in his left temple on Monday April 18, 2016, in his condominium in Charlotte, North Carolina. The police found 20 bottles of medications at his home, including Valium, Trileptal, Ascomp (a barbiturate), Desyrel, Wellbutrin, and Butalbital (another barbiturate). There were also seven suicide notes. The coroner's toxicology report showed that Fineburg had Butalbital (7.6 mcg), Valium (5,100 ng), codeine (3,300 ng), and morphine (330 ng) in his blood at the time of death.

After his Georgia businesses failed (he was a college graduate and had gone to law school), Fineburg moved to Charlotte and lived in a condo near his son. He had several heated arguments with other condo residents. Fineburg complained that "everything was wrong" with him. He had had quadruple bypass surgery, right-knee replacement, lumbar disc pain, and chest pain. His psychiatric diagnoses included altered mental state, a personality disorder, bipolar disorder, and major depressive disorder. His primary diagnosis was major depressive disorder.

When Fineburg moved to North Carolina, his family doctor in Georgia (Joseph Greenberg, whom he had known well and socialized with for many years) continued to write Fineburg prescriptions without seeing him face to face. The prescriptions were mainly for Valium and barbiturates. Greenberg also authorized 11 inappropriate early refills. Between February 2015 and February 2016, Greenberg gave Fineburg 1,610 Valium pills (10 mg), which amounted to about 4½ pills a day, even though his prescriptions specified one 10-mg pill each day.

The complaint alleged unreasonable ordering and filling of prescription medicine (especially Valium) by Fineburg's primary care doctor, which in turn caused or substantially contributed to Fineburg's suicidal death. Valium can initiate or exacerbate depressive disorder and have a disinhibiting effect. The complaint said that Fineburg's death was reasonably foreseeable under the circumstances. The case was settled.

Source: I testified in this case as an expert witness. Names, dates, and places have all been changed to protect the privacy of all parties.

CASE 27.2. John Roberts

John Roberts was a 25-year-old white male Iraq veteran who was found shot to death in his home on June 2, 2012. He had been out drinking the night before his death. His blood alcohol level at death was 0.232% (about four times the legal limit in South Carolina). He lived in Charleston. Recently John had been upset about getting a DUI citation and had been having girlfriend problems.

John had served a 7-month stint in Iraq, where he worked in a mortuary service. He later developed traumatizing memories, sleep problems, and nightmares, and was diagnosed with PTSD by the VA. Back home, he frequently got into bar fights and had to go to the emergency room for treatment.

John had 45 contacts with the VA in less than 1 year. However, he missed 47% of his hospital appointments. He had a long history of substance abuse, especially of alcohol. The VA treated John with Celexa, Vistaril, Ativan, Risperdal, Haldol, and Librium tapers for detox, plus individual psychotherapy.

In roughly 7 months of treatment, John saw the VA suicide prevention coordinator, psychiatrists, the Operation Iraqi Freedom coordinator, social workers, nurses, and psychologists. He was evaluated as a "high suicide risk" just 7 days before his suicide and had been given inpatient treatment for 8 days in the past. All guns were ordered removed from his home, which his grandfather in fact did.

John was kicked out of college for failing grades (some in repeat courses) and lost his job. He became increasingly depressed. While an inpatient at the VA, John was put on close observation. His primary VA diagnoses were alcohol dependence and anxiety and depressive disorders. The police and family reported that John might have died while playing Russian roulette.

The lawsuit claimed wrongful death, failure to monitor, failure to assess suicide risk, failure to protect, failure to properly train staff, improper policies and procedures, negligence and gross negligence, and recklessness/carelessness. The case was settled without a trial.

Source: This was a VA medical malpractice case in which I testified. Names, dates, and places have been changed.

Gross negligence is different from simple negligence. While *simple negligence* is a mere failure to exercise reasonable care, *gross negligence* is a carelessness and reckless disregard for the safety or lives of others, which is so great that it appears to be a conscious act of ignoring another person's safety. For example, there was a jail suicide in which an inmate was attempting to hang himself in his cell, and other inmates shouted out, "C. P. is trying to hang himself!" The jailer replied, "Shut the f— up," and then turned on the air conditioning to drown out the inmates' shouts. C. P. died from anoxic brain damage.

Finally, there can be other categories of derelictions. A clinician or jail/prison staff can be thought to exhibit *deliberate indifference* to the serious medical needs of a patient or inmate. Deliberate indifference, unlike negligence, implies at a minimum that defendants were placed on notice of a danger and chose to ignore it in spite of the notice (see *www.duhaime.org*). For example, suppose a psychiatric inpatient hospital was reviewed by the Joint Commission (an organization for the accreditation of hospitals; *www.jointcommission.org*) and was told in writing to remove phones with cords from the inpatient wards, but thereafter a patient hanged him- or herself with a phone cord.

Manner-of-Death Determination

Eventually, every one of us will have our own death certificate. Under manner of death, the coroner or medical examiner will have to check a box for *natural, accidental, suicidal,* or *homicidal*—the *NASH* classification. Other possibilities include *pending,* and *unknown* or *indeterminable.* Table 27.1 shows that the vast majority of all deaths are (1) natural (especially from heart disease, cancer, stroke, and respiratory failure), followed in order by (2) accidents, (3) suicides, and (4) homicides. In 5–20% of all deaths, the manner of death is uncertain (Scott & Resnik, 2012).

The manner of death can have major monetary and psychosocial implications. Accidents, suicides, and homicides are all unnatural and fairly sudden deaths. Accidents occur at a rate of 39.4 per 100,000 per year and are unintentional and unexpected for the most part. In Case 27.3, Daniella Steinhaus probably died by accident while performing an autoerotic act on herself. If her death was autoerotic, then suing for medical malpractice would become less tenable.

CASE 27.3. Daniella Steinhaus

Daniella Steinhaus was a 39-year-old white female from Jacksonville, Florida. College-educated and attractive, she worked as an event planner. In April 2014, she was found kneeling on her bed without underwear on, and her hands together beneath her vagina. She was hanged from a ceiling fan by a cord loosely fitted around her neck. It would not have obstructed her airways or arteries if she had not leaned forward. Her blood alcohol level was 0.251% when she was found the next day (Sunday). The question was whether to certify her death as a suicide or an accident (autoerotic asphyxia).

Daniella had been out drinking on a date at a local bar the Saturday night before her death and was brought home by her brother (she was temporarily living with her brother and his girlfriend). Although she was being treated for major depression, had also been diagnosed with DSM-IV alcohol dependence, and was taking the SNRI antidepressant Pristiq, she had no prior suicide attempts. In the past few years, she had also taken Prozac, Zoloft, and Wellbutrin. She did admit to intermittent suicide ideation. No suicide note was found.

Steinhaus had been married twice before and divorced once. She was separated from her second husband (who was living in Europe at the time) and was currently living with her brother. Daniella had a history of being very sexual and promiscuous, engaging in orgies, having a false "slut" name, watching porn, and using dildos.

At first, the coroner certified Daniella's death as an accident (autoerotic asphyxiation). But later (at the urging of her family), the manner of death was changed to *pending,* with none of the NASH boxes checked on the death certificate. The family believed that Daniella's death was a suicide and wanted to file a medical malpractice lawsuit against the treating advanced practice nurse and clinic.

Source: This was another case in which I testified as an expert witness. All names, dates, and places have been changed.

Suicide (12.3 per 100,000 in 2011) is intentional and is still widely stigmatized by the general public, in part due to its high association with mental disorder. Furthermore, a life insurance policy is usually null and void if suicide occurs within 2 years of the date of issuance, as noted earlier. An important forensic question in regard to manner of death is how to distinguish a suicide from either an accident or a homicide. Table 27.2 suggests several criteria for determining a suicide.

TABLE 27.1. Death Rates per 100,000 for Natural, Accidental, Suicidal, and Homicidal Manners of Death: United States, 2011

Manner or disease of death	Rate per 100,000
1. Heart	191.4
2. Cancer	184.6
3. Respiratory	46.0
4. Cardiovascular (incl. stroke)	41.4
5. **Accident**	39.4
6. Alzheimer's/other dementia	27.2
7. Diabetes	23.5
8. Influenza/pneumonia	17.2
9. Nephritis (kidney disease)	14.7
10. **Suicide**	12.3
11. Septicemia (infection)	11.4
12. Liver	10.8
13. Hypertension	8.8
14. Parkinson's	7.4
15. **Homicide**	4.6
16. All others	184.6

Source: Centers for Disease Control and Prevention (CDC; *www.cdc. gov*). Data in the public domain.

TABLE 27.2. Checklist for Possible Suicide, Behavior, and Mental State

1. Autopsy and death certificate indicates self-inflicted death.

2. Toxicology report specifies self-inflicted harm, such as toxic overdose levels of drugs.

3. Statements by witnesses of suicide intent.

4. Police conclude suicide was manner of death in incident report.

5. Behavior, lifestyle, personality suggest suicide.

6. Life conditions suggest suicide (being desperate, feeling boxed in, death or suicide of another, etc.).

7. Actions, if done, indicate high probability or lethality of death outcomes.

8. Presence of suicide ideation, especially repeated, prolonged ideation.

9. Sudden change in affect or emotion, especially anger, rage, or impulsivity.

10. Serious depression or other mental disorder (including intense anxiety and/or psychosis).

11. Oral or written (such as suicide notes) expressions of intent to die, including computer notes or searches and phone messages.

12. Expressed hopelessness to others.

13. Stressful events and/or significant losses, especially recently.

14. Family instability or turmoil.

15. Interpersonal conflict, including separation and/or divorce.

16. History of poor physical health, chronic pain, and/or abuse of pain medications.

Source: Adapted from Scott and Resnik (2012, p. 549). Adapted with permission from *The American Psychiatric Publishing Textbook of Suicide Assessment and Management,* Second Edition. (Copyright © 2012) American Psychiatric Association. All Rights Reserved.

A final thing to remember in determining suicide is that homicide (4.6 per 100,000) is normally contraintended; that is, the victim does not want to be killed or to die. A possible grey area is so-called "suicide by cop," which is a homicide but also can be a form of suicide. There was a trial in remote Alaska (*Sawyer v. State,* 2011) in which a young married woman appeared to have overdosed, but the jury ruled that her husband had in fact killed her and just made her death look like a suicide.

Contested Life Insurance

Average life expectancies for Americans in 2010 were about 79.7 years overall, 76.5 and 81.3 for white men and women, and 71.8 and 78.0 for black men and women. Monetary obligations and responsibilities tend to be based on the assumption that people will reach their approximate life expectancies. Such things as 30-year mortgages, multiyear college tuition commitments, long-term investments, and general lifestyle are predicated on living a certain number of years and reaping expected life incomes.

People can take out either *term* (in force for a limited time) or *whole* (like a savings account) life insurance to cover some of their unanticipated or premature financial losses. But they cannot profit from killing themselves (suicide) or others (homicide); for example, they cannot plan to have their families gain monetarily from their suicide, or to inherit an estate or others' life insurance proceeds after murdering them. For example, the 2-year suicide exclusion clause for most life insurance policies reads something like this: "If the insured, whether sane or insane, shall within two years from the date of issue hereof die as a result of suicide, the company's liability shall be limited to payment in one sum of the amount of premiums paid on the policy, less any debt owed to the company."

Because of this suicide clause, accurately determining a person's manner of death becomes very important. For example, if a car suicide is disguised to look like an accident, then the insurance beneficiaries may receive double indemnity (twice the policy value). But if it is clearly a suicide, then the beneficiaries may get virtually nothing. Furthermore, if a beneficiary murders the policy holder and tries to make it appear as an accident, then he or she may spend the rest of life in prison, or even be executed.

Not all exclusion clauses are for 2 years. Insurance companies know the average suicide rate of their policy holders, as well as the average amount of life insurance they take out and for how many years. It is then fairly easy to calculate the required number of years for a suicide exclusion (say, 2), in order to cover the company's unexpected losses.

With a 2-year suicide exclusion clause, a person can wait 2 years and 1 day before suiciding, and so turn a relatively small amount of money into (say) $1 million. For example, let us assume that a man age 25 has a 30-year term life policy that costs him about $650 a year ($800 per year if age 35, and $1,900 a year if 45). By suiciding in 2+ years, he could turn $1,300 into $1 million for his estate. Because of this suicide loophole, some insurance companies nullify a life policy if there is a suicide at any time.

It is hard to imagine a would-be suicide's being Machiavellian enough to hang in there for 2 years before suiciding. But it does happen. There was a case of a federal judge in the southeastern United States who was in major debt. A few days after 2 years of his purchasing a large term life insurance policy, his family said that he went out into his backyard early in the morning with a handgun to check for a possible intruder, only to trip, fall, and shoot himself right between his eyes (a contact wound). In another interesting life insurance case (see Case 27.4), the issue was whether a man named Arthur McClay Watkins died in a motor vehicle accident or suicided.

CASE 27.4. Arthur McClay Watkins

Arthur McClay ("Clay") Watkins was a 56-year-old white male who had graduated from UCLA, held a master's degree in psychology, and was a licensed marriage and family counselor. He was also the president of a local Rotary Club. Although he worked in the aerospace industry, he was also a very accomplished professional banjo player (he appeared on many YouTube videos, most of which seem to have been taken down in the years since his death). Over the years Clay suffered from depressive disorder, for which he variously took Celexa, Prozac, and Wellbutrin.

His therapist reported that Clay had serious financial problems. He embezzled large sums of money from a family trust fund intended for him and his siblings (he was the executor). In desperation, he donned a ski mask, got a .45 pistol, and committed armed robbery in daylight at a local Wells Fargo bank.

As his world was collapsing, he posted 18 videos on YouTube between January 29, 2014, and February 1, 2014. The February 1 YouTube post was a lengthy life review of his background and family history. That same day, he took out a large life insurance policy. The very next day (February 2, 2014), Clay drove his van over a seaside cliff and fell 450 feet to his death. A witness just behind Clay said that the vehicle accelerated into a barrier and that the driver did not apply the brakes. Later inspection found no mechanical failures in the van. Was this an accident or a suicide?

Source: All case information from public records, newspaper stories, and (now removed) YouTube videos.

Jail and Prison Suicides

Suicide is the leading cause of death in American jails (Hayes, 2010), but not in prisons (in part since the prison population tends to be older, stay there longer, and have a greater proportion of African Americans). Jail and prison suicides have been examined in great detail in Chapter 22 (above) and are not reexamined in depth here.

Legal issues for jail suicides tend to focus on (1) inadequate or poorly followed policy and procedures manuals (including substandard or too infrequent training in suicide standards and procedures; e.g., for South Carolina, see South Carolina Association of Counties, 2013); (2) poor suicide assessment (jail or prison personnel cannot just ask inmates if they are suicidal and then simply let them deny it); (3) substandard observation or suicide watch (a 15-minute watch is too long, since it takes only 4–5 minutes to hang oneself); (4) failure to suicide-proof jails or provide a safe environment; (5) substandard medical and psychiatric treatment (including failure to medicate appropriately); (6) violations of the Eighth (no cruel and unusual punishment) and Fourteenth (right to equal protection and due process) Amendments to the U.S. Constitution; and (7) deliberate indifference, negligence, and gross negligence.

For example, as described in Chapter 13, Case 13.2, inmate Franklyn Thornwell was not watched constantly as ordered; he was allowed to keep his street clothes (and was not given a suicide safety smock); and he was not given his antipsychotic medication.

Product Liability

All manufacturers can produce a product that may be dangerous, defective, or otherwise harmful to their consumers, and then fail to warn them, to protect them, or to withdraw the product from the market. If the products actually produce, cause, or substantially and proximately contribute to damages, then the consumers may be entitled to monetary compensation.

For example, on September 14, 2004 (for pediatric patients) and December 13, 2006 (for adults up to age 24), the U.S. FDA ordered black-box suicidality warnings for nine antidepressants to be placed at the very front of these products' package insert descriptions (Maris, 2015, p. 63). Similar FDA warnings have been issued for mood stabilizers and anxiolytics. *Suicidality* in this context refers to a suicidal outcome (both ideational and behavioral) rated on a 7-point scale (see Maris, 2015, p. 6); it ranges from completed suicide to suicide attempt, preparatory actions, self-injurious behavior with or without intent, suicide ideation, and other behaviors (like accidents).

Some of the alleged suicidogenic adverse drug effects include (1) *de novo* or increased suicide ideation after drug ingestion, (2) worsened or induced depressive disorders and anhedonia, (3) an inner and outer extreme restlessness called *akathisia,* (4) ego-dystonia or character change (i.e., the person is not his or her usual self after drug ingestion), (5) *de novo* or increased aggression and/or paradoxical rage, (6) emotional blunting or psychotic-like behavior, (7) feeling overly sedated and lethargic, (8) various sleep disorders, (9) new hypomanic episodes, (10) increased feeling of hopelessness, (11) sexual dysfunctions (such as lack of sexual desire or impotency), (12) addiction (especially to the benzodiazepines or pain medications), (13) impaired cognition, (14) chemical imbalances in the brain neurosystems (such as the serotonergic system), (15) nausea (especially early in drug use), and (16) behavioral changes (weight gain, withdrawal sensations [such as alleged shock sensations when stopping Paxil], etc.).

Clinical trial data have often shown that these adverse drug effects statistically significantly increase the probability of suicidality in a small, vulnerable minority of antidepressant drug users. For example, in Case 27.5 it was claimed that 18-year-old John Sterling became more depressed and anxious, more withdrawn and emotionally blunted, delusional, akathisic, tremorous, sleep-disordered, depersonalized, and hopeless after being treated for dysthymia with Lexapro, and that these alleged antidepressant adverse effects contributed significantly to his fatal suicide attempt.

CASE 27.5. John Sterling

John Sterling, a white male age 18, was a recent high school graduate who jumped to his death on June 18, 2015, from the Delaware Memorial Bridge near Wilmington. At the top of its towers, the bridge is 440 feet high. He had been visiting his brother the week before jumping and was now returning home on I-95.

John was on the bridge from about 11 P.M. on June 17 until 2:27 A.M. on June 18. The police spoke with John for about 15–20 minutes before he jumped. Curiously (was he ambivalent?), he was wearing a lifejacket and even began swimming the backstroke after he jumped. Sadly, John eventually drowned and was pronounced dead at 3:27 A.M. He left several suicide notes in his truck on the bridge.

John's toxicology report was negative for alcohol, but positive (48 ng/ml) for an antidepressant (and for some marijuana and a barbiturate). John had recently been diagnosed with dysthymia in his senior year of high school and had been missing many classes or being tardy at school. His physician prescribed 10 mg of an SSRI antidepressant. After taking it for 2 days,

John complained of nausea, dizziness, and headaches. His doctor cut the dose in half, but a week later resumed the 10-mg dose.

John's parents claimed that within 7 to 30 days after starting the SSRI, (1) John's depression and anxiety got worse, (2) he became withdrawn and unreachable, (3) his suicide notes reflected psychotic delusions and paranoia, (4) he became extremely agitated and starting pacing around the house (akathisia), (5) he had uncontrollable hand tremors, (6) he had trouble sleeping, (7) he became depersonalized and complained of feeling "dead," and (8) he became extremely hopeless.

After his death John's parents sued the manufacturer of the SSRI antidepressant, claiming that it caused or proximately and substantially contributed to the above-described serious adverse drug effects, which in turn contributed to or caused John's fatal suicide attempt. The case was settled.

Drug product liability suicide cases are hard to prove, since many other non-medication-related risk factors could cause suicide by themselves. In John's case, these included his depressive disorder itself, stress (John had been benched on his high school basketball team his senior year), anxiety, and substance abuse (he had marijuana and a barbiturate in his blood at death, not just the SSRI). Any of these risk factors could cause suicide, independently of any possible psychiatric drug effects.

Source: This was another case in which I testified as an expert witness. All names, places, and dates have been changed.

Products possibly related to suicide can include not only (1) drugs, but also (2) cars, (3) railroads, (4) airplanes, (5) seagoing vessels, (6) defective parts, (7) substandard services, and many more. For example, a surprising number (2.7% in one study; Huffine, 1971) of single-occupant motor vehicle fatal crashes may be disguised suicides in which the "accidents" are attributed to mechanical failures, road or weather conditions, not to suicide intent (Jenkins, 1980). Maris et al. (2000) described a case (under the fictitious names of *Wade v. Transcontinental Railroad*) in which a railroad company was sued for not locking its trains' exit doors and not warning passengers that they could fall out of the trains. In a case described in Chapter 21 (Case 21.12), EgyptAir Flight 990 crashed just outside Kennedy Airport in New York City. One issue in the ensuing litigation was the possible mechanical failure of a Boeing airplane versus murder–suicide by the pilot. There was also a suit against the owners of a Northwest-based crabbing boat (*Karmin v. The Valiant*, 2014) in which it was alleged that a crab pot hit a workman while at sea (giving him a concussion), and a claim that the injury later caused his serious suicide attempt: He shot himself in the face. In yet another case (service liability), a young girl got a deforming *Pseudomonas* ear infection from having her ear pierced and then later killed herself.

Workers' Compensation

Workers' compensation is a form of insurance providing wage replacement and medical benefits to employees injured during their employment, in exchange for the workers' relinquishing the right to sue their employers for negligence. Weekly deductions can be taken from the workers' wages to cover their compensation benefits. Dependents of workers killed or suiciding during their employment may be entitled to financial benefits similar to a kind of life insurance. Two workers' compensation cases in which employers were accused of responsibility for the suicides of employees are described in Cases 27.6 and 27.7.

CASE 27.6. *Wilson v. South Carolina Electric & Gas*

Over the years, I have had several workers' compensation cases in which employers were alleged to have caused or contributed to their employees' suicides. For example, in *Wilson v. South Carolina Electric & Gas* (1998), an electrical engineer killed himself in 1998 after months of extreme stress, work overload, and psychic strain. The company used to have two electrical engineers in the unit, but after one of the engineers died, the company refused to replace him and instead gave the entire workload of both previous engineers to the one who had continued working. When the remaining engineer suicided, his wife sued the company for workers' compensation for the death of her husband.

Source: This was another case in which I testified as an expert witness. All names, places, and dates have been changed.

CASE 27.7. *Credit Information Company v. Jones et al.*

In another workers' compensation case (*Credit Information Company v. Jones et al.,* 2005), a data-processing company in Salt Lake City had to update data for about 40% of all Visa and Mastercard transactions in the United States each night before the banks and markets opened the next day. There was a large wall of computer screens in what the company called the "War Room," which indicated computer programs that were processing properly (in green) and those that were not (in red). Some employees were at work 24 hours, 7 days a week. There was constant pressure not only to keep the system functioning properly, but also to increase the company's stock market value. When six company vice-presidents killed themselves within 8 weeks, several of their widows filed workers' compensation claims against the company for its alleged suicidogenic working conditions.

Source: This was another case in which I testified as an expert witness. All names, places, and dates have been changed.

School Suicides

A failure to implement and uphold policies and procedures designed to protect and safeguard students makes schools and their personnel vulnerable if a death (particularly a suicide) results. Case 27.8 describes a case in which a school band director was implicated in the suicide of a student with whom he had been having a sexual relationship.

CASE 27.8. Gillian Garrido-Lecca

In *Dade County v. Crear,* a 45-year-old African American band director at Palmetto High School, George Crear III, was accused of having sex with four of his teenage students—a violation of trust and exploitation of the student–teacher relationship with young, vulnerable adolescents.

One of the students, 16-year-old Gillian ("Gigi") Garrido-Lecca, shot herself in the chest in 1992, after Crear spurned her for another student. Gigi's parents blamed Crear for their daughter's suicide. Later, three other female students of Crear's testified that he also seduced them, with devastating psychological consequences. It turned out that Crear's background had not been properly investigated before he took the job at Palmetto High School; he had left his previous job in Flint, Michigan, due to similar suspicions. He had had a sexual affair with a 13-year-old middle school band member in Flint. The Michigan charges were originally dropped, since the 6-year statute of limitations had expired.

In Miami, Crear was put in jail for 2 years while awaiting trial. Surprisingly, on February 12, 1997, Crear was acquitted of three counts of sexual activity with a child. One family member at trial shouted, "May you rot in hell, Crear!" However, he was subsequently extradited to Michigan and retried there.

Source: All names, dates, and places have been previously published in the South Florida *Sun-Sentinel* newspaper (*http://articles.sun-sentinel.com/1997-02-12/news/9702120030_1_band-teacher-verdict-s-decision*). No confidential information has been cited here.

The next and concluding chapter, Chapter 28, summarizes the other chapters and states the major conclusions of the book.

PART VIII

SUMMARY
AND CONCLUSIONS

CHAPTER 28

What Have We Learned?

According to my lights, a last chapter should resemble a primitive
orgy after harvest. The work may have come to an end, but the worker
cannot let go all at once. He is still full of energy that will fester, if
it cannot find an outlet. Accordingly, he is allowed a time of license,
when he may say all sorts of things he would think twice before
saying in more sober moments, when he is no longer bound strictly by
logic and evidence but free to speculate on what he has done.

—GEORGE CASPER HOMANS

Most suicide textbooks (e.g., Maris et al., 2000; Hawton, 2005; Wasserman & Wasserman, 2009; and Simon & Hales, 2012; Nock et al., 2014) do not have much of a chapter providing a summary and conclusions. One reason for this is that they do not have an integrated, overarching theory of suicide or suicidology. Rather, they are mainly edited collections of disciplinary chapters on various suicide topics. Admittedly, in the last analysis readers will take home what they need or are interested in, not what they are told they should attend to. However, I have tried in this book to present a consistent, unified approach to suicidology, which makes it easier to attempt to summarize it.

Summary of the Book

This book is organized into sections and chapters that cover the following topics:

A. Foundations (Part I).
- Definitions.
- Concepts.
- Theories.
- Commonalities and Differences.
- Classification and Types (especially of suicide ideation, nonfatal suicide attempts, and completed suicides).
- Explanations and a General Model of Suicide.

487

B. Data, Research, and Assessment (Part II).
- Evidence-Based Suicidology.
- Measurement Issues: Risk Factors and Risk Assessment.

C. Sociodemographic Issues (Part III).
- Age, Lifespan, and Suicidal Careers.
- Sex, Gender, and Marital Status.
- Social Relations.
- International Variation, Ethnicity, and Race.
- Suicide Attempts, Methods, and Notes.

D. Mental Disorders, Biology, and Neurobiology (Part IV).
- Mental Disorders and Hopelessness.
- Major Depression.
- Bipolar Disorder.
- Schizophrenia. and Psychotic Disorders
- Personality Disorders.
- Alcoholism and Other Substance Abuse.
- Biogenics of the Brain.

E. Religion, Culture, History, Art, and Ethics (Part V).
- God, the Afterlife, Religious Factors, and Culture.
- Suicide in History and Art.
- Ethical Issues, Euthanasia, and Rational Suicide.

F. Special Topics (Part VI).
- Suicide in the Military: War, Aggression, and PTSD.
- Murder–Suicide.
- Jail and Prison Suicides.

G. Treatment and Prevention (Part VII).
- Treatment and Intervention: Pharmacology and Psychotherapy.
- Prevention.
- Postvention.
- Litigation.

H. Summary and Conclusions (Part VIII).

Major Issues Considered in the Assessment and Treatment of Suicide

In this section, I summarize the book's major research results and the theories that may explain them. Nevertheless, it is difficult to reduce the richness and diversity of an entire book to a few empirical generalizations. Here I focus is on some selected assessment and treatment issues raised by the book . They are the following::

- What is being assessed or treated?
- Multivariate interdisciplinary models and the comorbidity of suicide.
- Timing issues.
- The problem of rare behavior.
- False positives and false negatives.

- Tools for suicide assessment.
- Implications for treatment and suicide prevention.

What Is Being Assessed or Treated?

We can never predict individual suicides with any degree of accuracy, especially in the short run (Simon & Hales, 2006, 2012; Mundt et al., 2013; Green et al., 2015; Gilbert et al., 2011). We can only predict group suicide risk over fairly long time frames, usually years, says Motto (1992). We often settle for putting an individual into a "high-suicide-risk" group. For example, 10–15% of those with mood disorders (especially major depression or bipolar disorder) eventually suicide, particularly if they were hospitalized. Thus, lifetime suicide risk can go from 1 in 10,000 in the general population to 10–15% in those with mood disorders, though there is never more than about a 1% suicide risk per year, even in so-called "high-suicide-risk" groups. In individual suicide risk prediction, there are unacceptably high rates of false positives, that is, suicide is predicted but there is no suicide. Pokorny (1983, 1992) says there are about 30% false positives (see below) and 44% false negatives (in which no suicide is predicted but suicide occurs).

If no suicide was predicted for every individual assessed, the prediction would be right almost all of the time. Do not forget that a 1 in 10,000 suicide rate per year also means 9,999 *non*suicides (per 10,000) each year. When prediction settles for patient diagnostic groups with high or higher suicide risk (e.g., those with major depression or bipolar disorder), certain preferred treatments, medications, interventions, and suicide prevention strategies follow. For example, symptoms and assessment lead to diagnosis, which in turn leads to medications and treatment: $[Sx + Ax] \rightarrow Dx \rightarrow [Rx + Tx]$.

Most professionals see suicide assessment and treatment through their own disciplinary blinders (an "occupational psychosis," if you will). Remember that a suicidal outcome or dependent variable is not one single thing. For example, the FDA (cf. Posner et al., 2007) "suicidality" outcome is rated on a 7-point scale. One basic suicidality continuum is from (1) different types of completed suicides, to (2) types of nonfatal suicide attempts, to (3) preparatory actions, to (4 and 5) *parasuicides* (self-injurious behaviors with and without suicidal intent, respectively), to (6) suicide ideas with or without specific plans, and to (7) other behaviors (accidental death, natural death, not enough information, or no suicidal ideas or behaviors at all).

Multivariate Interdisciplinary Models and the Comorbidity of Suicide

The independent or explanatory variables of suicidality are complex and varied, too. How many risk and protective factors for suicide are there (Desjardins et al., 2016; Szanto et al., 2018; O'Neill et al., 2018)? I have listed 15 risk factors (see Chapters 3 and 4), but there could be hundreds (Plutchik, 2000; Jacobs et al., 2003, 2010). The more predictor variables one has and the rarer the suicidal outcomes, the larger and more well-designed the research sample has to be to guarantee what is termed *statistical power* (i.e., a targeted statistical probability of detecting true positives). Which independent variables are salient for which purposes? I have talked a lot in this book about my 15 suicide risk factors and Shneidman's 10 commonalities (which unfortunately are not operationally defined), but how are suicide risk factors weighted? What is their relative importance in contributing to a suicide outcome? How much variance (such as R^2) in suicidality does each factor explain in which models?

Psychiatric disorders like major depression and bipolar disorder are very important in determining suicide outcome. Forty-seven percent of my Chicago 5-year suicide sample was at least moderately depressed (Maris, 1981). Alcoholism and other substance abuse are also important; they were factors for 25% of Robins's (1981) St. Louis suicide sample. Prior suicide attempts are important for a suicide outcome in some groups, but not in others. For example, 88% of older white male suicides in Chicago made only one (fatal) suicide attempt. Having suicide ideas with a specific, rehearsed, lethal plan and available means are significant in determining a suicide outcome, although about 20% of the general population think about suiciding in a given year.

My general model of suicide (see Chapter 2, Figure 2.1) focuses on four overlapping interdisciplinary domains of suicide risk variables: (1) psychiatric diagnoses, (2) biology (including genetics and neurobiology), (3) personality/psychology, and (4) sociology/economics/culture. Both Joiner (2005, 2010) and I (Maris, 1981, 2015) think that suicides have what I have called "suicidal careers" over longish time frames (and what Joiner calls "the acquired ability to inflict lethal self-injury"), including a positive family history for suicide and/or mental disorder.

Timing Issues

Even if clinicians suspect with some certainty that a particular individual will eventually suicide or at least engage in self-destructive behaviors, they almost never know *when* this will occur (cf. Millner et al., 2017; Gilbert et al., 2011; Annor et al., 2018; Giner et al., 2014. Will it be this weekend, if the person isn't hospitalized? Will it be in the next 5 or 10 years? Or is the suicide going to happen at some vague time in the future? Most suicide prevention focuses on estimating group suicide risk over periods of years. For example, both Joiner and I concentrate more on chronic lethality than on acute lethality. This is not to deny that the probability of suicide is often higher in times of stress, trauma, or crucial negative life events, or that suicide can be triggered (Maltsberger & Stoklosa, 2012). However, the overall suicide rate cannot significantly be reduced simply by treating acutely at-risk individuals. Professionals must attempt to do primary prevention on a large scale before individuals ever become suicidal.

The Problem of Rare Behavior

It has been noted repeatedly that suicide is a rare behavior. With all rare behaviors, attempts at prediction tend to get false positives (in the present context, a suicide is predicted, but there is no suicide; Rothman et al., 2012). Perhaps the best that can be done is to utilize lists of suicide risk factors in specific situations, which identify groups at higher suicide risk. Ideally, the reduced size of these risk groups might allow better management of suicide. For example, such reduced size might permit closer supervision, more focused medication schedules, or more intense psychotherapy, or might give a clinician a better idea of when to hospitalize a patient. It is almost impossible to treat or prevent 1 suicide out of 10,000 people over a long time, but (say) treating 30 in 100 starts to become practical and promising.

Since suicide risk tends to be chronic, waxing and waning over prolonged periods of time, the treatment challenge is to be there over the long haul. Today may be *the* day, even though it may look like every other day. Having a caring, loving family member, friend, or therapist can be crucial when suicidality persists and most other people have gone away. Remember too, that some patients may need to remain on antidepressants (e.g., if they have "kindled" depression; Kramer, 1993) or to stay in psychotherapy indefinitely to guard against episodic, rare, unpredictable suicidal behaviors.

False Positives and False Negatives

I elaborate here on what I have said above about false positives and false negatives. Psychiatrist Alex Pokorny (1983, 1992) found that even after using the most sophisticated suicide risk factors and scales available, he still got about 30% *false positives* (i.e., predictions of suicides that never happened). The low base rate of completed suicide has led most suicidologists to conclude that individual suicides in short time frames are unpredictable (notice the implied reduced liability consequences). *Sensitivity* means correctly identifying true positives, and *specificity* means correctly identifying true negatives. A *true negative* means that we predict no suicide will happen and suicide then does not occur. To complete the predictive possibilities, a *true positive* means that we predict a suicide will happen and it does. A *false negative* means that we predict no suicide will happen, but the suicide happens anyway. False negatives in suicide prediction often result in medical malpractice lawsuits. Still, the biggest problem in suicide prevention is false positives, given the rarity of suicide outcomes.

Tools for Suicide Assessment

Throughout this book, I have noted that there are no valid or reliable psychological tests to predict suicide outcome (Eyman & Eyman, 1992; Rothberg & Geer-Williams, 1992; Simon, 2012). Does this mean that we should not try to measure suicidality? Not at all. Clinicians need all the help they can get in assessing suicidality. However, professionals should proceed with caution and not overinterpret their results.

Some of the tools utilized in assessing suicide are (1) self-reports on suicide ideation (although we must be careful not to commit the "I know a man who . . ." *ad hominem* fallacy), depression, suicide plans and methods (does the patient have a gun?), anxiety levels, a sense of urgency or desperation, feelings of rage, intense anger, agitation, hostility, and many more; (2) indirect evidence like notes, letters, calendar notations, computer searches, poems written, books read, incidents or life events; (3) scores on the MMPI-2, the BDI-II or HAM-D, the Cull and Gill SPS, the older LASPC scale, the Risk–Rescue Rating Scale by Weisman and Worden, Motto's scale, Lettieri's scale, and many more current up-to-date scales or tests; (4) psychiatric or nursing assessment, intake summaries, or discharge summaries at hospitals; (5) what the family and friends of the would-be suicide observe about the person's behavior and comments; (6) the individual's past medical, psychiatric, or psychological records; (7) the individual's results on a psychological autopsy questionnaire; and (8) the clinician's subjective feelings and clinical judgment about the individual right now or in the near future.

Implications for Treatment and Suicide Prevention

I have argued that at times suicide is Darwinian—that is, a failure of the relatively unfit to survive (see de Catanzaro, 1992, for his discussion of the ψ coefficient). That is, the person does not intend to die; he or she simply cannot keep going. People need to be able to live and have reasons for living (Linehan et al., 1983). These reasons usually involve someone or something outside themselves (Goodwin, 2003; Stanley et al., 2008; Zisook et al., 2018). Suicides tend to be narcissistically preoccupied with themselves and their own problems and pain. Normally, it takes a lot for most people to give up on their one and only life. Suicides usually have long-ish suicidal careers, with suicide risk increasing with age, especially for white males.

The median age for suicides in the Chicago study (Maris, 1981) was 51 (for more recent age data, see *https://afsp.org/about-suicide/suicide-statistics*). In 2014 in the United States, the highest suicide rate (19.3 per 100,000) was among people 85 years old or older, more recently exceeded by or virtually tied with rates of suicides ages 45–55. Suicides have many life experiences and conditions (including their genetics and biology) that conjointly contribute to suicidal acts over fairly long time periods; think of Ernest Hemingway, George Eastman, or even Thomas Joiner's and my own fathers. My father was an alcoholic who left his family, went off to Alaska, and died alone at age 43 in Anchorage.

Some younger celebrity suicides (like Kurt Cobain, John Belushi, Janis Joplin, Marilyn Monroe, Sylvia Plath, Vincent van Gogh, Judy Garland, Prince, Michael Jackson, Elvis Presley, and many others) lived on the edge, behaved impulsively, took many chances, and abused multiple substances (particularly stimulants, opiates, and prescribed painkillers). Few of them made it to age 40; their suicidal careers were compacted and "sparkler-like."

Summary of Research Results and Empirical Generalizations

Research results derived from well-designed studies (clinical trials, sample surveys, epidemiological studies, vital statistics, experiments, etc.) form the factual basis of a systematic theory of suicide (Maris, 1981). These statistically significant suicide facts, derived from properly controlled samples and appropriate analyses, are what a theory of suicide needs to be able to explain. For example, the general model of suicide in Figure 2.1 needs to be formulated as axioms, postulates, and definitions

(Maris, 1981), from which we are then able to deductively derive research results as theorems (i.e., hypotheses confirmed as research results) through the application of logic, rules of inference, mathematics, and statistics. If we can use the theory to deduce the research results, then they (the empirical results) are said to have been "explained." Note that systematic theories of suicide not only explain research results, but also suggest new candidates (via logical and mathematical inferences) for research, which can then be empirically tested, confirmed, or rejected. A systematic theory of suicide integrates and organizes all the disparate theoretical components of suicide into a coherent, unified whole.

Many of the following research results are from secondary data. That is, they are not all based on my own original studies (e.g., Maris, 1981); rather, they are major empirical findings reviewed earlier in this text. Note also that the following research results are a selection and do not represent all of the empirical generalizations in the book—and certainly not all in the scientific literature. Thus, the list below is not an exhaustive list of suicide research results. Each research result (designated RR in the list) is numbered to reflect the chapter in which it was reported. Most of the research results refer to U.S. populations, unless otherwise specified (of course, various studies may have different research result rates).[1] Different studies may yield other, different research results, and these differences need to be resolved.

- RR 1.1. The typical suicide is a middle-aged to older white male ("diathesis"). He is clinically depressed and is abusing alcohol and often other substances or drugs; is alone and socially isolated; uses a highly lethal method like a gun to attempt suicide; has grown ("achieved") increasingly hopeless and fearless about death and pain (including psychic pain) over a fairly long time; tends to engage in rigid, dichotomous thinking; often has nagging musculoskeletal pain (and may abuse painkillers) and physical illness or illnesses; has recurring work and marital or relationship problems; has experienced an accumulating series of negative life events ("stresses"); might have had another family member or friend who suicided; and comes to see suicide as the only real, permanent resolution to his persistent, perhaps escalating life problems, which are perceived to have become intolerable.
- RR 1.2. The typical nonfatal suicide attempter in the United States is a younger female with interpersonal problems, who overdoses or attempts suicide as many as four or five times over her lifetime.
- RR 1.3. Twenty-four percent of the American population thinks about suiciding at some time.
- RR 1.4. Most self-destructive acts are partial, chronic, and long-term.
- RR 3.1. In 2013 in the United States, there were 41,149 suicides, or a suicide rate of 13 per 100,000.
- RR 5.1. From 1900 to 2017 in the United States, the suicide rate has

---

[1]Most of these research results should have a notation of *ceteris paribus* ("holding other things constant" or "other things being equal") or *mutatis mutandis* ("necessary changes having been made"). For example, sometimes we may need to specify gender, age, country, mental status, or the like.

remained fairly constant, albeit with a few peaks and troughs and recent steady increases.

- RR 5.2. Only the suicide rates of U.S. white males go up virtually in a straight line with age (actually the pattern is bimodal, but generally upward).
- RR 5.3. Very few people under age 14 suicide.
- RR 5.4. The highest U.S. suicide rates are for those ages 45–54 or older.
- RR 5.5. The ratio of male to female suicide rates in the United States usually ranges from about 3:1 to 4:1.
- RR 5.6. African American male suicide rates tend to peak early (at about ages 25–34) but have increases later in life (ages 75–84) .
- RR 5.7. African American female suicide rates are very low throughout the life cycle.
- RR 5.8. Adolescent suicide rates rise dramatically by ages 15–24.
- RR 5.9. Since about 2007, the highest U.S. suicide rates have been in 45- to 54-year-olds (the middle-aged).
- RR 5.10. As one progresses through the age groups of young-old, old-old, and oldest-old, the group suicide rates tend to go straight up.
- RR 6.1. The U.S. male suicide rates exceed those of females at all ages.
- RR 6.2. Men and women tend to use different methods to attempt suicide.
- RR 6.3. Firearms are used to attempt suicide by 51.8% of U.S. men, but only by 38.3% of U.S. women.
- RR 6.4. About eighty percent (78%) of all suicides in the United States are committed by males.
- RR 6.5. The entire explanatory gestalt for suicide tends to be masculine (phallocentric).
- RR 6.6. In China, female suicide rates exceed those of males.
- RR 6.7. In general, marriage and family protect against suicide.
- RR 6.8. On average, homosexual males have a suicide rate about twice that of heterosexual males.
- RR 6.9. Suicide rates among males are much higher for the widowed and divorced than they are for the married.
- RR 7.1. The home is where 78.9% of U.S. suicides occur.
- RR 7.2. The U.S. suicide rate went up by 12% 7–10 days after the suicide of Marilyn Monroe.
- RR 7.3. Natural death controls in the Chicago study had twice as many close friends (even though they were older) as suicides did.
- RR 7.4. Nonfatal suicide attempters and completers in the Chicago study had higher negative interaction scores than the natural death controls did.
- RR 7.5. Perceived burdensomeness predicts the use of a more lethal method to attempt suicide.
- RR 7.6. The more similar a copying individual is to a stimulus suicide, the more likely the suicide is (to be copied).
- RR 7.7. Young people and teenagers are more likely to imitate a stimulus suicide.
- RR 7.8. Maybe 5% of all adolescent suicides occur in "clusters."

- RR 7.9. Physicians, dentists, and veterinarians have higher suicide rates than other professionals do.
- RR 7.10. Overall, SES and suicide rates have a negative association.
- RR 7.11. About one-third of all suicides are unemployed at the time of their death.
- RR 7.12. The median life expectancy for most business firms (organizational mortality or suicide) is 4 years.
- RR 8.1. The highest suicide rate for any country is Guyana's at 44.2 per 100,000, followed by South Korea's at 28.9.
- RR 8.2. The countries with the lowest suicide rates are Syria (0.4) and Saudi Arabia (0.4).
- RR 8.3. Asians typically do not have particularly high suicide rates.
- RR 8.4. For young females in southern India (ages 10–19 years), suicide accounts for 50–75% of all deaths.
- RR 9.1. From 10 to 15% of all nonfatal suicide attempters go on to complete suicide.
- RR 9.2. Eighty-two percent of handgun suicide wounds are to the head.
- RR 9.3. Twenty-five percent of female suicides are overdoses, but only 5.2% of male suicides are.
- RR 9.4. Firearm suicides are the number one method for both males (51.8%) and females (38.3%).
- RR 9.5. Seventy percent of all completed suicides make only one attempt.
- RR 9.6. From about 15 to 23% of suicides leave notes.
- RR 10.1. Over 90% of suicides have a diagnosable mental disorder.
- RR 10.2. The risk of suicide is highest in bipolar disorders, with major depression a close second.
- RR 11.1. About 60% of U.S. suicides occur in people with major depressive disorder.
- RR 11.2. The number of laughs per day is negatively correlated with completed suicide.
- RR 11.3. Remeron is the most effective and Zoloft the most acceptable antidepressant. Lexapro is second in both categories.
- RR 12.1. Lithium is one of the few mood stabilizers shown to reduce suicide risk.
- RR 13.1. From 5 to 10% of those with schizophrenia will eventually complete suicide.
- RR 13.2. All antipsychotic medications tend to block dopamine receptors (especially D_2 receptors).
- RR 14.1. Fifty-seven percent of suicides have one of the personality disorders.
- RR 14.2. As many as 84% of patients with borderline personality disorder have made at least one suicide attempt.
- RR 14.3. As many as 72% of males with antisocial personality disorder attempt suicide.
- RR 14.4. Perfectionism and suicide ideation are significantly positively correlated.

- RR 15.1. Alcohol intoxication is the second leading single suicide risk factor for a suicide outcome.
- RR 15.2. Substance-related disorders are involved in 17% of completed suicides worldwide.
- RR 15.3. Drunkenness is roughly twice as common in suicides as in natural deaths.
- RR 15.4. About 29% of New York City suicides ages 21–30 tested positive for cocaine.
- RR 16.1. Low levels of brain serotonin are associated with suicidal acts.
- RR 16.2. Suicides show decreased prefrontal cortex activity.
- RR 16.3. Persons with schizophrenia are thought to have an excess of dopamine in their brains and cerebrospinal fluid.
- RR 16.4. In one study, 11.3% of monozygotic twins were concordant for suicide, versus 1.8% of dizygotic twins.
- RR 16.5. Low-fat diets tend to increase or are related to aggressive behavior.
- RR 17.1. Religion tends to protect one from suicide.
- RR 17.2. Protestants have the highest suicide rates.
- RR 17.3. Some religious cults are death cults and do not protect their members from suicide.
- RR 17.4. Muslim countries typically have very low suicide rates.
- RR 17.5. The primary (82%) concept of death in suicides is escape from pain and suffering.
- RR 18.1. Among the first visual references to suicide is a vase that depicts Ajax falling on his sword.
- RR 19.1. Seventy-nine percent of assisted suicides had a malignant tumor (1998–2014).
- RR 19.2. Hospitals do not have to allow patients to starve themselves to death (1990, U.S. Supreme Court).
- RR 20.1. U.S. suicide rates dropped during World Wars I and II.
- RR 20.2. Suicides, homicides, and accidents are three out of the five leading causes of death from ages 15 to 45 and are violent and aggressive.
- RR 20.3. Military suicide rates and those of the white male general population are about the same.
- RR 20.4. Suicide rates of deployed combat veterans are not higher than those of soldiers who were never deployed.
- RR 20.5. Suicides constitute 2.1% of annual deaths overall, but 12.3% among 15- to 24-year-olds.
- RR 21.1. Murder–suicides account for 1–2% of all suicides.
- RR 22.1. The jail suicide rate is about three times higher than that of the general population.
- RR 22.2. Suicide is the number one cause of death in jails.
- RR 22.3. Almost half of all jail inmates who suicide do so within the first 6 hours of confinement.
- RR 22.4. Hanging is the preferred jail suicide attempt method.
- RR 23.1. Most of the treatment of suicidal individuals today is just pharmacological management of mood and anxiety disorders.

- RR 23.2. Lithium remains the drug of choice for the initial stabilization of mania (however, Latuda is an important newer augmenting drug for mood disorders).
- RR 23.3. For short-term, situational anxiety disorders, benzodiazepines are normally prescribed.
- RR 23.4. Clozaril is effective in treating a suicidal patient with psychosis.
- RR 23.5. If the suicidal crisis is acute, then the patient may receive electro-convulsive therapy.
- RR 24.1. About 17% of suicides are in therapy when they suicide.
- RR 24.2. Cognitive-behavioral therapy is the leading type of psychotherapy for suicidal patients.
- RR 24.3. Suicidal patients may need inpatient treatment, if they are not safe at home.
- RR 25.1. It is better to prevent a disease than it is to treat it.
- RR 25.2. Suicide prevention ought to be focused on middle-aged to elderly white males.
- RR 26.1. In 2014 in the United States, there were 256,638 to 1,924,785 new suicide survivors.
- RR 27.1. In the United States, assisting suicide remains a crime in all but seven states and the District of Columbia.
- RR 27.2. When someone suicides, family members tend to blame the care-givers.
- RR 27.3. The leading causes of death in the United States are, in order, heart disease, cancer, respiratory disease, cardiovascular problems, accident, and (10th) suicide.
- RR 27.4. There is a 2-year nullification clause for suicide in most life insurance policies.

These, then, are some of the main facts or research results that need to be explained in a systematic, comprehensive general theory of suicide. Some of our research results involve hypothetical claims that are tested.

Constructing a Systematic Theory of Suicide

The vast majority of suicide studies simply stop with statistically significant research results (e.g., confirmed by χ^2, odds ratios, relative risks, regression equations, and other statistical analyses, usually of clinical trial data) or probable empirical generalizations, as if these data themselves explained something (here, suicide). But in fact these research results are precisely what need to be explained. How is that done? It is done by constructing a systematic theory of suicide. A *theory* is a set of laws and definitions that are deductively interrelated, as in Figure 28.1.

Other definitions of *theory* include (1) a set of laws and definitions deductively interrelated—in short, an axiomatic system (as geometry is); (2) a connected set of propositions; and (3) sets of interrelated assumptions (single assumptions are ordinarily called *laws*). They require that definitions and postulates are not

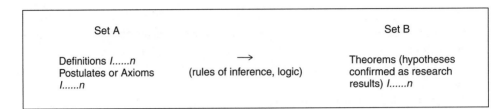

FIGURE 28.1. A model for constructing systematic theory. $l \ldots n$ = however many there are, e.g., 1–10, 1–1,000. *Source:* Maris, Ronald W. with Bernard Lazerwitz. *Pathways to Suicide: A Survey of Self-Destructive Behaviors.* © 1981 The Johns Hopkins University Press. Reprinted with permission of Johns Hopkins University Press.

self-contradictory. At least one of the derivable theorems of a system must apply to the facts of observation or research results (Maris, 1981, p. 288).

Thus, to formally and systematically explain suicide ideation and behavior, definitions and postulates or axioms have to be utilized to derive, infer, or deduce research results such as those stated in this chapter. A word is in order about *axioms.* Since this theory aspires to be interdisciplinary, its general propositions or axioms need to come from a combination of the professional disciplines of psychiatry, psychology, medicine, biology, chemistry, social sciences, public health, and many more. *Axioms* are highly general and abstract law-like propositions, while *hypotheses* are specific theorems deduced and supported or confirmed as research results.

Axioms can be formed from basic human needs and values, such as "Human beings tend to avoid pain and seek pleasure." Individual human needs, interests, values, or rewards can include (1) mundane biological or physical needs (the need for food, drink, shelter, sleep, sex, biological tension reduction, avoidance of pain, physical and mental health, etc.); and (2) more abstract interests or needs (the need for love, knowledge, social status, money, property, esteem, acceptability, etc.) (Maris, 1981; Maslow, 1963). There can also be corporate or societal interests, as well as individual interests.

Edwin Shneidman (1996), commenting on Henry Murray's (1938) *Explorations in Personality,* talked about the human needs for achievement, recognition, cognizance, succor, recognition, order, acquisition, construction, autonomy, aggression, sexual intercourse, reproduction, play, power, affection, information, materialism, and other things. Shneidman claimed that frustration of human needs leads to psychological pain or what he called "psychache," which in turn increases suicide risk.

Many years ago (Maris, 1981), I took a first step in constructing a systematic theory of suicide. However, to construct a truly comprehensive systematic theory of suicide is a daunting, presently unfinished task. For example, it is problematic to have a general model or theory of suicide (Figure 2.1) account for rare, specific individual events in a short time frame, especially across cultures.

What is usually proposed is a theory of group suicide risk over longish time periods. For example, can a theory narrow suicide and the risk factors down from (say) 1 in 10,000 people at risk to (say) 10–15 in 100 at risk? Suppose an inpatient treatment facility has 100 patients. All of them cannot be put on 24/7 suicide watch, but 10–15 of them might be. Such high-suicide-risk groups are more manageable, treatable, and protectable. Thus suicide theory should help us delineate small, vulnerable minority groups and individual types for prevention targets, as well as suggest how to approach them. Constructing a truly systematic theory of suicide is beyond the scope of this book. All I can hope to do here is to suggest what such a systematic theory might look like, and to construct a "skeletal" or "embryonic" theory of suicide.

In a systematic theory of suicide, all of our research results would need to be deduced (or able to be deduced) from axioms, which have not been fully formed and listed here. A series of deductive inferences would later have to be compiled into a whole, coherent theory. One example of a simplistic, deductive, syllogistic inference might be the following:

1. Axiom 1 = Completed suicide implies hopelessness and depression (Maris, 1981).
2. Axiom 2 = Hopelessness implies repeated depression, life failures over a suicidal career, negative interaction, and social isolation.
3. Theorem 1 = Hopelessness implies social isolation (simplification of axiom 2).
4. Therefore, completed suicide implies social isolation (hypothetical syllogism including axioms 2 and 3).

More formally, this might be stated as follows ($\supset$ = *implies*; $\bullet$ = *and*):

1. CS $\supset$ – H $\bullet$ D (axiom 1)
2. – H $\supset$ (D $\bullet$ F $\bullet$ NI $\bullet$ SI) (axiom 2)
3. – H $\supset$ SI (axiom 2, simplification)
4. CS $\supset$ SI (axioms 2 and 3, hypothetical syllogism)

Note that proposition 4 is close to one of our research results (viz., RR 7.3) that is now deduced. In a "valid" argument (which the one above is), if the premises are true, then the conclusion must be true. We have only done one deductive inference here. A general theory of suicide will require a much larger, complex list of axioms or law-like propositions, from which all of the theory's research results are or can be logically deduced and then related to each other in a coherent whole.

The General Model of Suicide Revisited

Figure 2.1, now reconsidered here, has sketched what a general theory of suicide might look like, the variables it should include, and the ways in which they are interrelated over a suicidal career. It is a skeletal outline of some of the essential characteristics that a theory of suicide should include, and it suggests how these characteristics or variables might be related to each other over the lifespan of a suicidal career. The following discussion reviews some of the salient characteristics of the general model of suicide, embellishing and elaborating them along the way. Notice that there are four rows and six columns in our model, with Postvention added as the heading to column 6 (Figure 28.2).

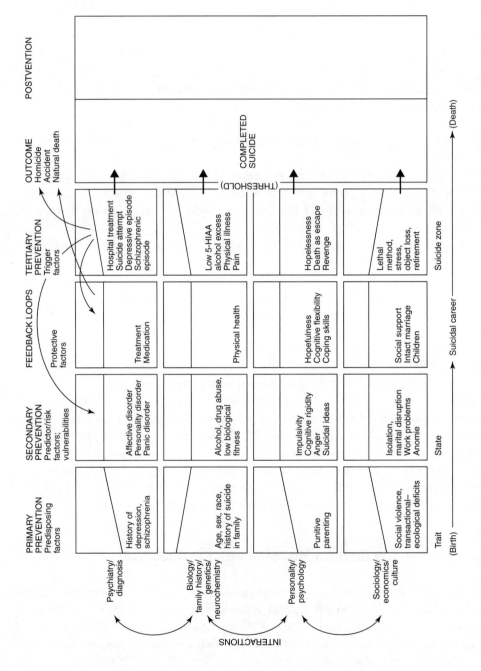

FIGURE 28.2. The general model of suicidal behaviors revisited. Not all interactions are depicted. The figure does not include suicide ideation. *Sources:* Maris et al. (1992, pp. 667–669); Maris et al. (2000, p. 58); Maris (2002, pp. 319–326).

The four rows in the model represent interdisciplinary explanatory domains: (1) psychiatry; (2) biology (including family history, genetics, neurobiology, and neurochemistry); (3) personality/psychology; and (4) sociology/economics/culture. These four domains interactively contribute to suicide outcomes, and thus my model of suicide is biopsychosocial. The ascending or descending lines in each of the four rows suggest the relative importance of the domains over the lifespan or suicidal career. For example, the model asserts that near the end of the suicidal life cycle, psychiatric and biological forces become more important; personality/psychological forces remains fairly constant; and social factors diminish somewhat in importance. Clearly, there could be more than just these four domains influencing suicide outcomes. Other domain candidates might include public health, medicine, forensics, criminal justice, education, counseling, religion, history, international variations, art, and many more

The columns in the model are labeled in at least two ways: First, from left to right, there are (1) predisposing factors (diathesis or traits), (2) risk or vulnerability factors, (3) protective factors, (4) triggers—precipitating, state, or situational factors (such as stress; note that most suicides are chronic, not acute or situationally triggered; healthy people usually absorb or deflect suicide triggers without suiciding); (5) outcomes (Blumenthal & Kupfer, 1990); and (6) postvention issues (note that at the time of the fourth column, natural, accidental, and homicidal death are also still possible outcomes). The second way the columns are labeled, particularly columns 1, 2, and 4, reminds us that suicide prevention varies over the life cycle. As discussed in Chapters 2 and 26, Gerald Caplan (1964) defined *primary prevention* (which reduces incidence, in this case by keeping suicide from ever developing), *secondary prevention* (which reduces prevalence or total cases), and *tertiary prevention* (which detects and limits damages of late-occurring disease processes—here, suicidality).

The fourth column in the model can be thought of as a "suicide zone." Predisposing and suicide risk factors over time can interact, compound, and potentiate each other leading either to suicide or (most likely) to feedback loops resulting in various treatments, interventions, or recurring episodes of suicidal disorders. Litman (1989) created the concept of a suicide zone with its heightened suicide risk, but also suggested that for perhaps every 100 people who enter the suicide zone, only 1 or 2 ever commit suicide. Suicide is a rare outcome.

There is also a "threshold" between heightened suicide risk (column 4) and completed suicide (column 5). Jerome Motto (1992) argued that every one of us has a personal threshold of pain tolerance beyond which suicide is likely, even necessary. Shneidman (1993, 1996), Joiner (2005), and others add the concepts of "psychache" and repeated painful life experiences leading to "the acquired ability" to breach the suicide threshold.

The vast majority of individuals in the suicide zone never commit suicide, but rather turn (via feedback loops) to psychotherapeutic and/or pharmacological treatment or to further suicide episodes and experiences. One big challenge in suicidology is to identify those individuals and their unique suicide risk factors that encourage or prod them to cross the suicide threshold. Even most suicidal individuals eventually die a natural death.

The particular suicide risk and protective factors listed in the various cells of Figures 2.1 and 28.2 have been defined and discussed in the earlier chapters of this text. Do not forget that there are many different types of suicide careers, each with its own dynamics, salient features, and idiosyncrasies. Suicidal careers are not linear, simple, or consistent. Most suicidal individuals' careers have many starts, stops, reversals, and restarts. Suicidal people do get better, and some even opt out of suicidal careers altogether, even if they fit the model at one time.

Epilogue

Sometimes we are lucky to avoid serious diathetic traits, misfortunes, injuries, or diseases, and we have others who care fiercely about us. To keep living and certainly to live well, we all need other people to sustain us. No doubt there are isolates who survive, but even they have a relationship with their work, art, or God. So I leave you with these words: Work hard; try your best to stay healthy and fit; sleep and eat well; beware of sexual indiscretions and callous aggression; think about the welfare of others; give your life back appropriately; be lucky, I hope; be persistent and keep trying; love at least one other person; have children and pets; and compromise.

Find something or someone meaningful to love or engage you until you die. Of course, we all have to die sooner or later, but not prematurely in a manner that diminishes the ideal of the good life and devastates those who love us and are left behind. We can have a good enough life for most of the time we are given. And if you are ever on the edge of the abyss, at least contact someone you respect and talk about it. You cannot undo a suicide.

We are now at the end of a long, arduous, and ambitious journey. Every book is an approach as much as it is an arrival. Here I have only been able to point broadly toward the understanding of suicide assessment, treatment, and prevention. Much remains to be done. My hope is that this book will inspire others to carry on this important work—to describe, with greater refinement, insight, and detail, the processes leading to suicide and suicide prevention. No one should have to throw away their one and only life to get relief from pain.

References

Aamodt, M, G., & Stalmaker, N. A. (2006, June 20). Police officer suicide: Frequency and officer profiles. Retrieved from *www.policeone.com/health-fitness/articles/137133-Police-Officer-Suicide-Frequency-and-officer-profiles*

Aaron, R., et al. (2004). Suicide in young people in rural southern India. *The Lancet, 363,* 1117–1118.

ABC [Australian Broadcasting Corporation] News. (2015, June 14). Australia's aboriginal suicide epidemic [Television broadcast].

Abdel Haleem, M. A. S., trans. (2004). *The Qur'an* (Oxford World's Classic Edition). New York: Oxford University Press.

Able, K. M., & Ramsey, R., eds. (2017). *The female mind: A user's guide.* London: Royal College of Physicians.

Abrutyn, S., & Mueller, A. S. (2014). Are suicidal behaviors contagious in adolescence? *American Sociological Review, 79*(2), 211–227.

Adacic-Gross, V., et al. (2008). Methods of suicide. *Bulletin of the World Health Organization, 86*(9), 728–732.

Allen, W. (Director/Writer). (1973). *Sleeper* [Motion picture]. United States: United Artists.

Alvarez, A. (1971). *The savage god.* New York: Random House.

American Association of Suicidology (AAS). (2008). National suicide statistics. Retrieved from *www.suicidology.org/resources/facts-statistics*

American Association of Suicidology (AAS). (2015, December 22). Suicide rates per 100,000 overall by age and gender, United States, 2004–2014. Retrieved from *www.suicidology.org/resources/facts-statistics*

American Association of Suicidology (AAS). (2016). Resources for clinicians who have lost a patient and/or family member to suicide. Retrieved from *www.suicidology.org/suicide-survivors/clinician-survivors*

American Heritage College Dictionary. (2010). Boston: Houghton Mifflin.

American Jail Association. (2010). *Statistics of note.* Hagerstown, MD: Author.

American Psychiatric Association. (1952). *Diagnostic and statistical manual of mental disorders.* Washington, DC: Author.

American Psychiatric Association. (1980). *Diagnostic and statistical manual of mental disorders* (3rd ed.). Washington, DC: Author.

American Psychiatric Association. (2000). *Diagnostic and statistical manual of mental disorders* (4th ed., text rev.). Washington, DC: Author.

American Psychiatric Association. (2013). *Diagnostic and statistical manual of mental disorders* (5th ed.). Arlington, VA: Author.

American Psychological Association. (2014, April 14). *Guidelines for psychological practice in healthcare delivery systems.* Washington, DC: Author.

American Psychological Association. (2015). Guidelines for psychological practice with transgender and gender nonconforming people. *American Psychologist, 70*(9), 832–864. Retrieved from *www.apa.org/practice/guidelines/transgender.pdf*

American Sociological Association. (n.d.). Race and ethnicity. Retrieved from *www.asanet.org/topics/race-and-ethnicity*

Anderson, I. M. (2018). Does electroconvulsive therapy damage the brain? *The Lancet Psychiatry, 5*(4), 294–295.

Andrade, C. (2017). Ketamine for depression: 2. Diagnostic and contextual indications. *Journal of Clinical Psychiatry, 78*(5), e555–e558.

Andreasen, N. C. (1984). *The broken brain.* New York: Harper & Row.

Andriessen, K. (2009). Can postvention be prevention? *Crisis, 30*(1), 43–47.

Anestis, M. D. (2018, April 19). *Guns and suicide: The time for change is now.* Paper presented at the 51st annual conference of the American Association of Suicidology, Washington, DC.

Anestis, M. D., & Houtsma, C. (2018). The association between gun ownership and statewide overall suicide rates. *Suicide and Life-Threatening Behavior, 48*(2), 204–217.

Anestis, M. D., et al. (2017). Treating the capability for suicide: A vital and understudied frontier in suicide prevention. *Suicide and Life-Threatening Behavior, 47*(5), 523–537.

Angell, M. (2011a, June 23). The epidemic of mental illness: Why? *New York Review of Books.* Retrieved from *www.nybooks.com/articles/2011/06/23/epidemic-mental-illness-why*

Angell, M. (2011b, July 14). The illusions of psychiatry. *New York Review of Books.* Retrieved from *www.nybooks.com/articles/2011/07/14/illusions-of-psychiatry*

Ann, C. S. (2016, March 29). Van Gogh, mental illness and the price of genius. *The Straits Times.* Retrieved from *www.straitstimes.com/opinion/van-gogh-mental-illness-and-the-price-of-genius*

Annor, F. B., et al. (2018). Characteristics of and participating circumstances surrounding suicide among persons aged 10–17 years—Utah, 2011–2015, *Morbidity and Mortality Weekly Report, 67*, 329–332.

Aristotle. (2002). *Nicomachean ethics.* New York: Oxford University Press.

Äsberg, M., et al. (1976). 5-HIAA in the cerebrospinal fluid: A biochemical predictor? *Archives of General Psychiatry, 136*, 559–562.

Äsberg, M., et al. (1986). Therapeutic effects of serotonin uptake in depression, *Journal of Clinical Psychiatry, 40*(4), 3–35.

Asch, S. (1955, November). Opinions and social pressure. *Scientific American*, pp. 31–35.

Ash, P. (2012). Children, adolescents, and college students. In R. I. Simon & R. E. Hales, eds., *The American Psychiatric Publishing textbook of suicide assessment and management* (2nd ed.). Washington, DC: American Psychiatric Publishing.

Ashby, H. (Director), & Higgins, C. (Writer). (1971). *Harold and Maude* [Motion picture]. United States: Paramount Pictures.

Babigian, H. M. (1975). Schizophrenia epidemiology. In A. M. Freedman et al., eds., *Comprehensive textbook of psychiatry* (2nd ed., Vol. 2). Baltimore: Williams & Wilkins.

Badham, J. (Director), & Clark, B. (Writer). (1981). *Whose life is it anyway?* [Motion picture]. United States: MGM.

Baechler, J. (1979). *Suicides.* New York: Basic Books.

Bagge, C. L., & Borges, G. (2017). Acute substance abuse as a warning sign for suicide attempts: A case-crossover examination of the 48 hours prior to a recent suicide attempt. *Journal of Clinical Psychiatry, 78*(6), 691–696.

Baldessarini, R. J. (2002). Treatment research in bipolar disorder: Issues and recommendations. *CNS Drugs, 16*, 721–729.

Baldessarini, R. J., & Tondo, L. (1999). Antisuicidal effects of lithium treatment in major depressive disorder. In D. Jacobs et al., eds., *Harvard Medical School guide to suicide assessment and intervention.* San Francisco: Jossey-Bass.

Baldessarini, R. J., et al. (2012). Bipolar disorder. In R. I. Simon & R. E. Hales, eds., *The American Psychiatric Publishing textbook of suicide assessment and management* (2nd ed.). Washington, DC: American Psychiatric Publishing.

Ballenger, J. C., et al. (1979). Alcohol and central serotonin metabolism in man. *Archives of General Psychiatry, 36*, 224–227.

Barnhill, J. W., ed. (2014). *DSM-5 clinical cases.* Washington, DC: American Psychiatric Publishing.

Barrows, S. B., with Novak, W. (1986). *Mayflower Madam: The secret life of Sydney Biddle Barrows.* New York: Arbor House.

Bates, M. J., et al. (2012). Clinical management of suicide risk with military and veteran personnel. In R. I. Simon & R. E. Hales, eds., *The American Psychiatric Publishing textbook of suicide assessment and management*

(2nd ed.). Washington, DC: American Psychiatric Publishing.

Battin, M. P. (1992). Dying in 559 beds: Efficiency, "best buys," and the ethics of standardized national health care. *Journal of Medicine and Philosophy, 17*(1), 59–77.

Battin, M. P., & Joiner, T. (2018, April 19). *Physician's aid-in-dying is not the same as suicide.* Paper presented at the 51st annual conference of the American Association of Suicidology, Washington, DC.

Battin, M. P., & Mayo, D. J., eds. (1980). *Suicide: The philosophical issues.* New York: St. Martin's Press.

Beautrais, A. L., et al. (1996). Prevalence and comorbidity of mental disorders in persons making serious suicide attempts. *American Journal of Psychiatry, 153*(8), 1007–1014.

Beck, A. T. (1990). Suicide Intent Scale. In S. J. Blumenthal & D. J. Kupfer, eds., *Suicide over the life cycle.* Washington, DC: American Psychiatric Press.

Beck, A. T., et al. (1974a). The measurement of pessimism: The Hopelessness Scale. *Journal of Consulting and Clinical Psychology, 42*(6), 861–865.

Beck, A. T., et al. (1974b). *The prediction of suicide.* Bowie, MD: Charles Press.

Beck, A, T., et al. (1979a). Assessment of suicide ideation: The Scale for Suicide Ideation. *Journal of Consulting and Clinical Psychology, 47,* 342–352.

Beck, A. T., et al. (1979b). *Cognitive therapy of depression.* New York: Guilford Press.

Beck, A. T., et al. (1985). Hopelessness and eventual suicide: A 10-year prospective study of patients hospitalized with suicidal ideation. *American Journal of Psychiatry, 142,* 559–563.

Beck, A. T., et al. (1996). *Manual for the Beck Depression Inventory–II.* San Antonio, TX: Psychological Corporation.

Becker, E. (1973). *The denial of death.* New York: Macmillan.

Behrman, A. (2002). *Electroboy.* New York: Random House.

Bender, T., et al. (2011). Impulsivity and suicidality: The mediating role of painful and provocative experiences. *Journal of Affective Disorders, 129,* 301–307.

Benson, T., et al. (2018). Use of prescription medicine by individuals who died by suicide in northern Irelan. *Archives of Suicide Research, 22*(1), 1–6.

Berk, M. S., et al. (2009). Beyond threats: Risk factors for suicide completion in borderline personality disorder. *Current Psychiatry, 8,* 33–41.

Berkowitz, L. (1962). *Aggression: A social psychological analysis.* New York: McGraw-Hill.

Berman, A. L. (1986). Notes on turning 18 (and 75): A critical look at our adolescence. *Suicide and Life-Threatening Behavior, 16,* 1–12.

Berman, A. L. (1996). Dyadic death: A typology. *Suicide and Life-Threatening Behavior, 26,* 342–350.

Berman, A. L. (2018, April 19). *Psychological autopsy certification training.* Workshop presented at the 51st annual conference of the American Association of Suicidology, Washington, DC.

Berman, A. L. (2018). Risk factors proximate to suicide and suicde risk assessment in the context of denied suicide ideation. *Suicide and Life-Threatening Behavior, 48,* 340–352.

Berman, A. L., & Jobes, D. A. (1995). Suicide prevention in adolescents (age 12–18). *Suicide and Life-Threatening Behavior, 25,* 143–154.

Berman, A. L., & Pompili, M., eds. (2011). *Medical conditions associated with suicide risk.* Washington, DC: American Association of Suicidology.

Berman, A. L., et al. (2006). *Adolescent suicide: Assessment and intervention* (2nd ed.). Washington, DC: American Psychological Association.

Berman, L., et al. (2015). Legal and liability issues in suicide care. Retrieved from *http://zerosuicide.sprc.org/webinar/legal-and-liability-issues-suicide-care*

Bettelheim, B. (1943). Individual and mass behavior in extreme situations. *Journal of Abnormal and Social Psychology, 38,* 417–452.

Black, D. W., & Andreasen, N. C. (2011). *Introductory textbook of psychiatry* (5th ed.). Washington, DC: American Psychiatric Publishing.

Black, D. W., & Andreasen, N. C. (2014). *Introductory textbook of psychiatry* (6th ed.). Washington, DC: American Psychiatric Publishing.

Black's law dictionary (B. A. Garner, ed.). (2009). St. Paul, MN: West.

Blasco-Fontecilla, H., et al. (2010). An exploratory study of the relationship between diverse life events and personality disorders in a sample of suicide attempters. *Journal of Personality Disorders, 24*(6), 773–784.

Blau, P. M. (1977). *Inequality and heterogeneity.* New York: Free Press.

Blumenthal, S. J., & Kupfer, D. J., eds. (1990). *Suicide over the life cycle.* Washington, DC: American Psychiatric Publishing.

Bohannan, P., ed. (1960). *African homicide and suicide.* Princeton, NJ: Princeton University Press.

Bolton, I. (2018, April 19). *Compassion for the deceased may lead to resolution of suicide loss.* Paper presented at the 51st annual conference of the American Association of Suicidology, Washington, DC.

Bolton, I., with Mitchell, C. (1983). *My son . . . my son . . . : A guide to healing after a suicide in the family.* Atlanta, GA: Bolton Press.

Bongar, B., et al., eds. (1998). *Risk management with suicidal patients.* New York: Guilford Press.

Bongar, B., et al. (2000). Marriage, family, family therapy, and suicide. In R. W. Maris et al., *Comprehensive textbook of suicidology.* New York: Guilford Press.

Borges, G., et al. (1996). Epidemiologia del suicidio en Mexico de 1970 a 1994. *Salud Publica de Mexico, 38,* 197–206.

Bostwick, J. M., & Pankratz, V. S. (2000). Affective disorder and suicide risk: A reexamination. *American Journal of Psychiatry, 157,* 1925–1932.

Bourget, D., et al. (2010). Domestic homicide and homicide–suicide: The older offender. *Journal of the American Academy of Psychiatry and the Law, 38,* 305–311.

Bowers, J. M. (1969). Cerebrospinal fluid 5-hydroyindoleacetic acid in psychiatric patients. *International Journal of Neuropharmacology, 8,* 255–262.

Bowlby, J. (1973). *Attachment and loss: Vol. 2. Separation: Anxiety and anger.* New York: Basic Books.

Bowlby, J. (1980). *Attachment and loss: Vol. 3. Loss: Sadness and depression.* New York: Basic Books.

Branas, C., et al. (2014, May). The impact of economic austerity and prosperity events on suicide in Greece. *British Medical Journal Open, 5*(1), e005619.

Brandt, R. B. (1975). The morality and rationality of suicide. In S. Perlin, ed., *A handbook for the study of suicide.* New York: Oxford University Press.

Breed, W. (1963). Occupational mobility and suicide among white males. *American Sociological Review, 28,* 179–188.

Brent, D. A., et al. (1987). Alcohol, firearms, and suicide among youth. *Journal of the American Medical Association, 257,* 3369–3372.

Brent, D. A., et al. (1988). Risk factors for adolescent suicide: A comparison of adolescent suicide victims with suicidal inpatients. *Archives of General Psychiatry, 45,* 581–588.

Brent, D. A., et al. (1994). Personality disorders, personality traits, impulsive violence, and completed suicide in adolescents. *Journal of the American Academy of Child and Adolescent Psychiatry, 3,* 1080–1086.

Brock, S. E. (2003). *School suicide prevention, intervention, and postvention.* Sacramento: California State University.

Brody, J. E. (2015, February 16). When grief won't relent. *The New York Times.* Retrieved from *https://well.blogs.nytimes.com/2015/02/16/when-grief-wont-relent*

Brown, G., & Goodwin, F. (1986). Human aggression and suicide. *Suicide and Life-Threatening Behavior, 16,* 223–243.

Brown, G., et al. (1992). Impulsivity, aggression, and associated effects: Relationship to self-destructive behavior and suicide. In R. W. Maris et al., eds., *Assessment and prediction of suicide.* New York: Guilford Press.

Brown, G. K., et al. (2012). Cognitive therapy for suicide prevention. In R. I. Simon & R. E. Hales, eds., *The American Psychiatric Publishing textbook of suicide assessment and management* (2nd ed.). Washington, DC: American Psychiatric Publishing.

Brown, S. L., et al. (2018, April 5). A psychometric investigation of the Painful and Provocative Events Scale: Moving forward. *Archives of Suicide Research.* [Epub ahead of print]

Bryan, C. J., & Morrow, C. E. (2011). Circumventing mental health stigma by embracing warrior culture: Lessons learned from the Defender's Edge program. *Professional Psychology: Research and Practice, 42*(1), 16–23.

Bryan, C. J., et al. (2012). Understanding and preventing military suicide. *Archives of Suicide Research, 16*(2), 95–110.

Bryan, C. J., et al. (2013). Reasons for suicide attempts in a clinical sample of active duty soldiers. *Journal of Affective Disorders, 144*(1), 148–152.

Bryan, C. J., et al. (2015). Combat exposure and risk for suicidal thoughts and behaviors among military personnel and veterans: A systematic review and meta-analysis. *Suicide and Life-Threatening Behavior, 45*(5), 633–649.

Bryan, C. J., et al. (2016). Evaluating potential iatrogenic suicide risk in trauma-focused group cognitive-behavioral therapy for the treatment of PTSD in active duty military personnel. *Depression and Anxiety, 33*, 549–557.

Bsigian, H. M. (1975). Schizophrenia epidemiology. In D. X. Freeman, J. Kaplan, & B. J. Sadock, eds., *Comprehensive textbook of psychiatry* (Vol. 2). Baltimore: Williams & Wilkins.

Burnett-Zeigler, I. E. (2018, April 25). The strong and stressed black woman. *The New York Times.* Retrieved from *www.nytimes. com/2018/04/25/opinion/strong-stressed-black-woman.html*

Cain, A. C., ed. (1972). *Survivors of suicide.* Springfield, IL: Charles C Thomas.

Caine, E., & Mann, J. J. (2017, November). *Debate: High risk versus population approaches to saving lives.* Paper presented at the IASP/AFSP International Summit on Suicide Research, Henderson, NV.

Callanan, V. J., & Davis, M. S. (2011). Gender and suicide method: Do women avoid facial disfiguration? *Sex Roles, 65*, 867–879.

Campbell, F. (2012). Aftermath of suicide: The clinician's role. In R. I. Simon & R. E. Hales, eds., *The American Psychiatric Publishing textbook of suicide assessment and management* (2nd ed.). Washington, DC: American Psychiatric Publishing.

Campbell, J., ed. (1971). *The portable Jung.* New York: Viking Press.

Camus, A. (1945). *The myth of Sisyphus.* London: Hamilton.

Canetto, S. S. (2008). Women and suicidal behavior: A cultural analysis. *American Journal of Orthopsychiatry, 78*, 259–266.

Canetto, S. S., & Sakinofsky, I. (1998). The gender paradox in suicide. *Suicide and Life-Threatening Behavior, 28*(1), 1–23.

Caollai, E. O. (2014, March 21). Ireland has 'exceptionally high rates' of suicide. *The Irish Times.* Retrieved from *www.irishtimes.com/news/social-affairs/ireland-has-exceptionally-high-rates-of-suicide-1.1732791*

Caplan, G. (1964). *Principles of preventive psychiatry.* New York: Basic Books.

Capote, T. (1966). *In cold blood.* New York: Vintage International.

Carballo, J. J., et al. (2012). Personality disorder. In R. I. Simon & R. E. Hales, eds., *The American Psychiatric Publishing textbook of suicide assessment and management* (2nd ed.). Washington, DC: American Psychiatric Publishing.

Card, J. J. (1974). Lethality of suicide methods and suicide risk: Two distinct concepts. *Omega, 5*, 37–45.

Carey, B. (2011, June 23). Expert on mental illness reveals her own fight. *The New York Times.* Retrieved from *www. nytimes.com/2011/06/23/health/23lives. html?pagewanted=all*

Carlat, D. (2010). *Unhinged: The trouble with psychiatry–a doctor's revelations about a profession in crisis.* New York: Simon & Schuster.

The Carlat Psychiatry Report. (2016, April). Thinking creatively about treatment-resistant depression: Q&A with J. Alexander Bodkin, MD. Retrieved from *https://pro.psychcentral.com/thinking-creatively-about-treatment-resistant-depression-qa-with-j-alexander-bodkin-md*

Centers for Disease Control. (CDC). (1992, September 1). *Youth suicide prevention programs and resource guide.* Atlanta, GA: Author.

Centers for Disease Control and Prevention (CDC). (2010). Fact sheets—alcohol use and your health. Retrieved from *www.cdc.gov/alcohol/fact-sheets/alcohol-use.htm*

Centers for Disease Control and Prevention (CDC). (2018). Leading causes of death reports, national and regional, 1999-2015. Retrieved from *https://webappa.cdc.gov/sasweb/ncipc/leadcaus10_us.html*

Cerel, J., et al. (2014). The continuum of "survivorship": Definitional issues in the aftermath of suicide. *Suicide and Life-Threatening Behavior, 44*(6), 591–600.

Cerel, J., et al. (2018, April 19). Presidential Address at the 51st annual conference of the American Association of Suicidology, Washington, DC.

Cha, C. B., et al. (2018). Accounting for diversity in suicide research: Sampling and reporting practices in the U.S. *Suicide and Life-Threatening Behavior, 48*(2), 131–139.

Chesin, M., et al. (2017, July 5). Combining mindfulness-based cognitive therapy with safety planning intervention to reduce suicidal behavior. American Foundation for Suicide Prevention. Retrieved from *https://afsp.org/combining-mindfulness-based-cognitive-therapy-safety-planning-intervention-reduce-suicidal-behavior*

Cipriani, A., et al. (2009). Comparative efficacy and acceptability of new-generation antidepressants. *The Lancet, 373,* 736–758.

Cipriani, A., et al. (2018). Comparative efficacy and acceptability of 22 antidepressant drugs for the acute treatment of adults with major depressive disorder: A systematic review sand network meta-analysis. *The Lancet, 391*(10128), 1357–1366.

Clark, D., & Horton-Deutsch, S. I. (1992). Assessment in absentia: The value of the psychological autopsy method for studying antecedents of suicide and predicting future suicides. In R. W. Maris et al., eds., *The assessment and prediction of suicide.* New York: Guilford Press.

Cleiren, M. R., et al. (1994). Mode of death and kinship in bereavement: Focusing on "who" rather than "how." *Crisis, 15,* 22–36.

Cobain, B., & Larch, J. (2006). *Dying to be free.* Center City, MN: Hazelden.

Coen, E., & Coen, J. (Directors/Writers). (2009). *A serious man* [Motion picture]. United States: Focus Features.

Coleman, J. S. (1962). *Centuries of childhood.* New York: Vintage Press.

Conwell, Y., & Heisel, M. J. (2012). The elderly. In R. I. Simon & R. E. Hales, eds., *The American Psychiatric Publishing textbook of suicide assessment and management* (2nd ed.). Washington, DC: American Psychiatric Publishing.

Cooper, J. E. (1994). *The ICD-10 classification of mental and behavioral disorders (pocket guide).* Geneva: World Health Organization.

Cooper, J. R., et al. (2003). *The biochemical basis of neuropharmacology* (8th ed.). New York: Oxford University Press.

Cousins, N. (1979). *Anatomy of an illness as perceived by the patient.* New York: Norton.

Cramer, R. J., et al. (2014). A trait-interpersonal analysis of suicide proneness among lesbian, gay, and bisexual community members. *Suicide and Life-Threatening Behavior, 44*(6), 601–615.

Cruzan v. Director, Missouri Department of Health, 497 U.S. 261 (1990).

Cull, J. G., & Gill, W. S. (1982). *Suicide Probability Scale.* Los Angeles: Western Psychological Services.

Cullen, A., & Hodgetts, D. (2001). Unemployment as illness. *Journal of Social Issues, 1-1,* 33–51.

Daigh, J., Jr. (2007, May 10). *Healthcare inspection: Implementing VHA's mental health strategic plan initiatives for suicide prevention.* Washington, DC: VA Office of Inspector General.

Daniel, A. E. (2007). Care of the mentally ill in prisons: Challenges and solutions. *Journal of the American Academy of Psychiatry and the Law, 35*(4), 406–410.

Daubert v. Merrill Dow Pharmaceuticals, 509 U.S. 579 (1993).

de Catanzaro, D. (1986). A mathematical model of evolutionary pressures and reflecting self-preservation and self-destruction. *Suicide and Life-Threatening Behavior, 16,* 84–99.

de Catanzaro, D. (1992). Prediction of self-preservation on the basis of quantitative evolutionary biology. In R. W. Maris et al., eds., *Assessment and prediction of suicide.* New York: Guilford Press.

Dean, P. J., et al. (1996). An escape theory of suicide in college students: Testing a model that includes perfectionism. *Suicide and Life-Threatening Behavior, 26,* 181–186.

Deaths by suicide per 100,000 resident population in the United States from 1950–2014 by gender. (n.d.) Retrieved from *www.statista.com/statistics/187478/death-rate-from-suicide-in-the-us-by-gender-since-1950*

Defense Suicide Prevention Office. (2017, December 31). *Department of Defense quarterly suicide report.* Washington, DC: Department of Defense.

DeLeo, D., et al. (1995). Lower suicide rates associated with a tele-help/tele-check service for elderly at home. *American Journal of Psychiatry, 152,* 632–634.

Desjardins, I., et al. (2016). Suicide risk assessment in hospitals: An expert systems-based triage tool. *Journal of Clinical Psychiatry, 77*(7), e874–e882.

DeSpelder, L. A., & Strickland, A. L. (2015). *The last dance: Encountering death and dying* (10th ed.). New York: McGraw-Hill Education.

Diekstra, R. F. W. (1986). The significance of Nico Speijer's suicide: How and when should suicide be prevented? *Suicide and Life-Threatening Behavior, 16,* 13–15.

DiMaio, V. J. M. (1999). *Gunshot wounds: Practical aspects of firearms, ballistics, and forensic techniques.* Boca Raton, FL: CRC Press.

Dollard, J., et al. (1939). *Frustration and aggression.* New Haven, CT: Yale University Press.

Donnelly, T. (2013, August 15). The military

epidemics that aren't. *The Wall Street Journal.* Retrieved from *www.wsj.com/articles/thomas-donnelly-the-military-epidemics-that-arent-1376606822*

Douglas, J. D. (1967). *The social meanings of suicide.* Princeton, NJ: Princeton University Press.

Drapeau, C. W., & McIntosh, J. L. (2015, April 24). *U.S.A. official final data, 2013.* Washington, DC: American Association of Suicidology.

Ducasse, D., et al. (2018). Psychological pain in suicidality: A meta-analysis. *Journal of Clinical Psychiatry, 79*(3). Retrieved from *www.psychiatrist.com/JCP/article/Pages/2017/v78n08/16r10732.aspx*

Dunne, E. J. (1987). *Suicide and its aftermath: Understanding and counseling the survivors.* New York: Norton.

Durkheim, E. (1951). *Suicide: A study in sociology.* Glencoe, IL: Free Press. (Original work published 1897)

Dwivedi, Y., ed. (2012). *The neurobiological basis of suicide.* Boca Raton: CRC Press/Taylor and Francis.

Early, K. E. (1992). *Religion and suicide in the African-American community.* Westport, CT: Greenwood Press.

Easterlin, R. A. (1987). *Birth and fortune: The impact of numbers on personal welfare.* New York: Basic Books.

Editorial. (2018). Suicide in prisons: NICE fights fires. *The Lancet, 391*(10124), 912.

Egeland, J., & Sussex, J. (1985). Suicide and family loading for affective disorders. *Journal of the American Medical Association, 254,* 915–918.

Egeland, J., et al. (1987). Bipolar affective disorders linked to DNA markers on chromosome 11. *Nature, 325,* 783–787.

Eisele, J. W., et al. (1981). Sites of suicidal gunshot wounds. *Journal of Forensic Sciences, 26,* 480–483.

Eitzen, D. S., with Zinn, M. B. (1989). *Social problems* (4th ed.). Boston: Allyn & Bacon.

Erikson, E. (1963). *Childhood and society* (2nd ed.). New York: Norton.

Erikson, K. (1969). *Wayward Puritans.* New York: Wiley.

Eyman, J. P., & Eyman, S. K. (1992). Personality assessment in suicide prediction. In R. W. Maris et al., eds., *Assessment and prediction of suicide.* New York: Guilford Press.

Fang, O., et al. (2015). Validation of Suicide Resilience Inventory–25 with American and Chinese college students. *Suicide and Life-Threatening Behavior, 45*(1), 51–64.

Farah, A. (2017). *Hemingway's brain.* Columbia: University of South Carolina Press.

Farberow, N. L., ed. (1975). *Suicide in different cultures.* Baltimore: University Park Press.

Farberow, N. L. (1980). *The many faces of suicide: Indirect self-destructive behavior.* New York: McGraw-Hill.

Farberow, N. L., & Shneidman, E. S., eds. (1961). *Cry for help.* New York: McGraw-Hill.

Favazza, A. R. (1996). *Bodies under siege.* Baltimore: Johns Hopkins University Press.

Fawcett, J. A. (2006). Depressive disorders. In R. I. Simon & R. E. Hales, eds., *The American Psychiatric Publishing textbook of suicide assessment and management.* Washington, DC: American Psychiatric Publishing.

Fawcett, J. A. (2012). Depressive disorders. In R. I. Simon & R. E. Hales, eds., *The American Psychiatric Publishing textbook of suicide assessment and management* (2nd ed.). Washington, DC: American Psychiatric Publishing.

Fawcett, J. A., et al. (1997). Acute versus long-term predictors of suicide. In D. Stoff & J. J. Mann, eds., *The neurology of suicide–from the bench to the clinic.* New York: New York Academy of Sciences.

Feeley, W. (2008, April 9). Deposition for *Veterans for Common Sense v. Peake,* 563 F. Supp. 2d 1049 (N.D. Ca. 2008).

Feigelman, W., et al. (2018, April 9). Identifying the social demographic correlated of suicide bereavement. *Archives of Suicide Research.* [Epub ahead of print]

Feinstein, R., & Plutchik, R. (1990). Violence and suicide risk assessment in the psychiatric emergency room. *Comprehensive Psychiatry, 31,* 337–343.

Felner, R. D., et al. (1992). Risk assessment and prevention of youth suicide in schools and educational contexts. In R. W. Maris et al., eds., *Assessment and prediction of suicide.* New York: Guilford Press.

Fincham, F., et al. (2011). *Understanding suicide: A sociological autopsy.* Houndsmill, UK: Palgrave Macmillan.

Fine, C. (1997). *No time to say goodbye.* New York: Doubleday.

Fiori, L. M., et al. (2014). Genetic and neurobiological approaches to understanding suicidal behavior. In M. K. Nock, ed., *The Oxford handbook of suicide and self-injury.* New York: Oxford University Press.

Firth, R. (1961). Suicide and risk-taking in Tikopia society. *Psychiatry, 24,* 1–17.

Fishbain, D. A., et al. (1984). A controlled study of suicide pacts. *Journal of Clinical Psychiatry, 45,* 154–157.

Folstein, M. F., et al. (1975). Mini-mental status: A practical method for grading the cognitive state of patients for the clinician. *Journal of Psychiatric Research, 12*(3), 189–198. (The exam itself is widely available online.)

Food and Drug Administration (FDA). (2006, August 31). *Safety review: Zolpidem, zaleplon, and eszopiclone.* Washington, DC: U.S. Department of Health and Human Services.

Fosse, B. (Director/Writer). (1979). *All that jazz* [Motion picture]. United States: Twentieth-Century Fox.

Freud, S. (1957). Mourning and melancholia. In J. Strachey, ed., & trans., *The standard edition of the complete works of Sigmund Freud* (Vol. 14). London: Hogarth Press. (Original work published 1917)

Frye v. United States, 293 F. 1013 (D.C. Cir. 1923).

Gabbard, G. O., et al. (2012). Psychodynamic treatment. In R. I. Simon & R. E. Hales (eds.), *Textbook of psychiatric assessment and management.* Washington, DC: American Psychiatric Publishing.

Gailiene, D. (2004). Suicidal behaviour in Lithuania. In A. Schmidtke et al., eds., *Suicidal behaviour in Europe.* Cambridge, MA: Hogrefe & Huber.

Gambino, M. (2018). Electroconvulsive therapy in America: The anatomy of a controversy. *American Journal of Psychiatry, 175*(1), 84.

Gananca, L., et al. (2017). Lipid correlations of antidepressant response to omega-3 polyunsaturated fatty acid supplements: A pilot study. *Prostaglandins, Leukotrienenes, and Essential Fatty Acids, 119,* 38–44.

Garrett Lee Smith Memorial Act, Pub. L. No. 108-355, 118 Stat. 1404 (2004).

Gay, P. (1988). *Freud: A life for our time.* New York: Norton.

Gibbs, J. P. (1994). Durkheim's heavy hand in the sociological study of suicide. In D. Lester, ed., *Emile Durkheim: Le suicide: One hundred years later.* Philadelphia: Charles Press.

Gibbs, J. P., & Martin, W. (1964). *Status integration and suicide.* Eugene: University of Oregon Press.

Gibbs, J. T. (1997). African-American suicide: A cultural paradox. *Suicide and Life-Threatening Behavior, 27,* 68–79.

Gibbs, N. (1994, November 14). Death and deceit. *Time.* Retrieved from *http://content.time.com/time/magazine/article/0,9171,981783,00.html*

Gibson, P. (1989). Gay male and lesbian youth suicide. In M. R. Feinleib, ed., *Report of the Secretary's Task Force on Youth Suicide: Vol. 3. Prevention and intervention in youth suicide* (DHHS Publication No. ADM 89-1623). Washington, DC: U.S. Government Printing Office.

Gilbert v. State, 487 So.2d 1185 (1986).

Gilbert, A. M., et al. (2011). Clinical and cognitive correlates of suicide attempts in bipolar disorder: Is suicide predictable? *Journal of Clinical Psychiatry, 72*(8), 1027–1033.

Giner, L., et al. (2014). Violent and serious suicide attempts: One step closer to suicide. *Journal of Clinical Psychiatry, 75*(3), e191–e197.

Ginn, S. (2011, November 3). Models of mental illness [Blog post]. Retrieved from *http://frontierpsychiatrist.co.uk/models-of-mental-illness/*

Ginsberg, A. (Director). (2003). *The iceman and the psychiatrist* [Motion picture]. United States: HBO Home Video.

Glennon, R. A., & Dukat, M. (1991). Serotonin receptors and their ligands: A lack of selective agents. *Pharmacology Biochemistry and Behavior, 40,* 1009–1017.

Goethe, J. W. von. (1774). *The sorrows of young Werther.* Leipzig: Weygand'sche Buchanlung.

Goffman, I. (1961). *Asylums.* Garden City, NY: Anchor Books.

Gold, L. H. (2006). Suicide and gender. In R. I. Simon & R. E. Hales, eds., *The American Psychiatric Publishing textbook of suicide assessment and management.* Washington, DC: American Psychiatric Publishing.

Gold, L. H. (2012). Suicide and gender. In R. I. Simon & R. E. Hales, eds., *The American Psychiatric Publishing textbook of suicide assessment and management* (2nd ed.). Washington, DC: American Psychiatric Publishing.

Goldblatt, M. J. (2000). Physical illness and suicide. In R. W. Maris et al., *Comprehensive textbook of suicidology.* New York: Guilford Press.

Goldsmith, S. K., et al. (2002). *Reducing*

suicide: A national imperative. Washington, DC: National Academies Press.

Goodwin, F. G. (2003). Commentary: Preventing inpatient suicide. *Journal of Clinical Psychiatry, 64*(1), 12–13.

Goodwin, F. G., & Jamison, K. R. (1990). *Manic-depressive illness.* New York: Oxford University Press.

Goodwin, F. G., & Jamison, K. R. (2007). *Manic-depressive illness* (2nd ed.). New York: Oxford University Press.

Gordon, R. S. (1983). An operational classification of disease prevention. *Public Health Reports, 98*, 107–109.

Gould, M. S., & Shaffer, D. (1986). The impact of suicide in television movies: Evidence of imitation, *New England Journal of Medicine, 315*, 690–694.

Gould, M. S., et al. (2018). Follow-up with callers to the National Suicide Prevention Lifeline: Evaluation of callers' perceptions of care. *Suicide and Life-Threatening Behavior, 48*(1), 75–86.

Graafsma, T., et al. (2006). High rates of suicide and attempted suicide using pesticides in Nickeri, Suriname. *Crisis, 27*(2), 77–81.

Gradus, J. L., et al. (2013). Treatment of PTSD reduces suicide ideation. *Depression and Anxiety, 30*(10), 1046–1053.

Green, K. L., et al. (2015). The predictive value of the Beck Depression Inventory suicide item. *Journal of Clinical Psychiatry, 76*(12), 683–686.

Griffiths, R. R., et al. (2011). Psilocybin occasional mystical-type experiences immediate and persisting dose-related effects. *Psychopharmacology, 218*(4), 649–665.

Grohol, J. M. (2017). Pharmacogenetic testing may change psychistric treatments for ADHD, depression. *PsychCentral.* Retrieved from *https://psychcentral.com/blog/pharmacogenetic-testing-may-change-psychiatric-treatments-for-adhd-depression*

Grunebaum, M. F., et al. (2018). Ketamine for rapid reduction of suicidal thoughts in major depression: A midazolam-controlled randomized clinical trial. *American Journal of Psychiatry, 175*(4), 327–335.

Guze, S. B., & Robins, E. (1970). Suicide in primary affective disorders. *British Journal of Psychiatry, 117*, 437–438.

Haberlandt, W. (1967). Aportacin a la genetica del suicidio. *Folia Clinica Internacional, 17*, 319–322.

Haddon, W., Jr., & Baker, S. P. (1981). Injury control. In D. W. Clark & B. MacMahon, eds., *Preventive and community medicine.* Boston: Little, Brown.

Hallinam, J. T. (2014, June 13). School shootings, suicide, and contagion. *Psychology Today.* Retrieved from *www.psychologytoday.com/blog/kidding-ourselves/201406/school-shootings-suicide-and-contagion*

Hamilton, M. (1960). A rating scale for depression. *Journal of Neurology, Neurosurgery and Psychiatry, 23*, 56–61.

Harris, G. (2017, March 2). State Department official praises Mexican efforts in war on drugs. *The New York Times.* Retrieved from *www.nytimes.com/2017/03/02/world/americas/drug-narcotics-mexico-state-department.html*

Harris, M. (1971), *Culture, man and nature.* New York: Crowell.

Harris, M., & Johnson, O. (2006). *Cultural anthropology* (7th ed.). Boston: Allyn & Bacon.

Harvard Injury Control Research Center. (2001). *Suicide.* Cambridge, MA: Harvard T. H. Chan School of Public Health.

Haw, C. M. (1994). A cluster of suicides at a London psychiatric unit. *Suicide and Life-Threatening Behavior, 24*(3), 256–266.

Hawton, K. (2005). *Prevention and treatment of suicidal behavior: From science to practice.* New York: Oxford University Press.

Hawton, K., et al. (2005). Suicide and attempted suicide in bipolar disorder: A systematic review of risk factors. *Journal of Clinical Psychiatry, 66*(6), 693–704.

Hayes, L. M. (2010). *National study of jail suicides, 20 years later.* Washington, DC: National Institute of Corrections.

Hayes, L, M., & Rowan, J, R. (1995, March). *Training curriculum on suicide detection and prevention in jails and lockups.* Alexandria, VA: National Center on Institutions and Alternatives.

Healy, D. (2012). *Pharmageddon.* Berkeley: University of California Press.

Healy, D., et al. (2006). Antidepressants increase suicide risk twenty times. *British Journal of Psychiatry, 188*, 223–228.

Hegel, G. W. F. (1874). *The logic of Hegel.* Oxford: Clarendon Press.

Hendin, H. (1964). *Suicide and Scandinavia.* New York: Grune & Stratton.

Hendin, H. (1969). *Black suicide.* New York: Basic Books.

Hendin, H. (1982). *Suicide in America*. New York: Norton.

Hendin, H. (1995). *Suicide in America* (new and expanded ed.). New York: Norton.

Hendin, H. (1997). *Seduced by death: Doctors, patients, and the Dutch cure*. New York: Norton.

Henry, A. F., & Short, J. (1954). *Suicide and homicide*. Glencoe, IL: Free Press.

Heyerdahl, T. (1950). *The Kon-Tiki expedition: By raft across the South Seas*. London: Allen & Unwin.

Hilker, R., et al. (2010). Concordance rates and early risk factors in schizophrenia: A twin study. *Schizophrenia Research, 2*(3), 199.

Hill, A. B. (1965). The environment and disease: Association or causation? *Proceedings of the Royal Society of Medicine, 58*(5), 295–300.

Hillman, J. (1977). Suicide as the soul's choice. In L. P. Carse & A. B. Dallery, eds., *Death and society*. New York: Harcourt Brace Jovanovich.

Hipple, E., et al. (2008). *Real men do cry*. Naples, FL: Quality of Life.

Hitchcock, A. (2001, July 4). Rising number of dowry deaths in India. *World Socialist Website*. Retrieved from *www.wsws.org/en/articles/2001/07/ind-j04.html*

Holland, S. S. (Director/Writer). (1985). *Better off dead* [Motion picture]. United States: CBS Entertainment Production.

Hollingshead, A. B., & Redlich, F. C. (1958). *Social class and mental illness*. New York: Wiley.

Holmes, T. H., & Rahe, R. H. (1967). The Social Readjustment Rating Scale. *Journal of Psychosomatic Research, 11*, 213–218.

Homans, G. C. (1974). *Social behavior: Its elementary forms*. New York: Harcourt Brace Jovanovich.

Hopkins Brain Wise. (2015, October 8). A nose for schizophrenia. Retrieved from *www.hopkinsmedicine.org/news/articles/a-nose-for-schizophrenia-risk*

Hor, K., & Taylor, M. (2010). Suicide and schizophrenia: A systematic of rates and risk factors. *Journal of Pharmacology, 24*(4), 81–90.

Horton, L. (2006). Social, cultural, and demographic factors in suicide. In R. I. Simon & R. E. Hales, eds., *The American Psychiatric Publishing textbook of suicide assessment and management*. Washington, DC: American Psychiatric Publishing.

Hotchner, A. E. (1966). *Papa Hemingway*. New York: Random House.

House, J. S. (1986). Occupational stress among men and women in the Tecumseh Community Health Study. *Journal of Health and Social Behavior, 27*, 62–77.

Howanitz, E., et al. (1999). The efficacy and safety of clozapine and chlorpromazine in geriatric schizophrenia. *Journal of Clinical Psychiatry, 60*(1), 41–44.

Huff, C. (2004, March). Where personality goes awry. *Monitor on Psychology, 35*(3), p. 42.

Huffine, C. L. (1971). Equivocal single-auto fatalities. *Suicide and Life-Threatening Behavior, 2*, 83–95.

Humphry, D. (2002). *Final exit: The practicalities of self-deliverance and assisted suicide for the dying*. New York: Dell. (Original work published 1991)

Humphry, D., & Wickett, A. (1986). *The right to die: Understanding euthanasia*. New York: Harper & Row.

Huxley, A. (1932). *Brave new world*. London: Chatto & Windus.

Iga, M. (1993). Japanese suicide. In A. A. Leenaars, ed., *Suicidology: Essays in honor of E. S. Shneidman*. Northdale, NJ: Jason Aronson.

Ikeda, R., et al. (2018, April 19). *Aligning efforts in the public sector: The national response to suicide*. Paper presented at the 51st annual conference of the American Association of Suicidology, Washington, DC.

Ilgen, M., et al. (2008). Pain and suicidal thoughts, plans, and attempts in the United States. *Hospital Psychiatry, 30*(6), 521–527.

Ilgen, M. A. (2010). Psychiatric diagnoses and the risk of suicide in veteran suicide. *Archives of Suicide Research, 67*(11), 1152–1158.

Institute of Medicine. (1994). *The mental health intervention spectrum*. Washington, DC: National Academy Press.

Interian, A., et al. (2018). Use of the Columbia-Suicide Severity Rating Scale (C-SSRS) to classify suicidal behaviors. *Archives of Suicide Research, 22*(2), 278–294.

Ishii, N., et al. (2015). Low risk of male suicide in drinking water. *Journal of Clinical Psychiatry, 76*(3), 319–326.

Isometsa, E. T., & Lönnqvist, J. E. (1998).

Suicide attempts preceding completed suicide. *British Journal of Psychiatry, 173,* 531–535.

Isometsa, E. T., et al. (1996). Suicide among children with personality disorders. *American Journal of Psychiatry, 153,* 667–673.

Jacobs, D. G., et al., eds. (2003, 2010). *Practice guideline for the assessment and treatment of patients with suicidal behaviors.* Washington, DC: American Psychiatric Press.

James, D. J., & Glaze, L. F. (2006). *Mental health problems of jail and prison inmates.* Washington, DC: Bureau of Justice Statistics.

Jamison, K. R. (Producer). (1991). *To paint the stars: The life and mind of Vincent Van Gogh* [Documentary]. Washington, DC: Georgetown Television Productions.

Jamison, K. R. (1993). *Touched with fire: Manic–depressive illness and the artistic temperament.* New York: Free Press.

Jamison, K. R. (1995). *An unquiet mind.* New York: Knopf.

Jenkins, J. (1980). Single car single driver fatalities. *British Medical Journal, 281,* 10–18.

Jobes, D. A. (2016). *Managing suicidal risk* (2nd ed.). New York: Guilford Press.

Jobes, D. A. (2018, April 19). *Innovations in clinical assessment and treatment of suicidal risk.* Paper presented at the 51st annual conference of the American Association of Suicidology, Washington, DC.

Jobes, D. A., et al. (1987). Improving the validity and reliability of medical–legal certification of death. *Suicide and Life-Threatening Behavior, 17,* 310–325.

Jobes, D. A., et al. (1996). The Kurt Cobain crisis. *Suicide and Life-Threatening Behavior, 26,* 260–271.

Jobes, D. A., et al. (2000). In the wake of suicide: Survivorship and postvention. In R. W. Maris et al., *Comprehensive textbook of suicide.* New York: Guilford Press.

Johnson, J. G., et al. (1999). Childhood maltreatment increases risk of personality disorder during early adulthood. *Archives of General Psychiatry, 56,* 600–606.

Joiner, T. (2005). *Why people die by suicide.* Cambridge, MA: Harvard University Press.

Joiner, T. (2010). *Myths about suicide.* Cambridge, MA: Harvard University Press.

Joiner, T. (2014). *Perversion of virtue.* New York: Oxford University Press.

Joiner, T., et al. (2017). A sociobiological explanation of the interpersonal theory of suicide. *Crisis, 38,* 69–72.

Jordan, J. R., & McIntosh, J. L., eds. (2011). *Grief after suicide.* New York: Routledge.

Joshua Omvig Veterans Suicide Prevention Act, Pub. L. No. 110-110, 121 Stat. 1031 (2007).

Jowett, B., ed., & trans. (1950). *Plato's dialogues* (3rd ed.). London: Oxford University Press.

Kachur, S. P., et al. (1995). *Suicide in the U.S., 1980–1992.* Atlanta, GA: National Center for Injury Prevention and Control.

Kallman, F. J. (1953). *Heredity and health in mental disorder.* New York: Norton.

Kang, H. K. (2007, December 11). *The risk of suicide among vets of OIF and OEF.* Unpublished manuscript.

Kaplan, A. G., & Klein, R. B. (1989). Women and suicide. In D. J. Jacobs & H. N. Brown, eds., *Suicide: Understanding and responding.* Madison, CT: International Universities Press.

Kar, N., et al. (2014, October). Scale for assessing lethality of suicide attempt risk. *Indian Journal of Psychiatry, 56*(4), 337–343.

Karp, D. A., & Sisson, G. E., eds. (2010). *Voices from the inside.* New York: Oxford University Press.

Kastenbaum, R. (1993). Avery D. Weisman, M.D.: An *Omega* interview. *Omega: Journal of Death and Dying, 27,* 97–103.

Katz, I. (2008, February 21). Deposition for *Veterans for Common Sense v. Peake,* 563 F. Supp. 2d 1049 (N.D. Ca. 2008).

Kaufman, P. (Director/Writer). (1993). *Rising sun* [Motion picture]. United States: Twentieth-Century Fox.

Kellerman, A. L., & Reay, D. T. (1986). Protection or peril: An analysis of firearm-related deaths in the home. *New England Journal of Medicine, 314,* 1557–1560.

Kesey, K. (1962). *One flew over the cuckoo's nest.* New York: Viking Press.

Kessler, R. (2005). Prevalence, severity, and comorbidity of DSM-IV disorders. *Archives of General Psychiatry, 62,* 617–627.

Kessler, R. C., et al. (2015). Predicting suicides after psychiatric hospitalization in U.S. Army soldiers (Army STARRS). *JAMA Psychiatry, 72*(1), 49–57.

Kettlewell, C. (1999). *Skin game.* New York: St. Martin's Press.

Kevorkian, J. (1991). *Prescription–medicide; The*

goodness of planned death. Amherst, NY: Prometheus Books.

Khan, M, M. (1995). *The translation of the meanings of summarized Sahih Al-Bukhari* [Arabic–English]. Chicago: Kazi.

Kime, P. (2015, April 1). Study: No link between combat deployment and suicides. *Military Times*. Retrieved from *www.militarytimes.com/pay-benefits/military-benefits/health-care/2015/04/01/study-no-link-between-combat-deployment-and-suicides*

King, C. A. (1997). Suicidal behavior in adolescence. In R. W. Maris et al., eds., *Review of suicidology, 1997*. New York: Guilford Press.

King, P. (2017, April 2). How many neurotransmitters are there in a human brain? *Quora*. Retrieved from *www.quora.com/how-many-types-of-neurotransmitters-are-there-in-a-human-brain*

Kinn, J. T., et al. (2011). *Department of Defense suicide event report: Calendar year 2010 annual report*. Washington, DC: National Center for Telehealth and Technology.

Kirsch, I. (2010). *The emperor's new drugs: Exploding the antidepressant myth*. New York: Basic Books.

Klausner, S. Z., ed. (1968). *Why man takes chances: Studies in stress-seeking*. Garden City, NY: Doubleday/Anchor.

Klonsky, J. D. (2015, April). *Edwin S. Shneidman award address*. Paper presented at the annual meeting of the American Association of Suicidology, Atlanta, GA.

Klonsky, J. D. (2018, April 19). *Suicide prevention is stalled*. Paper presented at the 51st annual conference of the American Association of Suicidology, Washington, DC.

Klonsky, J. D., & May, A. M. (2014). Differentiating suicide attempters from suicide ideators. *Suicide and Life-Threatening Behavior, 44*(1), 1–5.

Klonsky, J. D., & May, A. M. (2015). The three-step theory (3ST): A new theory of suicide rooted in the "ideation-to-action" framework. *International Journal of Cognitive Therapy, 8*, 114–129.

Koang, P. (2014, September 15). South Sudan has the highest suicide rates. Eye Radio. Retrieved from *www.eyeradio.org/south-sudan-highest-suicide-rates*

Koestler, A. (1940). *Darkness at noon*. London: Macmillan.

Kovacs, M., et al. (1975). Hopelessness: An indicator of suicide risk. *Suicide, 5*, 98–103.

Kraepelin, E. (1906). Über sprachtorungen im trauma. Leipzig, Germany: Egelmann.

Kramer, P. D. (1993). *Listening to Prozac*. New York: Viking.

Kreitman, N. (1976). The coal gas story: United Kingdom suicide rates, 1960–1971. *British Journal of Preventive and Social Medicine, 30*, 86–93.

Kübler-Ross, E. (1969). *On death and dying*. New York: Macmillan.

Kuehn, B. M. (2009). Solider suicide rates continue to rise. *Journal of the American Medical Association, 301*(11), 1111–1113.

Kuehn, B. M. (2014). Rate of suicide increases in middle-age. *Journal of the American Medical Association, 312*(17), 1727–1728.

Kulbarsh, P. (2014, December 11). The epidemiology of suicide: Who is most likely to take their own life? Retrieved from *www.officer.com/tactical/ems-hazmat/article/12026794/the-epidemiology-of-suicide-who-is-most-likely-to-take-their-own-life*

Kushner, H. I. (1989). *Self-destruction in the promised land*. New Brunswick, NJ: Rutgers University Press.

Lam, A. (2014, May 22). A hidden tragedy—mental illness and suicide among Asian-Americans. *New America Media*. Retrieved from *http://newamericamedia.org/2014/05/a-hidden-tragedy----mental-illness-and-suicide-among-asian-americans.php*

Lankford, A. (2009). *Human killing machines*. Lanham, MD: Lexington Books.

Lankford, A. (2013). *The myth of martyrdom: What really drives suicide bombers, rampage shooters, and other self-destructive killers*. New York: St. Martin's Press.

Leamon, M. H., & Bostwick, J. M. (2012). Substance-related disorders. In R. I. Simon & R. E. Hales, eds., *The American Psychiatric Publishing textbook of suicide assessment and management* (2nd ed.). Washington, DC: American Psychiatric Publishing.

LeardMann, C. A., et al. (2013). Risk factors associated with suicide in current and former U.S. military personnel. *Journal of the American Medical Association, 310*(5), 496–506.

Lee, E. H. M., et al. (2018). Suicide rates, psychiatric hospital bed numbers, and unemployment rates from 1999–2015: A population-based study in Hong Kong. *American Journal of Psychiatry, 175*(3), 285–286.

Lee, L., et al. (2015). Suicide. In M. Roser, ed., *Our world in data*. Oxford, UK: Oxford Martin Programme on Global Development. Retrieved from *https://ourworldindata.org/suicide*

Leenaars, A. (1988). *Suicide notes: Predictive clues and patterns*. New York: Human Sciences Press.

Leenaars, A. (1991). *Life-span perspectives of suicides: Time-lines in the suicide process*. New York: Plenum Press.

Lehman, A. F., et al. (1980). Recovery from schizophrenia. *Schizophrenia Bulletin, 6*, 606–618.

Leighton, A. H., & Hughes, C. C. (1955). Notes on Eskimo patterns of suicide. *Southwestern Journal of Anthropology, 11*, 327–338.

Lemert, E. M. (1951). *Social pathology*. New York: McGraw-Hill.

Lenzenweger, M. F., et al. (2007). DSM-IV personality disorders in the National Comorbidity Survey Replication. *Biological Psychiatry, 62*(6), 553–564.

Leo, J. (2003). The fallacy of the 50% concordance rate for schizophrenia in identical twins. *Human Nature Review, 3*, 406–415.

Lester, D. (1988). *The biochemical basis of suicide*. Springfield, IL: Charles C Thomas.

Lester, D. (1996). The sexual politics of double suicide. *Proceedings of the Parvese Society, 7*, 21–22.

Lester, D. (2000). Alcoholism, substance abuse, and suicide. In R. W. Maris et al., *Comprehensive textbook of suicidology*. New York: Guilford Press.

Lester, D. (2012). Suicide prevention by lethal means prevention. In R. I. Simon & R. E. Hales, eds., *The American Psychiatric Publishing textbook of suicide assessment and management* (2nd ed.). Washington, DC: American Psychiatric Publishing.

Lettieri, D. J., et al. (1974). *The prediction of suicide*. Bowie, MD: Charles Press.

Levinson, B. (Director). (2010). *You don't know Jack* [Motion picture]. United States: HBO Films.

Levinson, D. J., with Levinson, J. D. (1996). *The seasons of a woman's life*. New York: Knopf.

Levinson, D. J., et al. (1978). *The seasons of a man's life*. New York: Knopf.

Lifton, R. J. (1983). *The broken connection: On death and the continuity of life*. New York: Basic Books.

Linehan, M. M. (1997). Behavioral treatments of suicidal behaviors: Definitional obfuscation and treatment outcomes. *Annals of the New York Academy of Sciences, 836*, 302–308.

Linehan, M. M. (2015, April). *How I got out of hell*. Plenary address presented at the annual conference of the American Association of Suicidology, Atlanta, GA.

Linehan, M. M., & Laffaw, J. A. (1982). Suicidal behaviors among clients of an outpatient clinic versus the general population. *Suicide and Life-Threatening Behavior, 12*, 234–239.

Linehan, M. M., et al. (1983). Reasons for living when you are thinking of killing yourself: The Reasons for Living Inventory. *Journal of Consulting and Clinical Psychiatry, 51*, 276–286.

Linehan, M. M., et al. (2006). Two-year randomized controlled trial and follow up of dialectical behavioral therapy versus therapy by experts for suicidal behaviors and borderline personality disorder. *Archives of General Psychiatry, 7*, 757–766.

Linehan, M. M., et al. (2015). Dialectical behavior therapy for high suicide risk in individuals with borderline personality disorder. *JAMA Psychiatry, 72*(5), 475–482.

Linn-Gust, M. (2010). *Rocky roads*. Albuquerque, NM: Chellehead Books.

Lithium: Patient drug information. (2013). Retrieved from *http://sinalib.ir/uptodate/contents/mobipreview.htm?27/29/28117?source=see_link*

Litman, R. E. (1989). Suicides: What do they have in mind? In D. Jacobs & H. N. Brown, eds., *Suicide: Understanding and responding*. Madison, CT: International Universities Press.

Litman, R. E. (1992). Predicting and preventing hospital and clinic suicides. In R. W. Maris et al., eds., *Assessment and prediction of suicide*. New York: Guilford Press.

Loh, C., et al. (2012). Suicide in young Singaporeans aged 10–24 years between 2000–2004. *Archives of Suicide Research, 16*(2), 174–182.

Lubin, G., et al. (2010). Decrease in suicide rates after a change in policy reducing access to firearms in adolescents: A natural epidemiological study. *Suicide and Life-Threatening Behavior, 40*, 421–424.

Luxton, D. D., et al. (2012). *Department of Defense suicide event report: Calendar year*

2011 annual report. Washington, DC: National Center for Telehealth and Technology.

Mack, A. H., & Lightdale, H. A. (2006). Substance-related disorder. In R. I. Simon & R. E. Hales, eds., *The American Psychiatric Publishing textbook of suicide assessment and management*. Washington, DC: American Psychiatric Publishing.

MacRandle, J. H. (1965). *The track of the wolf*. Evanston, IL: Northwestern University Press.

Maguen, D., et al. (2011). Killing in combat, mental health symptoms, and suicide ideation in Iraq war veterans. *Journal of Anxiety Disorders, 25*(4), 563–567.

Malinowski, B. (1926). *Crime and custom in savage society*. London: Routledge & Kegan Paul.

Malmquist, C. P. (2012). Combined murder-suicide. In R. I. Simon & R. E. Hales, eds., *The American Psychiatric Publishing textbook of suicide assessment and management* (2nd ed.). Washington, DC: American Psychiatric Publishing.

Maltsberger, J. T. (1992). The psychodynamic formulation: An aid in assessing suicide risk. In R. W. Maris et al., eds., *Assessment and prediction of suicide*. New York: Guilford Press.

Maltsberger, J. T. (1998). Past consultation: Robert Salter, attempted suicide by jumping from a high bridge. *Suicide and Life-Threatening Behavior, 28*, 226–233.

Maltsberger, J. T. (2006). Outpatient therapy. In R. I. Simon & R. E. Hales, eds., *The American Psychiatric Publishing textbook of suicide assessment and management*. Washington, DC: American Psychiatric Publishing.

Maltsberger, J. T., & Buie, D. H. (1980). The devices of suicide: Revenge, riddance, and rebirth. *International Review of Psychoanalysis, 7*, 61–72.

Maltsberger, J. T., & Stoklosa, J. B. (2012). Outpatient treatment. In R. I. Simon & R. E. Hales, eds., *The American Psychiatric Publishing textbook of suicide assessment and management* (2nd ed.). Washington, DC: American Psychiatric Publishing.

Maltsberger, J. T., et al. (2003). Detection of precipitating events in the suicide of psychiatric patients. *Suicide and Life-Threatening Behavior, 33*(2), 111–119.

Manji, H. K., et al. (2003). The underlying neurobiology of bipolar disorder. *World Psychiatry, 2*(3), 136–146.

Mann, J. J. (2008, February 17). The neurobiology of suicide [Interview with ABC Radio, Australia].

Mann, J. J., & Currier, D. (2012). The neurobiology of suicide. In R. I. Simon & R. E. Hales, eds., *The American Psychiatric Publishing textbook of suicide assessment and management* (2nd ed.). Washington, DC: American Psychiatric Publishing.

Mann, J., & Rudd, D. (2018, April 19). *The 10-year billion dollar research challenge: What will make the difference?* Paper presented at the 51st annual conference of the American Association of Suicidology, Washington, DC.

Manning, M. (1995). *Undercurrents: a life beneath the surface*. New York: Harper One.

Marchalik, D., & Jurecic, A. (2018). Rethinking cures in Jessie Ball's *A Cure for Suicide*. *The Lancet, 391*(10127), 1252.

Maris, R. W. (1967). Suicide, status, and mobility in Chicago. *Social Forces, 46*, 246–256.

Maris, R. W. (1969). *Social forces in urban suicide*. Homewood, IL: Dorsey Press.

Maris, R. W. (1971). Deviance as therapy: The paradox of the self-destructive female. *Journal of Health and Social Behavior, 12*, 113–124.

Maris, R. W. (1972). Female suicidal careers. *Journal of Health and Social Behavior, 13*, 105–109.

Maris, R. W. (1981). *Pathways to suicide: A survey of self-destructive behaviors*. Baltimore: Johns Hopkins University Press.

Maris, R. W. (1982). Rational suicide. *Suicide and Life-Threatening Behavior, 12, 3–16*.

Maris, R. W. (1985). The adolescent suicide problem. *Suicide and Life-Threatening Behavior, 15*, 91–109.

Maris, R. W., ed. (1986). *The biology of suicide*. New York: Guilford Press.

Maris, R. W. (1988). *Social problems*. Belmont, CA: Wadsworth.

Maris, R. W. (1991). Suicide. In R. Dulbecco, ed., *Encyclopedia of human biology* (Vol. 7). San Diego, CA: Academic Press.

Maris, R. W. (1992a). [Book review of *Final exit* by D. Humphry]. *Suicide and Life-Threatening Behavior, 22*(4), 514–516.

Maris, R. W. (1992b). How are suicides different? In R. W. Maris et al., eds., *Assessment and prediction of suicide.* New York: Guilford Press.

Maris, R. W. (1993). The evolution of suicidology. In A. A. Leenaars, ed., *Suicidology: Essays in honor of Edwin S. Shneidman.* Northvale, NJ: Jason Aronson.

Maris, R. W. (1997a). Social and familial risk factors in suicidal behavior. In J. J. Mann, ed., *Psychiatric clinics of North America: Suicide.* Philadelphia: Saunders.

Maris, R. W. (1997b). Suicide. In R. Dulbecco, ed., *Encyclopedia of human biology* (2nd ed., Vol. 8). San Diego, CA: Academic Press.

Maris, R. W. (2002). Suicide. *The Lancet, 360,* 319–326.

Maris, R. W. (2007). A comment on Goldney: Suicide during the course of treatment for depression. *Suicide and Life-Threatening Behavior, 37,* 600–601.

Maris, R. W. (2008, May 6). Witness statement. In *The truth about veteran suicides: Hearing before the Committee on Veterans' affairs, U.S. House of Representatives, 110th Congress, second session.* Washington, DC: U.S. Government Printing Office.

Maris, R. W. (2010). Suicide within the dental profession. *The Nugget, 56*(6), 8–9.

Maris, R. W. (2015). *Pillaged: Psychiatric medications and suicide risk.* Columbia: University of South Carolina Press.

Maris, R. W. (2017). Suicide. In D. V. McQueen, ed., *Oxford bibliographies in public health.* New York: Oxford University Press.

Maris, R. W., et al., eds. (1992). *Assessment and prediction of suicide.* New York: Guilford Press.

Maris, R. W., et al. (2000). *Comprehensive textbook of suicidology.* New York: Guilford Press.

Martin, R. A., & Kuiper, N. A. (1999). Daily occurrence of laughter. *International Journal of Humor Research, 12*(4), 355–384.

Marver, J. E., et al. (2017). Friendship, depression, and suicide attempts in adults: Exploratory analysis of a longitudinal study. *Suicide and Life-Threatening Behavior, 47*(6), 660–671.

Marzuk, P. M., et al. (1992). Prevalence of cocaine use among residents of New York City who committed suicide. *American Journal of Psychiatry, 149,* 371–375.

Maslow, A. H. (1963). *Motivation and personality.* New York: Harper & Row.

Massey, J. T. (n.d.). *Suicide in the United States,* *1950–1964.* Rockville, MD: National Center for Health Statistics.

Mausner, J. S., & Baum, A. K. (1985). *Epidemiology: An introductory textbook.* Philadelphia: Saunders.

Mayhew, B. H. (1983). Hierarchical differentiation of imperatively coordinated associations. In S. B. Bacharach, ed., *Research in the sociology of organizations* (Vol. 2). Greenwich, CT: JAI Press.

Mayo, D. J. (1992). What is being predicted?: Definitions of "suicide." In R. W. Maris et al., eds., *Assessment and prediction of suicide.* New York: Guilford Press.

Mayo, D. J. (2015, April). Philosophy and suicide. Paper presented at the annual conference of the American Association of Suicidology annual conference, Atlanta, GA.

Mazower, M. (2000, January 2). A tormented life. Retrieved from *www.nytimes.com/ books/00/01/02/reviews/000102.02mazowet. html*

McCormick, C. G. (1992, January 31). Clinical review of gabapentin. *NDA # 20–235.*

McDowell, C. P., et al. (1994). Witnessed suicide. *Suicide and Life-Threatening Behavior, 24,* 213–223.

McIntosh, J. L. (1992). Methods of suicide. In R. W. Maris et al., eds., *Assessment and prediction of suicide.* New York: Guilford Press.

McIntosh, J. L. (2002). U.S. Official Suicide Rater, 2002. Retrieved from *www.suicidology.org/resources/facts-statistics*

McIntosh, J. L. (2005). U.S. Official Suicide Rater, 2005. Retrieved from *www.suicidology.org/resources/facts-statistics*

McIntosh, J. L. (2018a, April). *Observations on developmental trends in suicide and survivors of suicide loss issues.* Paper presented at the 51st annual conference of the American Association of Suicidology, Washington, DC.

McIntosh, J. L. (2018b, April). *Healing after suicide loss: Strength, hope, and connection.* Paper presented at the 51st annual conference of the American Association of Suicidology, Washington, DC.

Meltzer, H. Y. (1999). Suicide and schizophrenia: Clozapine and the IntersePT study. *Journal of Clinical Psychiatry, 12,* 47–50.

Melville, H. (1981). *Moby Dick.* Berkeley: University of California Press. (Original work published 1851)

Menninger, K. (1938). *Man against himself.* New York: Harcourt, Brace & World.

Merari, A. (2010). *Driven to death*. New York; Oxford University Press.

Metzner, J. L., & Hayes, L. M. (2012). Suicide prevention in jails and prisons. In R. I. Simon & R. E. Hales, eds., *The American Psychiatric Publishing textbook of suicide assessment and management* (2nd ed.). Washington, DC: American Psychiatric Publishing.

Meyer, D. (2012). Split treatment: Coming of age. In R. I. Simon & R. E. Hales, eds., *The American Psychiatric Publishing textbook of suicide assessment and management* (2nd ed.). Washington, DC: American Psychiatric Publishing.

Miller, A. L., et al. (2007). *Dialectical behavior therapy with suicidal adolescents*. New York: Guilford Press.

Miller, M., & Hemenway, D. (2008). Guns and suicide in the United States. *New England Journal of Medicine, 359*, 989–991.

Millner, A. J., et al. (2017). Describing and measuring the pathway to suicide attempts: A preliminary study. *Suicide and Life-Threatening Behavior, 47*(3), 353–369.

Milner, A., et al. (2013). Long-term unemployment and suicide: A systematic review and meta-analysis. *PLOS ONE, 8*(1), e51333.

Minkove, J. F. (2016, Winter). Combining genes, epigenetics, and stress response to study suicide and PTSD. *Hopkins Brain Wise*. Retrieved from *www.hopkinsmedicine.org/news/articles/combining-genes-epigenetics-and-stress-responses-to-study-suicide-and-ptsd*

Mishara, B. L., ed. (1995). *The impact of suicide*. New York: Springer.

Mishima, Y. (2012). Patriotism (G. W. Sargent, trans.). Retrieved from *www.mutant-frog.com/patriotism-by-yukio-mishima*. (Original work published 1960)

Mojtabai, R. (2013). Clinician identified depression in a community setting. *Psychotherapy and Psychometrics, 82*, 161–169.

Moksony, F. (1997, March 23). *Educational mobility and suicide in Hungary*. Paper presented at the 19th Congress of the International Association for Suicide Prevention, Adelaide, Australia.

Morgen, B. (Director/Writer). (2015). *Cobain: Montage of heck* [Motion picture]. United States: HBO Documentary Films.

Motto, J. A. (1992). An integrated approach to estimating suicide risk. In R. W. Maris et al., eds., *Assessment and prediction of suicide*. New York: Guilford Press.

Mueller, A. S., & Abrutyn, S. (2015). Suicidal disclosures among friends: Using social network data to understand suicide contagion. *Journal of Health and Social Behavior, 56*(1), 131–148.

Muncie, W. (1963, August). Depression or depressions. *Canadian Psychiatric Journal*, pp. 217–224.

Mundt, J. C., et al. (2013). Prediction of suicidal behavior in clinical research by lifetime suicidal ideation and behavior ascertained by the electronic Columbia-suicide severity rating scale. *Journal of Clinical Psychiatry, 74*(9), 887–893.

Murphy, G. E. (1992). *Suicide in alcoholism*. New York: Oxford University Press.

Murphy, G. E. (1998). Why women are less likely than men to commit suicide. *Comprehensive Psychiatry, 39*, 165–175.

Murphy, G. E., & Robins, E. (1967). Social factors in suicide. *Journal of the American Medical Association, 199*, 303–308.

Murray, H. A. (1938). *Explorations in personality*. New York: Oxford University Press.

Nasreddine, Z. S., et al. (2005). The Montreal Cognitive Assessment, MOCA. *Journal of the American Geriatric Society, 53*, 695–699.

National Commission on Correctional Health Care. (2015). *Standards for mental health services in correctional facilities* (2nd ed.). Chicago: Author.

National Institute on Drug Abuse. (2010, December 3). *Results of the 2010 Monitoring the Future survey*. Bethesda, MD: Author.

National Prevention Council. (2011, June). *National prevention strategy*. Washington, DC: U.S. Department of Health and Human Services, Office of the Surgeon General. Retrieved from *www.surgeongeneral.gov/priorities/prevention/strategy/report.pdf*

Nemeroff, C. B. (2018). Ketamine: Quo vadis? *American Journal of Psychiatry, 175*(4), 297–299.

Nemtsov, A. (2003). Suicides and alcohol consumption in Russia, 1965–1999. *Drug and Alcohol Dependence, 71*(2), 161–168.

Niederkrotenthaler, T., et al. (2015). Changes in suicide rates following media reports of celebrity suicides: A meta-analysis. *Journal of Epidemiology and Community Health, 66*, 1037–1042.

Nisbet, P. A. (1996). Protective factors for suicidal black females. *Suicide and Life-Threatening Behavior, 26*, 325–341.

Nock, M. K. (2009). Why do people hurt

themselves?: New insights into the nature and functions of self-injury. *Current Directions in Psychological Science, 18*(2), 78–83.

Nock, M. K., ed. (2014). *The Oxford handbook of suicide and self-injury.* New York: Oxford University Press.

Nock, M. K. (2018, April 19). *Future directions for suicide research.* Paper presented at the 51st Annual Conference of the American Association of Suicidology, Washington, DC.

Nock, M. K., et al. (2014). Prevalence and correlates of suicidal behavior among soldiers: Results from the Army STARRS. *JAMA Psychiatry, 71*(5), 514–522.

Noonan, M., et al. (2015, August 15). *Mortality in local jails and state prisons, 2000–2013–statistical tables.* Washington, DC: U.S. Bureau of Justice Statistics.

Nordt, C., et al. (2015). Modelling suicide and unemployment. *The Lancet Psychiatry, 2*(3), 239–245.

Oaklander, M. (2017, August 7). The anti antidepressant. *Time,* pp. 38–45.

O'Carroll, P. W., et al. (1996). Beyond the Tower of Babel: A nomenclature for suicidology. *Suicide and Life-Threatening Behavior, 26,* 237–252.

O'Connor, R. C. (2011). Towards an integrated motivational-volitional model of suicidal behavior. In R. C. O'Connor et al., eds., *International handbook of suicide prevention.* Chichester, UK: Wiley-Blackwell.

O'Connor, R. C. (2018, April 19). *The bridge between intention and behavior.* Paper presented at the 51st annual conference of the American Association of Suicidology, Washington, DC.

O'Connor, R. C., et al., eds. (2011). *International handbook of suicide prevention.* Chichester, UK: Wiley-Blackwell.

Ohnuki-Tierney, E. (2006). *Kamikaze diaries: Reflections of Japanese student soldiers.* Chicago: University of Chicago Press.

Olfson, M., et al. (2015). Trends in mental health care among children and adolescents. *New England Journal of Medicine, 372*(21), 2029–2038.

O'Neill, S., et al. (2018). Factors associated with suicides in four age groups: A population based study. *Archives of Suicide Research, 22*(1), 128–138.

Orwell, G. (1949). *1984.* London: Secker & Warburg.

Østergaard, S. D. (2018). Increasing male preponderance in suicide coinciding with a reduction by half in total suicides in the Danish population should raise awareness of male depression. *American Journal of Psychiatry, 175*(4), 381–382.

Ougrin, D., & Asarnow, J. R. (2018). The end of family therapy for self-harm, or a new beginning? *The Lancet Psychiatry, 5*(3), 188–189.

Parkin, R., & Dunne-Maxim, K. (1995). *Child survivors of suicide.* New York: American Foundation for Suicide Prevention.

Pasternick, M. A., et al. (2006). Naturalistic course in unipolar major depression in absence of somatic treatment. *Journal of Nervous and Mental Disease, 194,* 324–329.

Pearson, V., et al. (2002). Attempted suicides among young rural women in the People's Republic of China. *Suicide and Life-Threatening Behavior, 32*(4), 359–379.

People v. Roberts, 211 Mich. 187, 178 N.W. 2d 690 (1920).

Perry, F. (Director). (1962). *David and Lisa* [Motion picture]. United States: Vision Associates Productions.

Pescosolido, B. A. (1994). Bringing Durkheim into the twenty-first century: A network approach to unresolved issues in the sociology of suicide. In D. Lester, ed., *Emile Durkheim: Le suicide: One hundred years later.* Philadelphia: Charles Press.

Pescosolido, B. A., & Georgianna, S. (1989). Durkheim, suicide, and religion: Toward a network theory of suicide. *American Sociological Review, 54,* 33–48.

Petersen, A. (2016a, June 7). As suicide rates rise, scientists find new warning signs. *The Wall Street Journal.* Retrieved from *www.wsj.com/articles/as-suicide-rates-rise-scientists-find-new-warning-signs-1465235288*

Petersen, A. (2016b, June 20). Researchers study new ways to treat suicide risk. *The Wall Street Journal.* Retrieved from *www.wsj.com/articles/researchers-study-new-ways-to-treat-suicide-risk-1466447160*

Peterson, D. (1997, March 3). A lonely death in Texas: Pressures at the top drive a new CEO to suicide. *Newsweek,* p. 53.

Pfeffer, C. (1986). *The suicidal child.* New York: Guilford Press.

Pfeffer, C. (1989). *Suicide among youth.* Washington, DC: American Psychiatric Press.

Phillips, D. P. (1970). *Birthday and deathday.* Unpublished doctoral dissertation, Princeton University, Princeton, NJ.

Phillips, D. P. (1974). The influence of

suggestion on suicide: Substantive and theoretical implications of the Werther effect. *American Sociological Review, 39,* 340–354.

Phillips, D. P. (1980). Airplane accidents, murder, and the mass media. *Social Forces, 58,* 1001–1024.

Phillips, D. P., & Carstensen, L. L. (1986). Clustering of teenage suicides after television news stories about suicide. *New England Journal of Medicine, 315,* 685–689.

Phillips, D. P., et al. (1992). Suicide and the media. In R. W. Maris et al., eds., *Assessment and prediction of suicide.* New York: Guilford Press.

Phillips, M. R., et al. (2002). Risk factors for suicide in China: A national case–control psychological autopsy. *The Lancet, 360*(9247), 1728–1736.

Physicians' Desk Reference. (2013). (67th ed.). Montvale, NJ: PDR Network.

Piaget, J. (1929). *The child's conception of the world.* London: Routledge & Kegan Paul.

Pickert, K. (2014, February 3). The mindful revolution. *Time.* Retrieved from *http://content.time.com/time/subscriber/article/0,33009,2163560,00.html*

Plath, S. (1966). *Ariel.* New York: Harper & Row.

Plath, S. (2005). *The bell jar.* New York: HarperCollins. (Original work published 1963)

Platt, S. (1984). Unemployment and suicidal behavior: A review of the literature. *Social Science and Medicine, 19,* 93–115.

Plemmons, G., et al. (2018, May 16). Suicide attempts rising among American high schoolers. *Pediatrics.*

Plutchik, R. (2000). Agression, violence, and suicide. In R. L. Maris & A. L. Berman, eds., *Comprehensive textbook of suicidology.* New York: Guilford Press.

Pokorny, A. D. (1983). Prediction of suicide in psychiatric patients. *Archives of General Psychiatry, 40,* 249–257.

Pokorny, A. D. (1992). Prediction of suicide in psychiatric patients. In R. W. Maris et al., eds., *Assessment and prediction of suicide.* New York: Guilford Press.

Pompili, M., et al. (2014). Suicidality in DSM-IV Cluster B personality disorders. *Annali dell'Istituto Superiore di Senita, 40*(4), 475–483.

Porterfield, A. L., & Gibbs, J. P. (1960). Occupational prestige and social mobility of suicides in New Zealand. *American Journal of Sociology, 66,* 147–152.

Posner, K., et al. (2007). The Columbia Suicide Severity Scale. *American Journal of Psychiatry, 164,* 1035–1043.

Price, M. (2010, October). Suicide among preadolescents. *Monitor on Psychology, 41*(9), 52.

Pridemore, W. A., & Spivak, A. L. (2003). Patterns of suicide mortality in Russia. *Suicide and Life-Threatening Behavior, 33*(2), 132–150.

Prigerson, H. G., et al. (2009). Prolonged grief disorder: Psychometric validation of criteria proposed for DSM-V and ICD-11. *PLOS Medicine, 6*(8), 1–12.

Qiu, T. et al. (2017). Hopelessness predicts suicide ideation, but not attempts: A 10-year longitudinal study. *Suicide and Life-Threatening Behavior, 47*(6), 718–722.

Quan, H., et al. (2002). Association between physical illness and suicide among elderly. *Social Psychiatry and Psychiatric Epidemiology, 37,* 190–197.

Randall, E. (2013, May 8). Tattooing makes transition from cult to fine art. *The New York Times.* Retrieved from *www.nytimes.com/2013/05/10/arts/artsspecial/Tracing-the-transformation-of-tattoos-.html*

Range, L. M., & Goggin, W. C. (1990). Reactions to suicide: Does age of the victim make a difference? *Death Studies, 14,* 269–275.

Rapoport, J. (2010). The auto accident that never was. In D. A. Karp & G. E. Sisson, eds., *Voices from the inside.* New York: Oxford University Press.

Rappaport, N. (2009). *In her wake.* New York: Basic Books.

Rathbun, S. I. (2008, January 18 and February 22). Veteran suicides [Television broadcasts]. CBS News.

Reed, G. E. et al. (1990). Analysis of gunshot residue test results in 112 suicides. *Journal of Forensic Sciences, 35*(1), 62–68.

Reger, M. A., et al. (2015). Risk of suicide among U.S. military service members following Operation Enduring Freedom or Operation Iraqi Freedom deployment and separation for the U.S. military. *JAMA Psychiatry, 72*(6), 561–569.

Reynolds, G. (2012, April 18, 2012). How exercise could lead to a better brain. *The New York Times.* Retrieved from *www.nytimes.com/2012/04/22/magazine/how-exercise-could-lead-to-a-better-brain.html*

Ribeiro, J. D., et al. (2016). Self-injurious thoughts and behaviors as risk factors for future suicide ideation, attempts, and death: A meta-analysis of longitudinal studies. *Psychological Medicine, 66,* 225–236.

Rich, C. L., et al. (1986). San Diego Suicide Study: Young versus old subjects. *Archives of General Psychiatry, 43,* 577–582.

Richman, J. (1994). Psychotherapy with older suicidal adults. In A. A. Leenaars et al., eds., *Treatment of suicidal people.* Washington, DC: Taylor & Francis.

Rihmer, Z., et al. (2013). Suicide in Hungary. *Annals of General Psychiatry, 12,* 21.

Riley, A. (2003). *The book of bunny suicides.* London: Penguin Books.

Ringel, E. (1978). *Das Leben Wegwerfen?* Vienna: Freiburg.

Roberts, S. E., et al. (2013). High-risk occupations for suicide. *Psychological Medicine, 43*(6), 1231–1240.

Robins, E. (1981). *The final months: A study of the lives of 134 persons who committed suicide.* New York: Oxford University Press.

Robins, E., et al. (1959). Some clinical considerations in the prevention of suicide in older white men. *American Journal of Public Health, 49,* 888–889.

Robinson, E. A. (1897). Richard Cory. In E. A. Robinson, *The children of the night.* Whitefish, MT: Kessinger.

Roffman, J. L., et al. (2005). Neuroimaging and the functional anatomy of psychotherapy. *Psychological Medicine, 35,* 1385–1398.

Rojcewisz, S. J. (1971). War and suicide. *Suicide and Life-Threatening Behavior, 1*(1), 46–54.

Roman, J. (1992). *Exit house.* New York: Bantam Books. (Original work published 1980)

Rosenstein, H. C. (1973). *Sylvia Plath: 1932–1952.* Unpublished doctoral dissertation, Brandeis University, Waltham, MA.

Rothberg, J. M., & Geer-Williams, C. (1992). A comparison and review of suicide prevention scales. In R. W. Maris et al., eds., *Assessment and prediction of suicide.* New York: Guilford Press.

Rothberg, J. M., et al. (1987). Suicide in the U.S. military. *Psychiatric Annals, 17*(8), 545–548.

Rothman, K., et al. (2012). *Modern epidemiology.* Philadelphia: Lippincott, Williams & Wilkins.

Rothschild, A. J. (2017, October). Benzodiazepines do not cause suicide of suicide attempts. *Primary Care Companion, 19*(5), 17r02171.

Roy, A., & Linnoila, M. (1986). Alcoholism and suicide. *Suicide and Life-Threatening Behavior, 16,* 244–273.

Roy, A., et al. (1991). Suicide in twins. *Archives of General Psychiatry, 48,* 29–32.

Rudd, M. D. (2012). The clinical risk assessment interview. In R. I. Simon & R. E. Hales, eds., *The American Psychiatric Publishing textbook of suicide assessment and management* (2nd ed.). Washington, DC: American Psychiatric Publishing.

Rudd, M. D., et al. (2015). Brief cognitive-behavioral therapy effects on post-treatment suicide attempts in a military sample: Results of a randomized clinical trial with 2-year follow-up. *American Journal of Psychiatry, 172*(5), 441–449.

Rujescu, D., et al. (2007). Molecular genetic findings in suicidal behavior: What is beyond the serotonergic system? *Archives of Suicide Research, 11,* 17–40.

Sacks, O. (1973). *Awakenings.* London: Duckworth.

Sacks, O. (1985). *The man who mistook his wife for a hat.* New York: Touchstone.

Saghir, M., & Robins, E. (1971). *Male and female homosexuality: A comprehensive investigation.* Baltimore: Williams & Wilkins.

Sainsbury, P. (1955). *Suicide in London.* London: Chapman & Hall.

Saks, E. (2010). The center cannot hold. In D. A. Karp & G. E. Sisson, eds., *Voices from the inside.* New York: Oxford University Press.

Salin, Z. K., et al. (2013). Hopelessness, depression, and social support with end of life Turkish patients. *Asian-Pacific Journal of Cancer Prevention, 14*(5), 2823–2828.

Sample, I. (2011, November 14). Gene that raises suicide risk identified. *The Guardian.* Retrieved from *www.theguardian.com/science/2011/nov/14/gene-raises-suicide-risk*

Sanger-Katz, M. (2014, August 13). The science behind suicide contagion. *The New York Times.* Retrieved from *www.nytimes.com/2014/08/14/upshot/the-science-behind-suicide-contagion.html*

Sanger-Katz, M. (2016, October 6). Your surgeon is probably a Republican, your psychiatrist is probably a Democrat. *The New York Times.* Retrieved from *www.nytimes.com/2016/10/07/upshot/your-surgeon-is-probably-a-republican-your-psychiatrist-probably-a-democrat.html*

Sarasohn, J. (2017, April 3). Addressing public health crises: suicide and opiate addiction are preventable. *HHS Blog*. Retrieved from *www.hhs.gov/blog/2017/04/03/public-health-crisis-suicide-and-opioids.html*

Savitsky, J. (2009, December 8). A patient dies, and then the anguish of litigation. *The New York Times*. Retrieved from *http://query.nytimes.com/gst/fullpage.html?res=9C06E3DB1E3FF93AA15751C1A96F9C8B63*

Sawyer v. State, Alaska Court of Appeals No. A-10160, Opinion No. 2290 (2011).

Scheff, T. J. (1974). The labelling theory of mental illness. *American Sociological Review, 39*, 444–452.

Schmidtke, A., et al., eds. (2004). *Suicidal behaviour in Europe* Cambridge, MA: Hogrefe & Huber.

Schony W., & Grausgruber, A. (1987). Epidemiological data on suicide in upper Austria. *Crisis, 8*, 49–52.

Schwartz, C. (2016, October 12). Generation Adderall. *The New York Times Magazine*. Retrieved from *www.nytimes.com/2016/10/16/magazine/generation-adderall-addiction.html*

Scott, C. L., & Resnik, P. J. (2012). Patient suicide and litigation. In R. I. Simon & R. E. Hales, eds., *The American Psychiatric Publishing textbook of suicide assessment and management* (2nd ed.). Washington, DC: American Psychiatric Publishing.

Shaffer, D. (1974). Suicide in childhood and early adolescence. *Journal of Child Psychology and Psychiatry, 5*, 275–291.

Shea, S. G. (1999). *The practical art of suicide assessment*. New York: Wiley.

Shear, K. (2015). Complicated grief. *New England Journal of Medicine, 372*, 153–160.

Shepherd, D., & Barraclough, B. (1980). Work and suicide: An empirical investigation. *British Journal of Psychiatry, 136*, 469–478.

Sher, L. (2015). Suicide in men. *Journal of Clinical Psychiatry, 76*(3), v76n0320.

Shiang, J., et al. (1997). Suicide in San Francisco, California: A comparison of Caucasian and Asian groups. *Suicide and Life-Threatening Behavior, 27*, 80–91.

Shneidman, E. S. (1967). Can a mouse commit suicide? In E. S. Shneidman, ed., *Essays in self-destruction*. New York: Science House.

Shneidman, E. S. (1971). Prevention, intervention, and postvention. *Annals of Internal Medicine, 75*, 453–458.

Shneidman, E. S. (1973). Suicide notes reconsidered. *Psychiatry, 36*, 379–395.

Shneidman, E. S. (1985). *Definition of suicide*. New York: Wiley.

Shneidman, E. S. (1987). A psychological approach to suicide. In G. R. VandenBos & B. K. Bryant, eds., *Cataclysms, crises, and catastrophes*. Washington, DC: American Psychological Association.

Shneidman, E. S. (1993). *Suicide as psychache: A clinical approach to self-destructive behaviors*. Northvale, NJ: Jason Aronson.

Shneidman, E. S. (1996). *The suicidal mind*. New York: Oxford University Press.

Shneidman, E. S., & Farberow, N. L., eds. (1957). *Clues to suicide*. New York: McGraw-Hill.

Shneidman, E. S., & Farberow, N. L. (1957). *Cry for help*. New York: McGraw-Hill.

Shulgin, A. T., & Nichols, D. E. (1978). Characterization of three new psychotomimetics. In R. E. Willette & R. S. Stillman, eds., *The psychopharmacology of hallucinogens*. New York: Pergamon Press.

Silverman, M. M. (1997). Current controversies in suicidology. In R. W. Maris et al., eds., *Review of suicidology*. New York: Guilford Press.

Silverman, M. M., & Berman, A. L. (2014). Suicide risk assessment and risk formulation: Part I. A focus on suicide ideation in assessing suicide risk. *Suicide and Life-Threatening Behavior, 44*(4), 420–431.

Silverman, M. M., & Maris, R. W. (1995). The prevention of suicidal behavior: An overview. *Suicide and Life-Threatening Behavior, 25*, 10–21.

Simon, R. I. (2006). Suicide risk: Assessing the unpredictable. In R. I. Simon & R, E. Hales, eds., *The American Psychiatric Publishing textbook of suicide assessment and management*. Washington, DC: American Psychiatric Publishing.

Simon, R. I. (2012). Suicide risk assessment: Gateway to treatment and management. In R. I. Simon & R. E. Hales, eds., *The American Psychiatric Publishing textbook of suicide assessment and management* (2nd ed.). Washington, DC: American Psychiatric Publishing.

Simon, R. I., & Hales, R. E., eds. (2006). *The American Psychiatric Publishing textbook of suicide assessment and management*. Washington, DC: American Psychiatric Publishing.

Simon, R. I., & Hales, R. E., eds. (2012). *The American Psychiatric Publishing textbook of suicide assessment and management* (2nd ed.). Washington, DC: American Psychiatric Publishing.

Singer, P. (Producer & Director). (2013). *The last interview of Thomas Szasz* [Motion picture]. New York: Witness Films.

Sinyor, M. (2018, April 19). *Impact of Canadian media guidelines on suicide-related reporting and rates.* Paper presented at the 51st annual conference of the American Association of Suicidology/American Foundation for Suicide Prevention, Washington, DC.

Skinner, B. F. (1953). *Science and human behavior.* New York: Macmillan.

Slater, L. (1998). *Prozac diary.* London: Penguin Books.

Slater, L. (2010). Prozac diary. In D. A. Karp & G. E. Sisson, eds., *Voices from the inside.* New York: Oxford University Press.

Smith, K., et al. (1984). Lethality of Suicide Attempt Rating Scale. *Suicide and Life-Threatening Behavior, 14*, 215–242.

Smolenski, D. J., et al. (2014). *Department of Defense Suicide Event Report: Calendar year 2013 annual report.* Alexandria, VA: National Center for Telehealth and Technology.

Snider, J. E., et al. (2006). Standardizing the psychological autopsy: Addressing the *Daubert* standard. *Suicide and Life-Threatening Behavior, 36*, 511–516.

Soh, N. L., & Walter, G. (2011). Tryptophan and depression: Can diet alone be the answer? *Acta Neuropsychiatrica, 23*(1), 3–11.

Sokolov, G., et al. (2006). Inpatient treatment and partial hospitalization. In R. I. Simon & R. E. Hales, eds., *The American Psychiatric Publishing textbook of suicide assessment and management.* Washington, DC: American Psychiatric Publishing.

Sonntage, D. (2013, November 17). Addiction treatment with a dark side. *The New York Times,* 1, 22ff.

South Carolina Association of Counties. (2013, July 26). *Minimum standards for local detention facilities in South Carolina.* Columbia: Author. Retrieved from *www.sccounties. org/Data/Sites/1/media/publications/sc-jail-standards-final.pdf*

Speijer, N., & Diekstra, R. W. F. (1980). *Hulp bij zelfdoding [Aiding suicide].* Deventer, The Netherlands: Van Loghum Slaterus.

Spencer, A. J. (1988). *Death in ancient Egypt.* London: Penguin Books.

Spitzer, E. G., et al. (2018). Posttraumatic stress disorder symptom clusters and acquired capacity for suicide. *Suicide and Life-Threatening Behavior, 48*(1), 105–115.

Spuker, J., et al. (2002). Duration of major depression episodes in the general population. *British Journal of Psychiatry, 181*, 208–213.

Sridhar, V. (2001) The Indian situation. *Frontline, 18*(21).

Stack, S. (1982). Suicide: A decade review of the sociological literature. *Deviant Behavior, 4*, 41–66.

Stack, S. (1987). Celebrities and suicide: A taxonomy and analysis, 1848–1983. *American Sociological Review, 52*, 401–412.

Stack, S. (2000). Work and the economy. In R. W. Maris et al., *Comprehensive textbook of suicidology.* New York: Guilford Press.

Stack, S., & Bowman, B. (2011). *Suicide movies: Social patterns 1900–2009.* Cambridge, MA: Hogrefe.

Stagnetti, M. N. (2008, June). *Antidepressants prescribed by medical doctors in office based and outpatient settings by specialty for the U.S. civilian noninstitutionalized population, 2002 and 2005* (Statistical Brief No. 206). Rockville, MD: Agency for Healthcare Research and Quality.

Stanley, B., et al. (2008) *The safety plan treatment manual to reduce suicide risk: Veteran version.* Washington, DC: U.S. Department of Veterans Affairs.

Stone, G. (1999). *Suicide and attempted suicide.* New York: Carroll & Graf.

Styron, W. (1979). *Sophie's choice.* New York: Random House.

Styron, W. (1990). *Darkness visible.* New York: Random House.

Suicide Prevention Resource Center. (2017, May). Suicide prevention resources for adult corrections. Retrieved from *www.sprc. org/sites/default/files/resource-program/Adult-CorrectionsResourceSheet.pdf*

Summers, A. (1985). *Goddess: The secret lives of Marilyn Monroe.* New York: Open Road.

Szanto, K., et al. (2018). Pathways to late-life suicidal behavior: Cluster analysis and predictive validation of suicidal behavior in a sample of older adults with major depression. *Journal of Clinical Psychiatry, 79*(2).

Szasz, T. (1961). *The myth of mental illness.* New York: Harper & Row.

Szasz, T. (1977). *The theology of medicine.* New York: Harper & Row.

Szasz, T. (1985). *Suicide: What is the clinician's responsibility?* Paper presented at the Harvard Medical School.

Tandon, R., et al. (2013). Definition and description of schizophrenia in the DSM-5. *Schizophrenia Research, 150*(1), 3–10.

Tanney, B. L. (1995). After suicide: A helper's handbook. In B. J. Mishara, ed., *The impact of suicide.* New York: Springer.

Tanney, B. L. (2000). Psychiatric diagnoses and suicidal acts. In R. W. Maris et al., *Comprehensive textbook of suicidology.* New York: Guilford Press.

Tavernese, S. (2016, April 22). U.S. suicide rate surges to a 30-year high. *The New York Times,* pp. 1–5.

Tax Policy Center. (2016). *Briefing book.* Retrieved from *www.taxpolicycenter.org/briefing-book/what-are-major-federal-excise-taxes-and-how-much-money-do-they-raise*

Taymiyyah, T. D. A. (2001). *The religious and moral doctrine of jihad.* Birmingham, UK: Maktabah Al Ansaar.

Teicher, M. H., et al. (1990a). Antidepressant drugs and the emergence of tendencies. *Drug Safety, 8,* 186–212.

Teicher, M. H., et al. (1990b). Emergence of intense suicidal preoccupation during fluoxetine treatment. *American Journal of Psychiatry, 147,* 207–210.

Templeton, A. R. (2013). Biological races in humans. *Studies in the History and Philosophy of Biological and Biomedical Sciences, 44*(3), 262–271.

Tiesman, H. M., et al. (2015). Suicide in U.S. workplaces, 2003–2010: A comparison with non-workplace suicides. *American Journal of Preventive Medicine, 48*(6), 674–682.

Tiihonen, J., et al. (2006). Effectiveness of antipsychotic treatments in a nationwide cohort of patients in community care after first hospitalisation due to schizophrenia and schizoaffective disorder: Observational follow-up study. *British Medical Journal, 333,* 234.

Time. (n.d.). The big sleep: Karen Ann Quinlan. Retrieved from *http://content.time.com/time/specials/packages/article/0,28804,1864940_1864939_1864909,00.html*

Tishler, C. (1980). Intentional self-destruction behavior in children under 10. *Clinical Pediatrics,* 451–453.

Tolstoy, L. (2000). *Anna Karenina.* London: Penguin Books. (Original work published 1877)

Tondo, L., et al. (2001). Lower suicide risk with long-term lithium treatment in major affective illness. *Acta Psychiatrica Scandanavica, 104,* 163–172.

Tousignant, M., et al. (1998). Gender and suicide in India. *Suicide and Life-Threatening Behavior, 28,* 50–61.

Towner, B. (2009, October). The 50 most prescribed drugs. *AARP Bulletin,* pp. 38–39.

Treadway, D. (1996). *Dead reckoning.* New York: Basic Books.

Trimble, M. R. (2007, October 18 and December 11). Deposition taken in New York City for *In re Neurontin Mktg., & Sales Practices Litig.,* 244 F.R.D. 89 (D. Mass. 2007).

Trimble, M. R., & George, M. S. (2010). *Biological psychiatry* (3rd ed.). Chichester, UK: Wiley-Blackwell.

Tsaung, M. (1983). Risk of suicide in relatives of schizophrenics, manic depressives, and controls. *Journal of Clinical Psychiatry, 44,* 396–400.

Tuckman, J., & Youngman, W. F. (1968). A scale for assessing suicide risk of attempted suicides. *Journal of Clinical Psychiatry, 24,* 179–180.

Tuckman, J., et al. (1959). Emotional content of suicide notes. *American Journal of Psychiatry, 116,* 59–63.

Tylor, E. B. (1871). *Primitive culture.* London: Murray.

Ullman, K. (2007). Dieting can be depressing. *British Journal of Psychiatry, 177,* 534–539.

U.S. Committee on Veterans' Affairs. (2008, May 6). *The truth about veterans' suicides: Hearing before the Committee on Veterans' affairs, U.S. House of Representatives, 110th Congress, second session.* Washington, DC: U.S. Government Printing Office.

U.S. Department of Health and Human Services & National Action Alliance for Suicide Prevention (NAASP). (2012). *2012 national strategy for suicide prevention: Goals and objectives for action.* Washington, DC: U.S. Department of Health and Human Services. Retrieved from *www.surgeongeneral.gov/library/reports/national-strategy-suicide-prevention/full-report.pdf*

U.S. Department of Veterans Affairs. (2012, March). *Suicide risk assessment guide* [Card template]. Washington, DC: Author.

Retrieved from *www.mentalhealth.va.gov/docs/va029assessmentguide.pdf*

U.S. Public Health Service. (1999). *The Surgeon General's call to action to prevent suicide 1999.* Washington, DC: Author. Retrieved from *https://profiles.nlm.nih.gov/ps/access/nnbbbh.pdf*

U.S. Surgeon General. (1964). *The 1964 report on smoking and health.* Washington, DC: U.S. Public Health Service.

Vailliant, G. E., & Blumenthal, S. J. (1990). Introduction—Suicide over the life cycle: Risk factors and life-span development. In S. J. Blumenthal & D. J. Kupfer, eds., *Suicide over the life cycle.* Washington, DC: American Psychiatric Press.

Van Dongen, C. (1993). Social context of postsuicide bereavement. *Death Studies, 17,* 125–141.

van Hooff, A. J. L. (1998). *The image of ancient suicide.* Ames: University of Iowa Press.

van Hooff, A. J. L. (2000). A historical perspective on suicide. In R. W. Maris et al., *Comprehensive textbook of suicidology.* New York: Guilford Press.

van Praag, H., et al. (2005). Exercise enhances learning and hippocampal neurogenesis in aged mice. *Journal of Neuroscience, 25*(38), 8680–8685.

Van Putten, T. (1975). The many faces of akathisia. *Comprehensive Psychiatry, 16.* 43–46.

Vannoy, S. D. (2017, December). Under reporting of suicide ideation in U.S. Army population screening: An ogoing challenge. *Suicide and Life-Threatening Behavior, 47*(6), 723–728.

Vedantam, S. (2007, September 6). Youth suicides increased as antidepressant use fell. *The Washington Post.* Retrieved from *www.washingtonpost.com/wp-dyn/content/article/2007/09/05/AR2007090502303.html*

Velting, D. M., & Gould, M. S. (1997). Suicide contagion. In R. W. Maris et al., eds., *Review of suicidology.* New York: Guilford Press.

Veterans for Common Sense v. Peake, 563 F. Supp. 2d 1049 (N.D. Ca. 2008).

Vizzini, N. (2006). *It's a kind of funny story.* New York: Miramax Books.

Vonnegut, K. (1973). *Breakfast of champions.* New York: Delacourt Press.

Voracek, M., & Loibl, L. M. (2007). Genetics of suicide: A systematic review of twin studies. *Wiener Klinische Wochenschrift, 119,* 463–475.

Walker, R. L., et al. (2018). Religious coping style and cultural worldview are associated with suicide ideation among African-American adults. *Archives of Suicide Research, 22*(1), 1–27.

Wallace, D. F. (1998, January). The depressed person. *Harper's Magazine.* Retrieved from *https://harpers.org/wp-content/uploads/HarpersMagazine-1998-01-0059425.pdf*

Wasserman, A. (1989). The effects of war and alcohol consumption patterns on suicide: United States, 1910–1933. *Social Forces, 68,* 513–530.

Wasserman, D., & Varnik, A. (2001). Perestroika in the former U.S.S.R. In D. Wasserman, ed., *Suicide: An unnecessary death.* London: Martin Dunitz.

Wasserman, D., & Wasserman, C. (2009). *Textbook of suicidology and suicide prevention.* New York: Oxford University Press.

Wasserman, I. (1984). A reexamination of the Werther effect. *American Sociological Review, 49,* 427–436.

Watson, J. D., & Crick, F. H. C. (1953). Molecular structure of nucleic acids: A structure for deoxyribose nucleic acid. *Nature, 171,* 737–738.

Wayman, E. (2012, July 23). Rethinking modern human origins. Retrieved from *https://smithsonianmag.com/science-nature/rethinking-modern-human-origins-5370343*

Weishaar, M. E., & Beck, A. T. (1992). Clinical and cognitive predictors of suicide. In R. M. Maris et al. (eds.), *Assessment and prediction of suicide.* New York: Guilford Press.

Weisman, A. (1967). Self-destruction and sexual perversion. In E. S. Shneidman, ed., *Essays in self-destruction.* New York: Science House.

Weisman, A., & Worden, J. W. (1974). Risk-rescue rating in suicide assessment. In A. T. Beck et al., eds., *The prediction of suicide.* Bowie, MD: Charles Press.

Weisman, C. R., et al. (2018). Bilateral repetitive transcranial magnetic stimulation decreases suicide ideation in depression. *Journal of Clinical Psychiatry, 79*(3).

Werth, J. L., Jr. (1996). *Rational suicide: Implications for mental health professionals.* Washington, DC: Taylor & Francis.

Wertheimer, A. (2001). *A special scar* (2nd ed.). Philadelphia: Taylor & Francis.

West, D. J. (1966). *Murder followed by suicide.* Cambridge, MA: Harvard University Press.

West, H. C., et al. (2011, December 15). *Prisoners in 2009*. Washington, DC: Bureau of Justice Statistics.

Whitaker, R. (2010) *Anatomy of an epidemic*. New York: Crown.

White, L. T. (2014, July 18). Cultural values and the likelihood of suicide. *Psychology Today, 45*(7), 1145–1161.

Wickett, A. (1989). *Double exit: When aging couples commit suicide together*. Eugene, OR: Hemlock Society.

Woodward, B. (1984). *Wired*. New York: Simon & Schuster.

World Health Organization (WHO). (1992). *International classification of diseases* (10th rev.). Geneva: Author.

World Health Organization (WHO). (1996, 2008, 2012a). *The global burden of disease*. Geneva: Author.

World Health Organization (WHO). (1999). *Facts and figures about suicide*. Geneva: Author.

World Health Organization (WHO). (2012b). *Age-standardized suicide rates (per 100,000 population), both sexes, 2012*. Geneva: Author.

World Health Organization (WHO). (2015a). *International classification of diseases* (10th rev., 2015 update). Geneva: Author.

World Health Organization (WHO). (2015b). *International classification of diseases* (11th rev., 2015 draft). Geneva: Author.

World Health Organization (WHO). (2015c, June 13). *Suicide rates, age-standardized data by country*. Geneva: Author.

Wrobleski, A. (2002). *Suicide of a child*. Omaha, NE: Centering.

Xiong, G. L., et al. (2012). Inpatient psychiatric treatment. In R. I. Simon & R. E. Hales, eds., *The American Psychiatric Publishing textbook of suicide assessment and management* (2nd ed.). Washington, DC: American Psychiatric Publishing.

Xu, J., et al. (2016, February 16). *Deaths: Final data for 2013* (National Vital Statistics Reports, Vol. 64, No. 2). Hyattsville, MD: National Center for Health Statistics.

Yakeley, J. (2018). Treatment of complicated grief in survivors of suicide loss: A HEAL report. *Journal Clinical Psychiatry, 79*(2), 17m11592.

Yalom, I. D. (1992). *When Nietzsche wept*. New York: Basic Books.

Yates, G. L., et al. (1988). A risk profile comparison of runaway and nonrunaway youth. *American Journal of Public Health, 78*, 820–821.

Yeomans, F., & Kernberg, O. (2014). Fragile and angry. In J. W. Barnhill, ed., *DSM-5 clinical cases*. Washington, DC: American Psychiatric Publishing.

Yin, S. (2006, August). Elderly white men afflicted by high suicide rates. Population Reference Bureau. Retrieved from *www.prb.org/Publications/Articles/2006/ElderlyWhiteMenAfflictedbyHighSuicideRates.aspx*

Yoon, J. H., & Carter, C. S. (2012). Schizophrenia. In R. I. Simon & R. E. Hales, eds., *The American Psychiatric Publishing textbook of suicide assessment and management* (2nd ed.). Washington, DC: American Psychiatric Publishing.

Young, K. (2016, February 11). Physician-assisted suicide for psychiatric disorders examined. *NEJM Journal Watch*. Retrieved from *www.jwatch.org/fw111164/2016/02/11/physician-assisted-suicide-psychiatric-disorders-examined*

Yufit, R. I., & Bongar, B. (1992). Suicide, stress, and coping with life-cycle events. In R. W. Maris et al., eds., *Assessment and prediction of suicide*. New York: Guilford Press.

Zabihyan, K. (Director/Producer). *Death by hanging* [Motion picture]. United States: HBO Original Programming.

Zhang, J., et al. (2004). Culture, risk factors, and suicide in rural China. *Acta Psychiatrica Scandinavica, 110*(6), 430–437.

Zimmerman, M., et al. (2017). Identifying remission from depression on 3 self-report scales. *Journal of Clinical Psychiatry, 78*(2), 177–183.

Zisook, S., et al. (2018). Treatment of complicated grief in survivors of suicide loss: A HEAL report. *Journal of Clinical Psychiatry, 79*(2), e1–e7.

Zivin, K., et al. (2007). Suicide mortality among individuals receiving treatment for depression in the V.A. health system. *American Journal of Public Health, 97*, 2193–2197.

Author Index

Diekstra, R. F. W., 326, 327
Dietz, P., 247
DiMaggio, J., 465
DiMaio, V. J. M., 163
Dollard, J., 75, 117
Donne, J., 311, 312, 326, 363
Donnelly, T., 344, 346
Douglas, J. D., 45, 116, 119
Douglas, R., 366
Downey, R., Jr., 210, 366
Drapeau, C. W., 9, 10, 11, 53, 69, 71, 75, 85
Dreyfuss, R., 101, 334
Ducasse, D., 16, 62, 223, 394, 414
Dunne, E. J., 451, 454, 460
Dunne-Maxim, K., 461
Durkheim, E., 8, 9, 19, 34, 42, 43, 73, 103, 115, 117,
    118, 119, 120, 128, 129, 135, 139, 146, 147, 151, 172,
    290, 294, 300, 315, 318, 339, 341
Dwivedi, Y., 184, 194, 272

Early, K. E., 291
Easterlin, R. A., 88
Eastman, G., 7, 72, 95, 132, 304, 492
Eddy, M. B., 184
Egeland, J., 17, 182, 274
Eisele, J. W., 162, 163, 164
Eitzen, D. S., 183
El-Batouty, G., 372
El-Habashi, A., 372
Elkes, J., 269, 395
Enoch, M. A., 402
Erikson, E., 84, 93, 243, 420
Erikson, K., 106
Essen-Moller, E., 230
Eyman, J. P., 48, 491
Eyman, S. K., 48, 491

Falret, J.-P., 210
Fang, O., 146
Farah, A., 7
Farberow, N. L., 10, 12, 31, 144, 168
Farley, C., 166, 265
Favazza, A. R., 114
Fawcett, J. A., 177, 194, 195, 204, 222, 278, 401, 407,
    419
Fayad, R., 363
Feeley, W., 348, 356
Feigelman, W., 65, 115, 450, 452
Feinstein, R., 66
Felner, R. D., 124
Fincham, F., 121
Fine, C., 461
Fiori, L. M., 279
Firth, R., 302
Fishbain, D. A., 132
Flaherty, C., 53
Folstein, M. F., 47, 424
Forsyth, B., 364, 366
Forsyth, J., 364
Fosse, B., 12, 113, 132, 265, 318, 447
Frank, J., 395
Freedman, A. M., 229
Freud, A., 322, 323
Freud, S., 19, 29, 73, 74, 84, 100, 171, 179, 180, 182,
    183, 239, 243, 266, 321, 322, 323, 324, 325, 326, 335,
    340, 362, 420

Gabbard, G. O., 413
Gailiene, D., 142
Gale, H, 331
Gambino, M., 206, 395, 411
Gananca, L., 402, 414
Garland, J., 166, 213, 265, 492
Garrido-Lecca, G., 483
Gauguin, P., 213, 319
Gay, P., 29, 182, 201, 323
Geer-Williams, C., 56, 419, 491
George, M. S., 220, 222, 262, 272, 278, 398, 402, 403,
    407
Georgianna, S., 43
Gibbons, L., 375
Gibbs, J. P., 35, 43, 117, 118, 135
Gibbs, J. T., 51, 115
Gibbs, N., 370
Gibson, M., 210, 318
Gibson, P., 111
Gilbert, A. M., 10, 210, 489, 490
Gill, W. S., 48, 56, 181, 419, 492
Gilligan, V., 268
Giner, L., 24, 69, 74, 99, 341, 490
Ginn, S., 184
Ginsberg, A., 247
Glaze, L. F., 389
Glennon, R. A., 278
Gödel, K., 304
Goebbels, J., 304, 339
Goering, H., 271, 339
Goethe, J. W. von, 120, 465
Goffman, I., 183
Goggin, W. C., 252, 458
Gold, L. H., 101, 102
Goldblatt, M. J., 75
Goldsmith, S. K., 218, 236, 405
Goodwin, F., 260, 273, 341
Goodwin, F. G., 210, 214, 394, 423, 432, 443, 492
Gorbachev, M., 101, 141
Gordon, R., 92
Gordon, R. S., 436
Gould, M. S., 129, 131, 446
Graafsma, T., 140
Gradus, J. L., 354
Grausgruber, A., 136
Green, K. L., 67, 194, 198, 489
Griffiths, R. R., 271
Grohol, J. M., 205
Grunebaum, M. F., 202, 205, 272, 395
Guze, S. B., 194

Haberlandt, W., 181
Haddon, W., Jr., 437
Hales, R. E., xi, 4, 70, 77, 111, 210, 211, 217, 245, 246,
    266, 268, 487, 489
Hallinan, J. T., 129
Hamilton, M., 54, 349
Hannibal, 304
Harper, B., 361
Harper, V., 361
Harris, E., 362, 373
Harris, G., 263
Harris, M., 140, 300
Hartman, B., 365, 366
Hartman, P., 365, 366
Hartman, S., 365, 366

Subject Index

Note. *f* or *t* following a page number indicates a figure or table.

Health care deficiencies, 351–355
Heaven's Gate suicide, 12, 292, 293–294
Hebephrenia, 225
Helium, 157*t*
Helplessness, 27*t*, 29, 96, 169
Hemingway, Ernest, 5, 6–8, 16–18, 17*f*, 65, 72, 318
Hemlock Society, 131
Hendin, Herbert, 332
Heroin, 263–264
Heterogeneity, 184–185
High-risk groups, 438, 489
Hinduism, 121, 131
HIPAA (Health Insurance Portability and
    Accountability Act) rules, 463
Hippocratic Oath, 321
Histamine, 277
History, suicide in
    Age of Reason (18th century), 312, 313*f*
    from Christ to the Middle Ages, 309–310
    early modern times (16th and 17th centuries),
        310–312
    Greek and Roman antiquity, 306–308, 307*f*, 308*f*
    Metropolis (19th and 20th centuries), 314–317, 315*f*,
        316*f*, 317*f*
    nonhuman animal self-destructive behaviors,
        305–306
    overview, 303–305
    research results and, 496
History of suicide attempts. *See* Prior suicide attempts
Histrionic personality disorder, 242*t*. *See also* Mental
    disorders; Personality disorders
HIV/AIDS, 111
Hoffman, Philip Seymour, 263–264, 318
Homelessness, 352
Homes and Rahe test, 124–125, 126*t*
Homicide. *See* Murder–suicides
Hopelessness. *See also* Risk factors
    depression and, 195
    elderly suicides and, 95, 96
    general model of suicide and, 36–37, 36*f*
    goals of suicide and, 27*t*, 29
    jail and prison suicides and, 388
    outpatient therapy and, 419, 421
    overview, 71, 74, 342
    personality disorders and, 244, 252*t*, 254
    as a risk factor, 206–208, 207*t*, 208*t*
    substance-related disorders and, 257
    suicide risk assessment and, 79
    suicidogenic effects of treatment for bipolar
        disorder and, 222–223
    unemployment and, 136
    veteran suicide and, 349
Hopelessness Scale, 71
Hospital treatment. *See also* Inpatient treatment
    elderly suicides and, 96
    general model of suicide and, 36–37, 36*f*
    mental disorders and, 190–191, 190*t*
    outpatient therapy and, 419
    overview, 396*t*, 423–431, 429*f*
    research results and, 496, 497
    treatment records as a data source and, 46–48
Hostility, 428
Hotlines, 443, 446–447
Household chemicals, 167
HPA axis, 281–282
Human Genome Project, 279
Hume, David, 312

Humor, 200–201, 201*f*, 335, 495
Humphry, Derek, 131, 320–321, 333–334, 362
Hungary, 143–144, 289, 300
Hypnosis, 406
Hypnotics, 407. *See also* Medication
Hypomanic episodes. *See also* Bipolar disorder; Mania
    diagnosis and, 214–215
    overview, 209
    self-destructive female paradox and, 365
    suicide and, 211–214
    suicidogenic effects of treatment for, 220–223
    treatment and, 216–219
Hypothermia, 157*t*
Hypothesis, 20, 34–35

Idiographic states, 115
Illness, terminal. *See* Physical health; Terminal illness
Imipramine (Tofranil), 398, 399*t*, 408*t*. *See also*
    Antidepressants; Medication
Imitation, 127–129, 130*t*, 465–466, 494. *See also*
    Contagion
Immigrants, 123
Immolation, 157*t*
Impact of suicide. *See* Postvention; Survivors
The Impact of Suicide (Mishara, 1995), 454
Impulse-control disorders, 186*t*
Impulsivity. *See also* Risk factors
    artists' suicidality and, 319
    general model of suicide and, 36–37, 36*f*
    genetic factors and, 275
    isolation and, 121
    murder–suicide and, 362
    nonfatal suicide attempts and, 10
    overview, 74–75, 124
    personality disorders and, 243, 244
    selective serotonin reuptake inhibitor (SSRI) and,
        365
    serotonergic system and, 182, 273
    substance-related disorders and, 257
    suicide risk assessment and, 79
Incarceration. *See* Jail and prison suicides
India
    history of suicide and, 312, 313*f*
    overview, 104, 137, 147, 150
    religion and suicide data and, 289
    research results and, 495
Indicated interventions, 436. *See also* Prevention;
    Secondary prevention; Tertiary prevention;
    Treatment
Indifference, 380
Indirect evidence, 491–492
Indirect self-destructive behaviors (ISDBs), 12–14, 13*t*,
    31, 33. *See also* Self-destructive behaviors and ideas
Indirect suicides, 15, 23. *See also* Passive suicides
Individual facts, 115–116
Individual responsibilities, 325–329
Individual suicide risk assessment, 77–79. *See also*
    Assessment
Industrial Revolution, 314
Infanticide, 359. *See also* Murder–suicides
Inflammation, 281
Injury control strategies, 437, 437*t*
Inpatient treatment. *See also* Hospital treatment;
    Treatment
    interdisciplinary progress notes and, 429, 429*f*
    overview, 396*t*, 413, 423–431, 429*f*
    research results and, 497